Dosage Calculations

Dedication

To my parents, Tana and E.P., whose love, sacrifice, and encouragement have enabled me to use the resources necessary to make this text possible . . . and to Roger, Amy, Julie, and Sarah, who allowed me the time to make the first, second, third, fourth, fifth, and sixth editions possible.

Dosage Calculations

sixth edition

Gloria D. Pickar, RN, EdD
Seminole Community College
Sanford, Florida

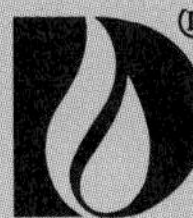

Delmar Publishers

an International Thomson Publishing company 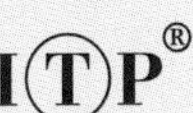

Albany • Bonn • Boston • Cincinnati • Detroit • London • Madrid
Melbourne • Mexico City • New York • Pacific Grove • Paris • San Francisco
Singapore • Tokyo • Toronto • Washington

NOTICE TO THE READER

Publisher does not warrant or guarantee any of the products described herein or perform any independent analysis in connection with any of the product information contained herein. Publisher does not assume, and expressly disclaims, any obligation to obtain and include information other than that provided to it by the manufacturer.

The reader is expressly warned to consider and adopt all safety precautions that might be indicated by the activities herein and to avoid all potential hazards. By following the instructions contained herein, the reader willingly assumes all risks in connections with such instructions.

The publisher makes no representation or warranties of any kind, including but not limited to, the warranties of fitness for particular purpose or merchantability, nor are any such representations implied with respect to the material set forth herein, and the publisher takes no responsibility with respect to such material. The publisher shall not be liable for any special, consequential, or exemplary damages resulting, in whole or part, from the readers' use of, or reliance upon, this material.

Cover Design: Timothy J. Conners

Delmar Staff

Publisher: William Brottmiller
Acquisitions Editor: Marion Waldman
Developmental Editor: Marah E. Bellegarde
Project Editor: Patricia Gillivan
Production Coordinator: Barbara A. Bullock
Art and Design Coordinator: Timothy J. Conners
Editorial Assistant: Diane Speece

an International Thomson Publishing company 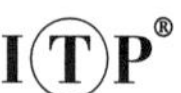

The ITP logo is a trademark under license
Printed in the United States of America

For more information contact:

Delmar Publishers
3 Columbia Circle, Box 15015
Albany, New York 12212-5015

International Thomson Publishing Europe
Berkshire House
168-173 High Holborn
London, WC1V7AA
United Kingdom

Nelson ITP, Australia
102 Dodds Street
South Melbourne,
Victoria, 3205 Australia

Nelson Canada
1120 Birchmont Road
Scarborough, Ontario
M1K 5G4, Canada

International Thomson Publishing France
Tour Maine-Montparnasse
33 Avenue du Maine
75755 Paris Cedex 15, France

International Thomson Editores
Seneca 53
Colonia Polanco
11560 Mexico D. F. Mexico

International Thomson Publishing GmbH
Königswinterer Strasse 418
53227 Bonn
Germany

International Thomson Publishing Asia
60 Albert Street
#15-01 Albert Complex
Singapore 189969

International Thomson Publishing Japan
Hirakawa-cho Kyowa Building, 3F
2-2-1 Hirakawa-cho, Chiyoda-ku,
Tokyo 102, Japan

ITE Spain/ Paraninfo
Calle Magallanes, 25
28015-Madrid, Espana

5 6 7 8 9 10 XXX 04 03 02 01

Library of Congress Cataloging-in-Publication Data

Pickar, Gloria D., 1946–
Dosage calculations / Gloria D. Pickar. — 6th ed.
p. cm.
Includes index.
ISBN 0-7668-0504-2
1. Pharmaceutical arithmetic. I. Title.
[DNLM: 1. Pharmaceutical Preparations—administration & dosage. 2. Mathematics. QV 748 P594d 1999]
RS57.P53 1999
615′.4—dc21
DNLM/DLC
for Library of Congress

98-32460
CIP

Contents

Preface

Introduction

Dosage Calculations, sixth edition, offers a clear and concise method of calculating medication (drug) dosages. The text is directed to the student or professional who feels uncomfortable with mathematics. The first through fifth editions have been classroom tested and reviewed by well over 600,000 faculty and students, who report that it helped them allay math anxiety and promoted confidence in their ability to perform accurate calculations. As one reviewer noted, "I have looked at others [texts] and I don't feel they can compare."

The only math prerequisite is the ability to do basic arithmetic. For those who need a review, Chapters 1 and 2 offer an overview of basic arithmetic procedures with extensive exercises for practice. The student is encouraged to use a 3-step method for calculating dosages:

1. convert measurements to the same system and same size units;
2. consider what dosage is reasonable; and
3. calculate using the formula method D/H × Q (*desired* over *have* times *quantity*) or the ratio-proportion method.

The sixth edition is based upon feedback from users of the previous editions and users of other calculations texts. The revision also responds to changes in the health care field and includes the introduction of new drugs, replacement of outdated drugs, and new or refined methods of administering medications. The importance of avoiding medication errors is highlighted by the incorporation of applied critical thinking skills based on patient care situations.

Full color is used to make the text user friendly. Chapter elements such as rules, math tips, cautions, remember boxes, quick reviews, and examples are color-coded for easy recognition and use. Color also highlights review sets and practice problems. All drug labels are reproduced in full color to provide greater clarity and readability for reference in solving problems.

All syringes are drawn to full size to provide accurate scale renderings to help students master the reading of injectable dosages. An amber color has been added to selected syringe drawings throughout the text to *simulate a specific amount of medication,* as indicated in the example or problem. Because the color used may not correspond to the actual color of the medications named, *it must not be used as a reference for identifying medications.*

In addition to the detailed table of contents, an extensive index is included as a tool to support the student's review of concepts and skills.

Organization of Content

The text is organized in a natural progression of basic to more complex information. Students gain self-confidence as they master content in small increments with ample review and reinforcement. Many students claim that while using this text it is the first time they haven't feared math.

The sixteen chapters are divided into four sections.

Section 1 includes a mathematics diagnostic evaluation and a mathematics review in Chapters 1 and 2. The *mathematics diagnostic evaluation* allows students to determine their computational strengths and weaknesses to guide them through the review of the Section 1 Chapters. *Chapters 1 and 2* provide a review of basic arithmetic procedures, with numerous examples and practice problems to ensure that students can apply the procedures.

Section 2 includes Chapters 3 through 8. This section provides a foundation of information essential for measuring drug dosages and understanding drug orders and labels. *Chapters 3* and *4* introduce the three systems of measurement (metric, apothecary, and household) and conversion from one system of measurement to another. The metric system of measurement is stressed because of its increased standardization in the health care field. The use of the apothecary and household system is further deemphasized. The ratio-proportion method of performing conversions is also included. International or 24-hour time and fahrenheit and centigrade temperature conversions are presented in *Chapter 5.*

In *Chapter 6* students learn to recognize and select appropriate equipment for the administration of medications based on the drug, dosage, and the method of administration. Emphasis is placed on interpreting syringe calibrations to ensure that the dosage to be administered is accurate. All photos and drawings have been enhanced for improved clarity.

Chapter 7 presents the common abbreviations used in health care so that students can become proficient in interpreting medical orders. Additionally, the section on computerized medication administration records has been updated and expanded.

It is essential that students be able to read medication labels to calculate dosages accurately. This ability is developed by having students interpret the medication labels provided beginning in *Chapter 8*. These labels represent current commonly prescribed medications and are presented in full color and actual size (except in a few instances where the label is enlarged to improve readability).

In *Section 3* the student learns and practices the skill of dosage calculations applied to patients across the life span. *Chapters 9 and 10* guide the student to apply all the skills mastered to achieve accurate oral and injectable drug dosage calculations. Students learn to think through the problem logically for the right answer and then to apply a simple formula to double-check their thinking. When this logical but unique system is applied every time to every problem, experience has shown that decreased math anxiety and increased accuracy result.

Insulin types, species, and manufacturers have been expanded with a description of insulin action time. The new 70-30 and 50-50 insulins are also thoroughly explained.

Chapter 11 introduces the ratio-proportion method of calculating dosages. Ample review sets and practice problems provide the opportunity to apply this method. Ratio-proportion is also applied in *Chapters 12* through *16*.

Chapter 12 covers the calculation of pediatric dosages and concentrates on the body weight method. Emphasis is placed on verifying safe dosages and applying concepts across the life span.

Advanced clinical calculations applicable to both adults and children are presented in *Section 4*. A new *Chapter 13* provides a segue to intravenous calculations by fully describing the preparation of solutions. With the increasing role of the nurse and other health care workers in the home setting, clinical calculations for home care are emphasized, such as nutritional feedings. Intravenous administration calculations have been expanded to three chapters (*14 through 16*). Coverage reflects the greater application of IVs in drug therapy. Shortcut calculation methods are presented and explained fully. More electronic infusion devices are included. Heparin and saline locks, types of IV solutions, IV monitoring, IV administration records, and IV push drugs are included in *Chapter 14*. Pediatric IV calculations are presented in *Chapter 15* and obstetric, heparin, and critical care IV calculations are covered in *Chapter 16*. Ample problems help students master the necessary calculations.

Procedures in the text are introduced using several examples. Key concepts are summarized and highlighted in quick review boxes before each set of review problems to give students an opportunity to review major concepts prior to working through the problems. Math tips provide memory joggers to assist students to accurately solve problems. Learning is reinforced by practice problems that conclude each chapter. The importance of calculation accuracy is emphasized by patient scenarios that apply critical thinking skills. Critical thinking skill scenarios have also been added to chapter practice problems to further emphasize accuracy.

Information to be memorized is identified in remember boxes and caution boxes alert students to critical procedures.

Section self-evaluations found at the end of each section provide students with an opportunity to test their mastery of chapter objectives prior to proceeding to the next section. Two *posttests* at the conclusion of the text serve to evaluate the student's overall skill in dosage calculations. The first posttest covers essential skills commonly tested by employers and the second serves as a comprehensive examination. Both are presented in a case study format to simulate actual clinical calculations.

An *answer key* at the back of the text provides all answers and selected solutions to problems in the Review Sets, Practice Problems, Section Self-Evaluations, and Posttests.

Features of the Sixth Edition

- Content is divided into four main sections to help students better organize their studies.
- The number of problems for students to practice their skills and reinforce their learning has been expanded to total over 2,050 problems.
- Critical thinking skills are applied to real-life patient care situations to emphasize the importance of accurate dosage calculations and the avoidance of medication errors.
- Photos and drug labels are presented in full color; color is used to highlight and enhance the visual presentation of content to improve readability. Special attention is given to visual clarity.
- The math review has been expanded to two chapters to bring students up to the required level of basic math competence.
- Measurable objectives at the beginning of each chapter emphasize the content to be learned.
- SI conventional metric system notation is used (apothecary and household system of measurement are deemphasized).
- RULE boxes draw the student's attention to pertinent instructions.

- REMEMBER boxes highlight information to be memorized.
- QUICK REVIEW boxes summarize critical information throughout the chapters.
- CAUTION boxes alert students to critical information.
- MATH TIPS serve to point out math short cuts and reminders.
- Content is presented from simple to complex concepts in small increments followed by Review Sets and Chapter Practice Problems for better understanding and to reinforce learning.
- Many problems are included involving the interpretation of syringe scales to ensure that the proper dosage is administered. Once the dosage is calculated, the student is directed to draw an arrow on a syringe at the proper value.
- Many more labels of current and commonly prescribed medications are included to help students learn how to select the proper information required to determine correct dosage.
- More solved examples are included to demonstrate the $D/H \times Q = X$ or ratio-proportion methods of calculating dosages.
- Ratio-proportion is included and expanded by popular demand, giving students and instructors a choice of which method they prefer to use.
- Additional and updated photographs of equipment commonly used in administering medications and IVs are included.
- Calculating pediatric dosages using both the body weight and body surface area (BSA) methods emphasizes the requirement for accurate dosages to prevent over- or under-medication of the pediatric patient.
- A new chapter on solutions and nutritional feedings applies calculations used in home health care.
- IV equipment and calculations have been expanded.
- Clear instructions are included for calculating IV medications administered in mg per kilogram per minute.
- Clinical situations are simulated using actual medication labels, syringes, physician order forms, and medication administration records.
- Case study format of posttests simulate actual clinical calculations and scenarios.
- New essential skills posttest simulates exams commonly administered by employers for new-hires.
- The index facilitates student and instructor access to content and skills.

Computer Software

With this edition of *Dosage Calculations,* Delmar continues to provide a companion study guide and testing CD-ROM for Windows95™. The CD-ROM is an interactive multimedia presentation that includes the complete text of the book, sample problems, review questions, and a testing component. The program provides scoring, helpful hints, animations, pronunciation of drug names, and color photos and illustrations. It is designed for individual, self-paced learning at home or in the computer lab.

Instructor's Manual

An *Instructor's Manual* is available for the sixth edition of the text. The *Instructor's Manual* includes solutions for all Review Sets, Practice Problems, Section Tests, and Posttests. In addition, extra problems are provided for each chapter for testing purposes. Transparency masters are available to help instructors highlight important concepts. The transparency masters also include additional drug labels.

Acknowledgments

Contributor

Rosemarie Westberg, RN, MSN
Northern Virginia Community College
Annandale, VA

Rosemarie expertly contributed to the research, updating, and expansion of the sixth edition.

Reviewers

The following people devoted considerable time and effort to reviewing this text in various stages. Appreciation is expressed to the instructors who reviewed the revised manuscript, verified accuracy or served as technical proofreaders.

Ann Bello, RN, MA
Norwalk Community Technical College
Norwalk, CT

Lou Ann Boose, RN, BSN, MSN
Harrisburg Area Community College
Harrisburg, PA

Christina Benson, RN, MSN
Naugatuck Valley Community-Technical College
Waterbury, CT

Dae Bugl, MSN, CS, APRN
Capital Community Technical College
Hartford, CT

Lynne Harris, RN, MSN
Northwestern Michigan College
Traverse City, MI

Barbara Lange
Indiana Vocational Technical College
Madison, IN

Frances Leahy, RNC, MS, Emerita
Quinisigamond Community College
Worcester, MA

Beverly Meyers, BA MEd
Jefferson College
St. Louis, MO

Patricia A. Roper, RN, MS
Columbus State Community College
Columbus, OH

Linda Jo Shelek, RNC, BSN
West Virginia Northern Community College
Wheeling, WV

Maureen Tremel, MSN, ARNP
Seminole Community College
Sanford, FL

Elda Vasquez, CMA
San Antonio College
San Antonio, TX

Manufacturers

The following companies provided technical data, photographs, syringes, drug labels, package inserts, package labels, or packaging to illustrate examples, problems, and posttests.

Abbott Laboratories, Abbott Park, IL 60064

Alaris Medical Systems, San Diego, CA

Amgen Inc., Thousands Oaks, CA 91320

Apothecon, Princeton, NJ 08543

Astra USA, Westborough, MA 01581

Baxter Healthcare Corporation, Deerfield, IL 60015

Bayer Corporation, West Haven, CT 06516

Becton Dickinson, Rutherford, NJ 07070

Boots Pharmaceuticals, Inc., Lincolnshire, IL 60069

Bristol Laboratories, Bristol-Myers Pharmaceutical and Nutritional Group, Evansville, IN 47221

Bristol-Myers Oncology Division, Evansville, IN 47721

Bristol-Myers Squibb Pharmaceutical Research Institute, Princeton, NJ 08543

CIBA Pharmaceutical Company, Division of CIBA-GEIGY Corporation, Summit, NJ 07901

Dista Products Company, Division of Eli Lilly & Co., Indianapolis, IN 46285

Eli Lilly and Company, Indianapolis, IN 46285

Elkins-Sinn, Inc., Cherry Hill, NJ 08003

GEIGY Pharmaceuticals, Division of CIBA-GEIGY Corporation, Ardsley, NY 10502

GlaxoWellcome, Research Triangle Park, NC 27709

Hoechst Marion Roussel Pharmaceuticals Inc., Cincinnati, OH 45215

Hoffman-LaRoche Inc., Nutley, NJ 07110

Jansson Pharmaceuticals, Titusville, NJ 08560

King Pharmaceuticals, Bristol, TN 37620

Lakeside Pharmaceuticals, Cincinnati, OH 45215

Lederle Parenterals, Inc., Carolina, Puerto Rico 00987

Luitpold Pharmaceuticals, Shirley, NY 11967

McNeil Consumer Products, Ft. Washington, PA 19034

Mead Johnson Nutritionals, Evansville, IN 47721

Mead Johnson Oncology Products, A Bristol-Myers Squibb Co., Evansville, IN 47721

Medex Inc., Dublin, OH 43017

Merck and Co., Inc., West Point, PA 19486

Muro Pharmaceutical, Inc., Tewksbury, MA 01876

Novartis Pharmaceutical Corp., Summit, NJ 07901

Novo Nordisk Pharmaceuticals Inc., Princeton, NJ 08540

Ortho-McNeil Pharmaceuticals, Raritan, NJ 08869

Parke-Davis Division of Warner-Lambert Company, Morris Plains, NJ 07950

Pfizer Pharmaceuticals, New York, NY 10017

Pharmacia and Upjohn Co., Kalamazoo, MI 49001

Proctor & Gamble, Cincinnati, OH 45201

Reed & Carnrick, Division of Block Drug Company, Inc., Jersey City, NJ 07302

Roche Products Inc., Manati, Puerto Rico 00701

Roxane Laboratories, Inc., Columbus, OH 43228

Sanofi Pharmaceuticals, New York, NY 10016

Schering Laboratories, Kenilworth, NJ 07033

G. D. Searle & Co., Chicago, IL 60680

SmithKline Beecham Pharmaceuticals, Philadelphia, PA 19101

Syntex Corporation, Palo Alto, CA 94303

UCB Pharma, Inc., Smyrna, GA 30080

Wallace Laboratories Division, Carter-Wallace, Inc., Cranbury, NJ 08512

Warner-Lambert Company, Morris Plains, NJ 07950

Wyeth-Ayerst Laboratories, Philadelphia, PA 19101

Zeneca Pharmaceuticals, Wilmington, DE 19850

From the Author

I wish to thank my many students and colleagues who have provided inspiration and made contributions to the production of the text. I am particularly grateful to Professors Rose Westberg and Maureen Tremel for their careful attention to researching and updating information, to Professor Beverly Meyers for her careful attention to accuracy, to Marah Bellegarde, Pat Gillivan, Barb Bullock, and Tim Conners for their careful attention to deadlines and details, and to Roger Pickar for his careful attention to me and our children.

Gloria D. Pickar

Introduction to the Student

The accurate calculation of drug dosages is an essential skill in health care. Serious harm to the patient can result from a mathematical error when calculating a drug dosage. It is the responsibility of those administering drugs to precisely and efficiently carry out medical orders.

Learning to calculate drug dosages need not be a difficult or burdensome process. *Dosage Calculations, 6E* provides an uncomplicated, easy-to-learn, easy-to-recall three-step method of dosage calculations. Once you master this method, you will be able to consistently compute dosages with accuracy, ease, and confidence.

The text is a self-study guide and it is divided into four main sections. The only mathematical prerequisite is the basic ability to add, subtract, multiply, and divide whole numbers. A review of fractions, decimals, percents, ratios, proportions, and Roman numerals is included. You are encouraged to work at your own pace and seek assistance from a qualified instructor as needed.

Each procedure in the text is introduced by several examples. Key concepts are summarized and highlighted before the practice problems. This gives you an opportunity to review the concepts before working the problems. Ample review and practice problems are given to reinforce your skill and confidence.

Before calculating the dosage, you are asked to consider the reasonableness of the computation. More often than not, the correct amount can be estimated in your head. Many errors can be avoided if you approach dosage calculation in this logical fashion. The mathematical computation can then be used to double-check your thinking. Answers to all problems and step-by-step solutions to select problems are included at the back of the text.

Many photos and drawings are included to demonstrate key concepts and equipment. Drug labels and measuring devices (for example, syringes) are included to give a simulated "hands on" experience outside of the clinical setting or laboratory. Critical thinking skills emphasize the importance of dosage calculation accuracy.

This text has helped hundreds of thousands of students just like you to feel at ease about math and to master dosage calculations. I am interested in your feedback. Please write to me to share your reactions and success stories.

Dr. Gloria D. Pickar, Dean
Seminole Community College
100 Weldon Boulevard
Sanford, FL 32773-6199

Using this Book . . .

- Content is presented from simple to complex concepts in small increments followed by a quick review and solved examples. Review sets and practice problems provide opportunities to reinforce learning.
- All syringes are drawn to full size to provide accurate scale renderings to help students master the reading of injectable dosages.

14. Administer 1.3 cc

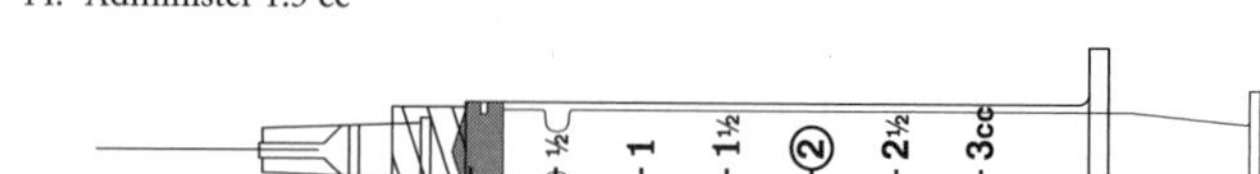

15. Administer 0.33 cc

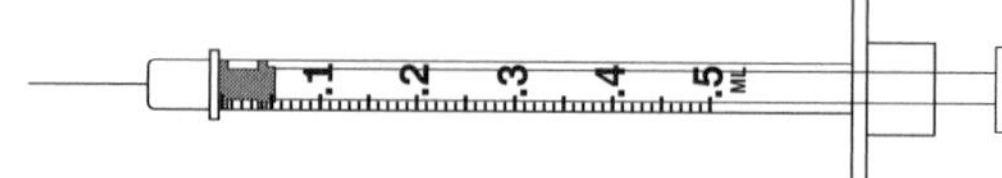

16. Administer 65 U of U-100 insulin

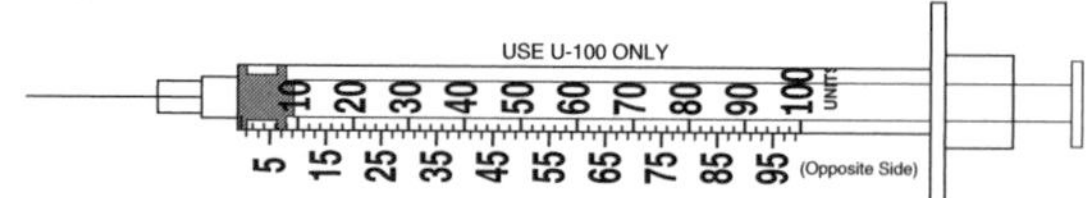

17. Administer 27 U of U-100 insulin

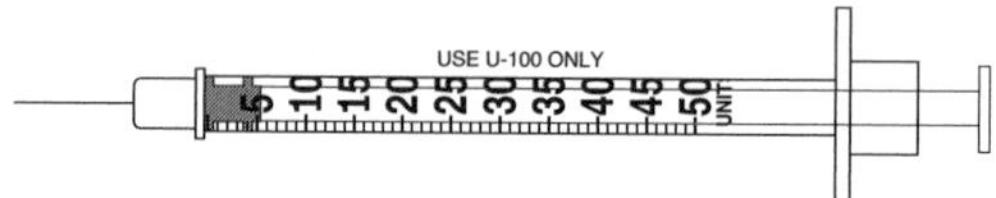

18. Administer 75 U of U-100 insulin

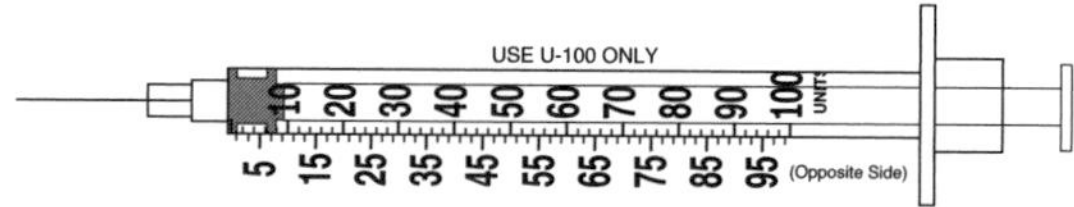

19. Administer 4.4 cc

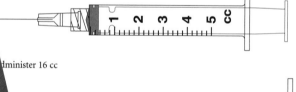

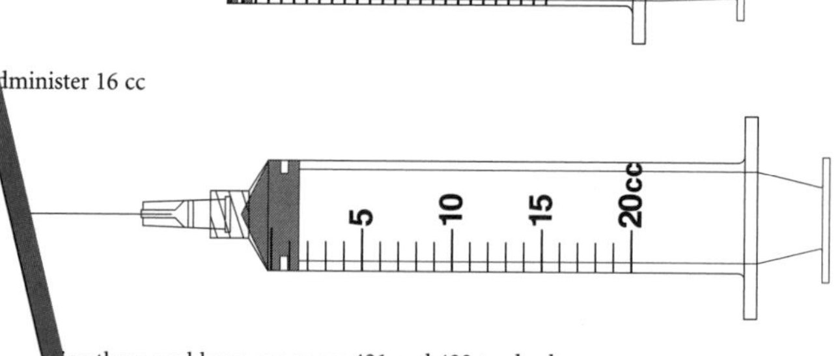

…dminister 16 cc

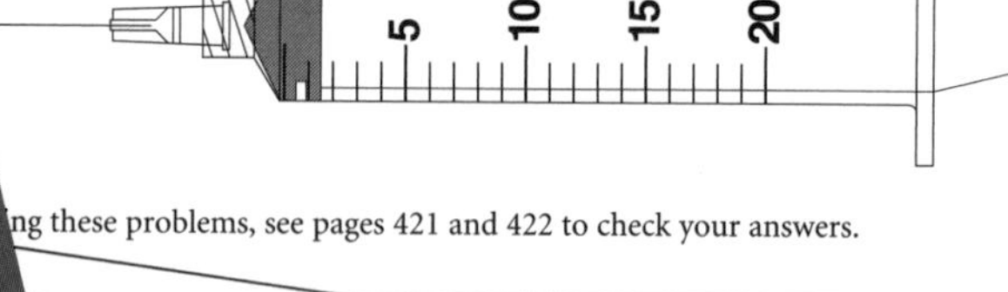

…ing these problems, see pages 421 and 422 to check your answers.

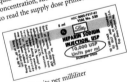

Supply dosage: This refers to both *dosage strength* and *form*. It is read "X measured units per some quantity." For solid form medications, such as tablets, the supply dosage is X measured units per tablet. For liquid medications, the supply dosage is the same as the medication's concentration, such as X measured units per milliliter. Take a minute to read the supply dose printed on the following labels.

HEPARIN SODIUM INJECTION, USP 10,000 USP Units per ml

10,000 units per milliliter

NUBAIN (nalbuphine HCl) 20 mg/ml injection 10 ml VIAL

20 milligrams per milliliter

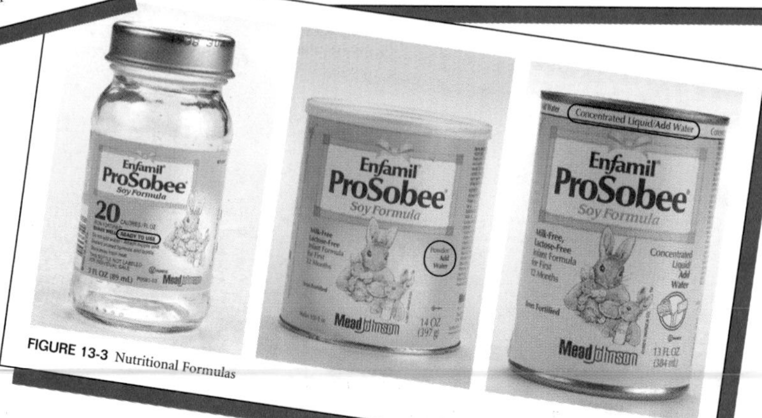

FIGURE 13-3 Nutritional Formulas

- Photos and drug labels are presented in full color; color is used to highlight and enhance the visual presentation of content and to improve readability. Special attention is given to visual clarity.

- ***critical thinking skills*** are applied to real-life patient care situations to emphasize the importance of accurate dosage calculations and the avoidance of medication errors. As an added benefit, critical thinking scenarios that allow students to present their own prevention strategy are included in end of chapter tests.
- ***rule*** boxes highlight and draw the students' attention to pertinent instructions.
- ***remember*** boxes highlight information to be memorized.
- ***quick review*** boxes summarize critical information.

critical thinking skills

It is important to know the equipment you are using. Let's look at an example in which the nurse was unfamiliar with the IV piggyback setup.

error

Failing to follow manufacturer's directions when using a new IV piggyback system.

possible scenario

Suppose the physician ordered Rocephin 1 g IV q.12h for an elderly patient with streptococcus pneumonia. The medication was sent to the unit by pharmacy utilizing the ADD-Vantage system. Rocephin 1 gram was supplied in a powder form and attached to a 50 mL IV bag of D_5W. The directions for preparing the medication were attached to the label. The nurse, who was unfamiliar with the new ADD-Vantage system, hung the IV medication, calculated the drip rate, and infused the 50 mL of fluid. The nurse cared for the patient for three days. During walking rounds on the third day, the on-coming nurse noticed that the Rocephin powder remained in the vial and never was diluted in the IV bag. The nurse realized that the vial stopper inside of the IV bag was not open. Therefore, the medication powder was not mixed in the IV fluid during this shift for the past three days.

potential outcome

The omission by the nurse resulted in the patient missing three doses of the ordered IV antibiotic. The delay in the medication administration could have serious consequence for the patient, such as worsening of the pneumonia, septicemia, and even death, especially in the elderly. The patient received only one-half of the daily dose ordered by the physician for three days. The physician would be notified of the error and likely order additional diagnostic studies, such as chest X ray, blood cultures, and an additional one-time dose of Rocephin.

prevention

This error could easily have been avoided had the nurse read the directions for preparing the medication or consulted with another nurse familiar with the system.

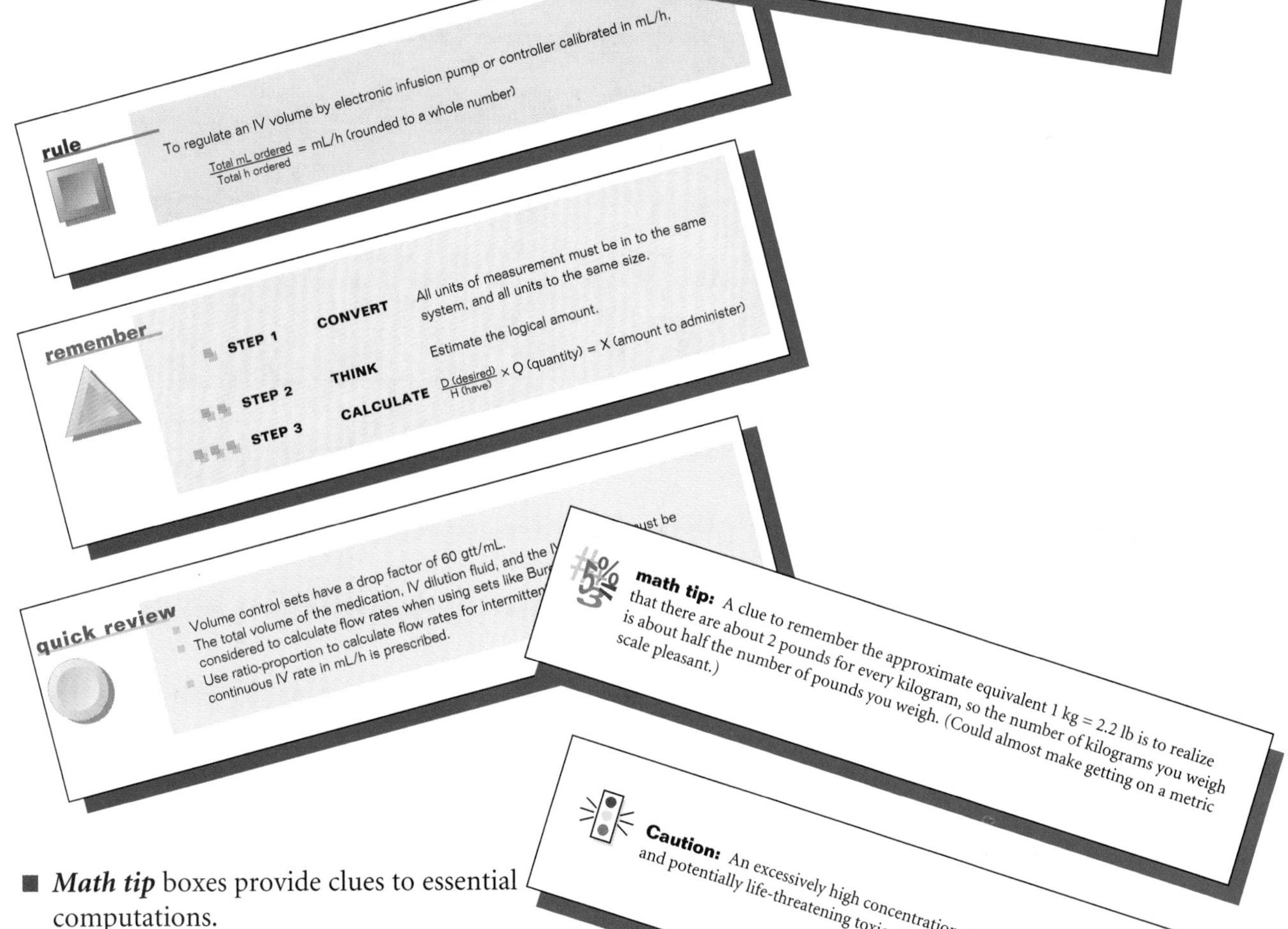
rule
To regulate an IV volume by electronic infusion pump or controller calibrated in mL/h,
Total mL ordered / Total h ordered = mL/h (rounded to a whole number)
remember
STEP 1 CONVERT All units of measurement must be in to the same system, and all units to the same size.
STEP 2 THINK Estimate the logical amount.
STEP 3 CALCULATE D (desired) / H (have) × Q (quantity) = X (amount to administer)
quick review
Volume control sets have a drop factor of 60 gtt/mL.
The total volume of the medication, IV dilution fluid, and the
considered to calculate flow rates when using sets like
Use ratio-proportion to calculate flow rates for
continuous IV rate in mL/h is prescribed.
math tip: A clue to remember the approximate equivalent 1 kg = 2.2 lb is to realize that there are about 2 pounds for every kilogram, so the number of kilograms you weigh is about half the number of pounds you weigh. (Could almost make getting on a metric scale pleasant.)
Caution: An excessively high concentration of an IV drug can cause vein irritation and potentially life-threatening toxic effects. Dilution calculations are critical skills.

- ***Math tip*** boxes provide clues to essential computations.
- ***Caution*** boxes alert students to critical information and safety concerns.

CD-ROM included!

With the sixth edition of Pickar's *Dosage Calculations*, Delmar Publishers includes a comprehensive learning program on CD-ROM for Windows 95™. The CD-ROM is an interactive multimedia presentation that has been designed to enhance self-paced learning.

Features include:

- Complete text
- Tutorial to help you get started
- 300-word glossary
- Audio pronunciation of drug names, including common sound-alike drug names
- Testing assessment tool with scoring capabilities
- Review questions with answers and rationales
- Chapter practice problems with answers and rationales
- Critical thinking skills
- Animations
- Color photographs
- 160 drug labels
- Intuitive and attractive interface
- Help feature
- Toll-free technical support
- Plus Flash!, an electronic flash card program

SECTION 1
Mathematics Review

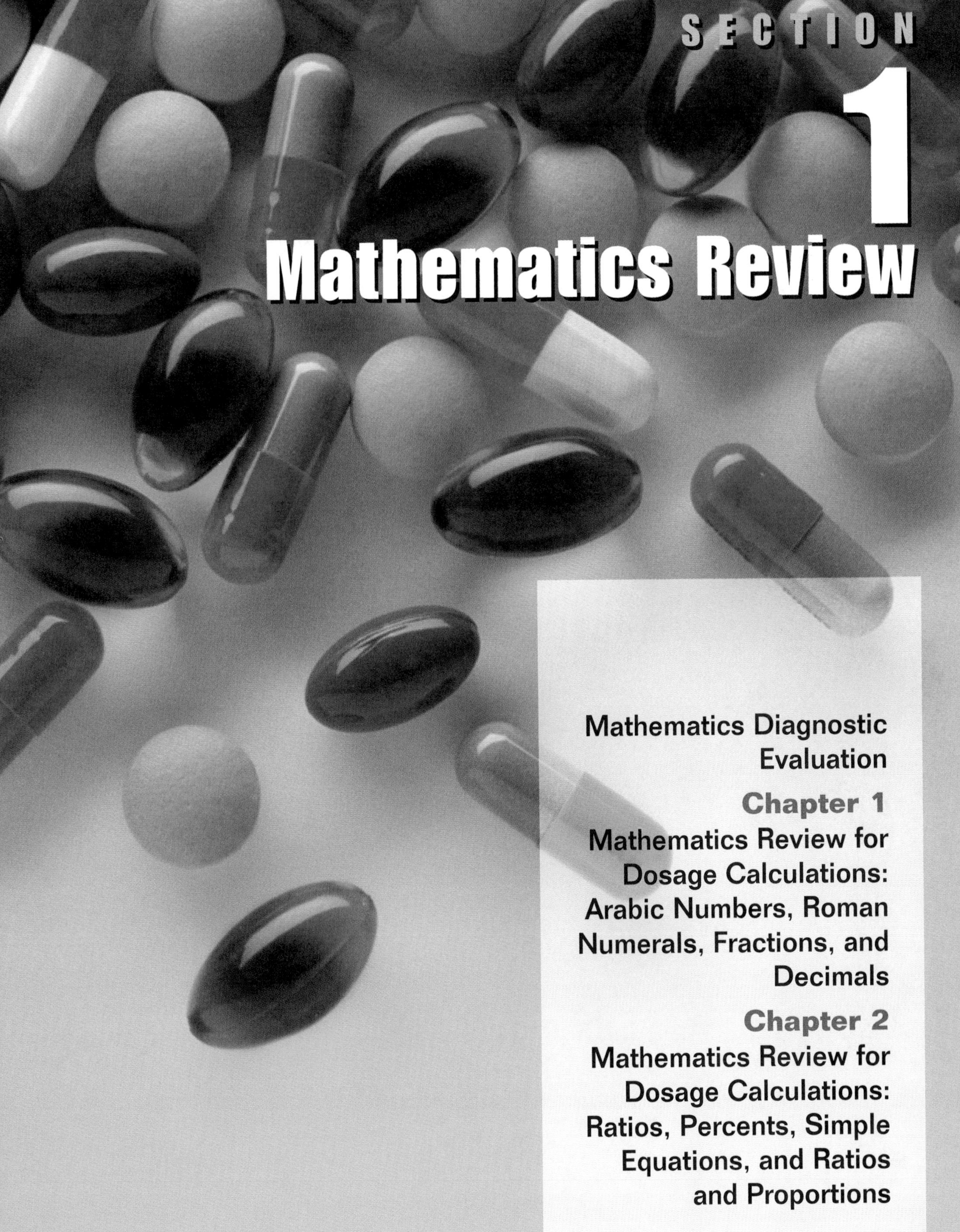

Mathematics Diagnostic Evaluation

As a prerequisite objective, *Dosage Calculations* takes into account that you can add, subtract, multiply, and divide whole numbers. You should have a working knowledge of fractions, decimals, ratios, percents, and basic problem solving as well. These elementary mathematical operations support all dosage calculations in health care.

Set aside $1\frac{1}{2}$ hours in a quiet place to complete the 50 items in the following diagnostic evaluation. You will need scratch paper and a pencil to work the problems.

Use your results to determine your current computational strengths and weaknesses to guide your review. A minimum score of 86 is recommended as an indicator of readiness for dosage calculations. If you achieve that score, you may proceed directly to Chapter 3. However, note any problems that you answered incorrectly, and use the related review materials in Chapters 1 and 2 to refresh your skills.

This mathematics diagnostic evaluation and the review that follows are provided to enhance your confidence and proficiency in arithmetic skills, thereby helping you to avoid careless mistakes later when you perform dosage calculations.

Good luck!

Directions:

1. Carry answers to three decimal places and round to two places.

   (Examples: 5.175 = 5.18; 5.174 = 5.17)

2. Express fractions in lowest terms.

   (Example: $\frac{6}{10} = \frac{3}{5}$)

Mathematics Diagnostic Evaluation

1. 1517 + 0.63 = ________
2. Express the value of XIX + VIII in Arabic numbers. ________
3. 9.5 + 17.06 + 32 + 41.11 + 0.99 = ________
4. $19.69 + $304.03 = ________
5. 93.2 – 47.09 = ________
6. 1005 – 250.5 = ________
7. Express the value of 6003 – 5995 in Roman numerals. ________
8. 509 × 38.3 = ________
9. $4.12 × 42 = ________
10. 17.16 × 23.5 = ________
11. 972 ÷ 27 = ________
12. 2.5 ÷ 0.001 = ________

13. Express the value of 176 ÷ 16 in Roman numerals. ________

14. Express $\frac{1500}{240}$ as a decimal. ________

15. Express 0.8 as a fraction. ________

16. Express $\frac{2}{5}$ as a percent. ________

17. Express 0.004 as a percent. ________

18. Express 5% as a decimal. ________

19. Express $33\frac{1}{3}\%$ as a ratio in lowest terms. ________

20. Express 1:50 as a decimal. ________

21. $\frac{1}{2} + \frac{3}{4} =$ ________

22. $1\frac{2}{3} + 4\frac{7}{8} =$ ________

23. $1\frac{5}{6} - \frac{2}{9} =$ ________

24. Express the value of $\frac{1}{100} \times 60$ as a fraction. ________

25. Express the value of $4\frac{1}{4} \times 3\frac{1}{2}$ as a fraction. ________

26. Identify the fraction with the greatest value: $\frac{1}{150}, \frac{1}{200}, \frac{1}{100}$ ________

27. Identify the decimal with the least value: 0.009, 0.19, 0.9 ________

28. $\frac{6.4}{0.02} =$ ________

29. $\frac{0.02 + 0.16}{0.4 - 0.34} =$ ________

30. Express the value of $\frac{3}{12+3} \times 0.25$ as a decimal. ________

31. 8% of 50 = ________

32. $\frac{1}{2}\%$ of 18 = ________

33. 0.9% of 24 = ________

Find the value of "X." Express your answer as a decimal.

34. $\frac{1:1000}{1:100} \times 250 = X$ ________

35. $\frac{300}{150} \times 2 = X$ ________

36. $\frac{2.5}{5} \times 1.5 = X$ ________

37. $\frac{1{,}000{,}000}{250{,}000} \times X = 12$ ________

38. $\frac{0.51}{1.7} \times X = 150$ ________

39. $X = (82.4 - 52)\frac{3}{5}$ ________

40. $\dfrac{\frac{1}{150}}{\frac{1}{300}} \times 1.2 = X$ __________

41. Express 2:10 as a fraction in lowest terms. __________

42. Express 2% as a ratio in lowest terms. __________

43. If 5 equal medication containers contain 25 tablets total, how many tablets are in each container? __________

44. If 1 pound of sugar equals 4 cups, how many pounds of sugar are in 1 cup? __________

45. If 1 kilogram equals 2.2 pounds, how many kilograms does a 66-pound child weigh? __________

46. If 1 kilogram equals 2.2 pounds, how many pounds are in 1.5 kilograms? (Express your answer as a decimal.) __________

47. If 1 centimeter equals $\frac{3}{8}$ inch, how many centimeters are in $2\frac{1}{2}$ inches? (Express your answer as a decimal.) __________

48. If you have a roll of quarters and you must pay $1.25, how many quarters will you use? __________

49. This diagnostic test has a total of 50 problems. If you incorrectly answer 5 problems, what percentage will you have answered correctly? __________

50. For every 5 female student nurses in a nursing class, there is 1 male student nurse. What is the ratio of female to male student nurses? __________

After completing these problems, see page 410 to check your answers. Give yourself two points for each correct answer.

Perfect score = 100 Readiness score = 86 or higher My score = ______

CHAPTER

1

Mathematics Review for Dosage Calculations: Arabic Numbers, Roman Numerals, Fractions, and Decimals

objectives

Upon mastery of Chapter 1, you will be able to perform basic mathematical computations that involve Arabic numbers, Roman numerals, fractions, and decimals. Specifically, you will be able to:

- Convert between Arabic numbers and Roman numerals from 1 to 30.
- Compare the sizes of fractions and decimals.
- Convert between mixed numbers and improper fractions, and between reduced and equivalent forms of fractions.
- Add, subtract, multiply, and divide fractions and decimals.
- Round a decimal to a given place value.
- Read aloud and write out the value of decimal numbers.

Arabic Numbers and Roman Numerals

Most of the medications you will administer will be ordered and measured by amounts expressed in *Arabic numbers:* the familiar system of whole numbers (0–9), fractions ($\frac{1}{2}$), and decimals (0.3) used widely in the United States and internationally. Some medication orders, however, will be expressed as Roman numerals. Interpreting Roman numerals is probably nothing new to you, as you most likely have used them frequently when reading chapter headings or preparing an outline.

The Roman system of counting dates back to ancient Rome. Alphabetic letters are used to designate numeric amounts. Specifically, the letters *I, V,* and *X* are the basic symbols of this system that you will use in dosage calculations.

A simple set of rules governs the Roman system of notation. The position of one letter to another is very important and determines the value of the Roman numeral.

rule

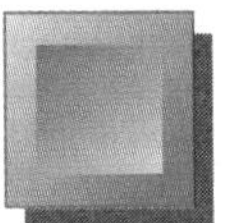

To repeat a Roman numeral twice doubles its value; to repeat a Roman numeral three times triples its value.

Examples:

I = 1 and II = 2

X = 10 and XXX = 30

rule

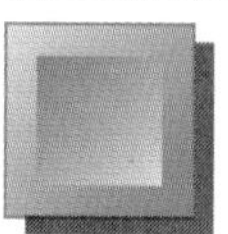

Roman numerals may not be repeated more than three times in succession.

Examples:

III = 3 is a correct notation; however, IIII = 4 is incorrect.

The Arabic number 4 is correctly written IV in Roman numerals.

rule

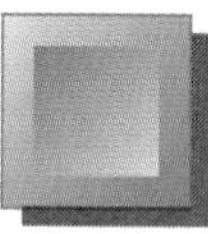

When a Roman numeral of a smaller value *follows* one of a larger value, the numerals are *added.*

Example:

VI = 5 + 1 = 6

rule

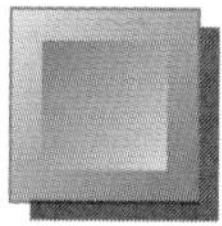

When a Roman numeral of a smaller value *precedes* one of a larger value, the smaller numeral is *subtracted* from the larger.

Example:

IV = 5 – 1 = 4

rule

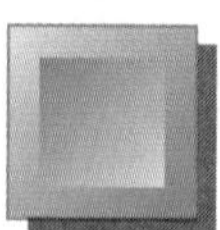

When a Roman numeral of a smaller value comes between two of larger values, it is subtracted from the value of the numeral that follows it; then the addition rule is applied.

Examples:

XIV = 10 + (5 – 1) = 10 + 4 = 14

XXIX = 10 + 10 + (10 – 1) = 10 + 10 + 9 = 29

In medical notation, lowercase letters are typically used to designate Roman numerals.

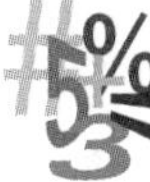

math tip: To decrease errors in interpretation of medical notation, a line can be drawn over the lowercase Roman numerals to distinguish them from other letters in a word or phrase. The lowercase *i* is dotted above, not below, the line.

Example:

3 = iii or $\overline{\dot{i}\dot{i}\dot{i}}$

Learn the following common Roman numerals and their Arabic equivalents. These are the values that you will use most frequently to interpret drug orders and read drug labels.

remember

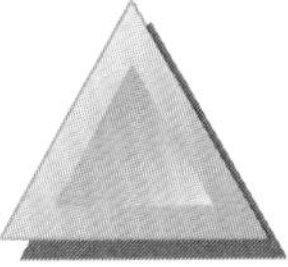

Roman Numeral	Arabic Number	Roman Numeral	Arabic Number
I, i, $\overline{\dot{i}}$	1	VIII, viii, $\overline{v\dot{i}\dot{i}\dot{i}}$	8
II, ii, $\overline{\dot{i}\dot{i}}$	2	IX, ix, $\overline{\dot{i}x}$	9
III, iii, $\overline{\dot{i}\dot{i}\dot{i}}$	3	X, x, $\overline{x}$	10
IV, iv, $\overline{\dot{i}v}$	4	XV, xv, $\overline{xv}$	15
V, v, $\overline{v}$	5	XX, xx, $\overline{xx}$	20
VI, vi, $\overline{v\dot{i}}$	6	XXV, xxv, $\overline{xxv}$	25
VII, vii, $\overline{v\dot{i}\dot{i}}$	7	XXX, xxx, $\overline{xxx}$	30

Let's review the major concepts from this section.

quick review

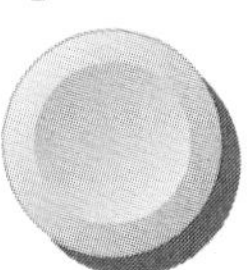

When interpreting Roman numerals:

- Letters are used to designate numbers. Example: I = 1, V = 5, X = 10
- Repeating a letter twice doubles its value. Example: II = 2
- Repeating a letter three times triples its value. Example: III = 3
- Roman numerals are only repeated up to three times. Example: III is correct, but IIII is not.
- When a smaller value Roman numeral follows a larger, add. Example: XI = 10 + 1 = 11
- When a smaller value Roman numeral comes before a larger, subtract. Example: IX = 10 − 1 = 9
- When a smaller value Roman numeral comes between two larger ones, it is subtracted from the value of the numeral that follows it; then addition is applied. Example: xix = 10 + (10 − 1) = 19

Work the following exercises to reinforce your understanding of this section.

review set 1

Convert the following Arabic numbers to Roman numerals.

1. 28 = ________
2. 13 = ________
3. 17 = ________
4. 15 = ________
5. 9 = ________
6. 12 = ________

Perform the indicated operations and record the results in Arabic numbers.

7. VII + XXIII = ________
8. XXVII − IV = ________
9. XIX − XIV = ________
10. XII × II = ________
11. XXIV ÷ VI = ________
12. IV × III = ________

Perform the indicated operations and record the results in Roman numerals:

13. $5 \times 4 =$ ________
14. $18 + 12 =$ ________
15. $16 \div 4 =$ ________
16. $4 \times 3 =$ ________
17. $625 \div 125 =$ ________
18. $17 + 14 - 11 + 4 =$ ________
19. $6 + 3 =$ ________
20. $20 - 16 + 3 =$ ________

After completing these problems, see page 410 to check your answers.

Fractions

Nurses need to understand fractions to be able to interpret and act on doctors' orders, read prescriptions, and understand patient records and information in health care literature. You will see fractions used in apothecary and household measures in dosage calculations. Proficiency with fractions will add to your success with medical applications.

A *fraction* indicates a portion of a whole number. There are two types of fractions: *common fractions*, such as $\frac{1}{2}$ (usually referred to simply as fractions) and *decimal fractions*, such as 0.5 (usually referred to simply as decimals).

A fraction is an expression of division, with one number placed over another number ($\frac{1}{4}$, $\frac{2}{3}$, $\frac{4}{5}$). The bottom number, or *denominator*, indicates the total number of parts into which the whole is divided. The top number, or *numerator*, indicates how many of those parts are considered. The fraction may also be read as the "numerator *divided* by the denominator."

Example:

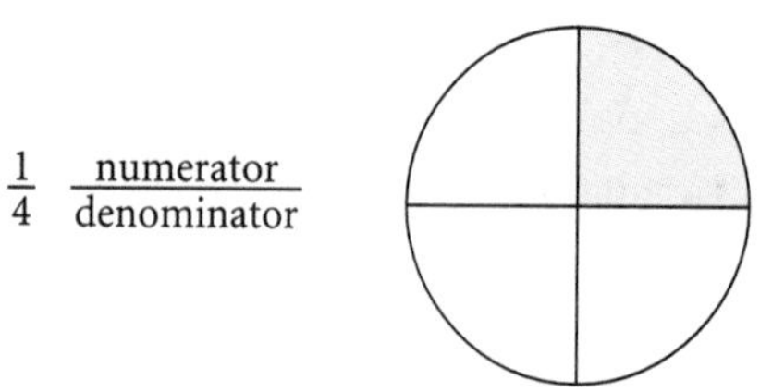

The whole is divided into four equal parts (denominator), and one part (numerator) is considered.

$\frac{1}{4}$ = 1 part of 4 parts, or $\frac{1}{4}$ of the whole.

The fraction $\frac{1}{4}$ may also be read as "1 divided by 4."

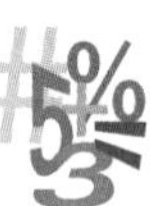

math tip: The *d*enominator begins with *d* and is *d*own below the line in a fraction.

There are four types of common fractions.

1. *Proper fractions*—in which the value of the numerator is *less* than the value of the denominator. The value of the proper fraction is also *less* than 1.

rule

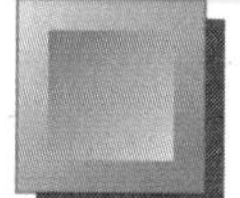

Whenever the numerator is less than the denominator, the value of the fraction must be less than 1.

Example:

$\frac{5}{8} \quad \frac{\text{numerator}}{\text{denominator}}$ = less than 1; $\frac{5}{8} < 1$

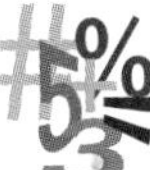

math tip: The symbol $<$ denotes "is less than," and the symbol $>$ denotes "is greater than." Notice that the point of the symbol always points toward the smaller number.

Examples:

$3 < 10$ means 3 "is less than" 10

$20 > 5$ means 20 "is greater than" 5

2. *Improper fractions*—in which the value of the numerator is *greater* than or *equal* to the value of the denominator. The value of the improper fraction is *greater* than or *equal* to 1.

rule

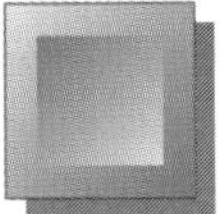

Whenever the numerator is greater than the denominator, the value of the fraction must be greater than 1.

Example:

$\frac{8}{5} > 1$

rule

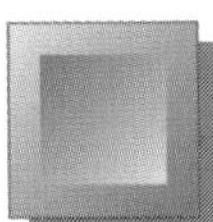

Whenever the numerator and denominator are equal, the value of the improper fraction is always equal to 1; a nonzero number divided by itself is equal to 1.

Example:

$\frac{5}{5} = 1$

3. *Mixed numbers*—in which a whole number and a proper fraction are combined. The value of the mixed number is always *greater* than 1.

Example:

$1\frac{5}{8} = 1 + \frac{5}{8}; 1\frac{5}{8} > 1$

4. *Complex fractions*—in which the numerator or the denominator or both may be a whole number, proper fraction, or mixed number. The value may be *less* than, *greater* than, or *equal to* 1.

Examples:

$$\frac{\frac{5}{8}}{\frac{1}{2}} > 1$$

$$\frac{\frac{5}{8}}{2} < 1$$

$$\frac{1\frac{5}{8}}{\frac{1}{5}} > 1$$

$$\frac{\frac{1}{2}}{\frac{2}{4}} = 1$$

To perform dosage calculations that involve fractions, you must be able to convert among these different types of fractions and reduce them to lowest terms. You must also apply the operations of addition, subtraction, multiplication, and division. Review these simple rules of working with fractions. Stay with it until the concepts are crystal clear and automatic.

Conversion

It is important to be able to convert among different types of fractions. Conversion allows you to perform various calculations with greater ease and permits you to express answers in simplest terms.

Converting Mixed Numbers to Improper Fractions

rule

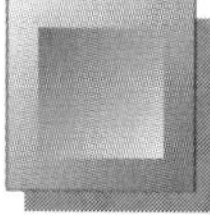

To change or convert a mixed number to an improper fraction with the same denominator, *multiply the whole number by the denominator and add the numerator.* Place that value in the numerator, and use the denominator of the fraction part of the mixed number.

Example:

$$1\frac{5}{8} = \frac{1 \times 8 + 5}{8} = \frac{13}{8}$$

Converting Improper Fractions to Mixed Numbers

rule

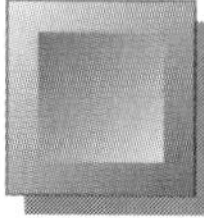

To change or convert an improper fraction to an equivalent mixed number or whole number, *divide the numerator by the denominator.* Any remainder is expressed as a proper fraction and reduced to lowest terms.

Examples:

$$\frac{8}{5} = 8 \div 5 = 1\frac{3}{5}$$

$$\frac{10}{4} = 10 \div 4 = 2\frac{2}{4} = 2\frac{1}{2}$$

Equivalent Fractions

The value of a fraction can be expressed in several ways. This is called *finding an equivalent fraction*. In finding an equivalent fraction, both terms of the fraction (numerator and denominator) are either multiplied or divided by the *same nonzero number*.

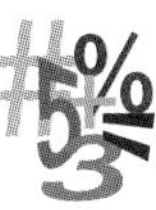

math tip: In an *equivalent fraction*, the form of the fraction is changed, but the value of the fraction remains the same.

Examples:

$$\frac{2 \div 2}{4 \div 2} = \frac{1}{2}$$

$$\frac{1 \times 3}{3 \times 3} = \frac{3}{9}$$

When calculating dosages, it is usually easier to work with fractions of the smallest numbers possible. Finding equivalent fractions is called *reducing the fraction to the lowest terms* or *simplifying the fraction*. The next section explains how to reduce or simplify fractions.

Reducing Fractions to Lowest Terms

rule

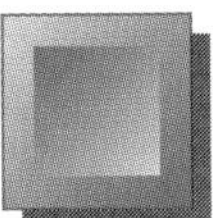

To reduce a fraction to lowest terms, *divide* both the numerator and denominator by the *largest nonzero whole number* that will go evenly into both the numerator and the denominator.

Example:

Reduce $\frac{6}{12}$ to lowest terms.

6 is the largest number that will divide evenly into both 6 (numerator) and 12 (denominator).

$\frac{6}{12} = \frac{6 \div 6}{12 \div 6} = \frac{1}{2}$ in lowest terms

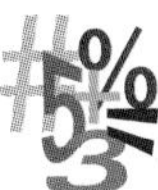

math tip: If *both* the numerator and denominator *cannot* be divided evenly by a nonzero number other than 1, then the fraction is in lowest terms.

Enlarging Fractions

rule

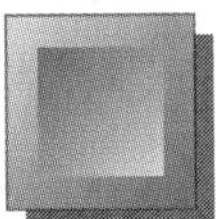

To find an equivalent fraction in which both terms are larger, *multiply both* the numerator and the denominator by the *same nonzero number*.

Example:

Enlarge $\frac{3}{5}$ to the equivalent fraction in tenths.

$$\frac{3}{5} = \frac{3 \times 2}{5 \times 2} = \frac{6}{10}$$

Comparing Fractions

In calculating some drug dosages, it is helpful to know when the value of one fraction is greater or less than another. The relative sizes of fractions can be determined by comparing the numerators when the denominators are the same or comparing the denominators if the numerators are the same.

rule

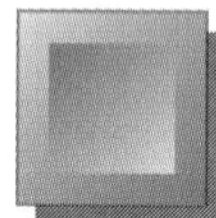

If the numerators are the same, the fraction with the smaller denominator has the greater value.

Example:

Compare $\frac{1}{2}$ and $\frac{1}{4}$.

Numerators are both 1.

Denominators: $2 < 4$.

$\frac{1}{2}$ has a greater value.

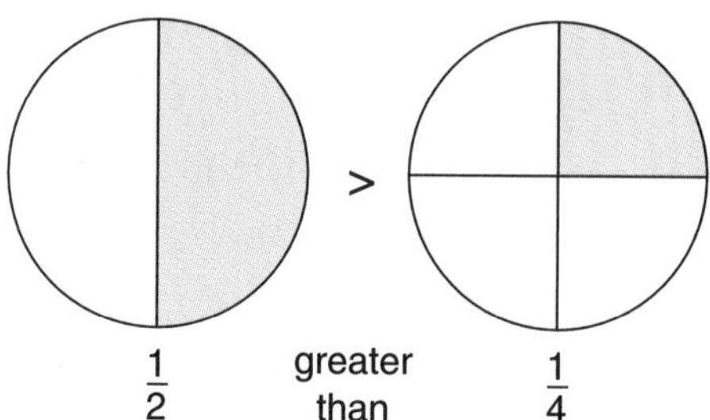

rule

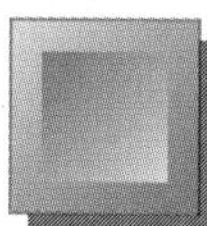

If the denominators are both the same, the fraction with the smaller numerator has the lesser value.

Example:

Compare $\frac{2}{5}$ and $\frac{3}{5}$.

Denominators are both 5.

Numerators: $2 < 3$

$\frac{2}{5}$ has a lesser value.

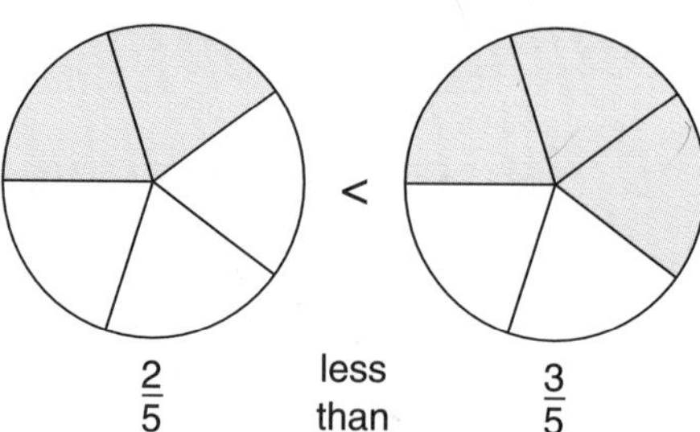

quick review

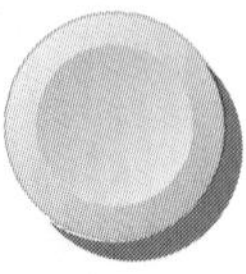

- Proper fraction: numerator $<$ denominator; value is < 1. Example: $\frac{1}{2}$
- Improper fraction: numerator $>$ denominator; value is > 1. Example: $\frac{4}{3}$. Or numerator = denominator; value = 1. Example: $\frac{5}{5}$
- Mixed number: whole number + a fraction; value is > 1. Example: $1\frac{1}{2}$
- Complex fraction: numerator and/or denominator composed of fractions; value is >, <, or = 1. Example: $\frac{\frac{1}{2}}{\frac{1}{50}}$
- Any nonzero number divided by itself = 1. Example: $\frac{3}{3} = 1$
- When numerators are equal, the fraction with the smaller denominator is greater. Example: $\frac{1}{2} > \frac{1}{3}$
- When denominators are equal, the fraction with the larger numerator is greater. Example: $\frac{2}{3} > \frac{1}{3}$

- To convert a mixed number to an improper fraction, multiply the whole number by the denominator and add the numerator; use original denominator in the fractional part. Example: $1\frac{1}{3} = \frac{4}{3}$
- To convert an improper fraction to a mixed number, divide the numerator by the denominator. Express any remainder as a proper fraction reduced to lowest terms. Example: $\frac{21}{9} = 2\frac{3}{9} = 2\frac{1}{3}$
- To reduce a fraction to lowest terms, divide both terms by the largest nonzero whole number that will divide both the numerator and denominator evenly. Value remains the same. Example: $\frac{6}{10} = \frac{6 \div 2}{10 \div 2} = \frac{3}{5}$
- To enlarge a fraction, multiply both terms by the same nonzero number. Value remains the same. Example: $\frac{1}{12} = \frac{1 \times 2}{12 \times 2} = \frac{2}{24}$

review set 2

1. Circle the *improper* fraction(s).

   $\frac{2}{3}$ $1\frac{3}{4}$ $\frac{6}{6}$ $\frac{7}{5}$ $\frac{16}{17}$ $\frac{\frac{1}{9}}{\frac{2}{3}}$

2. Circle the *complex* fraction(s).

   $\frac{4}{5}$ $3\frac{7}{8}$ $\frac{2}{2}$ $\frac{9}{8}$ $\frac{8}{9}$ $\frac{\frac{1}{100}}{\frac{1}{150}}$

3. Circle the *proper* fraction(s).

   $\frac{1}{4}$ $\frac{1}{14}$ $\frac{14}{1}$ $\frac{14}{14}$ $\frac{144}{14}$

4. Circle the *mixed* number(s) *reduced to the lowest terms.*

   $3\frac{4}{8}$ $\frac{2}{3}$ $1\frac{2}{9}$ $\frac{1}{3}$ $1\frac{1}{4}$ $5\frac{7}{8}$

5. Circle the pair(s) of *equivalent* fractions.

   $\frac{3}{4} = \frac{6}{8}$ $\frac{1}{5} = \frac{2}{10}$ $\frac{3}{9} = \frac{1}{3}$ $\frac{3}{4} = \frac{4}{3}$ $1\frac{4}{9} = 1\frac{2}{3}$

Change the following mixed numbers to improper fractions.

6. $6\frac{1}{2} =$ ________
7. $1\frac{1}{5} =$ ________
8. $10\frac{2}{3} =$ ________
9. $7\frac{5}{6} =$ ________
10. $102\frac{3}{4} =$ ________

Change the following improper fractions to whole numbers or mixed numbers; reduce to lowest terms.

11. $\frac{24}{12} =$ ________
12. $\frac{8}{8} =$ ________
13. $\frac{30}{9} =$ ________
14. $\frac{100}{75} =$ ________
15. $\frac{44}{16} =$ ________

Enlarge the following fractions to the number of parts indicated.

16. $\frac{3}{4}$ to eighths ________

17. $\frac{1}{4}$ to sixteenths ________

18. $\frac{2}{3}$ to twelfths ________

19. $\frac{2}{5}$ to tenths ________

20. $\frac{2}{3}$ to ninths ________

Circle the correct answer.

21. Which is larger? $\frac{1}{150}$, $\frac{1}{100}$

22. Which is smaller? $\frac{1}{1000}$, $\frac{1}{10,000}$

23. Which is larger? $\frac{2}{9}$, $\frac{5}{9}$

24. Which is smaller? $\frac{3}{10}$, $\frac{5}{10}$

25. You are serving pizza, and you give $\frac{1}{4}$ of it to each of 3 adults. You divide the remaining piece between 2 children. What portion of the whole pizza is each child's slice? (Think carefully. Hint: Draw yourself a picture.) ________

26. If 1 medicine bottle contains 12 doses, how many bottles are used up for 18 doses? ________

27. A nursing school class consists of 3 men and 57 women. What fraction of the students in the class are men? (Express your answer as a fraction reduced to lowest terms.) ________

28. A nursing student answers 18 out of 20 questions correctly on a test. Write a proper fraction (reduced to lowest terms) to represent the portion of the test questions which were answered correctly. ________

29. A typical dose of Children's Tylenol contains 160 milligrams of Tylenol per teaspoonful. Each 80 milligrams is what part of a typical dose? ________

30. In question 29, how many teaspoons of Tylenol would you need to give 80 milligrams? ________

After completing these problems, see pages 410 and 411 to check your answers. If you answered question 30 correctly, you can already calculate dosages!

Addition and Subtraction of Fractions

To add or subtract fractions, all the denominators must be the same.

rule

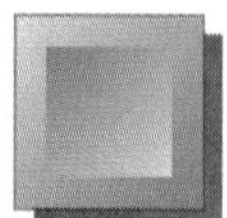

To add or subtract fractions:

1. Convert all fractions to equivalent fractions with the least common denominators; then
2. Add or subtract the numerators, place that value in the numerator, and use the least common denominator as the denominator; and,
3. Convert to a mixed number and/or reduce the fraction to lowest terms.

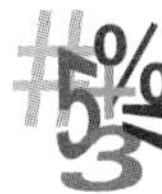

math tip: To *add or subtract fractions,* no calculations are performed on the denominators. Once they are all converted to common denominators, perform the mathematical operation (addition or subtraction) on the *numerators* only, and use the common denominator in your answer.

Example 1:

$\frac{3}{4} + \frac{1}{4} + \frac{2}{4}$

1. Find the least common denominator. This step is not necessary, because the fractions already have the same denominator.
2. Add the numerators: $\frac{3+1+2}{4} = \frac{6}{4}$
3. Convert to a mixed number and reduce to lowest terms: $\frac{6}{4} = 1\frac{2}{4} = 1\frac{1}{2}$

Example 2:

$\frac{1}{3} + \frac{3}{4} + \frac{1}{6}$

1. Find the least common denominator: 12.

   Convert to equivalent fractions in twelfths. This is the same as enlarging the fractions.

   $\frac{1}{3} = \frac{4}{12}$

   $\frac{3}{4} = \frac{9}{12}$

   $\frac{1}{6} = \frac{2}{12}$

2. Add the numerators: $\frac{4+9+2}{12} = \frac{15}{12}$
3. Convert to a mixed number, and reduce to lowest terms: $\frac{15}{12} = 1\frac{3}{12} = 1\frac{1}{4}$

Example 3:

$\frac{15}{18} - \frac{8}{18} = \frac{7}{18}$

1. Find the least common denominator. This is not necessary. The denominators are the same.
2. Subtract the numerators, and use the common denominator: $\frac{15-8}{18} = \frac{7}{18}$
3. Reduce to lowest terms. This is not necessary. No further reduction is possible.

Example 4:

$1\frac{1}{10} - \frac{3}{5}$

1. Find the least common denominator: 10

   Convert to equivalent fractions in tenths:

   $1\frac{1}{10} = \frac{11}{10}$

   $\frac{3}{5} = \frac{6}{10}$

   $\frac{11}{10} - \frac{6}{10}$

2. Subtract the numerators, and use the common denominator: $\frac{11-6}{10} = \frac{5}{10}$

3. Reduce to lowest terms: $\frac{5}{10} = \frac{1}{2}$

Let's review one more time how to add and subtract fractions.

quick review

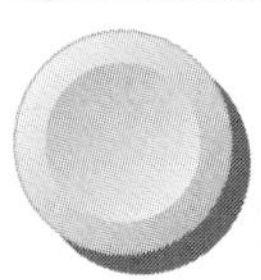

To add or subtract fractions:

- Convert to equivalent fractions with least common denominators.
- Add or subtract the numerators; place that value in the numerator. Use least common denominator as the denominator.
- Convert answer to mixed number and/or reduce to lowest terms.

review set 3

Add, and reduce the answers to lowest terms.

1. $7\frac{4}{5} + \frac{2}{3} =$ ______
2. $\frac{3}{4} + \frac{2}{3} =$ ______
3. $4\frac{2}{3} + 5\frac{1}{24} + 7\frac{1}{2} =$ ______
4. $\frac{3}{4} + \frac{1}{8} + \frac{1}{6} =$ ______
5. $12\frac{1}{2} + 20\frac{1}{3} =$ ______
6. $\frac{1}{4} + 5\frac{1}{3} =$ ______
7. $\frac{1}{7} + \frac{6}{11} + \frac{2}{5} =$ ______
8. $\frac{4}{9} + \frac{5}{8} + 4\frac{2}{3} =$ ______
9. $34\frac{1}{2} + 8\frac{1}{2} =$ ______
10. $\frac{12}{17} + 5\frac{2}{7} =$ ______
11. $\frac{6}{5} + 1\frac{1}{3} =$ ______
12. $\frac{1}{4} + \frac{5}{33} =$ ______

Subtract, and reduce the answers to lowest terms.

13. $\frac{3}{4} - \frac{1}{4} =$ ______
14. $8\frac{1}{12} - 3\frac{1}{4} =$ ______
15. $\frac{1}{8} - \frac{1}{12} =$ ______
16. $100 - 36\frac{1}{3} =$ ______
17. $355\frac{1}{5} - 55\frac{2}{5} =$ ______
18. $\frac{1}{3} - \frac{1}{6} =$ ______
19. $2\frac{3}{5} - 1\frac{1}{5} =$ ______
20. $14\frac{3}{16} - 7\frac{1}{8} =$ ______
21. $256 - 179\frac{7}{9} =$ ______
22. $4\frac{7}{10} - 3\frac{9}{20} =$ ______
23. $488\frac{6}{11} - 247 =$ ______
24. $1\frac{2}{3} - 1\frac{1}{12} =$ ______
25. A circle is divided into 12 equal parts, and 4 parts are shaded. Write a fraction reduced to lowest terms to express the unshaded parts. ______
26. A nursing student gave her patient $\frac{1}{4}$ ounce of medication at 8 A.M. and $\frac{1}{3}$ ounce of medication at 12 noon. What is the total amount of medication given? ______
27. An infant has grown $\frac{1}{2}$ inch during his first month of life, $\frac{1}{4}$ inch during his second month, and $\frac{3}{8}$ inch during his third month. How much did he grow? ______

28. The required margins for your term paper are $1\frac{1}{2}$ inches at the top and bottom of a paper that has 11 inches vertical length. How long is the vertical area available for written information? 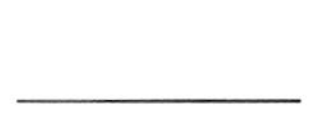

29. The central supply stock clerk finds there are $34\frac{1}{2}$ pints of hydrogen peroxide on the shelf. If the fully stocked shelf held 56 pints of hydrogen peroxide, how many pints were used? ________

30. Your one-year-old patient weighs $30\frac{1}{8}$ pounds. At birth, she weighed $10\frac{1}{16}$ pounds. How much weight has she gained in one year? ________

After completing these problems, see page 411 to check your answers.

Multiplication of Fractions

To multiply fractions, multiply numerators (for the numerator of the answer), and multiply denominators (for the denominator of the answer).

When possible, *cancellation of terms* simplifies and shortens the process of both multiplication and division of fractions. Cancellation (like reducing to lowest terms) is based on the fact that the division of both the numerator and denominator by the same whole number does not change the value of the resulting number. In fact, it makes the calculation simpler, because you are working with smaller numbers.

Example:

$\frac{1}{3} \times \frac{250}{500}$ (numerator and denominator of $\frac{250}{500}$ are both divisible by 250)

$$= \frac{1}{3} \times \frac{\overset{1}{\cancel{250}}}{\underset{2}{\cancel{500}}} = \frac{1}{3} \times \frac{1}{2} = \frac{1}{6}$$

Also, the numerators and denominators of any of the fractions involved in the multiplication may be canceled when they are like numbers. This is called *cross-cancellation*.

Example:

$$\frac{1}{8} \times \frac{8}{9} = \frac{1}{\underset{1}{\cancel{8}}} \times \frac{\overset{1}{\cancel{8}}}{9} = \frac{1}{1} \times \frac{1}{9} = \frac{1}{9}$$

rule

To multiply fractions:

1. Cancel terms, if possible;
2. Multiply numerators for the numerator of the answer, multiply denominators for the denominator of the answer, and
3. Reduce the result (*product*) to lowest terms.

Example 1:

$\frac{3}{4} \times \frac{2}{6}$

1. Cancel terms: Divide 2 and 6 by 2

   $\frac{3}{4} \times \frac{\overset{1}{\cancel{2}}}{\underset{3}{\cancel{6}}} = \frac{3}{4} \times \frac{1}{3}$

   Divide 3 and 3 by 3

   $\frac{\overset{1}{\cancel{3}}}{4} \times \frac{1}{\underset{1}{\cancel{3}}} = \frac{1}{4} \times \frac{1}{1}$

2. Multiply numerators and denominators:

   $\frac{1}{4} \times \frac{1}{1} = \frac{1}{4}$

3. Reduce to lowest terms: not neccesary. Product is in lowest terms.

Example 2:

$\frac{15}{30} \times \frac{2}{5}$

1. Cancel terms: Divide 15 and 30 by 15

   $\frac{\overset{1}{\cancel{15}}}{\underset{2}{\cancel{30}}} \times \frac{2}{5} = \frac{1}{2} \times \frac{2}{5}$

   Divide 2 and 2 by 2

   $\frac{1}{\underset{1}{\cancel{2}}} \times \frac{\overset{1}{\cancel{2}}}{5} = \frac{1}{1} \times \frac{1}{5}$

2. Multiply numerators and denominators:

   $\frac{1}{1} \times \frac{1}{5} = \frac{1}{5}$

3. Reduce to lowest terms: not necessary. Product is in lowest terms.

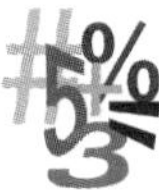

math tip: When multiplying a fraction by a nonzero whole number, the same rule applies for multiplying fractions. First convert the whole number to a fraction with a denominator of 1; the value of the number remains the same.

Example 3:

$\frac{2}{3} \times 4 = \frac{2}{3} \times \frac{4}{1}$

1. No terms to cancel. (You cannot cancel 2 and 4 since both are numerators. To do so would change the value.)

2. Multiply numerators and denominators:

   $\frac{2}{3} \times \frac{4}{1} = \frac{2}{3} \times \frac{4}{1} = \frac{8}{3}$

3. Convert to a mixed number.

   $\frac{8}{3} = 8 \div 3 = 2\frac{2}{3}$

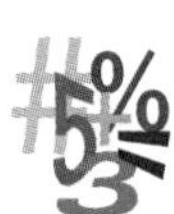

math tip: To multiply mixed numbers, first convert them to improper fractions, and then multiply.

Example 4:

$3\frac{1}{2} \times 4\frac{1}{3}$

1. Convert: $3\frac{1}{2} = \frac{7}{2}$

   $4\frac{1}{3} = \frac{13}{3}$

   Therefore, $3\frac{1}{2} \times 4\frac{1}{3} = \frac{7}{2} \times \frac{13}{3}$

2. Cancel: not necessary. No numbers can be canceled.
3. Multiply: $\frac{7}{2} \times \frac{13}{3} = \frac{91}{6}$
4. Convert to a mixed number: $\frac{91}{6} = 15\frac{1}{6}$

Division of Fractions

The division of fractions includes three terms: *dividend, divisor,* and *quotient*. The *dividend* is the fraction being divided or the first number. The *divisor,* the number to the right of the division sign, is the fraction the dividend is divided by. The *quotient* is the result of the division. To divide fractions, the divisor is inverted, and the operation is changed to multiplication. Once inverted, the calculation is the same as for multiplication of fractions.

Example:

$$\frac{1}{4} \div \frac{2}{7} = \frac{1}{4} \times \frac{7}{2} = \frac{7}{8}$$

Dividend ($\frac{1}{4}$) — Divisor ($\frac{2}{7}$) — ÷ changed to × — Inverted Divisor ($\frac{7}{2}$) — Quotient ($\frac{7}{8}$)

rule

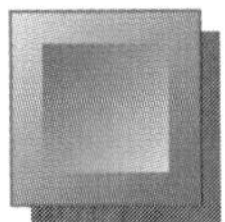

To divide fractions,

1. Invert the terms of the divisor, change ÷ to ×;
2. Cancel terms, if possible;
3. Multiply the resulting fractions; and
4. Convert the result (quotient) to a mixed number, and/or reduce to lowest terms.

Example 1:

$\frac{3}{4} \div \frac{1}{3}$

1. Invert divisor, and change ÷ to ×: $\frac{3}{4} \div \frac{1}{3} = \frac{3}{4} \times \frac{3}{1}$
2. Cancel: not necessary. No numbers can be canceled.
3. Multiply: $\frac{3}{4} \times \frac{3}{1} = \frac{9}{4}$
4. Convert to mixed number: $\frac{9}{4} = 2\frac{1}{4}$

Example 2:

$\frac{2}{3} \div 4$

1. Invert divisor, and change ÷ to ×: $\frac{2}{3} \div \frac{4}{1} = \frac{2}{3} \times \frac{1}{4}$

2. Cancel terms: $\frac{\overset{1}{\cancel{2}}}{3} \times \frac{1}{\underset{2}{\cancel{4}}} = \frac{1}{3} \times \frac{1}{2}$

3. Multiply: $\frac{1}{3} \times \frac{1}{2} = \frac{1}{6}$

4. Reduce: not necessary; already reduced to lowest terms.

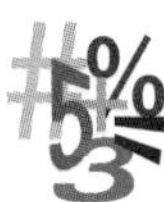

math tip: To divide mixed numbers, first convert them to improper fractions.

Example 3:

$1\frac{1}{2} \div \frac{3}{4}$

1. Convert: $\frac{3}{2} \div \frac{3}{4}$

2. Invert divisor, and change ÷ to ×: $\frac{3}{2} \times \frac{4}{3}$

3. Cancel: $\frac{\overset{1}{\cancel{3}}}{\underset{1}{\cancel{2}}} \times \frac{\overset{2}{\cancel{4}}}{\underset{1}{\cancel{3}}} = \frac{1}{1} \times \frac{2}{1}$

4. Multiply: $\frac{1}{1} \times \frac{2}{1} = \frac{2}{1}$

5. Reduce: $\frac{2}{1} = 2$

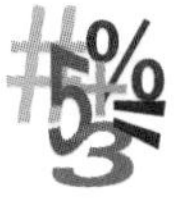

math tip: To multiply complex fractions also involves the division of fractions. Study this carefully.

Example 4:

$\frac{\frac{1}{150}}{\frac{1}{100}} \times 2$

1. Convert: Express 2 as a fraction. $\frac{\frac{1}{150}}{\frac{1}{100}} \times \frac{2}{1}$

2. Rewrite complex fraction as division: $\frac{1}{150} \div \frac{1}{100} \times \frac{2}{1}$

3. Invert divisor and change ÷ to ×: $\frac{1}{150} \times \frac{100}{1} \times \frac{2}{1}$

4. Cancel: $\frac{1}{\underset{3}{\cancel{150}}} \times \frac{\overset{2}{\cancel{100}}}{1} \times \frac{2}{1} = \frac{1}{3} \times \frac{2}{1} \times \frac{2}{1}$

5. Multiply: $\frac{1}{3} \times \frac{2}{1} \times \frac{2}{1} = \frac{4}{3}$

6. Convert to mixed number: $\frac{4}{3} = 1\frac{1}{3}$

This example appears difficult at first, but when solved logically, one step at a time, it is just like the others.

quick review

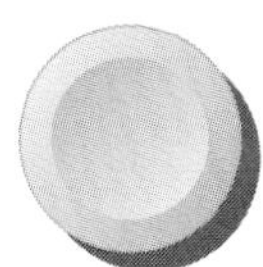

- *To multiply fractions,* cancel terms, multiply numerators, and multiply denominators.
- *To divide fractions,* invert the divisor, cancel terms, and multiply.
- Convert results to a mixed number and/or reduce to lowest terms.

review set 4

Multiply, and reduce the answers to lowest terms.

1. $\frac{3}{10} \times \frac{1}{12} =$ ______
2. $\frac{12}{25} \times \frac{3}{5} =$ ______
3. $\frac{5}{8} \times 1\frac{1}{6} =$ ______
4. $\frac{1}{100} \times 3 =$ ______
5. $\frac{\frac{1}{6}}{\frac{1}{4}} \times \frac{\frac{3}{2}}{3} =$ ______
6. $\frac{\frac{1}{150}}{\frac{1}{100}} \times 2\frac{1}{2} =$ ______
7. $\frac{30}{75} \times 2 =$ ______
8. $9\frac{4}{5} \times \frac{2}{3} =$ ______
9. $\frac{3}{4} \times \frac{2}{3} =$ ______
10. $4\frac{2}{3} \times 5\frac{1}{24} =$ ______
11. $\frac{3}{4} \times \frac{1}{8} =$ ______
12. $12\frac{1}{2} \times 20\frac{1}{3} =$ ______

Divide, and reduce the answers to lowest terms.

13. $\frac{3}{4} \div \frac{1}{4} =$ ______
14. $6\frac{1}{12} \div 3\frac{1}{4} =$ ______
15. $\frac{1}{8} \div \frac{7}{12} =$ ______
16. $\frac{1}{33} \div \frac{1}{3} =$ ______
17. $5\frac{1}{4} \div 10\frac{1}{2} =$ ______
18. $\frac{1}{60} \div \frac{1}{2} =$ ______
19. $2\frac{1}{2} \div \frac{3}{4} =$ ______
20. $\frac{\frac{1}{20}}{\frac{1}{3}} =$ ______
21. $\frac{1}{150} \div \frac{1}{50} =$ ______
22. $\frac{\frac{3}{4}}{\frac{7}{8}} \div \frac{1\frac{1}{2}}{2\frac{1}{3}} =$ ______
23. $\frac{\frac{3}{5}}{\frac{3}{4}} \div \frac{\frac{4}{5}}{1\frac{1}{9}} =$ ______
24. One large apple contains 80 calories. How many calories do you consume if you eat $\frac{3}{4}$ of an apple? ______
25. How many seconds are there in $9\frac{1}{3}$ minutes? ______

26. A bottle of Children's Tylenol contains 20 teaspoons of liquid. If each dose for a 2-year-old child is $\frac{1}{2}$ teaspoon, how many doses are available in this bottle? ________

27. You need to take $1\frac{1}{2}$ tablets of medication 3 times per day for 7 days. Over the 7 days, how many tablets will you take? ________

28. The nurse aide observes that the patient's water pitcher is still $\frac{1}{3}$ full. If he drank 850 milliliters of water, how many milliliters does the pitcher hold? (Hint: The 850 milliliters does not represent $\frac{1}{3}$ of the pitcher.) ________

29. A pharmacist weighs a tube of antibiotic eye ointment and discovers it weighs $\frac{7}{10}$ of an ounce. How much would 75 tubes weigh? ________

30. A patient is taking a liquid antacid from a 16-ounce bottle. If she takes $\frac{1}{2}$ ounce every 4 hours while awake beginning at 7 A.M. and ending with a final dose at 11 P.M., how many full days would this bottle last? (Hint: First, draw yourself a clock.) ________

After completing these problems, see pages 411 and 412 to check your answers.

Decimals

Decimal Fractions and Decimal Numbers

Decimal fractions are fractions with a denominator of 10, 100, 1000, or any multiple or power of 10. At first glance, they appear to be whole numbers because of the way they are written. But the numeric value of a decimal fraction is *always less than one.*

Examples:

$0.1 = \frac{1}{10}$

$0.01 = \frac{1}{100}$

$0.001 = \frac{1}{1000}$

These incremental multiples of 10 define the decimal system.

Decimal numbers are numeric values that include a whole number, a decimal point, and a decimal fraction.

Examples:

4.67 and 23.956

Nurses must have an understanding of decimals to be competent at dosage calculations. Medication orders and other measurements in health care primarily use metric measure, which is based on the decimal system. Decimals are a special shorthand for designating fractional values. They are simpler to read and faster to use when performing mathematical computations.

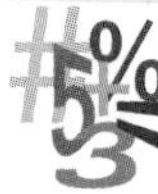

math tip: When dealing with decimals, think of the decimal point as the *center* that separates whole and fractional numbers. The position of the numbers in relation to the decimal point indicates the place value of the numbers.

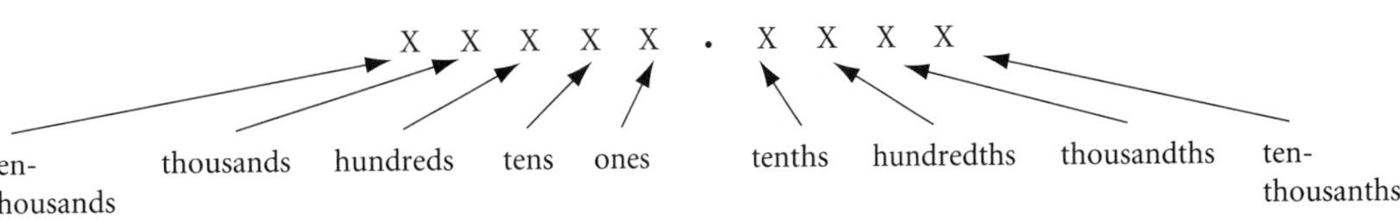

WHOLE NUMBERS DECIMAL FRACTIONS

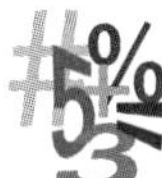

math tip: The words for all decimal fractions end in *th(s)*.

Examples:

0.001 = one-thousand*th*

0.02 = two-hundred*ths*

0.7 = seven-ten*ths*

Example:

Look carefully at the decimal fraction 0.125.

0 . 1 2 5

1 = Tenths
2 = Hundredths
5 = Thousandths

0.125 = $\frac{125}{1000}$ or one hundred twenty-five thousandths

0.125 is less than 0.25 (twenty-five hundredths) but greater than 0.0125 (one hundred twenty-five ten thousandths)

A set of rules governs the decimal system of notation.

rule

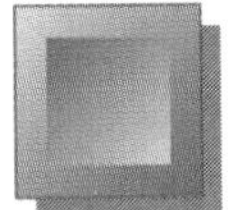

The whole number value is controlled by its position to the *left* of the decimal point.

Examples:

10.1 = ten and one-tenth. The whole number is *ten*.

1.01 = one and one-hundredth. The whole number is *one*.

(Notice that the decimal position completely changes the numeric value.)

rule

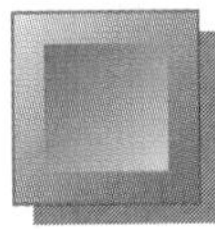

The decimal fraction value is controlled by its position to the *right* of the decimal point.

Examples:

25.1 = twenty five and one-tenth. The decimal fraction is *one-tenth.*

25.01 = twenty five and one-hundredth. The decimal fraction is *one-hundredth.*

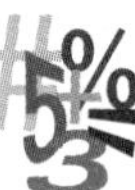

math tip: Each decimal place is counted off as a multiple of 10 to tell you which denominator is expected.

Example 1:

437.5 = four hundred thirty-seven and **five-tenths** ($437 + \frac{5}{10}$)
One decimal place indicates *tenths.*

Example 2:

43.75 = forty three and **seventy-five hundredths** ($43 + \frac{75}{100}$)
Two decimal places indicate *hundredths.*

Example 3:

4.375 = four and **three hundred seventy-five thousandths** ($4 + \frac{375}{1000}$)
Three decimal places indicate *thousandths.*

rule

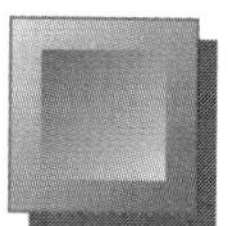

Zeros added *after* the last digit of a decimal fraction *do not* change its value.

Example:

0.25 = 0.25**0**

rule

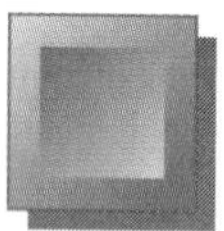

Zeros added *between* the decimal point and the first digit of a decimal fraction *do* change its value.

Example:

0.125 ≠ (is not equal to) 0.**0**125

rule

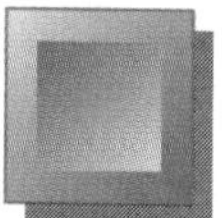

The decimal number is read by stating the whole number first, the decimal point as *and,* and then the decimal fraction by naming the value of the last decimal place.

Examples:

The number 6.2 is read as "six and two-tenths."

The number 10.03 is read as "ten and three hundredths."

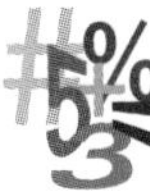

math tip: Given a *decimal fraction* (whose value is always less than one), the decimal number is read *alone,* without stating the zero.

Example:

0.125 is read as "one hundred twenty-five thousandths."

Comparing Decimals

It is important to be able to compare decimal amounts, noting which has a greater or lesser value.

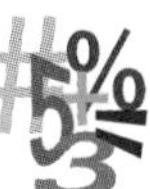

math tip: You can compare decimal amounts by aligning the decimal points and adding zeros, so that the numbers to be compared have the same number of decimal places.

Example 1:

Compare 0.125, 0.05, and 0.2 to find which decimal fraction is largest.

Align decimals and add zeros.

0.125 = one hundred twenty-five thousandths

0.05**0** = fifty thousandths

0.2**00** = two hundred thousandths

Now it is easy to see that 0.2 is the largest amount!

Example 2:

Suppose 0.5 microgram of a drug has been ordered. The recommended maximum dosage of the drug is 0.25 microgram, and the minimum recommended dosage is 0.125 microgram. Comparing decimals, you can see that the ordered dosage is not within the allowable range.

0.125 microgram (recommended minimum dosage)

0.25**0** microgram (recommended maximum dosage)

0.5**00** microgram (ordered dosage)

Now you can see that 0.5 microgram is outside the allowable limits of the safe dosage range of 0.125 to 0.25 microgram for this medication.

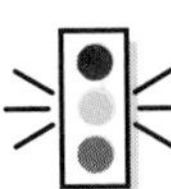

Caution: It is important to eliminate possible confusion and avoid errors in dosage calculation. To avoid overlooking a decimal point in a decimal fraction and thereby reading the numeric value as a whole number, *always place a zero to the left of the decimal point* to emphasize that the number has a value less than one.

Example:

0.425, **0**.01, or **0**.005

Conversion between Fractions and Decimals

For dosage calculations, you may need to convert decimals to fractions and vice versa.

rule

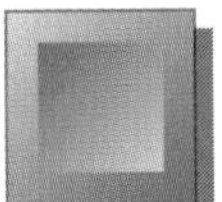

To convert a fraction to a decimal, divide the numerator by the denominator.

Example:

Convert $\frac{1}{4}$ to a decimal.

$$\frac{1}{4} = 4\overline{)1.00} = 0.25$$

$$\begin{array}{r} .25 \\ 4\overline{)1.00} \\ \underline{8} \\ 20 \\ \underline{20} \end{array}$$

rule

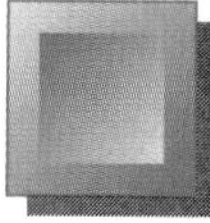

To convert a decimal to a fraction:

1. Express the decimal number as a whole number in the numerator of the fraction,
2. Express the denominator of the fraction as the number 1 followed by as many zeros as there are places to the right of the decimal point, and
3. Reduce the resulting fraction to lowest terms.

Example:

Convert 0.125 to a fraction.

1. Numerator: 125
2. Denominator: 1 followed by 3 zeros = 1000
3. Reduce: $\frac{125}{1000} = \frac{1}{8}$

quick review

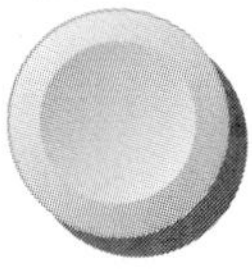

- In a decimal number, whole number values are to the left of the decimal point, and fractional values are to the right.
- Zeros added to a decimal fraction before the decimal point or after the decimal number *do not* change the value. Example: .5 = **0**.5 = 0.5**0**
- In a decimal number, zeros added after the decimal point *do* change the value. Example: 1.5 ≠ 1.**0**5
- To avoid overlooking the decimal point in a decimal fraction, *always* place a zero to the left of the decimal point. Example: **.**5 ← Avoid writing decimal fraction this way; it could be mistaken for the whole number *5*. Example: **0.**5 ← Preferred method of writing decimal fraction.
- The number of places in a decimal fraction indicate the power of 10.

  Examples:

  0.5 = five tenths

  0.05 = five hundredths

  0.005 = five thousandths
- Compare fractions by aligning decimal points and adding zeros.

  Example:

  Compare 0.5, 0.05, and 0.005

  0.500 = five hundred thousandths (largest)

  0.050 = fifty thousandths

  0.005 = five thousandths (smallest)

- To convert a fraction to a decimal, divide the numerator by the denominator.
- To convert a decimal to a fraction, express the decimal number as a whole number in the numerator and the denominator as the correct power of ten. Reduce the fraction to lowest terms.

Example:

$$0.04 = \frac{4 \text{ (numerator is a whole number)}}{100 \text{ (denominator is 1 followed by two zeros)}} = \frac{1}{25}$$

review set 5

Complete the following table of equivalent fractions and decimals. Reduce fractions to lowest terms.

	Fraction	Decimal	The decimal number is read as:
1.	$\frac{1}{5}$	______	______
2.	______	______	eighty-five hundredths
3.	______	1.05	______
4.	______	0.006	______
5.	$10\frac{3}{200}$	______	______
6.	______	1.9	______
7.	______	______	five and one-tenth
8.	$\frac{4}{5}$	______	______
9.	______	250.5	______
10.	$33\frac{3}{100}$	______	______
11.	______	0.95	______
12.	$2\frac{3}{4}$	______	______
13.	______	______	seven and five thousandths
14.	$\frac{21}{250}$	______	______
15.	______	12.125	______
16.	______	20.09	______
17.	______	______	twenty-two and twenty-two thousandths
18.	______	0.15	______
19.	$1000\frac{1}{200}$	______	______
20.	______	______	four thousand eighty-five and seventy-five thousandths

21. Change 0.017 to a four-place decimal. ________
22. Change 0.2500 to a two-place decimal. ________
23. Convert $\frac{75}{100}$ to a decimal. ________
24. Convert 0.045 to a fraction reduced to lowest terms. ________

Circle the correct answer.

25. Which is largest? 0.012 0.120 0.021
26. Which is smallest? 0.635 0.6 0.063
27. True or false? 0.375 = 0.0375
28. True or false? 2.2 grams = 2.02 grams
29. True or false? 6.5 ounces = 6.500 ounces
30. For a certain medication, the safe dose should be greater than or equal to 0.5 gram but less than or equal to 2 grams. Circle each dose that falls within this range.

    0.8 gram 0.25 gram 2.5 grams 1.25 grams

After completing these problems see page 412 to check your answers.

Addition and Subtraction of Decimals

The addition and subtraction of decimals are very similar to addition and subtraction of whole numbers. There are only two simple but essential rules that are different. Accurate dosage calculations for some medications rely on nurses using these two rules.

rule

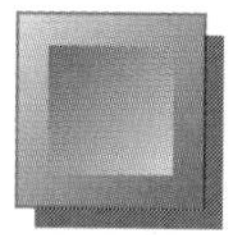

To add and subtract decimal fractions, line up the decimal points.

Example 1:

$$1.25 + 1.75 = \begin{array}{r} 1.25 \\ +\ 1.75 \\ \hline 3.00 \end{array} = 3$$

Example 2:

$$1.25 - 0.13 = \begin{array}{r} 1.25 \\ -\ 0.13 \\ \hline 1.12 \end{array}$$

rule

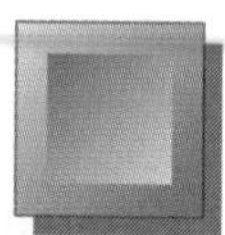

To add and subtract decimal fractions, add zeros at the end of any decimal fraction, making all decimal numbers of equal length.

Example 1:

$$\begin{array}{r} 3.75 \\ -\ 2.10 \\ \hline 1.65 \end{array}$$

3.75 − 2.1 = 3.75 − 2.10 = 1.65

Example 2:

Add 0.9, 0.65, 0.27, 4.712

$$\begin{array}{r} 0.900 \\ 0.650 \\ 0.270 \\ +\ 4.712 \\ \hline 6.532 \end{array}$$

quick review

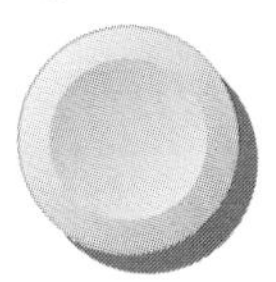

To add or subtract decimals, align the decimal points and add zeros, making all decimal numbers of equal length.

Examples:

$1.5 + 0.05 =$
$$\begin{array}{r} 1.50 \\ +\ 0.05 \\ \hline 1.55 \end{array}$$

$0.725 - 0.5 =$
$$\begin{array}{r} 0.725 \\ -\ 0.500 \\ \hline 0.225 \end{array}$$

review set 6

Find the result of the following problems

1. 0.16 + 5.375 + 1.05 + 16 = ________
2. 7.517 + 3.2 + 0.16 + 33.3 = ________
3. 13.009 − 0.7 = ________
4. 5.125 + 6.025 + 0.15 = ________
5. 175.1 + 0.099 = ________
6. 25.2 − 0.193 = ________
7. 0.58 − 0.062 = ________
8. $10.10 − $0.62 = ________
9. $19 − $0.09 = ________
10. $5.05 + $0.17 + $17.49 = ________
11. 4 + 1.98 + 0.42 + 0.003 = ________
12. 0.3 − 0.03 = ________

13. 16.3 – 12.15 = __________
14. 2.5 – 0.99 = __________
15. 5 + 2.5 + 0.05 + 0.15 + 2.55 = __________
16. 0.03 + 0.16 + 2.327 = __________
17. 700 – 325.65 = __________
18. 645.32 – 40.9 = __________
19. 18 + 2.35 + 7.006 + 0.093 = __________
20. 13.529 + 10.09 = __________
21. A dietitian calculates the sodium in a patient's breakfast: raisin bran cereal = 0.1 gram, 1 cup 2% milk = 0.125 gram, 6 ounces orange juice = 0.001 gram, 1 corn muffin = 0.35 gram, and butter = 0.121 gram. How many grams of sodium did the patient consume? __________
22. In a 24-hour period, an infant drank 3.6 oz, 4.2 oz, 3.9 oz, 3.15 oz, and 3.7 oz of formula. How many ounces did the infant drink in 24 hours? __________
23. A patient has a hospital bill for $16,709.43. Her insurance company pays $14,651.37. What is her balance due? __________
24. A patient's hemoglobin was 16.8 grams before surgery. During surgery, his hemoglobin dropped 4.5 grams. What is his current hemoglobin value? __________
25. A home health nurse accounts for her day of work. If she spent 3 hours 20 minutes at the office, 40 minutes traveling, $3\frac{1}{2}$ hours doing patient care, 24 minutes for lunch, and took a 12-minute break, what is her total number of hours including the break? Express your answer as a decimal. (HINT: First convert each time to hours and minutes.) __________

After completing these problems, see pages 412 and 413 to check your answers.

Multiplying Decimals

The procedure for multiplication of decimals is very similar to that used for whole numbers. The only difference is that the decimal point must be properly placed in the product or answer. Use the following simple rule.

rule

To multiply decimals:

1. Multiply the decimals without concern for decimal placement,
2. Count off the number of decimal places in the decimals multiplied, and
3. Place the decimal point in the product to the left of the total number of places counted.

Example 1:

$$1.5 \times 0.5 = \begin{array}{r} 1.5 \\ \times\ 0.5 \\ \hline 0.75. \end{array}$$

1.5 (1 decimal place)
× 0.5 (1 decimal place)
0.75. (The decimal point is located 2 places to the left, because a total of 2 decimal places are counted.)

Example 2:

$$1.72 \times 0.9 = \begin{array}{r} 1.72 \\ \times\ 0.9 \\ \hline 1.548 \end{array}$$

1.72 (2 decimal places)
× 0.9 (1 decimal place)
1.548 (The decimal point is located 3 places to the left, because a total of 3 decimal places are counted.)

Example 3:

$$5.06 \times 1.3 = \begin{array}{r} 5.06 \\ \times\ 1.3 \\ \hline 1\,518 \\ +\ 5\,06 \\ \hline 6.578 \end{array}$$

5.06 (2 decimal places)
× 1.3 (1 decimal place)
6.578 (The decimal point is located 3 places to the left, because a total of 3 decimal places are counted.)

rule

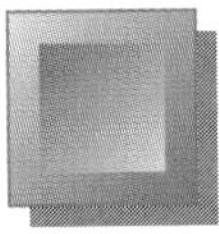

When multiplying a decimal by a multiplier of ten, move the decimal point as many places to the right as there are zeros in the multiplier.

Example 1:

1.25 × 10

The multiplier 10 has 1 zero; move the decimal point 1 place to the right.

1.25 × 10 = 1.2.5 = 12.5

Example 2:

2.3 × 100

The multiplier 100 has 2 zeros; move the decimal point 2 places to the right. (Note: Add zeros as necessary to complete the operation.)

2.3 × 100 = 2.30. = 230

Example 3:

0.001 × 1000

The multiplier 1000 has 3 zeros; move the decimal point 3 places to the right.

0.001 × 1000 = 0.001. = 1

Dividing Decimals

When dividing decimals, set up the problem the same as for the division of whole numbers. Follow the same procedure for dividing whole numbers after you apply the following rule.

rule

To divide decimals:

1. Move the decimal in the *divisor* (number divided by) and the *dividend* (number divided) the number of places needed to make the *divisor* a *whole number,* and
2. Place the decimal point in the *quotient* (answer) above the new decimal place in the dividend.

Example 1:

$$100.75 \div 2.5 = 2.5.\overline{)100.7.5} = 40.3$$

(dividend) (divisor)

```
          40.3   (quotient)
    2.5.)100.7.5
         100
         ----
           75
           75
           ==
```

Example 2:

$$56.5 \div 0.02 = 0.02.\overline{)56.50.} = 2825$$

```
          28 25.
    0.02.)56.50.
          4
          --
          16
          16
          --
           5
           4
           --
           10
           10
           ==
```

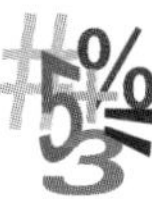

math tip: Recall that adding a zero after a decimal does not change its value (56.5 = 56.50).

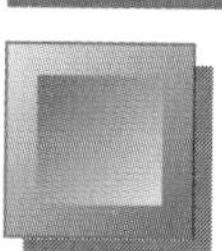

rule

When dividing a decimal by a power of ten, move the decimal point to the left as many places as there are zeros in the divisor.

Example 1:

0.65 ÷ 10

The divisor 10 has 1 zero; move the decimal point 1 place to the left.

0.65 ÷ 10 = .0.65 = 0.065

(Note: Place the zero to the left of the decimal point to avoid confusion and to emphasize that this is a decimal.)

Example 2:

7.3 ÷ 100

The divisor 100 has 2 zeros; move the decimal point 2 places to the left.

7.3 ÷ 100 = .07.3 = 0.073

(Note: Add zeros as necessary to complete the operation.)

Example 3:

0.5 ÷ 1000

The divisor 1000 has 3 zeros; move the decimal point 3 places to the left.

0.5 ÷ 1000 = .000.5 = 0.0005

Rounding Decimal Fractions

For many dosage calculations, it will be necessary to compute decimal calculations to *thousandths* (*three* decimal places) and round back to *hundredths* (*two* places) for the final answer. For example, pediatrics and critical care require this degree of accuracy. At other times, you will need to round to *tenths* (*one* place). Let's look closely at this important math skill.

rule

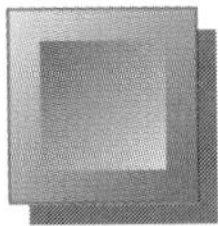

To round a decimal to hundredths, drop the number in thousandths place, and

1. Do not change the number in hundredths place, if the number in thousandths place is 4 or less;
2. Increase the number in hundredths place by 1, if the number in thousandths place is 5 or more.

Examples:

		Tenths	Hundredths	Thousandths		
0	.	1	2	3	= 0.12	Rounded to hundredths (two places)
1	.	7	4	4	= 1.74	
5	.	3	2	5	= 5.33	
0	.	6	6	6	= 0.67	

rule

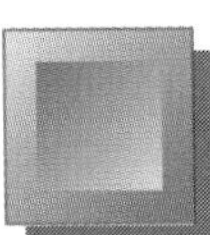

To round a decimal to tenths, drop the number in hundredths place, and

1. Do not change the number in tenths place, if the number in hundredths place is 4 or less;
2. Increase the number in tenths place by 1, if the number in hundredths place is 5 or more.

Examples:

		Tehths	Hundredths		
0	.	1	3	= 0.1	Rounded to tenths (one place)
5	.	6	4	= 5.6	
0	.	7	5	= 0.8	
1	.	6	6	= 1.7	

quick review

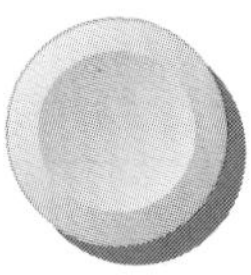

- To multiply decimals, place the decimal point in the product to the *left* as many decimal places as there are in the two decimals multiplied.

Example:

$0.25 \times 0.2 = 0.050 = 0.05$

- To divide decimals, move the decimal point in the divisor and dividend the number of decimal places that will make the divisor a whole number and align it in the quotient.

Example:

$$1.2 \overline{)24.0} = 20.$$

- To multiply or divide decimals by a multiplier of 10, move the decimal to the *right* (to *multiply*) or to the *left* (to *divide*) the number of decimal places as there are zeros in the multiplier of 10.

Examples:

$5.06 \times 10 = 5.0.6 = 50.6$; $2.1 \div 100 = .02.1 = 0.021$

- When rounding decimals, add 1 to the place value considered if the next decimal place is 5 or greater.

Examples:

Rounded to hundredths: 3.054 = 3.05; 0.566 = 0.57. Rounded to tenths: 3.05 = 3.1; 0.54 = 0.5

review set 7

Multiply, and round your answers to two decimal places.

1. $1.16 \times 5.03 =$ ________
2. $0.314 \times 7 =$ ________
3. $1.71 \times 25 =$ ________
4. $3.002 \times 0.05 =$ ________
5. $16.1 \times 25.04 =$ ________
6. $75.1 \times 1000.01 =$ ________
7. $16.03 \times 2.05 =$ ________
8. $55.50 \times 0.05 =$ ________
9. $23.2 \times 15.025 =$ ________
10. $1.14 \times 0.014 =$ ________

Divide, and round your answers to two decimal places.

11. $16 \div 0.04 =$ ________
12. $25.3 \div 6.76 =$ ________
13. $0.02 \div 0.004 =$ ________
14. $45.5 \div 15.25 =$ ________
15. $515 \div 0.125 =$ ________
16. $73 \div 13.40 =$ ________
17. $16.36 \div 0.06 =$ ________
18. $0.375 \div 0.25 =$ ________
19. $100.04 \div 0.002 =$ ________
20. $45 \div 0.15 =$ ________

Multiply or divide by the power of 10 indicated. Draw an arrow to demonstrate movement of the decimal point.

21. $562.5 \times 100 =$ ________
22. $16 \times 10 =$ ________
23. $25 \div 1000 =$ ________
24. $32.005 \div 1000 =$ ________
25. $0.125 \div 100 =$ ________
26. $23.25 \times 10 =$ ________

27. $717.717 \div 10 =$ ________

28. $83.16 \times 10 =$ ________

29. $0.33 \times 100 =$ ________

30. $14.106 \times 1000 =$ ________

After completing these problems, see page 413 to check your answers.

practice problems—chapter 1

Perform the indicated operation and record the results in Roman numerals (use uppercase).

1. $3 + 2 =$ ________
2. $43 - 18 =$ ________
3. $5\frac{1}{3} \times 4\frac{1}{8} =$ ________
4. $100 \div 6\frac{1}{4} =$ ________
5. $4 + 2 - 1 + 13 =$ ________
6. $6.2 + 5.3 + 1.5 =$ ________
7. $4.1 - 3 + 9.9 =$ ________
8. $7.5 \div 2.5 =$ ________
9. $273.6 \div 68.4 =$ ________
10. $75 \div 15 + 13.2 - 1.2 =$ ________

Convert the following Roman numerals to Arabic numbers.

11. XXX = ________
12. IX = ________
13. XVI = ________
14. XIV = ________
15. XXI = ________
16. XXIII = ________
17. VII = ________
18. XVI = ________
19. XX = ________
20. XIX = ________

Perform the indicated operation, and reduce fractions to lowest terms.

21. $1\frac{2}{3} + \frac{9}{5} =$ ________
22. $4\frac{5}{12} + 3\frac{1}{15} =$ ________
23. $\frac{7}{9} - \frac{5}{18} =$ ________
24. $5\frac{1}{6} - 2\frac{7}{8} =$ ________
25. $\frac{4}{9} \times \frac{7}{12} =$ ________
26. $1\frac{1}{2} \times 6\frac{3}{4} =$ ________
27. $7\frac{1}{5} \div 1\frac{7}{10} =$ ________
28. $8\frac{4}{11} \div 1\frac{2}{3} =$ ________
29. $\dfrac{9\frac{1}{2}}{1\frac{4}{5}} =$
30. $\dfrac{13\frac{1}{3}}{4\frac{6}{13}} =$
31. $\dfrac{\frac{1}{10}}{\frac{2}{3}} =$
32. $\frac{1}{125} \times \frac{1}{25} =$ ________
33. $\dfrac{\frac{7}{8}}{\frac{1}{3}} \div \dfrac{3\frac{1}{2}}{\frac{1}{3}} =$
34. $\frac{20}{35} \times 3 =$ ________

Perform the indicated operation, and round the answer to two decimal places.

35. $11.33 + 29.16 + 19.78 =$ ________
36. $93.712 - 26.97 =$ ________
37. $43.69 - 0.7083 =$ ________
38. $66.4 \times 72.8 =$ ________
39. $360 \times 0.53 =$ ________
40. $268.4 \div 14 =$ ________

41. $2974 \div 0.23 =$ ________

42. $51.21 \div 0.016 =$ ________

43. $0.74 \div 0.37 =$ ________

44. $1.5 + 146.73 + 1.9 + 0.832 =$ ________

45. A one-month-old infant drinks $3\frac{1}{2}$ ounces of formula every four hours. How many ounces will the infant drink in one week on this schedule? ________

46. There are 368 people employed at Riverview Clinic. If $\frac{3}{8}$ of the employees are nurses, $\frac{1}{8}$ are maintenance/cleaners, $\frac{1}{4}$ are technicians, and $\frac{1}{4}$ are all other employees, calculate the number of employees that each fraction represents. ________

47. True or false? A specific gravity of urine of $1\frac{2}{32}$ falls within the normal range of 1.01 to 1.025 for an adult patient. ________

48. Last week a nurse earning \$17.43 per hour gross pay worked 40 hours plus 6.25 hours overtime, which is paid at twice the hourly rate. What is the total regular and overtime gross pay for last week? ________

49. The instructional assistant is ordering supplies for the nursing skills laboratory. A single box of 12 urinary catheters costs \$98.76. A case of 12 boxes of these catheters costs \$975.00. Calculate the savings per catheter when a case is purchased. ________

50. If each ounce of a liquid laxative contains 0.065 gram of a drug, how much of the drug would be contained in 4.75 ounces? (Round answer to the nearest hundredth.) ________

After completing these problems, see page 413 to check your answers.

CHAPTER

2

Mathematics Review for Dosage Calculations: Ratios, Percents, Simple Equations, and Ratios and Proportions

objectives

Upon mastery of Chapter 2, you will be able to perform basic mathematical computations that involve ratios, percents, simple equations, and proportions. Specifically, you will be able to:

- Interpret values expressed in ratios.
- Convert among fractions, decimals, ratios, and percents.
- Compare the size of fractions, decimals, ratios, and percents.
- Determine the value of "X" in simple equations.
- Set up proportions for solving problems.
- Cross-multiply to find the value of "X" in a proportion.
- Calculate the percentage of a quantity.

Nurses need to understand ratios and percents to be able to accurately interpret, prepare, and administer a variety of medications and treatments. Let's take a look at each of these important ways of expressing ratios and percents and how they are related to fractions and decimals. It is important that you can convert quickly between equivalent ratios, percents, decimals, and fractions.

Ratios and Percents

Like a fraction, a *ratio* is used to indicate the relationship of one part of a quantity to the whole. When written, the two quantities are separated by a colon (:). The use of the colon is a traditional way to write the division sign within a ratio.

Example:

On an evening shift, if there are 5 nurses and 35 patients, what is the ratio of nurses to patients? 5 nurses to 35 patients = 5 nurses per 35 patients = $\frac{5}{35} = \frac{1}{7}$. This is the same as a ratio of 5:35 or 1:7.

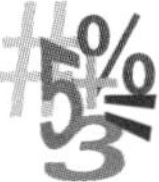

math tip: The terms of a ratio are the *numerator* (always to the left of the colon) and the *denominator* (always to the right of the colon) of a fraction. Like fractions, ratios should be stated in lowest terms.

If you think back to the discussion of fractions and parts of a whole, it is easy to see that a ratio is *actually the same as* a fraction and its equivalent decimal fraction. It is just a different way of *expressing the same quantity*. Recall from Chapter 1 that to convert a fraction to a decimal fraction, you simply divide the numerator by the denominator.

Example:

Adrenalin 1:1000 for injection = 1 part Adrenalin to 1000 total parts of solution. It is a fact that 1:1000 is the same as $\frac{1}{1000}$ and 0.001.

In drug solutions such as Adrenalin 1:1000, the ratio is used to indicate the drug's concentration. This will be covered in more detail later.

Percent

A type of ratio is a percent. *Percent* comes from the Latin phrase *per centum*, translated *per hundred.* This means per hundred parts or hundredth part.

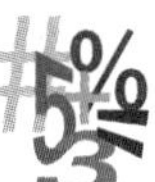

math tip: To remember the value of a given percent, replace the % symbol with / for *per* and *100* for *cent*. THINK: *Percent* means */100.*

Example:

$3\% = 3 \text{ percent} = 3/100 = \frac{3}{100} = 0.03$

rule

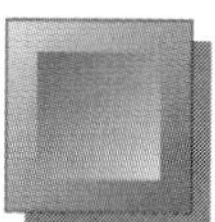

To convert a percent to a fraction:

1. Delete the % sign,
2. Write the remaining number as the numerator,
3. Write 100 as the denominator, and
4. Reduce the result to lowest terms.

Example:

$5\% = \frac{5}{100} = \frac{1}{20}$

It is also easy to express a percent as a ratio.

rule

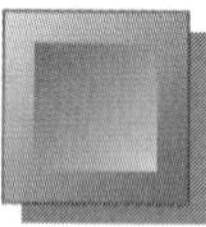

To convert a percent to a ratio:

1. Delete the % sign,
2. Write the remaining number as the numerator,
3. Write "100" as the denominator,
4. Reduce the result to lowest terms, and
5. Express the fraction as a ratio.

Example:

$25\% = \frac{25}{100} = \frac{1}{4} = 1{:}4$

Because the denominator of a percent is always 100, it is easy to find the equivalent decimal. Recall that to divide by 100, you move the decimal point two places to the left, the number of places equal to the number of zeros in the denominator. This is the hundredths place.

rule

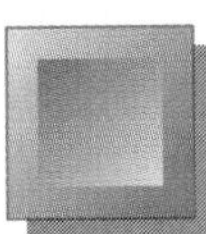

To convert a percent to a decimal:

1. Delete the % sign; and
2. Divide the remaining number by 100, which is the same as moving the decimal point 2 places to the left.

Example:

$25\% = \frac{25}{100} = 25 \div 100 = .25. = 0.25$

Conversely, it is easy to change a decimal to a percent.

rule

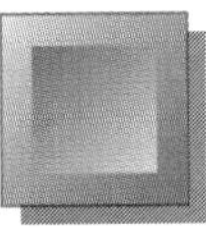

To convert a decimal to a percent:

1. Multiply the decimal number by 100 (move the decimal point 2 places to the right), and
2. Add the % sign.

Example:

$0.25 \times 100 = 0.25. = 25\%.$

Now you know all the steps to change a ratio to the equivalent percent.

rule

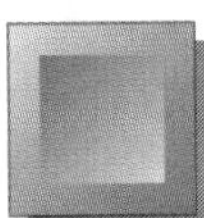

To convert a ratio to a percent:

1. Convert the ratio to a fraction,
2. Convert the fraction to a decimal, and
3. Convert the decimal to a percent.

Example:

Convert 1:1000 Adrenalin solution to the equivalent concentration expressed as a percent.

1. $1{:}1000 = \frac{1}{1000}$ (ratio converted to fraction)

2. $\frac{1}{1000} = .001. = 0.001$ (fraction converted to decimal)

3. $0.001 = 0.001 \times 100 = 0.00.1 = 0.1\%$ (decimal converted to percent)

Thus, 1:1000 Adrenalin solution = 0.1% Adrenalin solution.

Review the preceding example again slowly until it is clear. Ask your instructor for assistance, as needed. If you go over this one step at a time, you can master these important calculations. You need never fear fractions, decimals, ratios, and percents again.

Comparing Percents

In health care, nurses frequently administer solutions with the concentration expressed as a percent. Consider two intravenous solutions given directly into a person's vein: one that is 0.9%; the other 5%. It is important to be clear that 0.9% is *smaller* than 5%. A 0.9% solution means that there are 0.9 parts of drug per 100 total parts (0.9 parts is less than one whole part, so it is less than 1%). Compare this to the 5% solution, with 5 parts of drug (or more than 5 times 0.9 parts) per 100 total parts. Therefore, the 5% solution is much more concentrated, or stronger, than the 0.9% solution. A misunderstanding of these numbers and the quantities they represent can have dire consequences.

Likewise, you may see a solution concentration expressed as $\frac{1}{3}$% and another expressed as 0.45%. Convert these amounts to equivalent fractions to clarify values and compare concentrations.

$$\frac{1}{3}\% = \frac{\frac{1}{3}}{100} = \frac{1}{3} \div \frac{100}{1} = \frac{1}{3} \times \frac{1}{100} = \frac{1}{300} = 0.0033$$

$$0.45\% = \frac{0.45}{100} = 0.0045 \text{ (greater value, stronger concentration)}$$

quick review

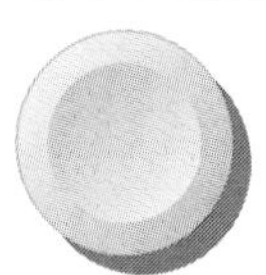

- Fractions, decimals, ratios, and percents are related equivalents.

  Example: $1:2 = \frac{1}{2} = 0.5 = 50\%$

- Like fractions, ratios should be reduced to lowest terms.

  Example: $2:4 = 1:2$

- To express a ratio as a fraction, the number to the left of the colon becomes the numerator, and the number to the right of the colon becomes the denominator. The colon in a ratio is equivalent to the division sign in a fraction.

  Example: $2:3 = \frac{2}{3}$

- To change a ratio to a decimal fraction, convert the ratio to a fraction, and divide the numerator by the denominator.

  Example: $1:4 = \frac{1}{4} = 1 \div 4 = 0.25$

- To change a percent to a common fraction, drop the % sign and place the remaining number as the numerator over the denominator 100. Reduce the fraction to lowest terms. THINK: per (/) cent (100)

  Example: $75\% = \frac{75}{100} = \frac{3}{4}$

- To change a percent to a ratio, first convert the percent to a fraction in lowest terms. Then, place the numerator to the left of a colon and the denominator to the right of that colon.

  Example: $35\% = \frac{35}{100} = \frac{7}{20} = 7:20$

- To change a percent to a decimal fraction, drop the % sign, and divide by 100.

  Example: 4% = .04. = 0.04

- To change a decimal to a percent, multiply by 100, and add the % sign.

  Example: 0.5 = 0.50. = 50%

- To change a ratio to a percent, first convert the ratio to a fraction. Convert the resulting fraction to a decimal and then to a percent.

  Example: $1:2 = \frac{1}{2} = 1 \div 2 = 0.5 =$ 0.50. = 50%

review set 8

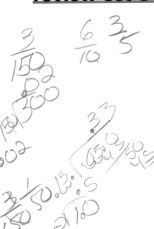

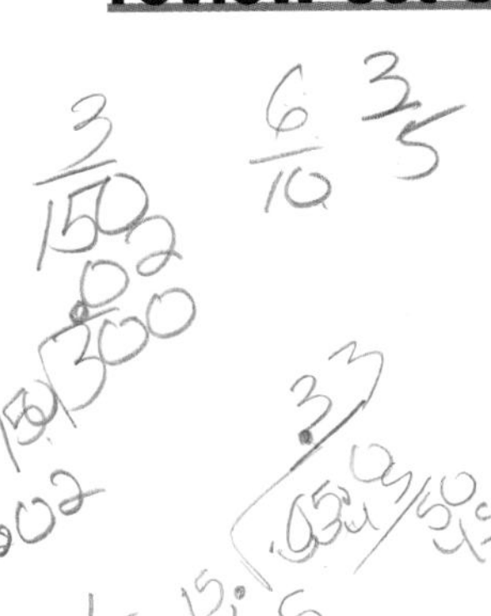

Change the following ratios to fractions; reduce to lowest terms.

1. 3:150 = ______
2. 6:10 = ______
3. 0.05:0.15 = ______
4. 4:7 = ______
5. 6:8 = ______

Change the following ratios to decimal fractions; round to two decimal places.

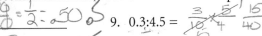

6. 20:40 = ______
7. $\frac{1}{1000} : \frac{1}{150}$ = ______
8. 0.12:0.88 = ______
9. 0.3:4.5 = ______
10. $1\frac{1}{2}:6\frac{2}{9}$ = ______

Change the following ratios to percents.

11. 12:48 = ______
12. 2:5 = ______
13. 0.08:0.64 = ______
14. 7:10 = ______
15. 50:100 = ______

Change the following percents to fractions; reduce to lowest terms.

16. 45% = ______
17. 60% = ______
18. 0.5% = ______
19. 1% = ______
20. $66\frac{2}{3}$% = ______

Change the following percents to decimal fractions, round to two decimal places.

21. 2.94% = ______
22. 4.5% = ______
23. 6.32% = ______
24. 33% = ______
25. 0.9% = ______

Change the following percents to ratios; reduce to lowest terms.

26. 16% = ______
27. 25% = ______
28. 50% = ______
29. 45% = ______
30. 6% = ______

Which of the following is largest? Circle your answer.

31. 0.9% 0.9 1:9 $\frac{1}{90}$
32. 0.05 $\frac{1}{5}$ 0.025 1:25
33. 0.0125% 0.25% 0.1% 0.02%
34. $\frac{1}{150}$ $\frac{1}{300}$ 0.5 $\frac{2}{3}$%
35. 1:1000 0.0001 $\frac{1}{100}$ 0.1%

After completing these problems, see pages 413 and 414 to check your answers.

Solving Simple Equations for "X"

The dosage calculations you will perform can be set up and solved in different ways. One way is to use a simple equation form. The following examples demonstrate the various forms of this equation. Learn to express your answers in decimal form, because decimals will be used most often in dosage calculations and administration. Round decimals to hundredths or to two places.

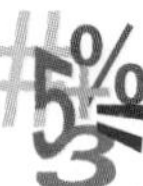

math tip: The unknown quantity is represented by "X."

Example 1:

$\frac{100}{200} \times 1 = X$

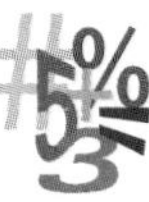

math tip: You can drop the 1, because a number multiplied by 1 is the same number. Therefore, $\frac{100}{200} = X$

1. Reduce to lowest terms: $\frac{100}{200} = \frac{\overset{1}{\cancel{100}}}{\underset{2}{\cancel{200}}} = \frac{1}{2} = X$

2. Convert to decimal form: $\frac{1}{2} = 0.5 = X$

3. You have your answer. $X = 0.5$

Example 2:

$\frac{3}{5} \times 2 = X$

1. Convert: Express 2 as a fraction. $\frac{3}{5} \times \frac{2}{1} = X$

2. Multiply fractions: $\frac{3}{5} \times \frac{2}{1} = \frac{6}{5} = X$

3. Convert to a mixed number: $\frac{6}{5} = 1\frac{1}{5} = X$

4. Convert to decimal form: $1\frac{1}{5} = 1.2 = X$

5. You have your answer. $X = 1.2$

Example 3:

$\frac{\frac{1}{6}}{\frac{1}{4}} \times 5 = X$

1. Convert: Express 5 as a fraction. $\frac{\frac{1}{6}}{\frac{1}{4}} \times \frac{5}{1} = X$

2. Divide fractions: $\frac{1}{6} \div \frac{1}{4} \times \frac{5}{1} = X$

3. Invert the divisor, and multiply. $\frac{1}{6} \times \frac{4}{1} \times \frac{5}{1} = X$

4. Cancel terms: $\frac{1}{\underset{3}{\cancel{6}}} \times \frac{\overset{2}{\cancel{4}}}{1} \times \frac{5}{1} = \frac{1}{3} \times \frac{2}{1} \times \frac{5}{1} = \frac{10}{3} = X$

5. Convert to a mixed number: $\frac{10}{3} = 3\frac{1}{3} = X$

6. Convert to decimal form: $3\frac{1}{3} = 3.33\overline{3} = X$

7. Round to hundredths place: $3.333 = 3.33 = X$

8. Easy, when you take it one step at a time. $X = 3.33$

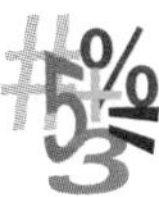

math tip: The line over the last 3 in step 6 ($3.33\overline{3}$) indicates the number repeats indefinitely.

Example 4:

$$\frac{\frac{1}{100}}{\frac{1}{150}} \times 2.2 = X$$

1. Convert: Express 2.2 in fraction form. $\dfrac{\frac{1}{100}}{\frac{1}{150}} \times \frac{2.2}{1} = X$

2. Divide fractions: $\frac{1}{100} \div \frac{1}{150} \times \frac{2.2}{1} = X$

3. Invert the divisor, and multiply. $\frac{1}{100} \times \frac{150}{1} \times \frac{2.2}{1} = X$

4. Cancel terms: $\frac{1}{\underset{2}{\cancel{100}}} \times \frac{\overset{3}{\cancel{150}}}{1} \times \frac{2.2}{1} = \frac{1}{2} \times \frac{3}{1} \times \frac{2.2}{1} = X$

5. Multiply: $\frac{1}{2} \times \frac{3}{1} \times \frac{2.2}{1} = \frac{6.6}{2} = X$

6. Divide: $\frac{6.6}{2} = 3.3 = X$

7. That's it! $X = 3.3$

Example 5:

$$\frac{0.125}{0.25} \times 1.5 = X$$

1. Convert: Express 1.5 in fraction form. $\frac{0.125}{0.25} \times \frac{1.5}{1} = X$

2. Convert: Add a zero to thousandths place for 0.25 for easier comparison. $\frac{0.125}{0.250} \times \frac{1.5}{1} = X$

3. Cancel terms: $\frac{\overset{1}{\cancel{0.125}}}{\underset{2}{\cancel{0.250}}} \times \frac{1.5}{1} = \frac{1}{2} \times \frac{1.5}{1} = X$

4. Multiply: $\frac{1}{2} \times \frac{1.5}{1} = \frac{1.5}{2} = X$

5. Divide: $\frac{1.5}{2} = 0.75 = X$ 6.

6. You've got it! $X = 0.75$

Example 5 can also be solved by computing with common fractions instead of decimal fractions.

Try this: $\frac{0.125}{0.25} \times 1.5 = X$

1. Convert: Express 1.5 in fraction form. $\frac{0.125}{0.25} \times \frac{1.5}{1} = X$
2. Convert: Add zeros for easier comparison, making *both* decimal fractions of equal length. $\frac{0.125}{0.250} \times \frac{1.5}{1.0} = X$
3. Cancel terms: $\frac{\overset{1}{\cancel{0.125}}}{\underset{2}{\cancel{0.250}}} \times \frac{\overset{3}{\cancel{1.5}}}{\underset{2}{\cancel{1.0}}} = \frac{1}{2} \times \frac{3}{2} = X$ (It is easier to work with whole numbers.)
4. Multiply: $\frac{1}{2} \times \frac{3}{2} = \frac{3}{4} = X$
5. Convert: $\frac{3}{4} = 0.75 = X$
6. You've got it again! X = 0.75

   Which way do you find easier?

Example 6:

$\frac{3}{4} \times 45\% = X$

1. Convert: Express 45% as a fraction reduced to lowest terms: $45\% = \frac{45}{100} = \frac{9}{20}$
2. Multiply fractions: $\frac{3}{4} \times \frac{9}{20} = X$

   $\frac{27}{80} = X$
3. Divide: $\frac{27}{80} = 0.337 = X$
4. Round to hundredths place: 0.34 = X
5. You have your answer. X = 0.34

quick review

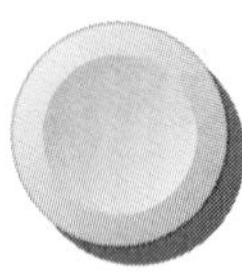

- To solve simple equations, perform the mathematical operations indicated to find the value of the unknown "X."
- Express the result (value of X) in decimal form.

review set 9

Solve the following problems for "X." Express answers as decimals; round to two places.

1. $\frac{75}{125} \times 5 = X$ ________
2. $\frac{\frac{3}{4}}{\frac{1}{2}} \times 2.2 = X$ ________
3. $\frac{150}{300} \times 2.5 = X$ ________
4. $\frac{40\%}{60\%} \times 8 = X$ ________
5. $\frac{0.35}{2.5} \times 4 = X$ ________
6. $\frac{0.15}{0.1} \times 1.2 = X$ ________

7. $\frac{0.4}{2.5} \times 4 = X$ ________

8. $\frac{1,200,000}{400,000} \times 4.2 = X$ ________

9. $\frac{\frac{2}{3}}{\frac{1}{6}} \times 10 = X$ ________

10. $\frac{30}{50} \times 0.8 = X$ ________

11. $\frac{200,000}{300,000} \times 1.5 = X$ ________

12. $\frac{0.08}{0.1} \times 1.2 = X$ ________

13. $\frac{7.5}{5} \times 3 = X$ ________

14. $\frac{250,000}{2,000,000} \times 7.5 = X$ ________

15. $\frac{600}{150} \times 2.5 = X$ ________

16. $\frac{600,000}{750,000} \times 0.5 = X$ ________

17. $\frac{75\%}{60\%} \times 1.2 = X$ ________

18. $\frac{0.25}{0.125} \times 5 = X$ ________

19. $\frac{1,000,000}{250,000} \times 5 = X$ ________

20. $\frac{\frac{1}{100}}{\frac{1}{150}} \times 1.2 = X$ ________

After completing these problems, see page 414 to check your answers.

Ratio-Proportion: Cross-Multiplying to Solve for "X"

A *proportion* is two ratios that are equal or an equation between two equal ratios.

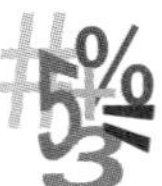

math tip: A proportion is written as two ratios separated by an equal sign, such as 5:10 = 10:20. The two ratios in a proportion may also be separated by a double colon sign, such as 5:10 :: 10:20.

Some of the calculations you will perform will have the unknown "X" as a different term in the equation. To determine the value of the unknown "X," you must apply the rule for cross-multiplying used in a proportion.

rule

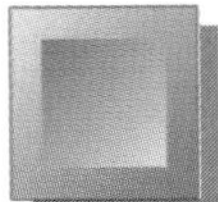

In a proportion, the product of the *means* (two inside numbers) equals the product of the extremes (two outside numbers). Finding the product of the means and the extremes is called *cross-multiplying*.

Example:

Extremes

5:10 = 10:20

Means

$5 \times 20 = 10 \times 10$

$100 = 100$

Because ratios are the same as fractions, the same proportion can be expressed like this: $\frac{5}{10} = \frac{10}{20}$. The fractions are *equivalent*, or equal. The numerator of the first fraction and the denominator of the second fraction are the extremes, and the denominator of the first fraction and the numerator of the second fraction are the means.

Example:

Extreme	$\frac{5}{10} = \frac{10}{20}$	Mean
Mean		Extreme

Cross-multiply to find the equal products of the means and extremes.

rule

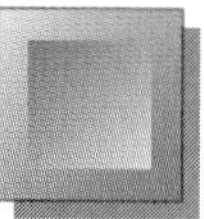

If two fractions are *equivalent*, or equal, their cross-products are also equal.

Example:

$$\frac{5}{10} = \frac{10}{20}$$

$5 \times 20 = 10 \times 10$

$100 = 100$

When one of the quantities in a proportion is unknown, a letter, such as "X," may be substituted for this unknown quantity. You would solve the equation to find the value of "X." In addition to cross-multiplying, there is one more rule you need to know to solve for "X" in a proportion.

rule

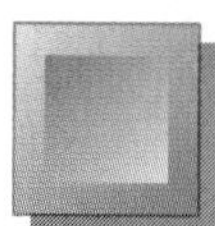

Dividing or multiplying each side (*member*) of an equation by the same nonzero number produces an equivalent equation.

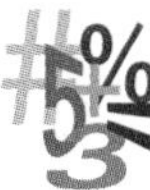

math tip: Dividing each side of an equation by the same nonzero number is the same as reducing or simplifying the equation. Multiplying each side by the same nonzero number enlarges the equation.

Let's examine how to simplify an equation.

Example:

$25X = 100$ (25X means $25 \times X$)

$\frac{25X}{25} = \frac{100}{25}$ Simplify the equation to find "X." Divide both sides by 25, the number before "X."

$X = 4$

Replace "X" with 4 in the same equation, and you can prove that the calculations are correct.

$25 \times \mathbf{4} = 100$

Now you are ready to apply the concepts of cross-multiplying and simplifying an equation to solve for "X" in a proportion.

Example 1:

$\frac{90}{2} = \frac{45}{X}$

You have a proportion with an unknown quantity "X" in the denominator of the second fraction. Find the value of "X."

1. Cross-multiply: $\frac{90}{2} \times \frac{45}{X}$

2. Multiply terms: $90 \times X = 2 \times 45$

   $90X = 90$ (90X means $90 \times X$)

3. Simplify the equation: Divide both sides of the equation by the number before the unknown "X." You are equally reducing the terms on both sides of the equation.

   $\frac{90X}{90} = \frac{90}{90}$

   $X = 1$

Try another one. The unknown "X" is a different term.

Example 2:

$\frac{80}{X} \times 60 = 20$

1. Convert: Express 60 as a fraction.

   $\frac{80}{X} \times \frac{60}{1} = 20$

2. Multiply fractions: $\frac{80}{X} \times \frac{60}{1} = 20$

   $\frac{4800}{X} = 20$

3. Convert: Express 20 as a fraction.

   $\frac{4800}{X} = \frac{20}{1}$

   You now have a proportion.

4. Cross-multiply: $\frac{4800}{X} \times \frac{20}{1}$

   $20X = 4800$

5. Simplify: Divide both sides of the equation by the number before the unknown "X."

   $\frac{20X}{20} = \frac{4800}{20}$

   $X = 240$

Example 3:

$\frac{X}{160} = \frac{2.5}{80}$

1. Cross-multiply: $\frac{X}{160} \times \frac{2.5}{80}$

   $80 \times X = 2.5 \times 160$

   $80X = 400$

2. Simplify: $\frac{80X}{80} = \frac{400}{80}$

$X = 5$

Example 4:

$$\frac{3}{\frac{1}{4}} = \frac{X}{\frac{1}{2}}$$

1. Cross-multiply: $\frac{3}{\frac{1}{4}} \times \frac{X}{\frac{1}{2}}$

$\frac{1}{4}X = 3 \times \frac{1}{2}$

$\frac{1}{4}X = \frac{3}{1} \times \frac{1}{2}$

$\frac{1}{4}X = \frac{3}{2}$

2. Simplify terms: $\frac{\frac{1}{4}X}{\frac{1}{4}} = \frac{\frac{3}{2}}{\frac{1}{4}}$

$X = \frac{\frac{3}{2}}{\frac{1}{4}}$

3. Divide fractions; invert and multiply: $X = \frac{3}{2} \div \frac{1}{4} = \frac{3}{2} \times \frac{4}{1}$

4. Cancel: $X = \frac{3}{\not{2}_1} \times \frac{\not{4}^2}{1} = \frac{3}{1} \times \frac{2}{1}$

5. Multiply: $X = \frac{3}{1} \times \frac{2}{1} = \frac{6}{1}$

$X = 6$

Calculations that result in an amount less than 1 should be expressed in decimal fractions. Most medications are ordered and supplied in metric measure. Metric measure is a decimal-based system.

quick review

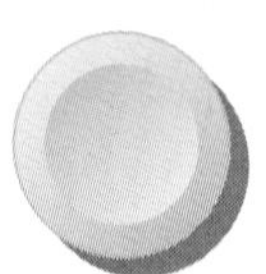

- A *proportion* is an equation of two equal ratios. The ratios may be expressed as fractions.

  Example: 1:4 = X:8 or $\frac{1}{4} = \frac{X}{8}$

- In a proportion, the product of the means equals the product of the extremes.

  Example: 1:4 = X:8 (Extremes: 1 and 8; Means: 4 and X) Therefore, $4 \times X = 1 \times 8$

- If two fractions are equal, their cross-products are equal. This operation is referred to as cross-multiplying.

  Example: $\frac{1}{4} \times \frac{X}{8}$ Therefore, $4 \times X = 1 \times 8$

- Dividing each side of an equation by the same number produces an equivalent equation. This operation is referred to as *simplifying the equation*.

Example: If $4X = 8$, then $\frac{4X}{4} = \frac{8}{4}$, and $X = 2$.

review set 10

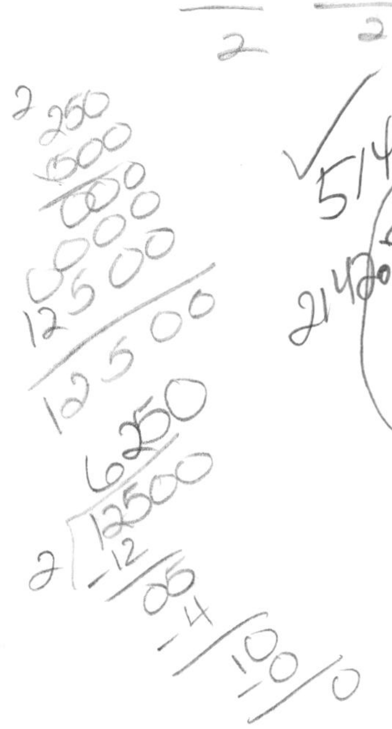

Find the value of "X." Express answers as decimals, round to two places.

1. $\frac{1000}{2} = \frac{125}{X}$ _____
2. $\frac{500}{2} = \frac{250}{X}$ _____
3. $\frac{500}{1} = \frac{280}{X}$ _____
4. $\frac{0.5}{2} = \frac{250}{X}$ _____
5. $\frac{75}{1.5} = \frac{35}{X}$ _____
6. $\frac{1200}{X} \times 12 = 28$ _____
7. $\frac{1000}{X} \times 60 = 28$ _____
8. $\frac{2}{2000} \times X = 0.5$ _____
9. $\frac{15}{500} \times X = 6$ _____
10. $\frac{5}{X} = \frac{10}{21}$ _____
11. $\frac{250}{1} = \frac{750}{X}$ _____
12. $\frac{80}{5} = \frac{10}{X}$ _____
13. $\frac{5}{20} = \frac{X}{40}$ _____
14. $\frac{\frac{1}{100}}{1} = \frac{\frac{1}{150}}{X}$ _____
15. $\frac{2.2}{X} = \frac{8.8}{5}$ _____
16. $\frac{60}{15} = \frac{125}{X}$ _____
17. $\frac{60}{10} = \frac{100}{X}$ _____
18. $\frac{80}{X} \times 60 = 20$ _____
19. $\frac{X}{0.5} = \frac{6}{4}$ _____
20. $\frac{5}{2.2} = \frac{X}{1}$ _____
21. $\frac{\frac{1}{4}}{15} = \frac{X}{60}$ _____
22. $\frac{25\%}{30\%} = \frac{5}{X}$ _____
23. In any group of 100 nurses, you would expect to find 45 nurses who will specialize in a particular field of nursing. In a class of 240 graduating nurses, how many would you expect to specialize? _____
24. Low-fat cheese has 48 calories per ounce. How many calories are in a $1\frac{1}{2}$ ounce portion? _____
25. If a patient receives 450 milligrams of a medication given evenly over 5.5 hours, how many milligrams did the patient receive per hour? _____

After completing these problems, see page 415 to check your answers.

Finding a Percentage of a Quantity

An important computation that nurses need for dosage calculations is to find a given percentage or part of a quantity. *Percentage* is a term that describes a *part* of a whole quantity. A *known percent* determines the part in question. Said another way, the percentage (or part in question) is equal to some known percent multiplied by the whole quantity.

rule

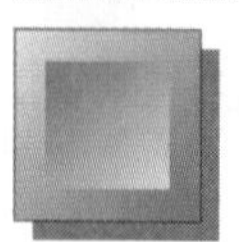

Percentage (Part) = Percent × Whole Quantity

Finding the Percentage

To find a percentage or part of a whole quantity:

1. Change the percent to a decimal fraction, and
2. Multiply the decimal fraction by the whole quantity.

Example:

A patient reports that he drank 75% of his 8-ounce cup of coffee for breakfast. He drank only part or a percentage of the whole 8 ounces. To record this in his chart, you must determine what amount 75% is of 8 ounces.

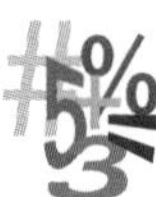

math tip: In a mathematical expression, the word *of* means *times* and indicates that you should multiply.

To continue with the example:

Percentage (Part) = Percent × Whole Quantity

Let X represent the unknown.

1. Change 75% to a decimal fraction: $75\% = \frac{75}{100} = .75. = 0.75$
2. Multiply 0.75 × 8 ounces: $X = 0.75 \times 8 = 6$ ounces

Therefore, 75% of 8 ounces is 6 ounces.

You also need to know how to find the other two quantities related to percentage.

Finding the Percent

Example:

What percent of 10 ounces is 4 ounces? You would be looking for the percent in this case. Using the previous formula, let X represent the percent.

Percentage (Part) = Percent × Whole Quantity

$4 = X \times 10$

$4 = 10X$ or $10X = 4$

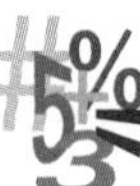

math tip: Learn to express the unknown "X" on the *left* side of the equation.

To continue, $10X = 4$

$\frac{10X}{10} = \frac{4}{10}$

$X = \frac{4}{10} = 40\%$

Finding the Whole Quantity

Example:

3 ounces is 5% of what number of ounces? In this example, the unknown "X" is the whole quantity. The *3 ounces* is the percentage or part. You are looking for the whole quantity of ounces.

Percentage (Part) = Percent × Whole Quantity

$3 = 5\% \times X$

$3 = 0.05X$ or $0.05X = 3$

$\frac{0.05X}{0.05} = \frac{3}{0.05}$

$X = 60$

quick review

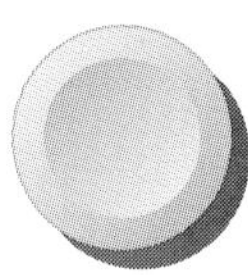

- Percentage (Part) = Percent × Whole Quantity

  Example: What is 12% of 48? $X = 12\% \times 48 = 0.12 \times 48 = 5.76$

- To find the percent one part is of a whole quantity, the unknown X (in the same equation) is the *percent.*

  Example: What percent of 20 is 5? $5 = X \times 20$; $5 = 20X$ or $20X = 5$; $\frac{20X}{20} = \frac{5}{20}$; $X = \frac{1}{4} = 25\%$

- To find what whole quantity a given percent is of a part of that quantity, let X represent the whole quantity in the same formula.

  Example: 4 feet is 50% of how many feet? $4 = 50\% \times X$; $50\%X = 4$; $0.5X = 4$; $\frac{0.5X}{0.5} = \frac{4}{0.5}$; $X = 8$

review set 11

Perform the indicated operation; round decimals to hundredths place.

1. What is 0.25% of 520? ______
2. What is 5% of 95? ______
3. What is 40% of 140? ______
4. What is 0.7% of 62? ______
5. What is 3% of 889? ______
6. What percent of 75 is 6.3? ______
7. What percent of 20 is $\frac{3}{5}$? ______
8. What percent of 34 is 8? ______
9. What percent of 5.4 is 1.2? ______
10. What percent of 92 is 4? ______
11. 8 ounces are 64% of what total number of ounces? ______
12. 12 cups are 10% of what total number of cups? ______
13. $2\frac{1}{2}$ teaspoons are 10% of what total number of teaspoons? ______
14. $\frac{1}{4}$ quart is 13% of what total number of quarts? ______
15. 100 pills are 10% of what total number of pills? ______

16. During a one year period, a hospital admitted 2048 women who gave birth. If this represents 40% of the total patients admitted during the year, how many total number of patients were admitted to the hospital? __________

17. The human body is made up of 206 bones. What percent of the bones of the body are:

    A. the 24 rib bones? __________ B. the 38 foot bones? __________

18. A patient's hospital bill for surgery is $17,651.07. Her insurance company pays 80%. How much will the patient owe? __________

19. Table salt (sodium chloride) is 40% sodium by weight. If a box of salt weighs 18 ounces, how much sodium is in the box of salt? __________

20. If a patient who has an average daily intake of 3500 calories per day consumes a 675 calorie breakfast, what percent of the total daily caloric intake has been consumed? __________

After completing these problems, see pages 415 and 416 to check your answers.

practice problems—chapter 2

Find the equivalent decimal, fraction, percent, and ratio forms. Reduce fractions and ratios to lowest terms; round decimals to two places.

	Decimal	Fraction	Percent	Ratio
1.	0.4	$\frac{2}{5}$	40%	2:5
2.	0.05	$\frac{1}{20}$	5%	1:20
3.	0.17	$\frac{17}{100}$	17%	17:100
4.	0.25	$\frac{1}{4}$	25%	1:4
5.	0.06	$\frac{3}{50}$	6%	3:50
6.	0.17	$\frac{1}{6}$	17%	1:6
7.	______	______	50%	______
8.	______	______	______	1:100
9.	0.09	______	______	______
10.	______	$\frac{3}{8}$	______	______
11.	______	______	______	2:3
12.	______	$\frac{1}{3}$	______	______
13.	0.52	______	______	______
14.	______	______	______	9:20
15.	______	$\frac{6}{7}$	______	______

16.	______	______	______	3:10
17.	______	$\frac{1}{50}$	______	______
18.	0.6	______	______	______
19.	0.04	______	______	______
20.	______	______	10%	______

Convert as indicated.

21. 1:25 to a decimal ______
22. $\frac{10}{400}$ to a ratio ______
23. 0.075 to a percent ______
24. 17:34 to a fraction ______
25. 75% to a ratio ______

Perform the indicated operation. Round decimals to hundredths.

26. What is 35% of 750? ______
27. What is 7% of 52? ______
28. What is 8.2% of 24? ______
29. What percent of $\frac{2}{3}$ is $\frac{1}{6}$? ______
30. What percent of 6.2 is 1.2? ______

Find the value of X in the following equations. Express your answers as decimals rounded to the nearest hundredth.

31. $\frac{20}{400} = \frac{X}{1680}$ ______
32. $\frac{75}{X} = \frac{\frac{1}{300}}{4}$ ______
33. $\frac{X}{5} = \frac{3}{15}$ ______
34. $\frac{500}{250} = \frac{2.2}{X}$ ______
35. $\frac{0.6}{1.2} = \frac{X}{200}$ ______
36. $\frac{\frac{1}{200}}{\frac{1}{4}} \times 125 = X$ ______
37. $\frac{\frac{1}{8}}{\frac{1}{3}} \times 2 = X$ ______
38. $\frac{X}{7} = \frac{12}{4}$ ______
39. $\frac{1,000,000}{425,000} \times 7.35 = X$ ______
40. $\frac{4\%}{1\%} \times 62.1 = X$ ______
41. A portion of meat totaling 125 grams contains 25 grams of protein and 6 grams of fat. What percent of the portion is: (A) protein? 20% (B) fat? 4.8%
42. You took a test that contained 150 questions, and you correctly answered 131 questions. What is your score as a percent? 87.33%
43. To work off 90 calories, Angie must walk for 27 minutes. How many minutes would she need to walk to work off 200 calories? ______
44. A multivitamin tablet provides 28.75 milligrams of a certain vitamin for which the recommended daily allowance (RDA) is 60 milligrams. What percent of the RDA is supplied by the tablet? ______
45. An 80 gram tube of ointment contains 1.75 grams of a certain drug. What percent of the total weight of the ointment is the drug? 2.2%

46. A label on a dinner roll wrapper reads, "2.7 grams of fiber per $\frac{3}{4}$ ounce serving." If you eat 1.5 ounces of dinner rolls, how many grams of fiber will you consume? ________

47. A patient received an intravenous medication at a rate of 6.75 milligrams per minute. After 42 minutes, how much medication had he received? ________

48. Mrs. Brown tells you she thinks her 3-day-old baby has lost too much weight. The baby weighed $6\frac{1}{2}$ pounds at birth and lost $\frac{1}{2}$ pound. What percent of the birth weight has the baby lost? ________

49. The cost of a certain medication is expected to decrease by 17% next year. If the cost is $12.56 now, how much would you expect it to cost at this time next year? ________

50. A patient is to be started on 150 milligrams of a medication and then decreased by 10% of the original dose for each dose until he is receiving 75 milligrams. When he takes his 75 milligram dose, how many total doses will he have taken? HINT: Be sure to count his first (150 milligrams) and last (75 milligrams) doses. ________

After completing these problems, see page 416 to check your answers.

Section 1 Self-Evaluation

Directions:

1. Round decimals to two places.
2. Express fractions in lowest terms.

Chapter 1 and Chapter 2 Mathematics Review for Dosage Calculations

Convert to Roman numerals:

1. 14 ________
2. 25 ________
3. 8 ________
4. 20 ________

Convert to Arabic numbers:

5. VII ________
6. XXIV ________
7. XIX ________
8. XXX ________

Complete the operations indicated:

9. $\frac{1}{4} + \frac{2}{3} =$ ________
10. $\frac{6}{7} - \frac{1}{9} =$ ________
11. $1\frac{3}{5} \times \frac{5}{8} =$ ________
12. $\frac{3}{8} \div \frac{3}{4} =$ ________
13. $13.2 + 32.55 + 0.029 =$ ________
14. $80.3 - 21.06 =$ ________
15. $0.3 \times 0.3 =$ ________
16. $1.5 \div 0.125 =$ ________
17. $\frac{1}{150} \div \frac{1}{100} =$ ________
18. $\dfrac{\frac{1}{120}}{\frac{1}{60}} =$ ________
19. 20% of 0.09 = ________
20. $\dfrac{16\%}{\frac{1}{4}} =$ ________

Arrange in order from smallest to largest:

21. $\frac{1}{3}$ $\frac{1}{2}$ $\frac{1}{6}$ $\frac{1}{10}$ $\frac{1}{5}$ ________
22. $\frac{3}{4}$ $\frac{7}{8}$ $\frac{5}{6}$ $\frac{2}{3}$ $\frac{9}{10}$ ________

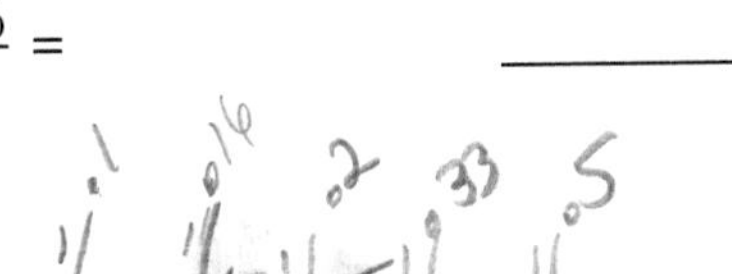

23. 0.25 0.125 0.3 0.009 0.1909 ________
24. 0.9% $\frac{1}{2}$% 50% 500% 100% ________

Convert as indicated:

25. 1:100 to a decimal ________
26. $\frac{6}{150}$ to a decimal ________
27. 0.009 to a percent ________
28. $33\frac{1}{3}$% to a fraction ________
29. $\frac{5}{9}$ to a ratio ________
30. 0.05 to a fraction ________
31. $\frac{1}{2}$% to a ratio ________
32. 2:3 to a fraction ________

33. 3:4 to a percent ________

34. $\frac{2}{5}$ to a percent ________

35. $\frac{1}{6}$ to a decimal ________

Find the value of "X" in the following equations. Express your answers as decimals; round to the nearest hundredth.

36. $\frac{0.35}{1.3} \times 4.5 = X$ ________

37. $\frac{0.3}{2.6} = \frac{0.15}{X}$ ________

38. $\frac{1,500,000}{500,000} \times X = 7.5$ ________

39. $\frac{\frac{1}{6}}{\frac{1}{4}} \times 1 = X$ ________

40. $\frac{1:100}{1:4} \times 2500 = X$ ________

41. $\frac{0.25}{0.125} \times 2 = X$ ________

42. $\frac{10\%}{\frac{1}{2}\%} \times 1000 =$ ________

43. $\frac{\frac{1}{100}}{\frac{1}{150}} \times 2.2 = X$ ________

44. X:15 = 150:7.5 ________

45. $\frac{1,000,000}{600,000} \times 5 = X$ ________

46. The unit has 30 patients and each nurse is assigned 6 patients. What percent of the total patients does each nurse care for? ________

47. If you have a roll of dimes and you must pay $1.10, how many dimes will you use? ________

48. If 1 pound of apples costs $0.69, how much do $3\frac{1}{2}$ pounds cost? ________

49. To prepare orange juice from frozen concentrate, you mix 3 cans of water to every 1 can of juice concentrate. How many cans of water will you need to prepare juice from 4 cans of frozen concentrate? ________

50. If 1 centimeter equals $\frac{3}{8}$ inch, how many centimeters are there in 3 inches? ________

After completing these problems, see page 417 to check your answers. Give yourself two points for each correct answer.

Perfect score = 100 Readiness score = 86 or higher My score = ______

For more practice, go back to the beginning of this text and repeat the Mathematics Diagnostic Evaluation.

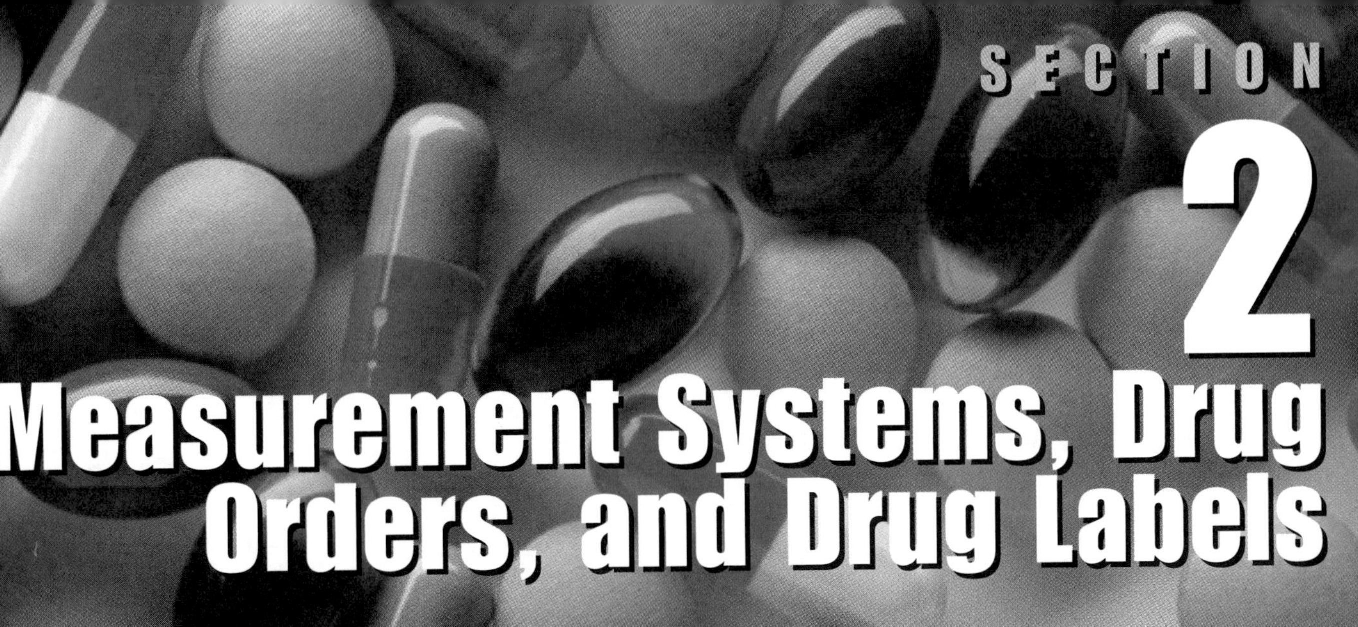

SECTION 2

Measurement Systems, Drug Orders, and Drug Labels

CHAPTER 3

Systems of Measurement

objectives

Upon mastery of Chapter 3, you will be able to recognize and express the basic systems of measurement used to calculate dosages. To accomplish this you will also be able to:

- Interpret and properly express metric, apothecary, and household notation.
- Recall metric, apothecary, and household equivalents.
- Explain the use of milliequivalent (mEq), international unit (IU), unit (U), and milliunit (mU) in dosage calculation.

To administer the correct amount of the prescribed medication to the patient, you must have a thorough knowledge of the weights and measures used in the prescription and administration of medications. The three systems used by health professionals are the metric, the apothecary, and the household systems.

It is necessary for you to understand each system and how to convert from one system to another. Most prescriptions are written using the metric system, and all U.S. drug labels today provide metric measurements. The household system uses measurement found in familiar containers such as teaspoons, cups, and quarts. Prescriptions for older drugs may still be written in the apothecary system, usually by physicians trained in this system. Until the metric system completely replaces the apothecary and household systems, nurses must be familiar with each system.

Three essential parameters of measurement are associated with the prescription and administration of drugs within each system of measurement: weight, volume, and length. *Weight* is the most utilized parameter. It is very important as a dosage unit. Most drugs are ordered and supplied by the weight of the drug. Keep in mind that the metric weight units, such as gram and milligram, are the most accurate and are preferred for health care usage. Occasionally you will also use the apothecary unit of weight referred to as the grain.

Think of capacity, or how much a container holds, as you contemplate *volume*, which is the next most important parameter. Volume usually refers to liquids. Volume also adds two additional parameters to dosage calculations: *quantity* and *concentration*. The milliliter is the most common metric volume unit for dosage calculations. Much less frequently you will use household and apothecary measures, such as teaspoon and ounce.

Length is the least utilized parameter for dosage calculations, but linear measurement is still essential to learn for health care situations. A person's height, the circumference of an infant's head, body surface area, and the size of lacerations and tumors are examples of important length measurements. You are probably familiar with the household measurements of inches and feet. Typically in the health care setting, length is measured in millimeters and centimeters.

The Metric System

The metric system was first adopted in 1799 in France. It is the most widely used system of measurement in the world today and is preferred for prescribing and administering medications.

The metric system is a decimal system, which means it is based on multiples of ten. The base units (the primary units of measurement) of the metric system are *gram* for weight, *liter* for volume, and *meter* for length. In this system, prefixes are used to show which portion of the base unit is being considered. It is important that you learn the most commonly used prefixes.

remember

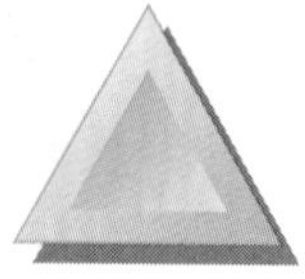

METRIC PREFIXES

micro = one millionth or 0.000001 or $\frac{1}{1,000,000}$ of the base unit

milli = one thousandth or 0.001 or $\frac{1}{1000}$ of the base unit

centi = one hundredth or 0.01 or $\frac{1}{100}$ of the base unit

kilo = one thousand or 1000 times the base unit

Figure 3-1 demonstrates the relationship of metric units. Notice that the values of most of the common prefixes used in health care and the ones applied in this text are highlighted: **kilo-, base, milli-,** and **micro-**. These units are three places away from the next place. Often you can either multiply or divide by 1000 to calculate an equivalent quantity. The only exception is *centi-*. It is easy to remember, though, if you think the relationship between one cent and one U.S. dollar as a clue to the relationship of centi- to the base.

The international standardization of metric units was adopted throughout much of the world in 1960 with the International System of Units or SI (from the French *Système International*). The abbreviations of this system of metric notation are the most widely accepted. The metric units of measurement and the SI abbreviations most often used for dosage calculations and measurements of health status are given in the following units of weight, volume, and length. Other acceptable abbreviations are given in parentheses. While these alternate abbreviations are still in use, they are considered confusing. This text uses SI standardized abbreviations throughout. It is recommended that you learn and practice these notations primarily.

remember

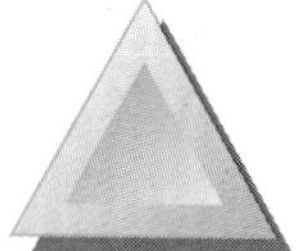

INTERNATIONAL SYSTEM (SI) OF METRIC UNITS AND ABBREVIATIONS

Weight
- gram (base unit)—g
- milligram—mg
- microgram—mcg (μg)
- kilogram—kg

Volume
- liter (base unit)—L (ℓ)
- milliliter—mL (mℓ) *or*
- cubic centimeter—cc

Length
- meter (base unit)—m
- centimeter—cm
- millimeter—mm

PREFIX	KILO-	HECTO-	DEKA-	BASE	DECI-	CENTI-	MILLI-	DECIMILLI-	CENTIMILLI-	MICRO-
Common Units	kilogram			gram liter meter		centimeter	milligram milliliter millimeter			microgram
Value to Base	**1000**	100	10	**1.0**	0.1	**0.01**	**0.001**	0.0001	0.00001	**0.000001**

FIGURE 3-1 Comparison of Common Metric Units Used in Health Care

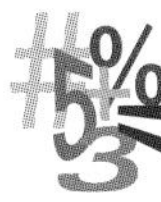

math tip: A cubic centimeter is the amount of space occupied by one milliliter of liquid. 1 cc = 1 mL.

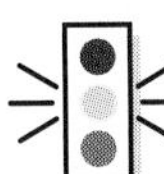

Caution: You may see gram abbreviated as *Gm* or *gm*, liter as lowercase *l*, or milliliter as *ml*. These abbreviations are considered obsolete and too easily misinterpreted. You should only use the standardized SI abbreviations. Use *g* for gram, *L* for liter, and *mL* for milliliter.

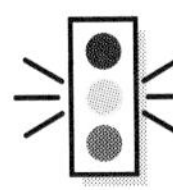

Caution: The SI abbreviations for milligram (*mg*) and milliliter (*mL*) appear to be somewhat similar, but in fact mg is a weight unit and mL is a volume unit. Confusing these two units can have dire consequences in dosage calculations. Learn to clearly differentiate them now.

In addition to learning the metric units, their values, and their abbreviations, it is important to use the following rules of metric notation.

rules of metric notation

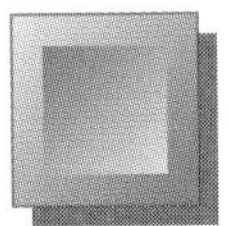

1. The unit or abbreviation always follows the amount. Example: 5 g, NOT g 5.
2. Decimals are used to designate fractional metric units. Example: 1.5 mL, not $1\frac{1}{2}$ mL.
3. Use a zero to emphasize the decimal point for fractional metric units of less than 1. Example: 0.5 mg, NOT .5 mg. This is a critical rule as it will prevent confusion and potential dosage error. Consider for a moment if you overlooked the decimal point and misinterpreted the medication order as 5 mg instead of 0.5 mg. The dosage would be 10 times too much.
4. Omit unnecessary zeros. Example: 1.5 g, NOT 1.50 g. This is another critical rule.
5. When in doubt, double check. Ask the writer for clarification.

The following table represents the basic metric units, abbreviations, and equivalents that are important for you to know. Learn the prefixes, and you will find the metric system easy to understand and use. Notice that most calculations of equivalents you will use are derived simply by multiplying or dividing by 1000. See Chapter 1 to review the rules for multiplying and dividing decimals by a power of ten.

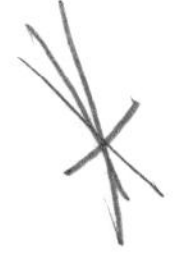

remember

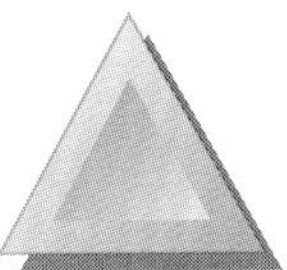

METRIC

	Unit	Abbreviation	Equivalents
Weight	gram	g	1 g = 1000 mg
	milligram	mg	1 mg = 1000 mcg, or 0.001 g
	microgram	mcg (μg)	1 mcg = 0.001 mg = 0.000001 g
	kilogram	kg	1 kg = 1000 g
Volume	liter	L (or ℓ)	1 L = 1000 mL
	milliliter	mL (or mℓ)	1 mL = 0.001 L, or 1 cc
	cubic centimeter	cc	1 cc = 1 mL, or 0.001 L
Length	meter	m	1 m = 100 cm, or 1000 mm
	centimeter	cm	1 cm = 0.01 m, or 10 mm
	millimeter	mm	1 mm = 0.001 m, or 0.1 cm

The metric system is the most common and the only standardized system of measurement in health care. Take a few minutes to review these essential points.

quick review

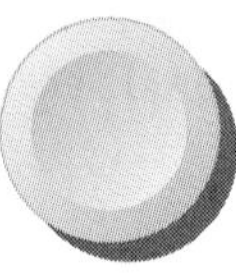

In the metric system:

- The metric base units are gram, liter, and meter.
- Subunits are designated by the appropriate prefix and the base unit (such as *milli*gram) and standardized abbreviations (such as mg).
- The unit or abbreviation always follows the amount.
- Decimals are used to designate fractional amounts.
- Use a zero to emphasize the decimal point for fractional amounts of less than 1.
- Omit unnecessary zeros.
- Multiply or divide by 1000 to derive most equivalents needed for dosage calculations.
- 1 cc = 1 mL.
- When in doubt about the exact amount or the abbreviation used, do not guess. Ask the writer to clarify.

review set 12

1. The system of measurement most commonly used for prescribing and administering medications is the ______ system.
2. Liter and milliliter are metric units that measure ______.
3. Gram and milligram are metric units that measure ______.
4. Meter and millimeter are metric units that measure ______.
5. 1 mg is ______ of a g.
6. There are ______ mL in a liter.
7. 10 mL = ______ cc
8. Which is largest, kilogram, gram or milligram? ______
9. Which is smallest, kilogram, gram, or milligram? ______
10. 1 liter = ______ cc
11. 1000 mcg = ______ mg
12. 1 kg = ______ g
13. 1 cm = ______ mm

Select the *correct* metric notation.

14. .3 g, 0.3 Gm, 0.3 g, .3 Gm, 0.30 g ______
15. $1\frac{1}{3}$ ml, 1.33 mL, 1.33 ML, $1\frac{1}{3}$ ML, 1.330 mL ______
16. 5 Kg, 5.0 kg, kg 05, 5 kg, 5 kG ______
17. 1.5 mm, $1\frac{1}{2}$ mm, 1.5 Mm, 1.50 MM, $1\frac{1}{2}$ MM ______
18. mg 10, 10 mG, 10.0 mg, 10 mg, 10 MG ______

Interpret these metric abbreviations.

19. mcg ________
20. mL ________
21. cc ________
22. g ________
23. mm ________
24. kg ________
25. cm ________

After completing these problems, see page 417 to check your answers.

The Apothecary and Household Systems

It seems likely that within a few years the metric system will be used exclusively in the measurement of medicines. However, as long as prescriptions are being written with apothecary notation, it is necessary that health care workers be knowledgeable about this system. Likewise, the household system persists and nurses need to be familiar with the equivalent measurements that patients or clients use at home.

It is interesting to realize the historic interconnection between the apothecary and household systems. The apothecary system was the first system of medication measurement used by pharmacists (apothecaries) and physicians. It originated in Greece and made its way to Europe via Rome and France. The English used it during the late 1600s, and the colonists brought it to America. A modified system of measurement for everyday use evolved, which is now recognized as the household system. Large liquid volumes were based on familiar trading measurements, such as *pints*, *quarts*, and *gallons*, which originated as apothecary measurements. Vessels to accommodate each measurement were made by craftsmen and widely circulated in colonial America.

Units of weight, such as the *grain*, *ounce*, and *pound*, also are rooted in the apothecary system. The grain originated as the standard weight of a single grain of wheat, which happens to be approximately 60 milligrams. This one equivalency of weight (one grain = 60 milligrams) is recognized in drug orders. Celebrating over 100 years as the world's most popular pill, aspirin is still prescribed and dispensed in grains.

The Apothecary System

Apothecary notation is unusual. Exercise caution when using this system. Apothecary notation uses Roman numerals, common fractions, special symbols, and units of measure that precede numeric values. The common units are grain (gr) and ounce (℥). Let's outline the rules and examine what this notation looks like.

rules of apothecary notation

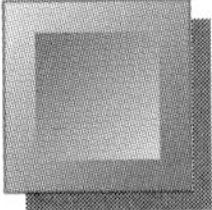

1. The unit or abbreviation precedes the amount. Example: gr v, NOT: v gr
2. Lowercase Roman numerals are used to express whole numbers, 1–10, 20, and 30. Arabic numbers are used for other quantities. Examples: ℥ iii (three ounces), gr 12 (twelve grains), and gr xx (twenty grains)
3. Fractions are used to designate amounts less than 1. Example: gr $\frac{1}{4}$, NOT: 0.25 gr
4. The fraction $\frac{1}{2}$ is designated by the symbol *ss*. Example: ℥ iiss (two and one-half ounces)

The apothecary units of measurement and essential equivalents for volume are given in the following table. There are no essential equivalents of weight or length to learn for this system.

remember

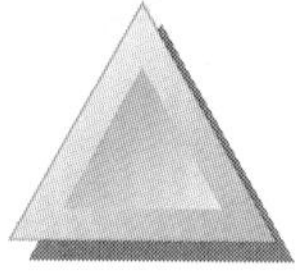

APOTHECARY

Unit	Abbreviation	Equivalents
grain	gr	
quart	qt	qt i = pt ii
pint	pt	qt i = ℥ 32
ounce or fluidounce	℥	pt i = ℥ 16
dram	ʒ	
minim	♏	

NOTE: The minim (♏) and fluid dram (ʒ) are given only so that you will be able to recognize them. Many syringes still have the minim scale identified, and the medicine cup continues to show the dram scale. However, their use is discouraged.

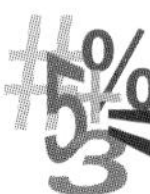

math tip: The ounce (℥) is a larger unit, and its symbol has one more loop than the dram (ʒ).

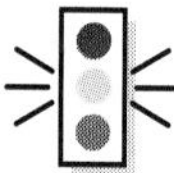

Caution: Notice that the abbreviations for the apothecary grain (gr) and the metric gram (g) can be confusing. The rule of indicating the abbreviation or symbol before the quantity in apothecary measurement further distinguishes it from a metric measurement. If you are ever doubtful about the meaning that is intended, be sure to ask the writer for clarification.

quick review

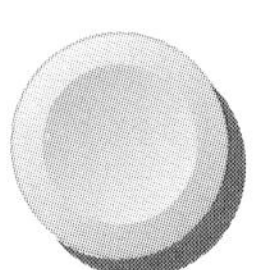

In the apothecary system:

- The common units for dosage calculation are grain and ounce.
- The quantity is best expressed in lowercase Roman numerals. Amounts greater than ten may be expressed in Arabic numbers, *except* 20 (xx) and 30 (xxx).
- Quantities of less than one are expressed as fractions, *except* $\frac{1}{2}$. One-half ($\frac{1}{2}$) is expressed by the symbol *ss.*
- The abbreviation or unit symbol is clearly written *before* the quantity.
- If you are unsure about the exact meaning of any medical notation, do not guess or assume. Ask the writer for clarification.

review set 13

Interpret the following apothecary symbols.

1. ʒ ______
2. ℥ ______
3. ♏ ______
4. ss ______
5. gr ______

Correctly write the following quantities in the apothecary system.

6. one-half ounce ______
7. one-sixth grain ______
8. four ounces ______
9. two pints ______

10. one and one-fourth quarts ______
11. ten grains ______
12. eight and one-half ounces ______
13. two grains ______
14. sixteen pints ______
15. three grains ______
16. thirty-two ounces ______
17. seven and one-half grains ______

Give the equivalent units.

18. qt i = ℥ ______
19. ℥ 16 = pt ______
20. qt i = pt ______

After completing these problems, see page 417 to check your answers.

The Household System

Household units are likely to be used by the patient at home where hospital measuring devices are not usually available. You should be familiar with the household system of measurement so that you can explain take-home prescriptions to your patient at the time of discharge. There is no standardized system of notation, but preferably the quantity is expressed in Arabic numbers and common fractions with the abbreviation following the amount. The common household units and abbreviations are given in the following table.

remember

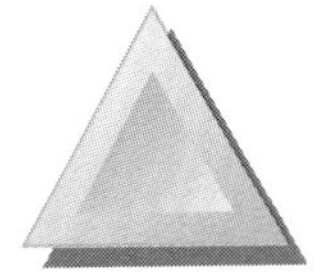

HOUSEHOLD

Unit	Abbreviation	Equivalents
drop	gtt	
teaspoon	t (or tsp)	
tablespoon	T or (tbs)	1 T = 3 t
ounce	oz (℥)	2 T = 1 oz
ounce (weight)	oz	1 pound (lb) = 16 oz
cup	cup	1 cup = 8 oz

NOTE: Like the minim (♏) and dram (ʒ), the drop (gtt) unit is given only for the purpose of recognition. There are no standard equivalents for drop to learn. The amount of each drop varies according to the diameter of the utensil used for measurement. (See Figure 6-2 Calibrated Dropper and Figure 14-16 Intravenous Drip Chambers.)

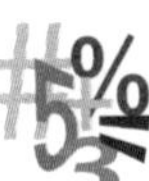

math tip: Tablespoon is the larger unit, and its abbreviation is expressed with a capital *T*. Teaspoon is the smaller unit, and its abbreviation is expressed with a lowercase or small *t*.

quick review

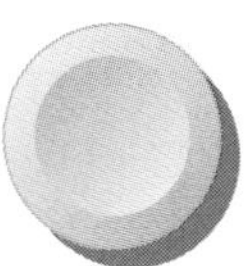

In the household system:

- The common units used in health care are teaspoon, tablespoon, ounce, cup, and pound.
- The quantity is typically expressed in Arabic numbers with the unit abbreviation following the amount. Example: 5 t
- Quantities of less than one are preferably expressed as common fractions. Example: $\frac{1}{2}$ cup
- When in doubt about the exact amount or the abbreviation used, do not guess or assume. Ask the writer to clarify.

Other Common Drug Measurements: Units and Milliequivalents

Four other measurements may be used to indicate the quantity of medicine prescribed: international unit (IU), unit (U), milliunit (mU), and milliequivalent (mEq). The quantity is expressed in Arabic numbers with the symbol following. The *international unit* (IU) represents a unit of potency used to measure such things as vitamins and chemicals. The *unit* (U) is a standardized amount needed to produce a desired effect. Medications such as penicillin, heparin, and insulin have their own meaning and numeric value related to the type of unit. One-thousandth ($\frac{1}{1000}$) of a unit (U) is a *milliunit* (mU). The equivalent of 1 U is 1000 mU. Pitocin is a drug measured in mU. The *milliequivalent* (mEq) is one-thousandth ($\frac{1}{1000}$) of an equivalent weight of a chemical. The mEq is the unit used when referring to the concentration of serum electrolytes, such as calcium, magnesium, potassium, and sodium.

It is not necessary to learn conversions for the international unit, unit, or milliequivalent because medications prescribed in these measurements are also prepared and administered in the same system.

Example 1:

Heparin 7500 U is ordered, and *heparin 10,000 units per mL* is the stock drug.

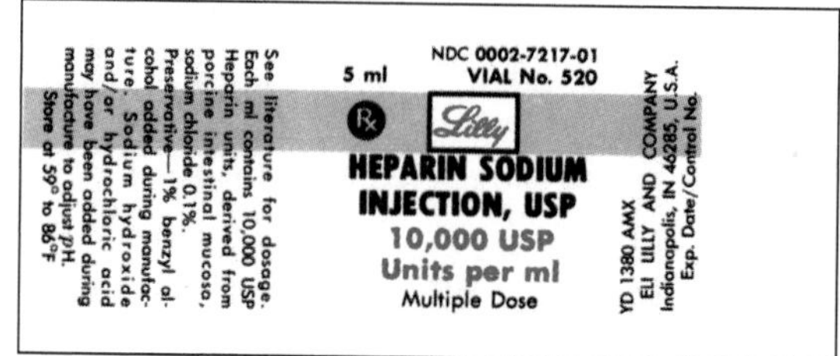

Example 2:

Potassium chloride 10 mEq is ordered, and *potassium chloride 20 mEq per 15 mL* is the stock drug.

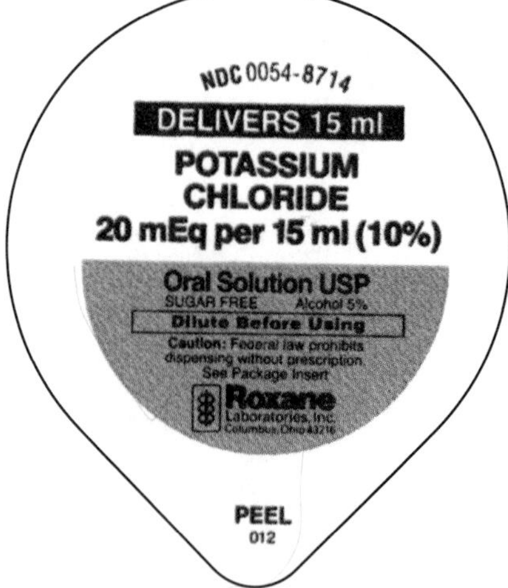

Example 3:

Syntocinon 2 mU (0.002 U) intravenous per minute is ordered and *Syntocinon 10 U/mL* to be added to 1,000 mL intravenous solution is available.

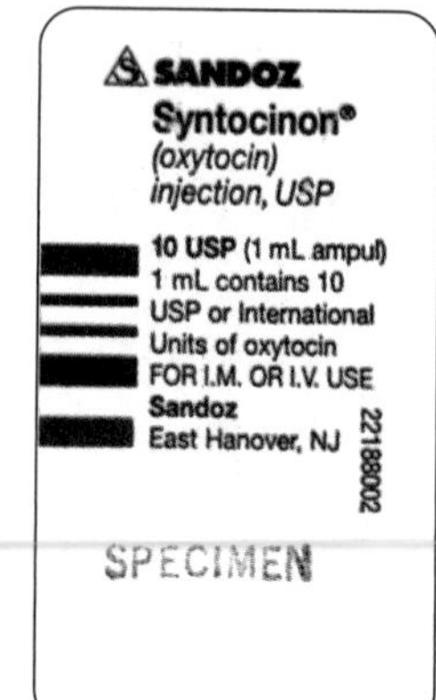

quick review

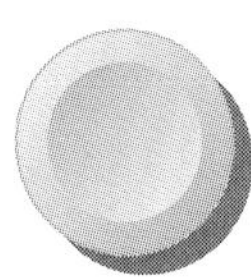

- The international unit (IU), unit (U), milliunit (mU), and milliequivalent (mEq) are special measured quantities expressed in Arabic numbers followed by the unit symbol.
- No conversion is necessary for IU and mEq, because the ordered dosage and supply dosage are in the same system.
- 1 U = 1000 mU.

review set 14

Interpret the following notations.

1. 20 gtt ______
2. 1000 U ______
3. 10 mEq ______
4. 4 t ______
5. 10 T ______

Express the following using correct notation.

6. four drops ______
7. 30 milliequivalents ______
8. 5 tablespoons ______
9. 1500 units ______
10. 10 teaspoons ______
11. The household system of measurement is commonly used in hospital dosage calculations. (True) (False)
12. The drop is a standardized unit of measure. (True) (False)
13. Drugs such as heparin and insulin are commonly measured in ______, abbreviated ______.
14. 1 T = ______ t
15. 3 T = ______ t
16. 32 oz = ______ lb
17. 4 T = ______ oz
18. 2 oz = ______ t
19. 15 t = ______ T
20. The unit of potency used to measure vitamins and chemicals is the ______ ______ and is abbreviated ______.

After completing these problems, see page 417 to check your answers.

critical thinking skills

The importance of the placement of the decimal point cannot be overemphasized. Let's look at some examples of potential medication errors related to the placement of the decimal point.

error 1

Not placing a zero before a decimal point on medication orders.

possible scenario

An emergency room physician wrote an order for the bronchodilator terbutaline for a patient with asthma. The order was written as follows:

Terbutaline .5 mg subcutaneously now, repeat dose in 30 minutes if no improvement

Suppose the nurse, not noticing the faint decimal point, administered 5 mg of terbutaline subcutaneously instead of 0.5 mg. The patient would receive ten times the dose intended by the physician.

potential outcome

Within minutes of receiving the injection the patient would likely complain of headache, and develop tachycardia, nausea, and vomiting. The patient's hospital stay would have been lengthened due to the need to recover from the overdose.

prevention

This type of medication error is avoided by remembering the rule to place a 0 in front of a decimal to avoid confusion regarding the dosage: 0.5 mg. Further, remember to question orders that are unclear or seem unreasonable.

critical thinking skills

Many medication errors occur by confusing mg and mL. Remember that mg is the weight of the medication, and mL is the volume of the medication preparation.

error 2

Confusing mg and mL.

possible scenario

Suppose a physician ordered Prelone (prednisolone, a steroid) 15 mg by mouth twice a day for a patient with cancer. Prelone syrup is supplied in a concentration of 15 mg in 5 mL. The pharmacist supplied a bottle of Prelone containing a total volume of 240 mL with 15 mg of Prelone in every 5 mL. The nurse, in a rush to give her medications on time, misread the order as 15 mL and gave the patient 15 mL of Prelone instead of 5 mL. Therefore, the patient received 45 mg of Prelone, or three times the correct dosage.

potential outcome

The patient could develop a number of complications related to a high dosage of steroids: gastrointestinal bleeding, headaches, seizures, and hypertension, to name a few.

prevention

Mg is the weight of a medication, and mL is the volume you prepare. Do not allow yourself to get rushed or distracted so that you would confuse milligrams with milliliters. When you know you are distracted or stressed, have another nurse double check the calculation of the dose.

practice problems—chapter 3

Give the metric prefix for the following parts of the base units.

1. 0.001 ________
2. 0.000001 ________
3. 0.01 ________
4. 1000 ________

Identify the equivalent unit with a value of 1 that is indicated by the following amounts (such as 1000 mU:1 U).

5. 0.001 gram ________
6. 1000 grams ________
7. 0.001 milligram ________
8. 0.01 meter ________

Identify the metric base unit for the following.

9. length ________
10. weight ________
11. volume ________

Interpret the following notations.

12. gtt ________
13. ℥ ________
14. oz ________
15. gr ________
16. mg ________
17. mcg ________
18. U ________
19. mEq ________
20. t ________
21. mU ________
22. mL ________
23. cc ________
24. pt ________
25. T ________
26. mm ________
27. g ________
28. cm ________
29. L ________
30. m ________
31. kg ________
32. IU ________

Express the following amounts in proper notation.

33. one-half grain ________
34. two teaspoons ________
35. one-third ounce ________
36. five hundred milligrams ________
37. one-half liter ________
38. one-fourth dram ________
39. one two-hundredths of a grain ________
40. five-hundredths of a milligram ________

Express the following numeric amounts in words.

41. $8\frac{1}{4}$ oz ________
42. 375 IU ________
43. gr $\frac{1}{125}$ ________
44. 2.6 mL ________
45. 20 mEq ________
46. 0.4 L ________
47. gr ivss ________
48. 0.17 mg ________

49. Critical Thinking Skill: Describe the strategy that would prevent the medication error.

possible scenario

Suppose a physician ordered oral Coumadin (an anticoagulant) for a patient with a history of phlebitis. The physician wrote an order for 1 mg, but while writing the order placed a decimal point after the 1 and added a 0:

Coumadin 1.0 mg orally once per day

Coumadin 1.0 mg was transcribed on the medication record as Coumadin 10 mg. The patient received ten times the correct dose.

potential outcome

The patient would likely begin hemorrhaging. An antidote, such as vitamin K, would be necessary to reverse the effects of the overdose. However, it is important to remember that not all drugs have antidotes.

prevention

____

____

50. Critical Thinking Skill: Describe the strategy that would prevent the medication error.

possible scenario

Suppose a physician ordered oral Codeine (a potent narcotic analgesic) for an adult patient recovering from extensive nasal surgery. The physician wrote the following order for 1 grain (equivalent to about 60 mg), but while writing the order placed the 1 before the abbreviation gr. The gr smeared and the abbreviation gr is unclear. Is it *grains* or *grams*?

Codeine 1 gr orally every four to six hours as needed for pain.

Codeine 1 gram was transcribed on the medication record. Because 1 gram is equivalent to 1000 mg or about 15 grains, this erroneous dosage is about 15 times more than the intended amount.

potential outcome

Even though the nurse was in a rush to help ease the patient's pain, she realized that the available codeine pills would not be dispensable in this amount. She would have to give the patient 15 tablets to equal the 1 gram amount. Rechecking the original order, the nurse saw the questionable order and called the physician for clarification. The nurse correctly concluded it was unlikely that the physician would have ordered such an excessive number of pills or dose.

prevention

____

____

After completing these problems, see pages 417 and 418 to check your answers.

CHAPTER 4

Conversions: Metric, Apothecary, and Household Systems

objectives

Upon mastery of Chapter 4, you will be able to complete step 1, conversions, in the three-step process of dosage calculations. To accomplish this, you will also be able to:

- Recall from memory the metric, apothecary, and household approximate equivalents.
- Convert between units of measurement within the same system.
- Convert units of measurement from one system to another.

Medications are usually prescribed or ordered in a unit of weight measurement such as grams or grains. The nurse must interpret this order and administer the correct number of tablets, capsules, teaspoons, milliliters, or some other unit of volume or capacity measurement, which will deliver the prescribed amount of medication.

Example 1:

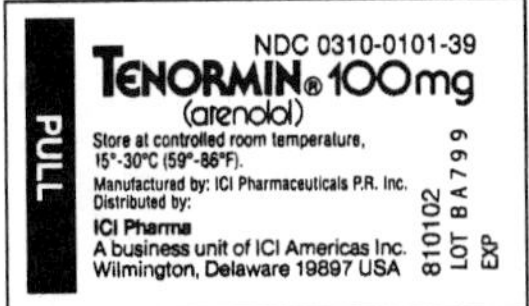

NDC 0310-0101-39
TENORMIN® 100mg
(atenolol)
PULL
ICI Pharma

A prescription notation may read:

Tenormin 200 mg to be given orally

The nurse has on hand unit dose blister packets labeled *100 mg of Tenormin in each tablet.* To administer the correct amount of the drug, the nurse must convert the prescribed weight of 100 mg to the correct number of tablets. In this case, the nurse gives the patient two of the 100-mg tablets, which equals 200 mg of *Tenormin.* To give the prescribed dosage, the nurse must be able to calculate the order in weight to the correct amount of tablets of the drug on hand or in stock. (THINK: If one tablet equals 100 mg, then two tablets equal 200 mg.)

Example 2:

5 mg/mL 5 mL Vial
VERSED®
(midazolam HCl)
For I.M. or I.V. Use.
FACSIMILE

A prescription notation may read:

Versed 2.5 mg by intramuscular injection

The nurse has on hand a vial of *Versed* labeled *5 mg/mL.* To administer the correct amount of the drug, the nurse must be able to fill the injection syringe with the correct number of milliliters. As the nurse, how many milliliters would you give? (THINK: If 5 mg = 1 mL, then 2.5 mg = 0.5 mL. Therefore, 0.5 mL should be administered.)

Sometimes a drug order may be written in a unit of measurement that is different from the supply of drugs the nurse has on hand.

Example 1:

Medication order: *Keflex 0.5 g orally*

Supply on hand: *Keflex 250 mg capsules*

The drug order is written in grams, but the drug is supplied in milligrams.

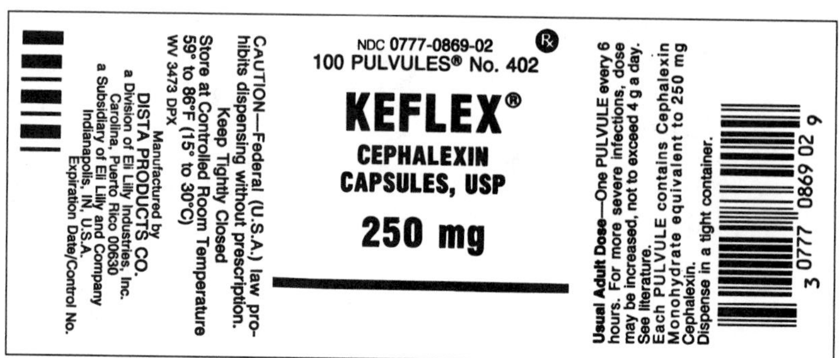

Example 2:

Medication order: *Codeine gr ss orally*

Supply on hand: *Codeine 30 mg tablets*

The drug order is written in grains (apothecary measurement), but the drug is supplied in milligrams (metric measurement).

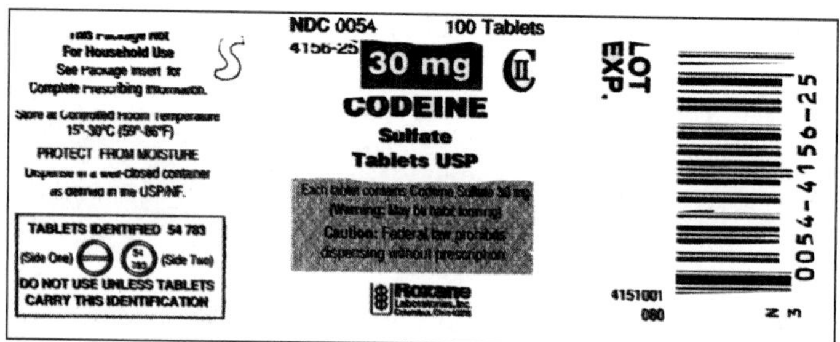

In such cases, the prescribed quantities must be converted into the units as supplied. The nurse can then calculate the correct dosage to prepare and administer to the patient. Thus, conversion is the first step in the calculation of dosages.

In this chapter you will learn two methods to do conversions: the *conversion factor* method and the *ratio-proportion* method. Study them both and then choose to use whichever one is easier and more logical to you.

Converting from One Unit to Another Using the Conversion Factor Method

After learning the systems of measurement common for dosage calculations and their equivalents (Chapter 3), the next step is to learn how to use them. First, you must be able to convert or change from one unit to another within the same measurement system. To accomplish this simple operation you need to:

- recall the equivalents, and
- multiply or divide.

The following information will help you remember when to multiply and when to divide.

The *conversion factor* is a number used with either multiplication or division to change a measurement from one unit of measurement to its *equivalent* in another unit of measurement.

rule

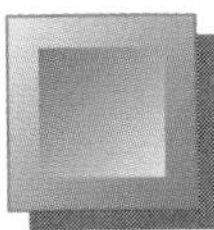

To convert from a larger to a smaller unit of measurement, multiply by the conversion factor. THINK: Larger → Smaller: (×)

This is true because it takes *more* parts of a *smaller* unit to make an equivalent amount of a larger unit. To get *more* parts, *multiply*.

Example 1:

Let's examine units already familiar to you. How many cups are in 2 quarts? In units of measurement, 1 quart = 4 cups. It takes 4 of the cup units to equal 1 of the quart units. Cups are *smaller* than quarts. THINK: Larger → Smaller: (×). The conversion factor for the cup and quart units is 4. Multiply by the conversion factor.

Therefore, 3 quarts (the larger unit) = 3 × 4 = 12 cups (the smaller unit).

Example 2:

How many inches are in 2 feet?

To convert 2 feet to the equivalent number of inches, multiply by the conversion factor of 12, because 1 foot = 12 inches. Multiplication is used because it takes *more* inches to represent the same amount in feet. Inches are smaller units than feet. THINK: Larger → Smaller: (×)

Therefore, 2 feet = 2 × 12 = 24 inches.

rule

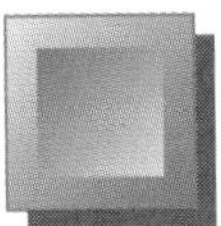

To convert from a smaller to a larger unit of measurement, divide by the conversion factor. THINK: Smaller → Larger: (÷)

This is true because it takes *fewer* parts of the *larger* unit to make an equivalent amount of a smaller unit. To get *fewer* parts, *divide*.

Example 1:

How many feet are in 36 inches?

1 foot = 12 inches. Feet are larger units than inches. To convert 36 inches to the equivalent number of feet, divide by the conversion factor of 12. Division is used because it takes *fewer* feet to represent the same amount in inches. THINK: Smaller → Larger: (÷)

Therefore, 36 inches (the smaller unit) = 36 ÷ 12 = 3 feet (the larger unit).

Example 2:

How many quarts are in 8 cups?

You know that 1 quart = 4 cups. The conversion factor is 4. Quarts are larger units than cups.

Divide by the conversion factor because it takes *fewer* of the quart units to equal the same amount in the cup units. THINK: Smaller → Larger: (÷)

Therefore, 8 cups = 8 ÷ 4 = 2 quarts.

quick review

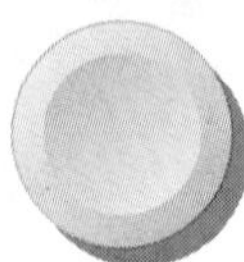

Use the conversion factor method to convert from one unit of measurement to another.

- Recall the equivalents.
- Identify the conversion factor.
- MULTIPLY by the conversion factor to convert to a smaller unit. THINK: Larger → Smaller: (×)
- DIVIDE by the conversion factor to convert to a larger unit. THINK: Smaller → Larger: (÷)

review set 15

Use the following common household equivalents to answer these items. Express amounts that are less than one as common fractions.

1 gallon = 4 quarts	1 foot = 12 inches
1 quart = 2 pints = 4 cups	1 yard = 3 feet

1. To convert from a smaller unit of measurement (such as inches) to a larger unit of measurement (such as feet), you would ________. (multiply or divide?)
2. To convert from gallons to quarts, you would ________. (multiply or divide?)

3. 12 cups =	________	quarts	12. 10 yards =	________	feet
4. 36 inches =	________	feet	13. 10 feet =	________	yards
5. 14 quarts =	________	gallons	14. $3\frac{1}{2}$ quarts =	________	cups
6. 32 cups =	________	pints	15. 3 cups =	________	quart
7. 6 feet =	________	inches	16. 1 inch =	________	foot
8. $\frac{1}{2}$ yard =	________	feet	17. 2 feet =	________	yard
9. 8 inches =	________	foot	18. 1 cup =	________	quart
10. $3\frac{1}{4}$ gallons =	________	cups	19. $2\frac{1}{2}$ gallons =	________	cups
11. 3 inches =	________	foot	20. 126 inches =	________	yards

21. A fruit punch recipe requires 2 quarts of orange juice, $\frac{1}{2}$ gallon of soda water, and 4 cups of cranberry juice. How many 1-cup servings will this make? ________
22. If you have 16 pints, you have the equivalent of how many quarts? ________
23. Milk costs \$1.56 per $\frac{1}{2}$ gallon at Store A; at Store B, milk costs \$0.94 per quart. How much do you save by buying 1 gallon of milk at Store A? ________

Using the prices in question 23, calculate the cost of 1 cup of milk bought at Store A and at Store B.

24. Store A cost = ________
25. Store B cost = ________

After completing these problems, see page 418 to check your answers.

Converting Within the Metric System Using the Conversion Factor Method

The most common conversions in dosage calculations are within the metric system. As you recall, most metric conversions are simply derived by multiplying or dividing by 1000. Recall from Chapter 1 that multiplying by 1000 is the same as moving the decimal point three places to the right. Also recall that dividing by 1000 is the same as moving the decimal point three places to the left.

To convert 2 grams to the equivalent number of milligrams, you would first determine that gram is the larger unit. Therefore, you would multiply to convert to milligrams, the smaller unit. THINK: Larger → Smaller: (×)

The equivalent is: 1 g = 1000 mg. Multiply 2 by the conversion factor of 1000.

1 g = 1000 mg (equivalent). Therefore,

2 g = 2 × 1000 = 2000 mg (multiplying by 1000) or

2.000. = 2000 mg (moving decimal 3 places to the right)

Thus, you know that a medicine container labeled *2 grams per tablet* is the same as *2000 milligrams per tablet*. Let's look at more examples.

Example 1:

Convert 0.3 g to mg.

Equivalent: 1 g = 1000 mg. Conversion factor is 1000.

THINK: Larger → Smaller: (×)

Multiply by 1000: 0.3 g = 0.3 × 1000 = 300 mg

or move decimal point 3 places to the right: 0.3 g = 0.300. = 300 mg

Example 2:

Convert 2.5 g to mg.

Equivalent: 1 g = 1000 mg. Conversion factor is 1000.

THINK: Larger → Smaller: (×)

Multiply by 1000: 2.5 g = 2.5 × 1000 = 2500 mg

or move decimal point 3 places to the right: 2.5 g = 2.500. = 2500 mg

Example 3:

Convert 0.15 kg to g.

Equivalent: 1 kg = 1000 g. Conversion factor is 1000.

THINK: Larger → Smaller: (×)

Multiply by 1000: 0.15 kg = 0.15 × 1000 = 150 g

or move decimal point 3 places to the right: 0.15 kg = 0.150. = 150 g

Example 4:

Convert 0.04 L to mL.

Equivalent: 1 L = 1000 mL. Conversion factor is 1000.

THINK: Larger → Smaller: (×)

Multiply by 1000: 0.04 L = 0.04 × 1000 = 40 mL

or move decimal point 3 places to the right: 0.04 L = 0.040. = 40 mL

Example 5:

An infant's head circumference is 40.5 cm. How many millimeters is that?

Convert 40.5 cm to mm.

Equivalent: 1 cm = 10 mm. Conversion factor is 10. THINK: Larger → Smaller: (×). Notice that, in this example, you are multiplying by 10 (not 1000).

40.5 cm = 40.5 × 10 = 405 mm

or move decimal point 1 place to the right: 40.5 cm = 40.5. = 405 mm

To convert a smaller unit to its equivalent larger unit, such as *milliliters to liters*, divide. THINK: Smaller → Larger: (÷). Recall the equivalent of 1 L = 1000 mL and then divide the number of milliliters by 1000. Thus, if you have a bottle that contains 2000 milliliters of boric acid solution, you know that this is the same as 2 liters. Dividing by 1000 is the same as moving the decimal point three places to the left.

Example 1:

Convert 5000 mL to L.

Equivalent: 1 L = 1000 mL. Conversion factor is 1000.

THINK: Smaller → Larger: (÷)

Divide by 1000: 5000 mL = 5000 ÷ 1000 = 5 L

or move decimal point 3 places to the left: 5000 mL = 5.000. = 5 L

Example 2:

Convert 500 mL to L.

Equivalent: 1 L = 1000 mL. Conversion factor is 1000.

THINK: Smaller → Larger: (÷)

Divide by 1000: 500 mL = 500 ÷ 1000 = 0.5 L

or move decimal point 3 places to the left: 500 mL = 0.500. = 0.5 L

Example 3:

Convert 50 mL to L.

Equivalent: 1 L = 1000 mL. Conversion factor is 1000.

THINK: Smaller → Larger: (÷)

Divide by 1000: 50 mL = 50 ÷ 1000 = 0.05 L

or move decimal point 3 places to the left: 50 mL = 0.050. = 0.05 L

Example 4:

Convert 5 mL to L.

Equivalent: 1 L = 1000 mL. Conversion factor is 1000.

THINK: Smaller → Larger: (÷)

Divide by 1000: 5 mL = 5 ÷ 1000 = 0.005 L

or move decimal point 3 places to the left: 5 mL = 0.005. = 0.005 L

Example 5:

A patient's wound measures 31 millimeters. How many centimeters is that? Convert 31 mm to cm.

Equivalent: 1 cm = 10 mm. Conversion factor is 10.

THINK: Smaller → Larger: (÷). Notice that in this example, you are dividing by 10 (not 1000).

31 mm = 31 ÷ 10 = 3.1 cm

or move decimal point 1 place to the left: 31 mm = 3.1. = 3.1 cm

In time you will probably do these calculations in your head with little difficulty. If you feel you do not understand the concept of conversions within the metric system, review the decimal section in Chapter 1 and the metric section in Chapter 3 again. Get help from your instructor before proceeding further.

quick review

To use the conversion factor method to convert between units in the metric system:

- Recall the metric equivalents and appropriately multiply or divide by the conversion factor.
- MULTIPLY to convert from a *larger unit to a smaller unit,* or move the decimal point to the right. Example: 3 L = ? mL. THINK: Larger → Smaller: (×). Equivalent: 1 L = 1000 mL; 3 L = 3 × 1000 or 3.000. = 3000 mL.
- DIVIDE to convert from a *smaller unit to a larger unit,* or move the decimal point to the left. Example: 400 mg = ? g. THINK: Smaller → Larger: (÷). Equivalent: 1 g = 1000 mg; 400 mg = 400 ÷ 1000 or .400. = 0.4 g.

review set 16

Convert each of the following to the equivalent unit indicated.

1. 500 cc = ________ L
2. 0.015 g = ________ mg
3. 8 mg = ________ g
4. 10 mg = ________ g
5. 60 mg = ________ g
6. 300 mg = ________ g
7. 0.2 mg = ________ g
8. 1.2 g = ________ mg
9. 0.0025 kg = ________ g
10. 0.065 g = ________ mg
11. 0.005 L = ________ mL
12. 1.5 L = ________ cc
13. 2 mL = ________ cc
14. 250 cc = ________ L
15. 2 kg = ________ g
16. 56.08 cc = ________ mL
17. 79,200 mL = ________ L
18. 1 L = ________ mL
19. 1 g = ________ mg
20. 1 mL = ________ L

21. 23 mcg = __________ mg
22. 1.05 g = __________ kg
23. 18 mcg = __________ mg
24. 0.4 mg = __________ mcg
25. 25 g = __________ kg
26. 50 cm = __________ m
27. 10 L = __________ mL
28. 450 cc = __________ L
29. 5 mL = __________ L
30. 30 mg = __________ mcg

After completing these problems, see page 418 to check your answers.

Approximate Equivalents

Fortunately, the use of the apothecary and household systems is becoming less and less frequent. But until they are obsolete, the nurse must be familiar with conversions between the metric, apothecary, and household systems of measurement.

Approximate equivalents are used for conversions from one system to another. Exact equivalents are not practical and, therefore, rarely used by health care workers. For example, the exact equivalent of one gram as measured in grains is: 1 gram = 15.432 grains. This is rounded to give the approximate equivalent of 1 g = gr 15.

Approximate equivalents that are used for dosage calculations are listed in the accompanying Remember box. Learn the equivalents so that you can change from one system to another quickly and accurately. The equivalents should be committed to memory. Review them often. When you learn these essential equivalents in addition to the other equivalents you learned in Chapter 3, you are on your way to mastering the skill of dosage calculations.

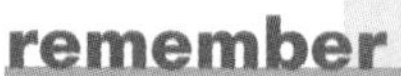

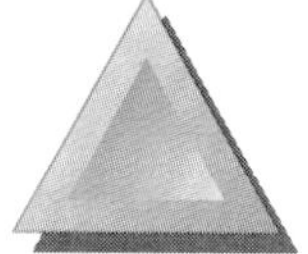

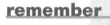

APPROXIMATE EQUIVALENTS

1 g = gr 15
gr i = 60 mg
1 t = 5 mL
1 T = 3 t = 15 mL = ℥ss
℥i = 30 mL = 6 t
1 L = qt i = ℥32 = pt ii = 4 cups
pt i = 500 mL = ℥16 = 2 cups
1 cup = 250 mL = ℥viii
1 kg = 2.2 lb
1 in = 2.5 cm

Look at Figure 4-1 for additional equivalents for metric and apothecary weight measurement of grains to milligrams. They are the most common ones still in use. You know how to convert between grains and milligrams, so you do not need to memorize these equivalents.

Figures 4-2 and 4-3 are visual aids that associate most of the base equivalents. You may find these diagrams easier to remember than the tables.

Look at the first triangle of weight equivalents (Figure 4-2). Beginning at the top of the triangle, use your finger to trace the arrow from *g* (gram) down to *gr* (grain). The arrow indicates that *1 g = gr 15*. On the other side, trace down from *g* (gram) to *mg* (milligram). This arrow indicates that *1 g = 1000 mg*. Likewise, the bottom arrow goes from *gr* to *mg* to remind you that *gr i = 60 mg*. In summary, the triangle simply says:

1 g = gr 15, 1 g = 1000 mg, and gr i = 60 mg.

APPROXIMATE EQUIVALENTS: gr to mg

Apothecary	Metric	Conversion Calculation
gr i	60 mg	gr i = 60 mg
gr $\frac{3}{4}$	45 mg	$\frac{3}{\cancel{4}_{1}} \times \frac{\cancel{60}^{15}}{1}\text{ mg} = 45\text{ mg}$
gr ss	30 mg	$\frac{1}{\cancel{2}_{1}} \times \frac{\cancel{60}^{30}}{1}\text{ mg} = 30\text{ mg}$
gr $\frac{1}{4}$	15 mg	$\frac{1}{\cancel{4}_{1}} \times \frac{\cancel{60}^{15}}{1}\text{ mg} = 15\text{ mg}$
gr $\frac{1}{8}$	7.5 mg	$\frac{1}{\cancel{8}_{2}} \times \frac{\cancel{60}^{15}}{1}\text{ mg} = 7.5\text{ mg}$
gr $\frac{1}{60}$	1 mg	$\frac{1}{\cancel{60}_{1}} \times \frac{\cancel{60}^{1}}{1}\text{ mg} = 1\text{ mg}$
gr $\frac{1}{100}$	0.6 mg	$\frac{1}{\cancel{100}_{10}} \times \frac{\cancel{60}^{6}}{1}\text{ mg} = \frac{6}{10}\text{ mg} = 0.6\text{ mg}$
gr $\frac{1}{120}$	0.5 mg	$\frac{1}{\cancel{120}_{2}} \times \frac{\cancel{60}^{1}}{1}\text{ mg} = \frac{1}{2}\text{ mg} = 0.5\text{ mg}$
gr $\frac{1}{150}$	0.4 mg	$\frac{1}{\cancel{150}_{5}} \times \frac{\cancel{60}^{2}}{1}\text{ mg} = \frac{2}{5}\text{ mg} = 0.4\text{ mg}$
gr $\frac{1}{200}$	0.3 mg	$\frac{1}{\cancel{200}_{10}} \times \frac{\cancel{60}^{3}}{1}\text{ mg} = \frac{3}{10}\text{ mg} = 0.3\text{ mg}$
gr $\frac{1}{300}$	0.2 mg	$\frac{1}{\cancel{300}_{5}} \times \frac{\cancel{60}^{1}}{1}\text{ mg} = \frac{1}{5}\text{ mg} = 0.2\text{ mg}$

FIGURE 4-1 Common Grain to Milligram Approximate Equivalents

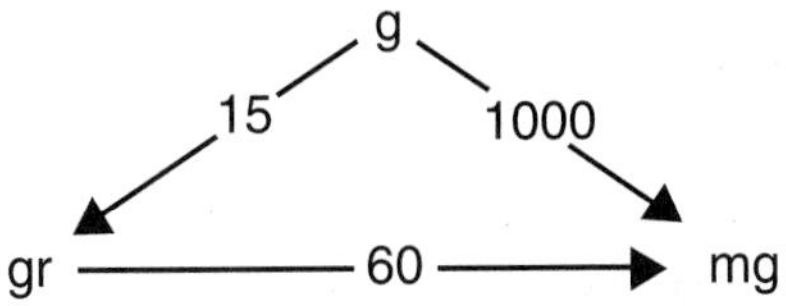

FIGURE 4-2 Weight Equivalents

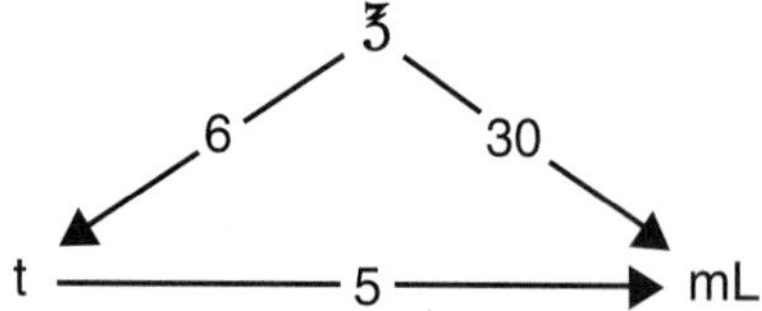

FIGURE 4-3 Volume Equivalents

Look at the second triangle of volume equivalents (Figure 4-3). Beginning at the top of the triangle, use your finger to trace the arrow from ʒ (ounce) down to *t* (teaspoon). The arrow indicates that *ʒ i = 6 t*. On the other side, trace down from ʒ (ounce) to *mL* (milliliter). This arrow reminds you that *ʒ i = 30 mL*. Likewise, the bottom arrow goes from *t* (teaspoon) to *mL* (milliliter). This arrow reminds you that *1 t = 5 mL*. In summary this triangle simply says:

ʒ i = 6 t, ʒ i = 30 mL, and 1 t = 5 mL.

Converting Between Systems of Measurement Using the Conversion Factor Method

Now let's convert units between systems of measurement using approximate equivalents and the conversion factor method. Recall that to convert from a larger to a smaller unit of measure, you must multiply by the conversion factor. Larger → Smaller: (×).

Example 1:

Convert 0.5 g to gr.

Approximate equivalent: 1 g = gr 15. Conversion factor is 15.

THINK: Larger → Smaller: (×)

0.5 g = 0.5 × 15 = 7.5 = gr viiss

Example 2:

Convert ʒii to mL.

Approximate equivalent: ʒi = 30 mL. Conversion factor is 30.

THINK: Larger → Smaller: (×)

ʒii = 2 × 30 = 60 mL

Example 3:

Convert gr $\frac{1}{300}$ to mg.

Approximate equivalent: gr i = 60 mg. The conversion factor is 60.

THINK: Larger → Smaller: (×)

$$\text{gr } \frac{1}{300} = \frac{1}{\cancel{300}_{5}} \times \frac{\cancel{60}^{1}}{1} = \frac{1}{5} = 0.2 \text{ mg}$$

Example 4:

The scale weighs the child at 40 kilograms. The mother wants to know her child's weight in pounds.

Convert 40 kg to lb.

Approximate equivalent: 1 kg = 2.2 lb. The conversion factor is 2.2.

THINK: Larger → Smaller: (×)

40 kg = 40 × 2.2 = 88 lb

Recall that to convert from a smaller to a larger unit of measure, you must divide by the conversion factor. THINK: Smaller → Larger: (÷)

Example 1:

Convert 120 mg to gr.

Approximate equivalent: gr i = 60 mg. Conversion factor is 60.

THINK: Smaller → Larger: (÷)

120 mg = 120 ÷ 60 = 2 = gr ii

Example 2:

Convert 45 mL to t.

Approximate equivalent: 1 t = 5 mL. Conversion factor is 5.

THINK: Smaller → Larger: (÷)

45 mL = 45 ÷ 5 = 9 t

Example 3:

Convert 66 lb to kg.

Approximate equivalent: 1 kg = 2.2 lb. Conversion factor is 2.2.

THINK: Smaller → Larger: (÷)

66 lb = 66 ÷ 2.2 = 30 kg

Example 4:

Convert 40 cm to in (inches).

Approximate equivalent: 1 in = 2.5 cm. Conversion factor is 2.5.

THINK: Smaller → Larger: (÷)

40 cm = 40 ÷ 2.5 = 16

NOTE: Because inches are a household measurement, amounts less than 1 are preferably expressed in fractions.

Try this: Convert your weight in pounds to kilograms rounded to hundredths or two decimal places.

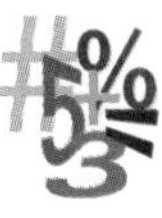

math tip: A clue to remember the approximate equivalent 1 kg = 2.2 lb is to realize that there are about 2 pounds for every kilogram, so the number of kilograms you weigh is about half the number of pounds you weigh. (Could almost make getting on a metric scale pleasant.)

quick review

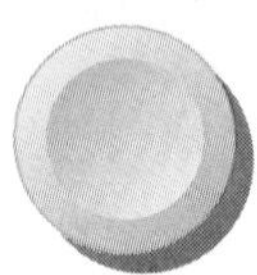

In order to perform dosage calculations, you must be able to convert between systems of measurement. To use the *conversion factor method,* recall the approximate equivalent, identify the conversion factor, and

- MULTIPLY by the conversion factor to convert to a SMALLER unit.
- THINK: Larger → Smaller: (×)
- DIVIDE by the conversion factor to convert to a LARGER UNIT.
- THINK: Smaller → Larger: (÷)

review set 17

Use the conversion factor method to convert each of the following amounts to the unit indicated. Indicate the approximate equivalent used in the conversion.

	Approximate Equivalent		Approximate Equivalent
1. gr ss = ________ mg	________	21. 0.4 mg = gr ________	________
2. gr $\frac{3}{4}$ = ________ mg	________	22. 0.6 mg = gr ________	________
3. 0.03 g = gr ________	________	23. pt i = ________ mL	________
4. gr $\frac{1}{150}$ = ________ mg	________	24. gr x = ________ mg	________
5. gr viiss = ________ g	________	25. 300 mg = gr ________	________
6. 15 mg = gr ________	________	26. 30 cm = ________ in	________
7. 13 t = ________ cc	________	27. 90 mg = gr ________	________
8. 15 cc = ℥ ________	________	28. 60 mL = ℥ ________	________
9. ℥ iiss = ________ mL	________	29. gr $\frac{1}{6}$ = ________ mg	________
10. 750 mL = pt ________	________	30. 30 mg = gr ________	________
11. 20 mL = ________ t	________	31. 32 in = ________ cm	________
12. 4 T = ________ cc	________	32. 350 mm = ________ in	________
13. 9 kg = ________ lb	________	33. 7.5 cm = ________ in	________
14. qt iv = pt ________	________	34. 2 in = ________ mm	________
15. 3 L = ℥ ________	________	35. 40 kg = ________ lb	________
16. 55 kg = ________ lb	________	36. 7.16 kg = ________ g	________
17. 12 in = ________ cm	________	37. 110 lb = ________ kg	________
18. qt ii = ________ L	________	38. 3.5 kg = ________ lb	________
19. 3 t = ________ mL	________	39. 63 lb = ________ kg	________
20. 99 lb = ________ kg	________		

40. A newborn infant is $21\frac{1}{2}$ inches long. Her length is ________ cm.

41. The label for a granular medicine recommends mixing it with at least 120 mL of water or juice. At the time of discharge, the nurse should advise the patient to mix the medicine with ________ ounce(s) or ________ cup(s) of water or juice.

42. A patient starts an exercise program and walks 0.75 kilometer on the first day. Each day he increases his distance by 500 meters. How many kilometers does he walk on the seventh day? __________ kilometers

43. Calculate the total fluid intake in mL for 24 hours.

Breakfast	8 ounces milk
	6 ounces orange juice
	4 ounces water with medication
Lunch	8 ounces iced tea
Snack	10 ounces coffee
	4 ounces gelatin dessert
Dinner	8 ounces water
	6 ounces tomato juice
	6 ounces beef broth
Snack	5 ounces pudding
	12 ounces diet soda
	4 ounces water with medication

Total = __________ mL

44. A child who weighs 55 lb is to receive 0.05 mg of a drug per kg of body weight per dose. How much of the drug should the child receive for each dose? __________ mg

45. A child takes 12 mL of a medication four times per day. If the full bottle contains 16 ounces of the medication, how many days will the bottle last? __________ day(s)

46. The doctor prescribes 60 mL of Epsom Salts crystals in 1000 mL of warm water as a soak for a sprained ankle. Using measures commonly found in the home, how would you instruct the patient to prepare the solution?

____

47. The patient is to receive 10 mL of a drug. How many teaspoonsful should the patient take? __________ t

48. An infant is taking a ready-to-feed formula. The formula comes in quart containers. If the infant usually takes 4 ounces of formula every 3 hours during the day and night, how many quarts of formula should the mother buy for a 3-day supply? __________ qt

49. An infant's head circumference is 40 cm. The parents ask for the equivalent in inches. You tell the parents their infant's head circumference is __________ in.

50. The patient tells you he was weighed in the doctor's office and was told he is 206 pounds. What is his weight in kilograms? __________ kg

After completing these problems, see pages 418 and 419 to check your answers.

Converting Using the Ratio-Proportion Method

An alternate method of performing conversions is to set up a proportion of two ratios expressed as fractions. Refer to Chapter 2 to review ratios and proportions if needed. To use ratio-proportion to convert from one unit to another, you need to:

- recall the equivalents,
- set up a proportion of two equivalent ratios, and
- cross-multiply to solve for an unknown quantity, X.

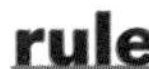

rule

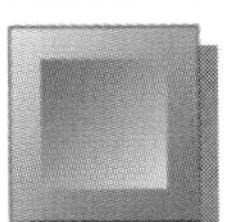

Ratio for known equivalent equals ratio for unknown equivalent.

Each ratio in a proportion must have the same relationship and follow the same sequence. A proportion compares like things to like things. Be sure the units in the numerators match and the units in the denominators match. Label the units in each ratio.

Example 1:

How many grams are equivalent to 3.5 kg?

The first ratio of the proportion contains the *known equivalent,* for example 1 kg : 1000 g. The second ratio contains the *desired unit of measure* and the *unknown equivalent* expressed as "X," for example 3.5 kg : X g. This proportion in fractional form looks like this:

$$\frac{1 \text{ kg}}{1000 \text{ g}} = \frac{3.5 \text{ kg}}{\text{X g}}$$

Notice that the ratios follow the same sequence. **THIS IS ESSENTIAL.** The proportion is set up so that like units are across from each other. The units in the numerators match (kg) and the units in the denominators match (g).

Cross-multiply to solve the proportion for "X." Refer to Chapter 2 to review this skill if needed.

$$\frac{1 \text{ kg}}{1000 \text{ g}} = \frac{3.5 \text{ kg}}{\text{X g}}$$

$\text{X} = 3.5 \times 1000 = 3.500. = 3500 \text{ g}$

You know the answer is in grams, because grams is the unknown equivalent.

3.5 kg = 3500 g

In Example 2 the unknown "X" is in the numerator. It doesn't matter, as long as the sequence is the same (numerator units match and denominator units match). Remember, a proportion must compare like things to like things. In the next example it is gr : mg = gr : mg.

Example 2:

Convert 45 milligrams to grains

Known equivalent: gr i = 60 mg

$$\frac{\text{gr i}}{60 \text{ mg}} = \frac{\text{gr X}}{45 \text{ mg}}$$

$$60\text{X} = 45$$

$$\frac{60\text{X}}{60} = \frac{45}{60}$$

$$\text{X} = \frac{45}{60} = \text{gr } \frac{3}{4}$$

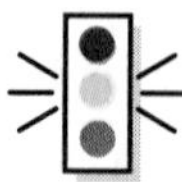

Caution: As is customary, the capital letter "X" is consistently used in this text to denote the unknown quantity in an equation and proportion. It is important that you do not confuse the unknown "X" with the value of gr x, which designates ten grains.

Example 3:

Convert 10 milliliters to teaspoons

Known equivalent: 1 t = 5 mL

$$\frac{1 \text{ t}}{5 \text{ mL}} = \frac{\text{X t}}{10 \text{ mL}}$$

$$5\text{X} = 10$$

$$\frac{5X}{5} = \frac{10}{5}$$

$$X = \frac{10}{5} = 2 \text{ t}$$

Example 4:

Convert 150 pounds to kilograms

Known equivalent: 1 kg = 2.2 lb

$$\frac{1 \text{ kg}}{2.2 \text{ lb}} = \frac{X \text{ kg}}{150 \text{ lb}}$$

$$2.2X = 150$$

$$\frac{2.2X}{2.2} = \frac{150}{2.2}$$

$$X = \frac{150}{2.2} = 68.18 \text{ kg}$$

quick review

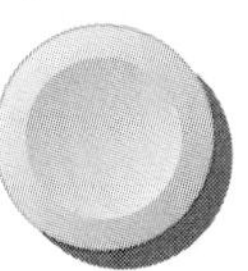

To use the ratio-proportion method to convert from one unit to another or between systems of measurement:

- Recall the equivalent.
- Follow the rule: Ratio for known equivalent equals ratio for unknown equivalent.
- Label the units and match the units in the numerators and denominators.
- Cross-multiply to find the value of the unknown "X" equivalent.

review set 18

Use the ratio-proportion method to convert each of the following amounts to the unit indicated. Indicate the approximate equivalent used in the conversion.

	Approximate Equivalent		Approximate Equivalent
1. 50 mL = ______ L	______	11. 2.5 mL = ______ t	______
2. 3 g = gr ______	______	12. gr ss = ______ mg	______
3. 84 lb = ______ kg	______	13. 7.5 mg = gr ______	______
4. gr xx = ______ g	______	14. 0.6 mg = gr ______	______
5. gr $\frac{1}{8}$ = ______ mg	______	15. 7.5 cm = ______ in	______
6. 75 mL = ℥ ______	______	16. 16 g = ______ mg	______
7. 750 mL = pt ______	______	17. 15 mL = ℥ ______	______
8. ℥iss = ______ mL	______	18. ℥16 = qt ______	______
9. 15 mg = gr ______	______	19. qt ii = ______ L	______
10. 625 mcg = ______ mg	______	20. pt i = qt ______	______

21. The medicine order states to administer a potassium chloride supplement added to at least 150 mL of juice. How many ounces of juice should you pour? ℥ ______

22. A child should have 5 mL of liquid Children's Tylenol (acetaminophen) every 4 hours as needed for fever above 100°F. To relate these instructions to the child's mother, you should advise her to give her child ______ teaspoon(s) of Tylenol per dose.

23. The doctor advises his patient to drink at least 2000 mL of fluid per day. The patient should have at least __________ 8-ounce glasses of water per day.

24. A child needs 15 mL of a drug. How many teaspoonsful should he receive? __________ t

25. The doctor orders codeine gr $\frac{1}{4}$. This is equivalent to how many milligrams? __________ mg

After completing these problems, see pages 419 and 420 to check your answers.
For more practice rework Review Sets 15, 16, and 17 using the ratio-proportion method.

critical thinking skills

error

Incorrectly interpreting grains as milligrams.

possible scenario

A physician ordered a single dose of 15 grains of aspirin for a patient complaining of a severe headache. Aspirin was available in 500 mg aspirin tablets. While preparing the medication, the nurse was distracted by a visitor who fell by the nurses' station. The nurse returned to read the order as *1.5 grams* and calculated the dose this way:

If: 1 g = 1000 mg

then: 1.5 g = 1000 mg + 500 mg = 1500 mg, so the patient was given 3 tablets.

You know that 15 grains is equivalent to 1 g or 1000 mg. By misreading the dose, the nurse gave 500 mg more than ordered, overdosing the patient.

potential outcome

The patient received $1\frac{1}{2}$ times, or 150% of the dosage ordered. This larger dose, 1500 mg, could cause nausea, heartburn, and gastric upset. In aspirin-sensitive patients it could result in gastric bleeding.

prevention

This type of medication error is avoided by carefully checking the drug orders at least three times: before pouring a medication, once the dose is prepared, and prior to giving the patient the medication. Also, the nurse should recognize that the ordered dose is in *apothecary* measurement, while the supply dosage is in *metric* measurement, and carefully convert between systems.

Summary

At this point, you should be quite familiar with the equivalents for converting within the metric, apothecary, and household systems, and from one system to another. From memory, you should be able to recall quickly and accurately the equivalents for conversions. If you are having difficulty understanding the concept of converting from one unit of measurement to another, review this chapter and seek additional help from your instructor.

Work the practice problems for Chapter 4. Concentrate on accuracy. One error can be a serious mistake when calculating the dosages of medicines or performing critical measurements of health status.

practice problems—chapter 4

Give the following equivalents without consulting conversion tables.

1. 0.5 g = ______ mg
2. 0.01 g = ______ mg
3. 7.5 cc = ______ mL
4. qt iii = ______ L
5. 4 mg = ______ g
6. 500 mL = ______ L
7. 250 mL = pt ______
8. 300 g = ______ kg
9. 28 in = ______ cm
10. 68 kg = ______ lb
11. gr iii = ______ mg
12. ℥ iiiss = ______ mL
13. gr $\frac{1}{200}$ ______ mg
14. gr $\frac{1}{4}$ = ______ mg
15. gr $\frac{1}{10}$ = ______ mg
16. gr iss = ______ mg
17. 70$\frac{1}{2}$ lb = ______ kg
18. 3634 g = ______ lb
19. 8 mL = ______ L
20. gr xxx = ______ g
21. 237.5 cm = ______ in
22. 0.5 g = gr ______
23. 0.6 mg = gr ______
24. gr x = ______ g
25. 150 lb = ______ kg
26. 60 mg = gr ______
27. gr 15 = ______ g
28. 2 cups = ______ cc
29. 6 t = ______ T
30. 90 mL = ℥ ______
31. 1 ft = ______ cm
32. 2 T = ______ cc
33. 2.2 lb = ______ kg
34. 5 cc = ______ t
35. 1000 mL = ______ L
36. 1.5 g = ______ mg
37. ℥ iss = ______ cc
38. 1500 mL = qt ______
39. 10 mg = gr ______
40. 25 mg = ______ g
41. 4.3 kg = ______ g
42. 60 mg = ______ g
43. 0.015 g = ______ mg
44. 45 cc = ______ mL
45. gr 12 = ______ g
46. As a camp nurse for 9- to 12-year-old children, you are administering 2$\frac{1}{2}$ teaspoonsful of oral liquid Tylenol to 6 feverish campers every 4 hours for oral temperatures above 100°F. You have on hand a 4-ounce bottle of liquid Tylenol. How many complete or full doses are available from this bottle? ______ full doses
47. At this same camp, the standard dosage of Pepto-Bismol for 9- to 12-year-olds is 1 tablespoonful. How many full doses are available in a 120-mL bottle? ______ full doses
48. Calculate the total fluid intake in mL of this clear liquid lunch:

apple juice	4 ounces
chicken broth	8 ounces
gelatin dessert	6 ounces
hot tea	10 ounces
TOTAL =	____ mL

49. An ampule contains 10 mg of morphine. The doctor orders *morphine gr $\frac{1}{6}$ intramuscularly every 4 hours as needed for pain.* What percentage of the solution in the ampule should the patient receive?__________

50. Critical Thinking Skill: Describe the strategy you would implement to prevent this medication error.

possible scenario

An attending physician ordered *Claforan 2 g intravenously immediately* for a patient with a leg abscess. The supply dosage available is 1000 mg per 10 mL. The nurse was in a rush to give the medication and calculated the dose this way:

If: 1 g = 1000 mg

then: 2 g = 1000 ÷ 2 = 500 mg or 5 cc

potential outcome

The patient received only $\frac{1}{4}$ or 25% of the dosage ordered. The patient should have received 2000 mg or 20 mL of Claforan. The leg abscess could progress to osteomyelitis (a severe bone infection) because of underdosage.

prevention

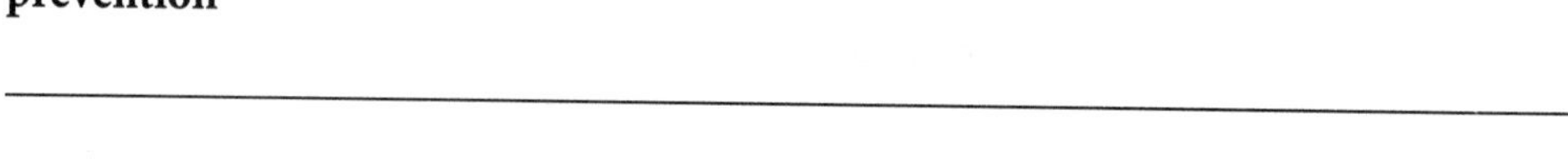

After completing these problems, see page 420 to check your answers.

CHAPTER

5

Conversions for Other Clinical Applications: Time and Temperature

objectives

Upon mastery of Chapter 5, you will be able to:

- Convert between traditional and international time.
- Convert between Celsius and Fahrenheit temperature.

This chapter focuses on two other conversions applied in health care. *Time* is an essential part of the drug order. *Temperature* is an important measurement of health status.

Converting Between Traditional and International Time

It is becoming increasingly popular in health care settings to keep time with a more straightforward system using the *24-hour clock.* In use around the world and in the U.S. military for many years, this system is known as *international time* or *military time.*

Look at the 24-hour clock (Figure 5–1). Each time designation is comprised of a unique four-digit number. Notice there is an inner and outer circle of numbers that identify the hours from 0100 to 2400. The inside numbers correlate to traditional AM time (12:00 midnight to 11:59 AM). AM time represents time periods that are *ante meridian* or "before noon." The outside numbers correlate to traditional PM time (12:00 noon to 11:59 PM); time periods that are *post meridian* or "after noon."

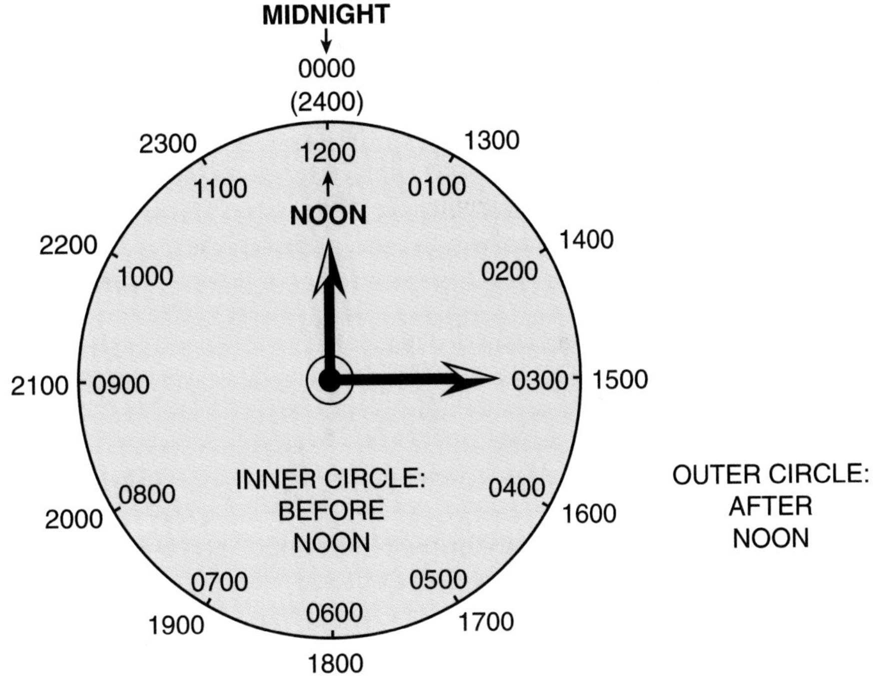

FIGURE 5–1 24-Hour Clock Depicting 0015 (12:15 AM) and 1215 (12:15 PM)

Hours on the 24-hour clock after 0059 minutes ("zero zero fifty-nine") are stated in hundreds. The word *zero* precedes single-digit hours.

Example 1:

0400 is stated as "zero four hundred."

Example 2:

1600 is stated as "sixteen hundred."

Between each hour, the time is read simply as the hour and the number of minutes, preceded by "zero" as needed.

Example 1:

0421 is stated as "zero four twenty-one."

Example 2:

1659 is stated as "sixteen fifty-nine."

The minutes between 2400 (12:00 midnight) and 0100 (1:00 AM) are written as 0001, 0002, 0003 . . . 0058, 0059. Each zero is stated before stating the number of minutes.

Example 1:

0009 is stated as "zero-zero-zero nine."

Example 2:

0014 is stated as "zero-zero fourteen."

Midnight can be written two different ways in international time:

- 2400 and read as "twenty-four hundred," or
- 0000 (used by the military) and read as "zero hundred."

Use of the 24-hour clock decreases the possibility for error in administering medications and documenting time, because no two times are expressed by the same number. There is less chance for misinterpreting time using the 24-hour clock.

Example 1:

13 minutes after 1 AM is written "0113."

Example 2:

13 minutes after 1 PM is written "1313."

The same cannot be said for traditional time. The AM or PM are the only things that differentiate traditional times.

Example 1:

13 minutes after 1 AM is "1:13 AM."

AM	Int'l. Time	PM	Int'l. Time
12:00 midnight	2400	12:00 noon	1200
1:00	0100	1:00	1300
2:00	0200	2:00	1400
3:00	0300	3:00	1500
4:00	0400	4:00	1600
5:00	0500	5:00	1700
6:00	0600	6:00	1800
7:00	0700	7:00	1900
8:00	0800	8:00	2000
9:00	0900	9:00	2100
10:00	1000	10:00	2200
11:00	1100	11:00	2300

FIGURE 5–2 Comparison of Traditional and International Time

Example 2:

13 minutes after 1 PM is "1:13 PM."

Careless notation in a medical order or in patient records can create misinterpretation about when a therapy is due or actually occurred. Figure 5–2 shows the comparison of traditional and international time. Notice that international time is less ambiguous.

rules

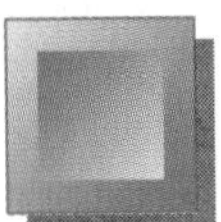

1. Traditional time and international time are the same hours starting with 1:00 AM (0100) through 12:59 PM (1259).
2. Minutes after 12:00 AM (midnight) and before 1:00 AM are 0001 through 0059 in international time.
3. Hours starting with 1:00 PM through 12:00 AM (midnight) are 12:00 hours greater in international time (1300 through 2400).

Let's apply these rules to convert between the two time systems.

Example 1:

3:00 PM = 3:00 + 12:00 = 1500

Example 2:

2212 = 2212 – 1200 = 10:12 PM

Example 3:

12:45 AM = 0045

Example 4:

0004 = 12:04 AM

Example 5:

0130 = 1:30 AM

Example 6:

11:00 AM = 1100

quick review

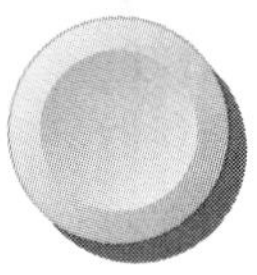

- International time is designated by 0001 through 1259 for 12:01 AM through 12:59 PM, and 1300 through 2400 for 1:00 PM through 12:00 midnight.
- The hours from 1:00 PM through 12:00 midnight are 12:00 hours greater in international time (1300 through 2400).

review set 19

Convert international time to traditional AM/PM time.

1. 0032 = ______
2. 0730 = ______
3. 1640 = ______
4. 2121 = ______
5. 2359 = ______
6. 1215 = ______
7. 0220 = ______
8. 1010 = ______
9. 1315 = ______
10. 1825 = ______

Convert traditional to international time.

11. 1:30 PM = ______
12. 12:04 AM = ______
13. 9:45 PM = ______
14. 12:00 noon = ______
15. 11:15 PM = ______
16. 3:45 AM = ______
17. 12:00 midnight = ______
18. 3:30 PM = ______
19. 6:20 AM = ______
20. 5:45 PM = ______

Fill in the blanks by writing out the words as indicated.

21. 24-hour time 0623 is stated "______."
22. 24-hour time 0041 is stated "______."
23. 24-hour time 1903 is stated "______."
24. 24-hour time 2311 is stated "______."
25. 24-hour time 0300 is stated "______."

After completing these problems, see page 420 to check your answers.

Converting Between Celsius and Fahrenheit Temperature

Another important conversion in health care involves Celsius and Fahrenheit temperatures. Simple formulas are used for converting between the two temperature scales. It is easier to remember the formulas when you understand how they have been developed.

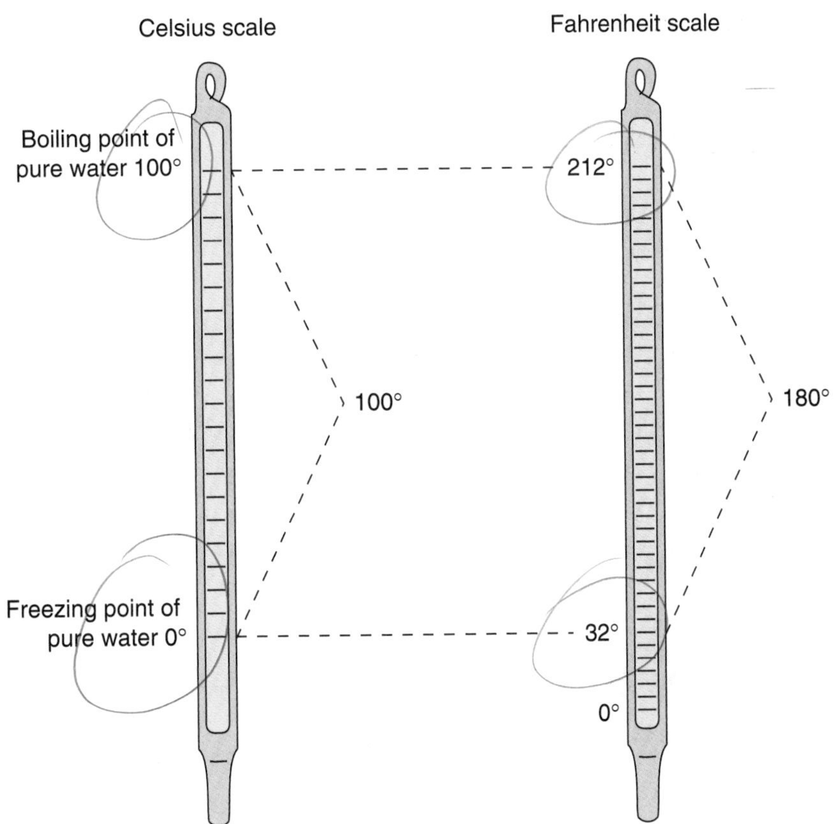

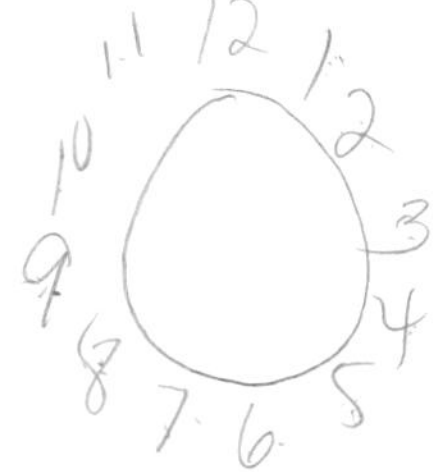

FIGURE 5–3 Comparison of Celsius and Fahrenheit Temperature Scales

The Fahrenheit (F) scale establishes the freezing point of pure water at 32° and the boiling point of pure water at 212°. The Celsius (C) scale establishes freezing point of pure water at 0° and boiling point of pure water at 100°.

Look at Figure 5–3. Note that there is 180° difference between the boiling and freezing points on the Fahrenheit thermometer, and 100° between the boiling and freezing points on the Celsius thermometer. Each Celsius degree is $\frac{180}{100}$ or 1.8 the size of a Fahrenheit degree. Therefore, every one Celsius degree is equivalent to 1.8 Fahrenheit degrees. Taken the other way, each Fahrenheit degree is $\frac{100}{180}$ (or $\frac{5}{9}$) of the size of a Celsius degree.

NOTE: Glass thermometers pictured in Figure 5–3 are for demonstration purposes. Electronic digital temperature devices are more commonly used in health care settings. Most electronic devices can instantly convert between the two scales, freeing the nurse from the actual calculations. However, the nurse's ability to understand the difference between Celsius and Fahrenheit remains important.

To convert between Fahrenheit and Celsius temperature, formulas have been developed based on the differences between the freezing and boiling points on each scale.

rule

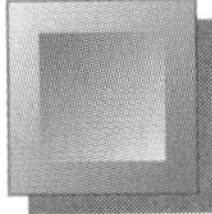

To convert a given Fahrenheit temperature to Celsius, first subtract 32 and then divide the result by 1.8.

$$°C = \frac{°F - 32}{1.8}$$

Example:

Convert 98.6°F to °C

$$°C = \frac{98.6 - 32}{1.8}$$

$$°C = \frac{66.6}{1.8}$$

$$°C = 37°$$

rule

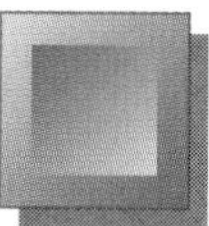

To convert Celsius temperature to Fahrenheit, multiply by 1.8 and add 32.

$$°F = 1.8°C + 32$$

Example:

Convert 35°C to °F

$$°F = 1.8 \times 35 + 32$$

$$°F = 63 + 32$$

$$°F = 95°$$

quick review

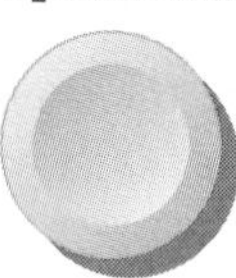

Use these formulas to convert between Fahrenheit and Celsius temperatures:

- $°C = \frac{°F - 32}{1.8}$
- $°F = 1.8\ °C + 32$

review set 20

Convert these temperatures as indicated. Round your answers to tenths.

1. 0°F = ________ °C
2. 85°C = ________ °F
3. 100°C = ________ °F
4. 32°C = ________ °F
5. 72°F = ________ °C
6. 99°F = ________ °C
7. 103.6°F = ________ °C
8. 40°C = ________ °F
9. 80°C = ________ °F
10. 36.4°C = ________ °F
11. 100°F = ________ °C
12. 19°C = ________ °F
13. 4°C = ________ °F
14. 94.2°F = ________ °C
15. 102.8°F = ________ °C

For each of the following statements, substitute the given temperature in °F or °C to its corresponding equivalent in °C or °F.

16. An infant has a body temperature of 95.5°F. 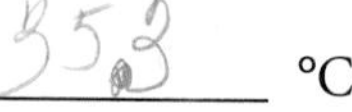 ________ °C

17. Store the vaccine serum at 7°C. ________ °F
18. Do not expose medication to temperatures > 88°F. ________ °C
19. Normal body temperature is 37°C. ________ °F
20. If Mr. Rose's temperature is > 103.5°F, call MD. ________ °C

After completing these problems, see page 420 to check your answers.

critical thinking skills

error

Incorrect interpretation of order due to misunderstanding of traditional time.

possible scenario

A physician ordered a mild sedative for an anxious patient who is scheduled for a colonoscopy in the morning. The order read "*Valium 5 mg orally at 6:00 × 1 dose.*" The evening nurse interpreted that single-dose order to be scheduled for 6 o'clock PM along with the enema to be given to the patient. The doctor meant for the Valium to be given at 6 o'clock AM to help the patient relax prior to the actual test.

potential outcome

Valium certainly would help the patient relax during the enema and make the patient sleepy. But because of the omission of the AM designation, the patient would not benefit from this mild sedative at the intended time, just before the test. The patient would have likely experienced unnecessary anxiety both before and during the test.

prevention

This scenario emphasizes the benefit of the 24-hour clock. If international time had been in use at this facility, the order would have been written as "*Valium 5 mg orally at 0600 × 1 dose*" clearly indicating the exact time of administration. Be careful to verify AM and PM times if your facility uses traditional time.

practice problems—chapter 5

Give the following time equivalents as indicated.

AM/PM Clock	24-Hour Clock	AM/PM Clock	24-Hour Clock
1. ________	0257	11. 7:31 PM	________
2. 3:10 AM	________	12. 12:00 midnight	________
3. 4:22 PM	________	13. 6:45 AM	________
4. ________	2001	14. ________	0915
5. ________	1102	15. ________	2107
6. 12:33 AM	________	16. ________	1823
7. 2:16 AM	________	17. ________	0540
8. ________	1642	18. 11:55 AM	________
9. ________	2356	19. 10:12 PM	________
10. 4:20 AM	________	20. 9:06 PM	________

Find the length of each time interval.

21. 0200 to 0600 ________
22. 1100 to 1800 ________
23. 1500 to 2330 ________
24. 0935 to 2150 ________
25. 0003 to 1453 ________
26. 2316 to 0328 ________
27. 8:22 AM to 1:10 PM ________
28. 4:35 PM to 8:16 PM ________
29. 1:00 AM to 7:30 AM ________
30. 10:05 AM Friday to 2:43 AM Saturday________
31. The 24-hour clock is imprecise and not suited to health care. (True) (False)
32. Indicate whether these international times would be AM or PM when converted to traditional time.
    a. 1030 ________
    b. 1920 ________
    c. 0158 ________
    d. 1230 ________

Give the following temperature equivalents as indicated.

33. 99.6°F ________ °C
34. 36.5°C ________ °F
35. 39.2°C ________ °F
36. 100.2°F ________ °C
37. 98°F ________ °C
38. 37.4°C ________ °F
39. 0°C ________ °F
40. 104°F ________ °C
41. 97.8°F ________ °C
42. 35.4°C ________ °F
43. 103.5°F ________ °C
44. 25°C ________ °F
45. 100°C ________ °F
46. 42°F ________ °C
47. 18°F ________ °C
48. 41°C ________ °F
49. Four temperature readings in °C for Mrs. Baskin are 37.6, 35.5, 38.1, and 37.6. Find her average (or mean) °C temperature and convert it to °F. ________°C, or ________°F
50. The freezing and boiling points of pure water on the Fahrenheit and Celsius temperature scales were used to develop the conversion formulas. (True) (False)

After completing these problems, see page 421 to check your answers.

CHAPTER

6

Equipment Used In Dosage Measurement

objectives

Upon mastery of Chapter 6, you will be able to correctly measure the prescribed dosages that you calculate. To accomplish this, you will also be able to:

- Recognize and select the appropriate equipment for the medication, dosage, and method of administration ordered.
- Read and interpret the calibrations of each utensil presented.

Now that you are familiar with the systems of measurement used in the calculation of dosages, let's take a look at the common measuring utensils. In this chapter you will learn to recognize and read the calibrations of devices used in both oral and parenteral (other than gastrointestinal) administration. The oral utensils include the medicine cup, pediatric oral devices, and calibrated droppers. The parenteral devices include the 3-cc syringe, prefilled syringes, variety of insulin syringes, 0.5 and 1 mL tuberculin syringes, and special safety and intravenous syringes.

Oral Administration

Medicine Cup

Figure 6-1 shows the 30-milliliter or 1-ounce medicine cup that is used to measure most liquids for oral administration. Two views are presented to show all of the scales. Notice that the approximate equivalents of the metric, apothecary, and household systems of measurement are indicated on the cup. The medicine cup can serve as a great study aid to help you learn the volume equivalents of the three systems of measurement. Look at the calibrations for milliliters, teaspoons, tablespoons, ounces, and drams. You can see that 30 milliliters equal 1 ounce, 5 milliliters equal 1 teaspoon, and so forth. For volumes less than 2.5 mL, a smaller, more accurate device should be used (see Figures 6-2, 6-3, and 6-4).

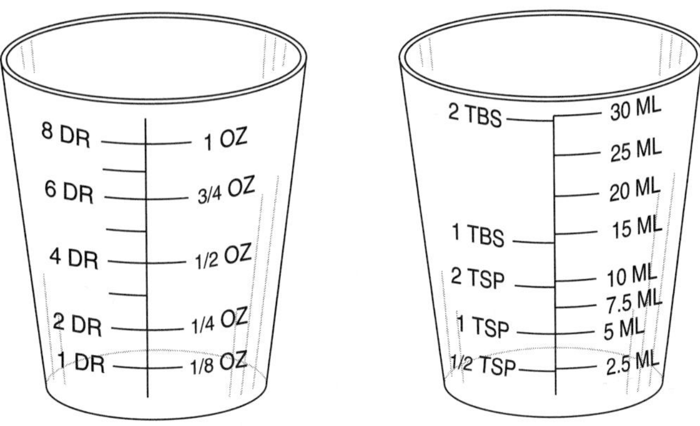

FIGURE 6-1 Medicine Cup with Approximate Equivalent Measures

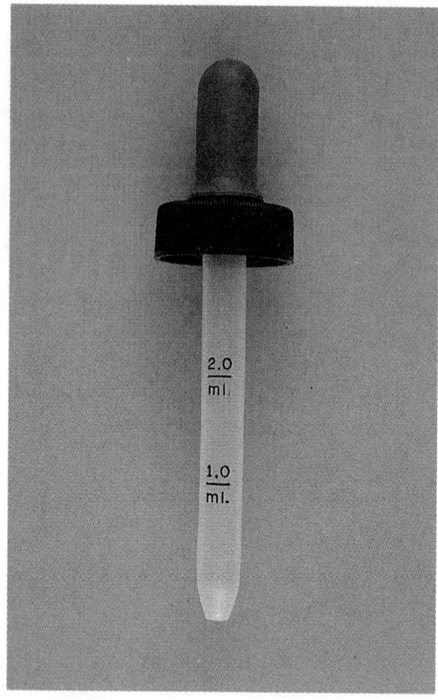

FIGURE 6-2 Calibrated Dropper

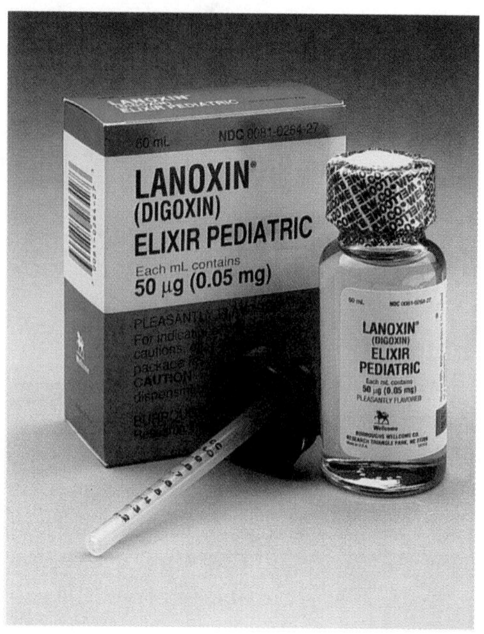

FIGURE 6-3 Digoxin Dropper (Reproduced with permission of Burroughs Wellcome Co.)

Calibrated Dropper

Figure 6-2 shows the calibrated dropper, which is used to administer some small quantities. A dropper is used when giving medicine to children and when adding small amounts of liquid to water or juice. Eye and ear medications are also dispensed from a medicine dropper or squeeze drop bottle.

The amount of the drop varies according to the diameter of the hole at the tip of the dropper. For this reason, a properly calibrated dropper usually accompanies the medicine (Figure 6-3). It is calibrated according to the way that drug is prescribed. The calibrations are usually given in milliliters, cubic centimeters, or drops.

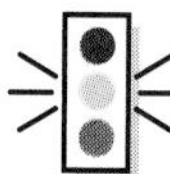

Caution: To be safe, never interchange droppers between medications, because drop size varies from one dropper to another.

Pediatric Oral Devices

Various types of calibrated equipment are available to administer oral medications to children. Several devices intended only for oral use are shown in Figure 6-4. Parents and child care givers should be taught to always use calibrated devices when administering medications to children. Household spoons vary in size and are not reliable for accurate dosing.

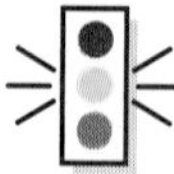

Caution: To be safe, do not use syringes intended for injections in the administration of oral medications. Confusion about the route of administration may occur.

Parenteral Administration

The term *parenteral* is used to designate routes of administration other than gastrointestinal. However, in this text, parenteral always means injection routes.

3-cc Syringe

Figures 6-5(a) and (b) show a 3-cc syringe assembled with needle unit. The parts of the syringe are identified in Figure 6-6. Notice the black rubber tip of the suction plunger is visible.

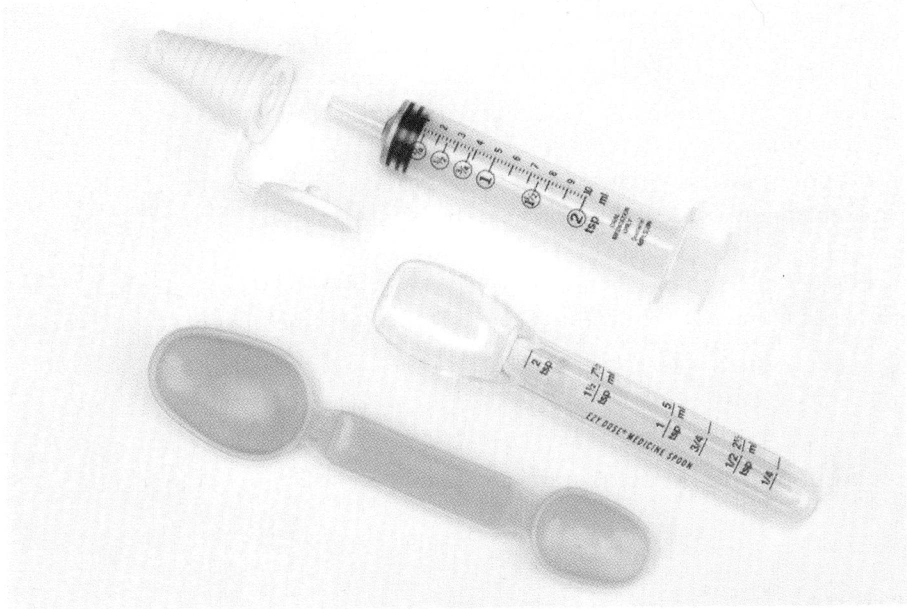

FIGURE 6-4 Devices for Administering Oral Medications to a Child

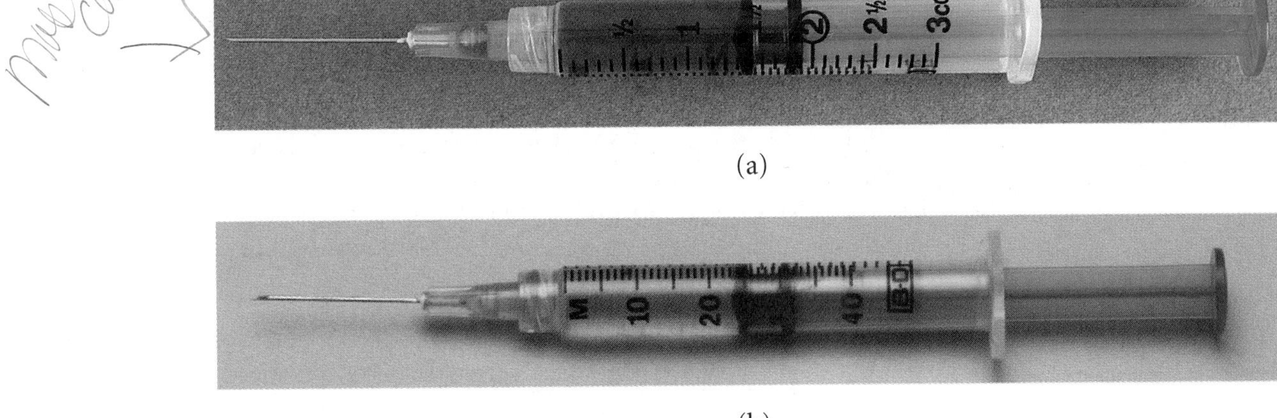

(a)

(b)

FIGURE 6-5 (a) 3-cc Syringe with Needle Unit Measuring 1.5 cc; (b) Reverse Side of 3-cc Syringe with Minim Scale View

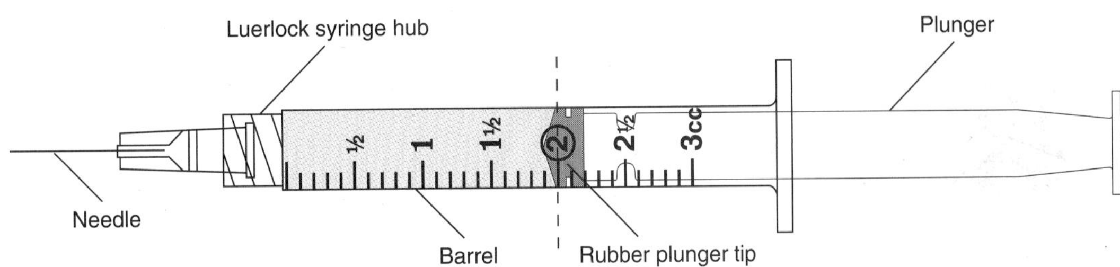

FIGURE 6-6 3-cc Syringe with Needle Unit Measuring 2 cc

The nurse pulls back on the plunger to withdraw the medicine from the storage container. The calibrations are read from the top black ring, NOT the raised middle section and NOT the bottom ring. Look closely at the metric scale in Figure 6-5(a), which is calibrated in cubic centimeters (cc) for each tenth (0.1) of a cubic centimeter. Each $\frac{1}{2}$ cubic centimeter is marked up to the maximum volume of 3 cubic centimeters.

Figure 6-5(b) shows the apothecary scale calibrated in minims. You may disregard this scale, because it has become obsolete. It will not be used for the measurement of dosages.

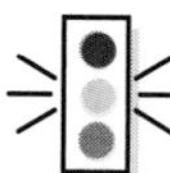

Caution: Take care to distinguish the minim (m) markings from the cubic centimeter (cc) calibrations. Failure to do so can lead to medication errors. Figures 6-5(a) and (b) picture both sides of a 3-cc syringe. Do not use the minim scale to measure parenteral doses. It is shown here only for recognition.

Standard drug dosages of 1 mL or greater are to be rounded to the nearest tenth (0.1) of a mL or cc and measured on the cc scale. Refer to Chapter 1 to review the rules of decimal rounding.

Example:

1.45 cc is rounded to 1.5 cc. Notice that the colored liquid in Figure 6-5(a) identifies 1.5 cc.

Prefilled Syringe

Figure 6-7 is an example of a prefilled, single-dose syringe. Such syringes contain the usual single dose of a medication and are to be used once and discarded.

If you are to give *less than the full single dose* of a drug provided in a prefilled, single-dose syringe, you should discard the extra amount *before* injecting the patient.

Example:

The drug order prescribes 7.5 mg of Valium to be administered to a patient. You have a prefilled, single-dose syringe of Valium containing 10 mg per 2 mL of solution (as in Figure 6-7). You would discard 2.5 mg (0.5 mL) of the drug solution; then, 7.5 mg would be remaining in the syringe. You will learn more about calculating drug dosages beginning in Chapter 9.

Figure 6-8 is an example of the Carpuject brand injection syringe system. The disposable system contains a single-dose cartridge-needle unit. The cartridge-needle unit is to be used only once and discarded. The medication contained in the cartridge is measured and supplied in the usual single dose. However, if the medication order is for *less than the full single dose,* you should discard the extra amount *before* injecting the patient.

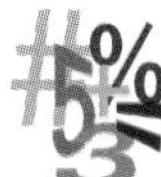

math tip: Most syringes are marked in cubic centimeters (cc), whereas most drugs are prepared and labeled with the strength given per milliliter (mL). Remember that the cubic centimeter and milliliter are equivalent measurements in dosage calculations (1 cc = 1 mL).

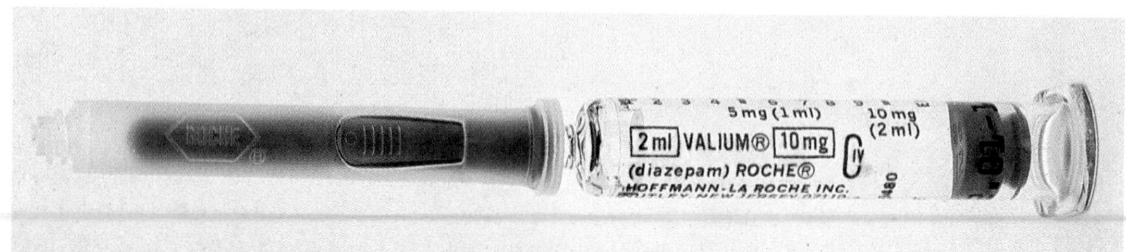

FIGURE 6-7 Prefilled, Single Dose Syringe (Courtesy Roche Laboratories, Inc.)

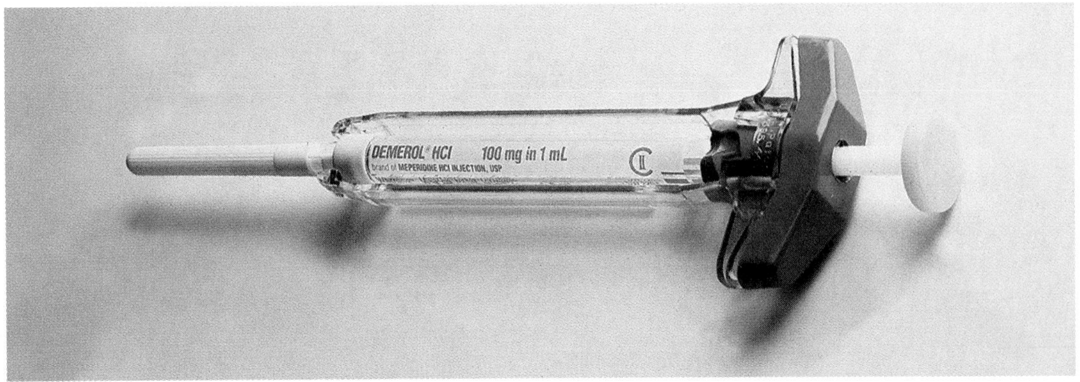

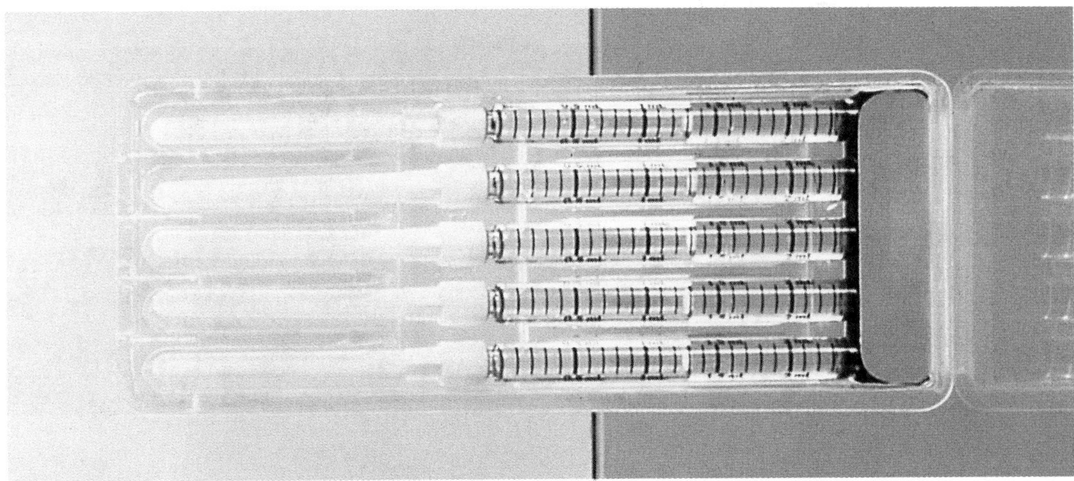

FIGURE 6-8 Carpuject Sterile Cartridge-Needle Unit and a Package of Prefilled Cartridges (Courtesy of Sanofi Winthrop Pharmaceuticals)

Insulin Syringe

Figure 6-9(a), shows *both sides* of a standard U-100 syringe. This syringe is to be used for the measurement and administration of U-100 insulin *only*. It must not be used to measure other medications that are measured in units.

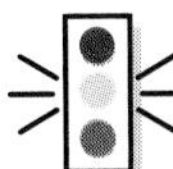

Caution: U-100 insulin should only be measured in a U-100 insulin syringe.

Notice that Figure 6-9(a) pictures one side of the insulin syringe calibrated in odd two-unit increments and the other side calibrated in even two-unit increments. The plunger in Figure 6-10(a) simulates the measurement of 70 units of U-100 insulin. It is important to note that for U-100 insulin, 100 units equal 1 mL.

Figure 6-9(b) shows two U-100 Lo-Dose insulin syringes. The enlarged scale is easier to read and is calibrated for each 1 unit (U) up to 50 units per 0.5 mL or 30 units per 0.3 mL. Every 5 units are labeled. The 30 unit syringe is commonly used for pediatric administration of insulin. The plunger in Figure 6-10(b) simulates the measurement of 19 units of U-100 insulin.

Tuberculin Syringe

Figure 6-11(a) on page 105 shows the 1 mL tuberculin syringe. Figure 6-11(b) shows the 0.5 mL tuberculin syringe. This syringe should be used when a small dose of a drug must be measured, such as an allergen extract, vaccine, or child's medication. Notice that the tuberculin syringe is calibrated in hundredths (0.01) of a milliliter with each one-tenth (0.1) milliliter labeled on the metric scale. The apothecary scale on the reverse side of the syringe (not shown in

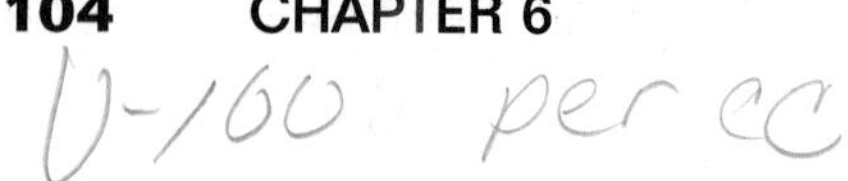

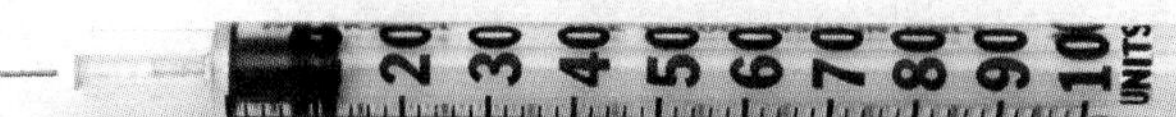

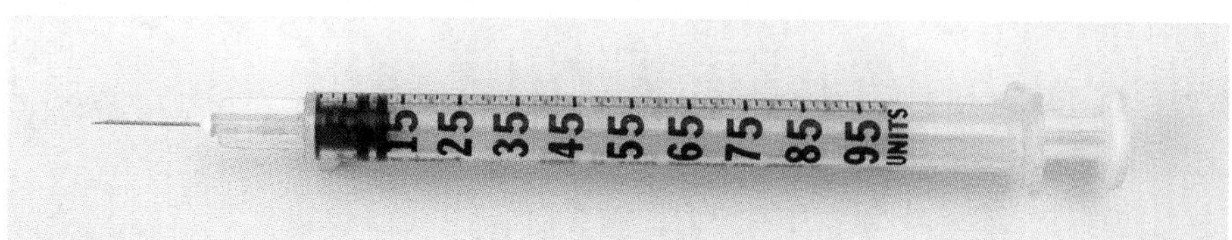

(a)

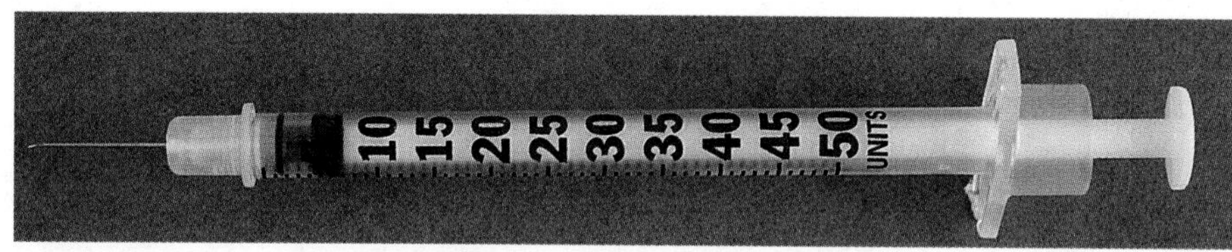

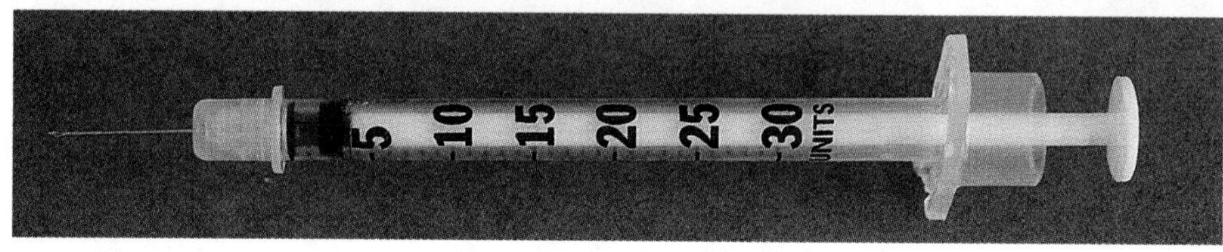

(b)

FIGURE 6-9 (a) Standard U-100 Insulin Syringe; (b) Lo-Dose Insulin Syringes, 50 and 30 Units (Courtesy Becton-Dickinson Consumer Products)

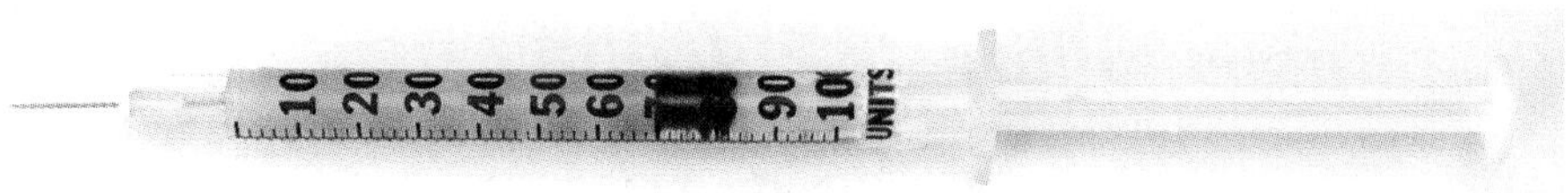

(a)

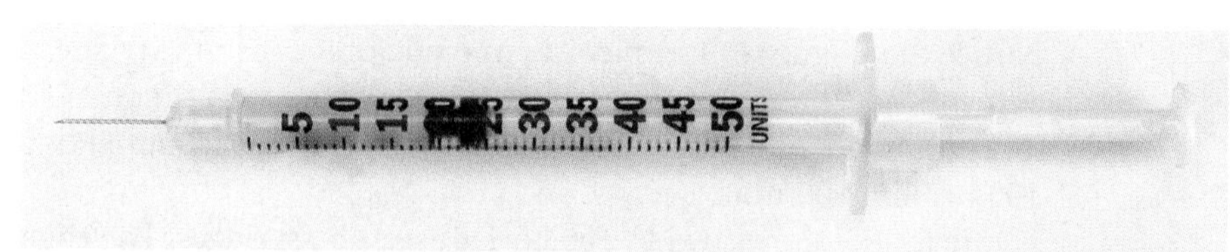

(b)

FIGURE 6-10 (a) Standard U-100 Insulin Syringe Measuring 70 Units of U-100 Insulin; (b) U-100 Lo-Dose Insulin Syringe Measuring 19 Units of U-100 Insulin

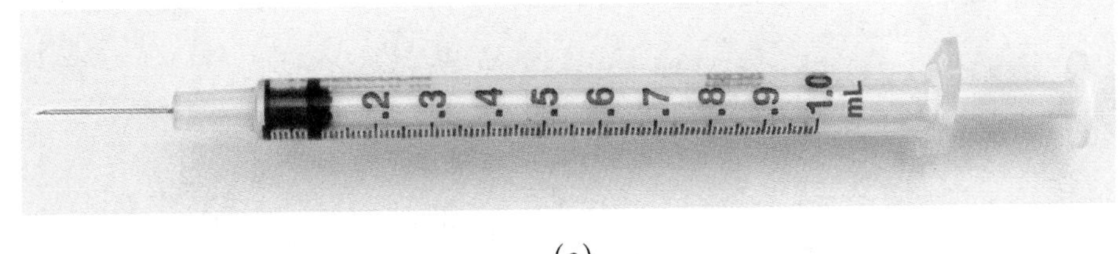

(a)

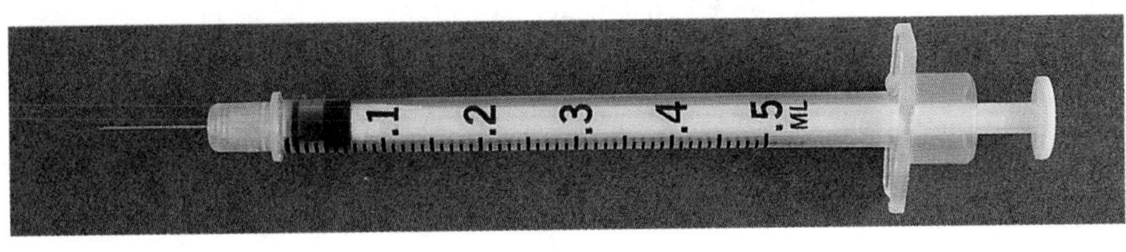

(b)

FIGURE 6-11 (a) 1-mL Tuberculin Syringe; (b) 0.5-mL Tuberculin Syringe (Courtesy Becton Dickinson and Company)

photo), calibrated in minims, is seldom used. It should be disregarded. Amounts of less than 1 mL should be rounded to hundredths and measured in the 0.5 or 1 mL tuberculin syringe.

Example:

The amount 0.766 mL is rounded to 0.77 and measured in the 1 mL tuberculin syringe.

Safety Syringe

Figure 6-12 shows (top to bottom) the safety 3-cc syringe, insulin syringe, and tuberculin syringe. Notice that the needle is protected by a shield to prevent accidental needlestick injury to the nurse while administering an injectable medication.

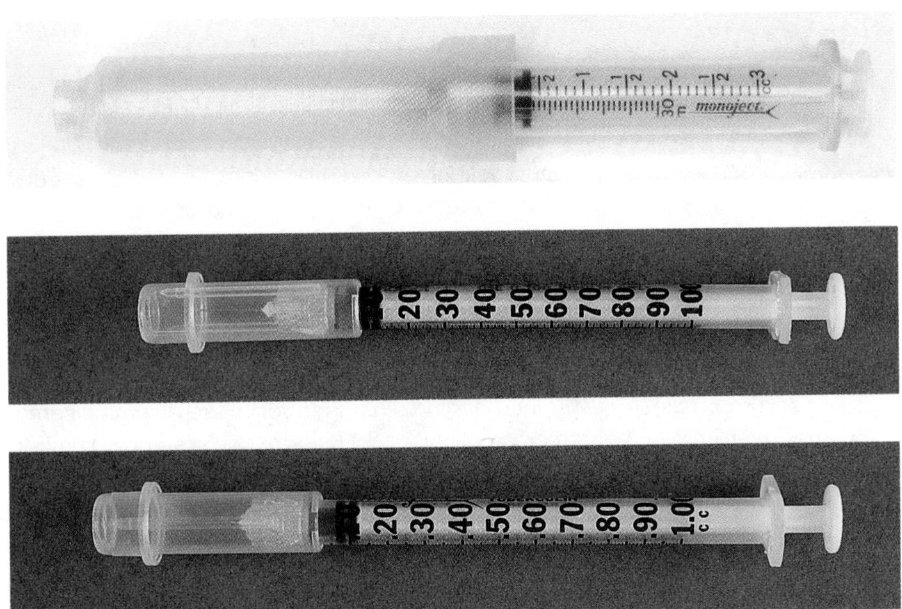

FIGURE 6-12 Safety Syringes

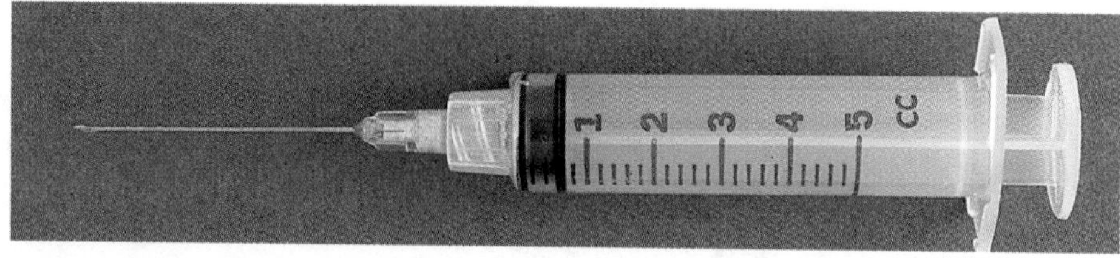

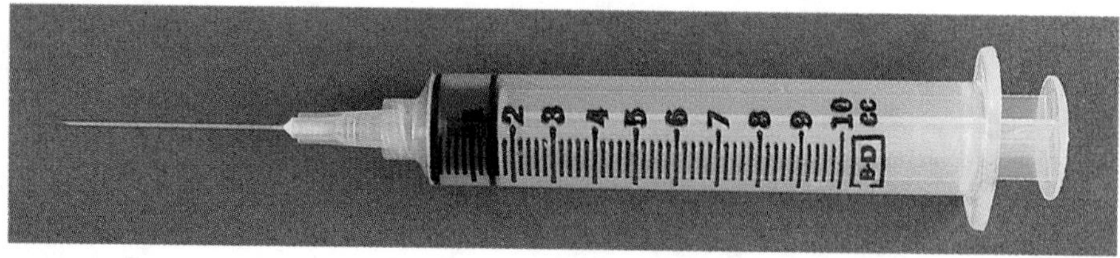

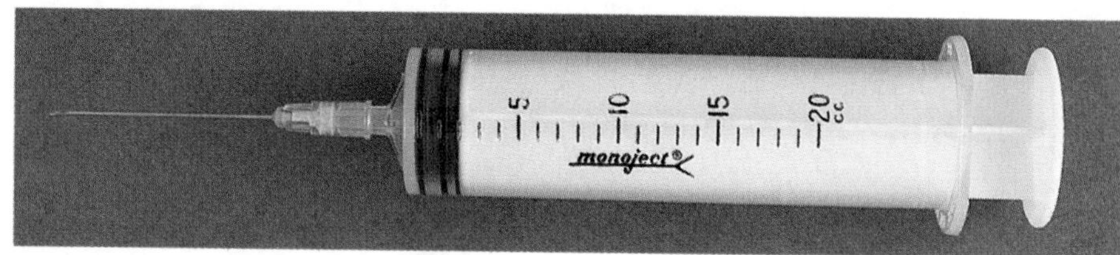

FIGURE 6-13 Intravenous Syringes

Intravenous Syringes

Figure 6-13 shows common large syringes used to prepare medications for intravenous administration. The volume and calibration of these syringes vary. To be safe, examine the calibrations of the syringes, and select the one that is best suited for the volume to be administered.

Needleless Syringes

Figure 6-14 pictures a needleless syringe system designed to prevent accidental needlesticks during intravenous administration.

quick review

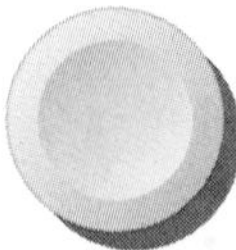

- The medicine cup has a 1-ounce or 30-milliliter capacity for oral liquids. It is also calibrated to measure teaspoons, tablespoons, and drams. Amounts less than 2.5 milliliters should be measured in a smaller device, such as an oral syringe.
- The calibrated dropper measures small amounts of oral liquids. The size of the drop varies according to the diameter of the tip of the dropper.
- The standard 3-cc syringe is used to measure most injectable drugs. It is calibrated in tenths of a cc.
- The prefilled, single-dose syringe is to be used once and discarded.
- The standard U-100 insulin syringe is used to measure U-100 insulin only. It is calibrated for a total of 100 units, or equivalent to 1 mL.
- The Lo-Dose U-100 insulin syringe is used for measuring small amounts of U-100 insulin. It is calibrated for a total of 50 units per 0.5 mL or 30 units per 0.3 mL. The smaller syringe is commonly used for administering insulin to children.
- The 0.5 or 1 mL tuberculin syringe is used to measure small or critical amounts of injectable drugs. It is calibrated in hundredths of a mL.
- Do not use syringes intended for injections when measuring and administering oral medications.

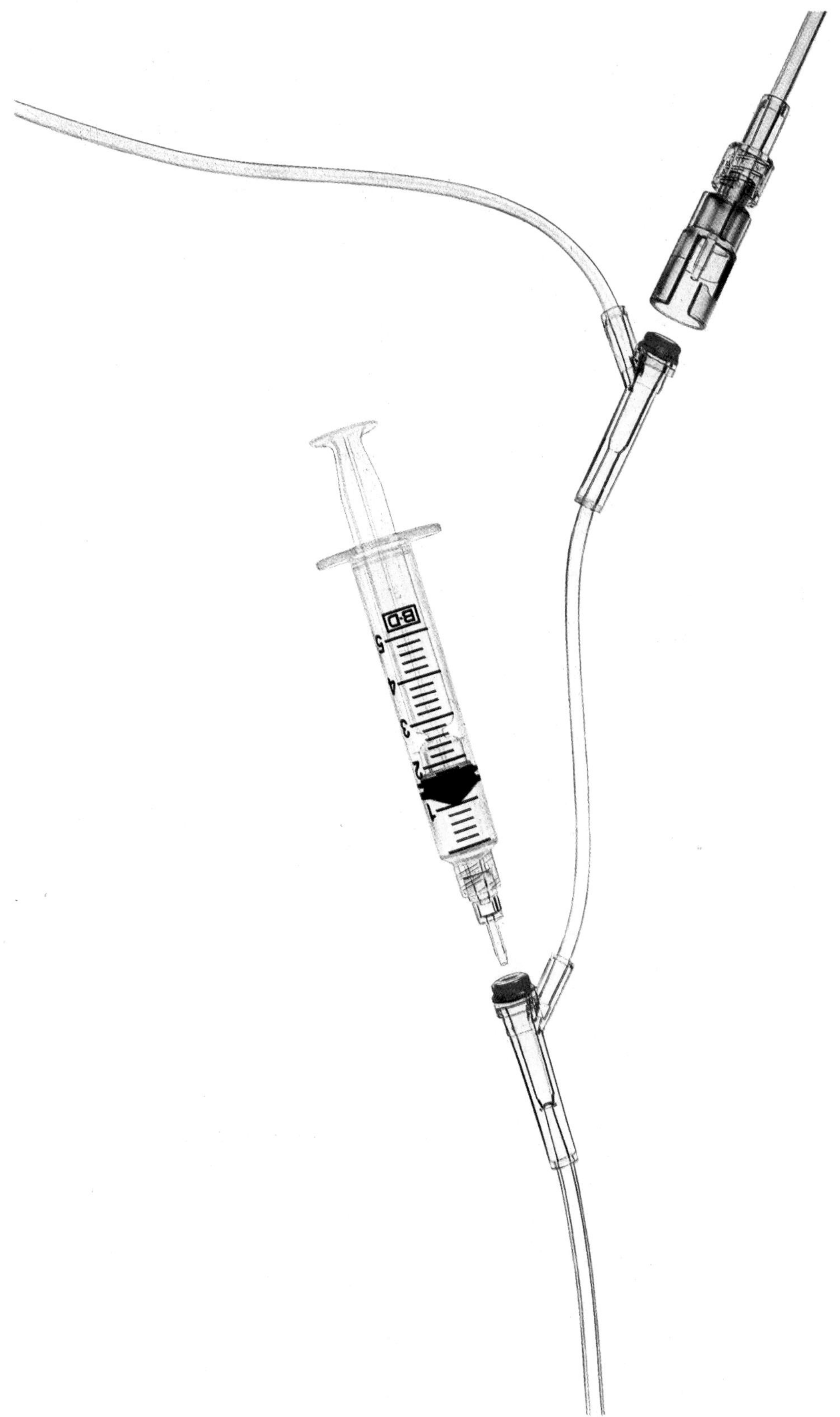

FIGURE 6-14 Needleless Syringe System (Courtesy of Becton Dickinson and Company)

review set 21

1. In which syringe should 0.25 mL of a drug solution be measured? ________
2. a. Can 1.25 mL be measured in the regular 3-cc syringe? ________

   b. How? ________
3. Should insulin be measured in a tuberculin syringe? ________
4. Fifty (50) units of U-100 insulin equals how many cubic centimeters? ________
5. a. The gtt is considered a consistent quantity for comparisons between different droppers. (True) (False)

   b. Why? ________
6. Can you measure 3 mL in a medicine cup? ________
7. How would you measure 3 mL of oral liquid to be administered to a child? ________
8. The medicine cup indicates that each teaspoon is the equivalent of ________ mL.
9. Describe your action if you are to administer less than the full amount of a drug supplied in a prefilled, single-dose syringe. ________
10. What is the primary purpose of the safety and needleless syringes? ________

Note to Learner

The drawings on subsequent pages of the syringes represent actual sizes.

Draw an arrow to point to the calibration that corresponds to the dose to be administered.

11. Administer 0.75 cc

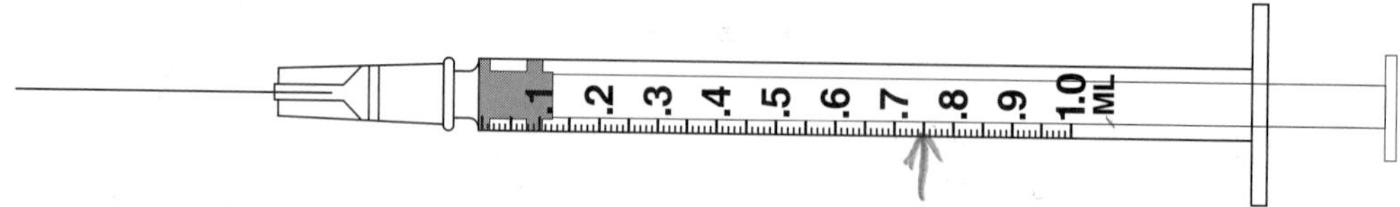

12. Administer 1.33 cc

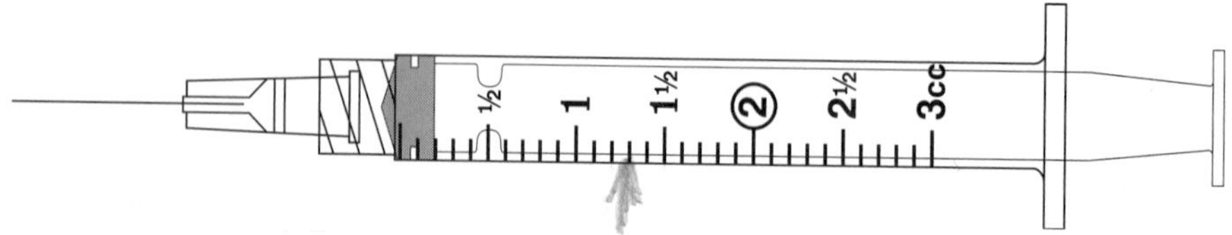

13. Administer 2.2 cc

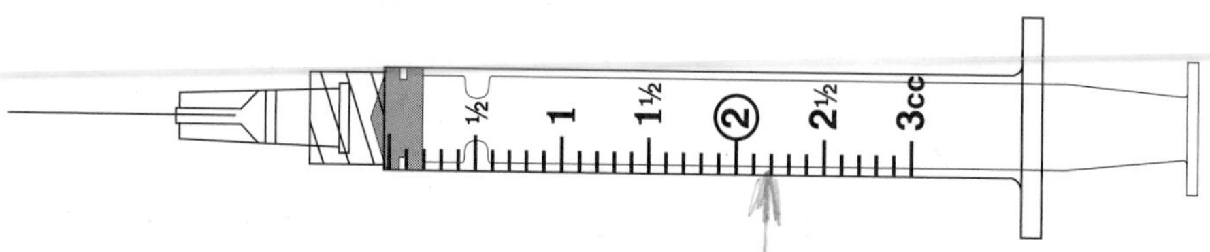

14. Administer 1.3 cc

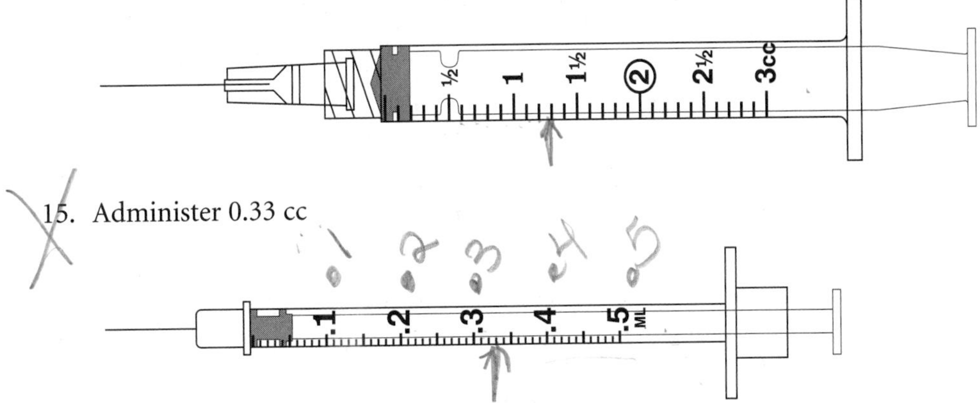

15. Administer 0.33 cc

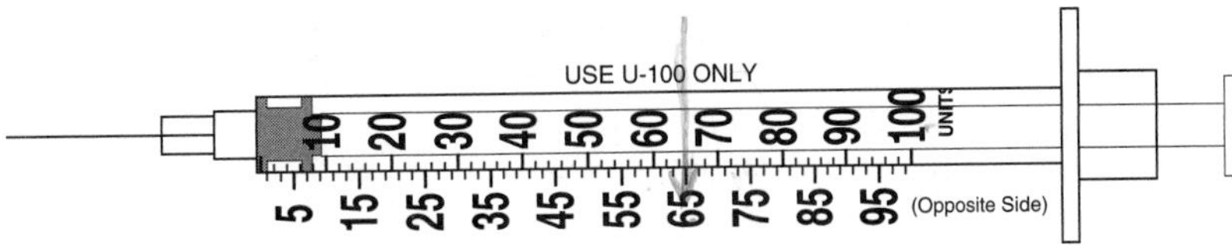

16. Administer 65 U of U-100 insulin

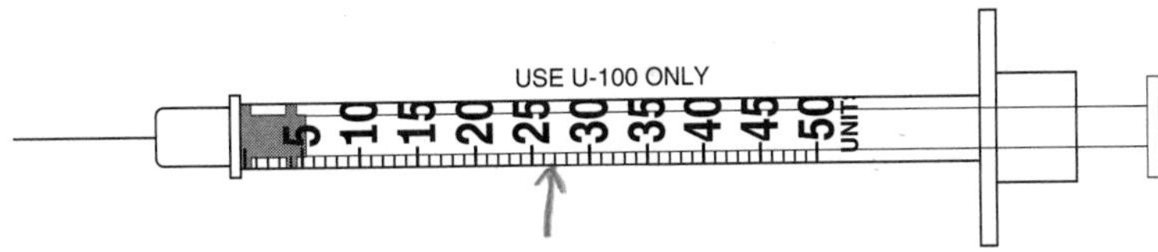

17. Administer 27 U of U-100 insulin

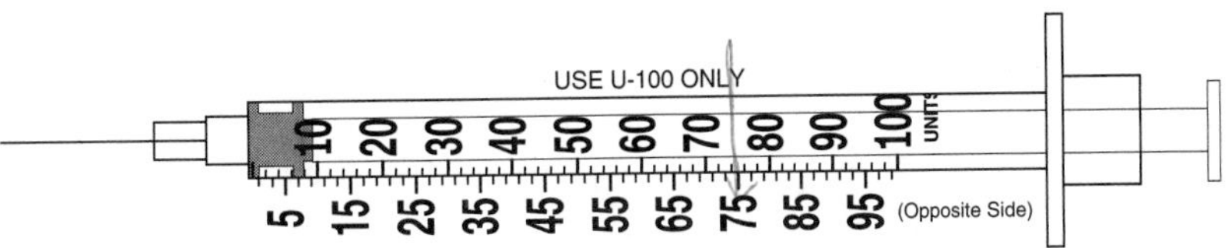

18. Administer 75 U of U-100 insulin

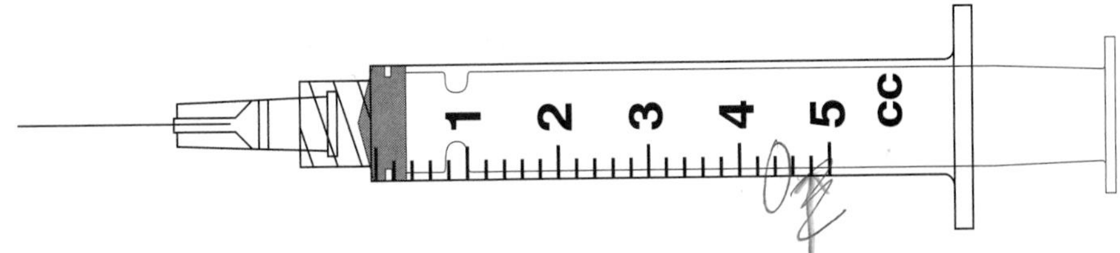

19. Administer 4.4 cc

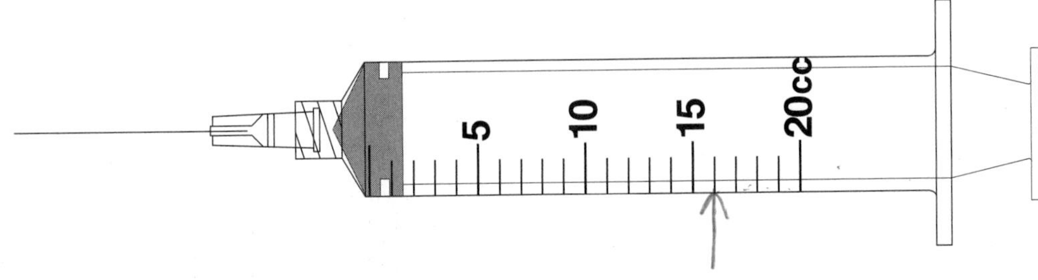

20. Administer 16 cc

After completing these problems, see pages 421 and 422 to check your answers.

critical thinking skills

Select correct equipment to prepare medications. In the following situation the correct dosage was not given because an incorrect measuring device was used.

error

Using an inaccurate measuring device for oral medications.

possible scenario

Suppose a pediatrician ordered Amoxil suspension (250 mg/5 mL), 1 teaspoon, every 8 hours, to be given to a child seen in the pediatric clinic. The child should receive the medication for 10 days for otitis media, an ear infection. The pharmacy dispensed the medication in a bottle containing 150 mL, or a 10-day supply. The nurse did not clarify for the mother how to measure and administer the medication. The child returned to the clinic in ten days for routine follow-up. The nurse asked whether the child had taken all the prescribed Amoxil. The child's mother stated, "No, we have almost half of the bottle left." When the nurse asked how the medication had been given, the mother showed the bright pink plastic teaspoon she obtained from the local ice cream parlor. The nurse measured the spoon's capacity and found it to be less than 3 mL. (Remember, 1 tsp = 5 mL.) The child would have received only $\frac{3}{5}$, or 60%, of the correct dose.

potential outcome

The child would not have been receiving a therapeutic dosage of the medication and was actually underdosed. The child could develop a super infection, which could lead to a more severe illness like meningitis.

prevention

Teach family members (and patients, as appropriate) to use calibrated measuring spoons or specially designed oral syringes to measure the correct dosage of medication. The volumes of serving spoons may vary considerably as in this situation.

practice problems—chapter 6

1. In the U-100 insulin syringe, 100 U = _____ cc.
2. The tuberculin syringe is calibrated in _____ of a cc.
3. Can you measure 1.25 cc in a single tuberculin syringe? _____ Explain._____
4. How would you measure 1.33 mL in a 3-cc syringe? _____
5. The medicine cup has a _____ capacity.
6. To administer exactly 0.52 cc to a child, select a _____ syringe.
7. 75 U of U-100 insulin equals _____ mL.
8. All droppers are calibrated to deliver standardized drops of equal amounts regardless of the dropper used. (True) (False)
9. The prefilled syringe is a multiple-dose system. (True) (False)
10. Insulin should be measured in an insulin syringe *only*. (True) (False)

11. The purpose of needleless syringes is ______________________.

12. Medications are measured in syringes by aligning the calibrations with the __________ of the black rubber tip of the plunger. (top ring, raised middle, or bottom ring)

13. The medicine cup calibrations indicate that 2 teaspoons are approximately __________ milliliters.

14. The __________ scale has become obsolete on syringes and should not be used to measure medications. (milliliter, cubic centimeter, or minim?)

15. The __________ syringe(s) is(are) intended to measure parenteral doses of medications. (standard 3-cc, tuberculin, or insulin?)

Draw an arrow to indicate the calibration that corresponds to the dose to be administered.

16. Administer 0.45 cc

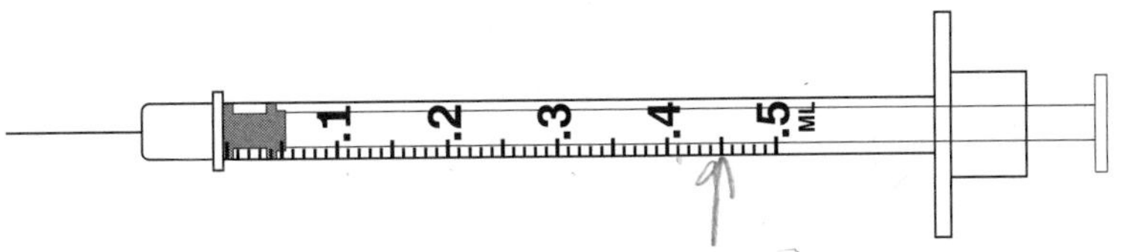

17. Administer 80 U of U-100 insulin

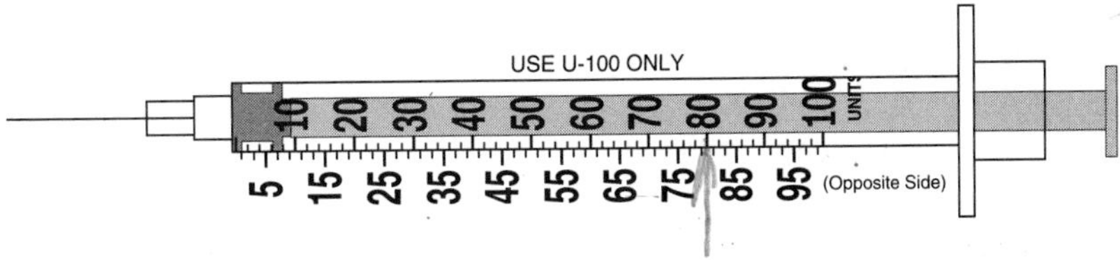

18. Administer ℥ ss

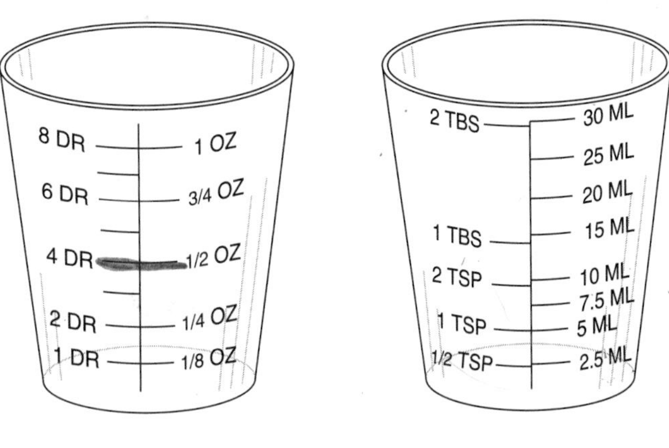

19. Administer 2.4 cc

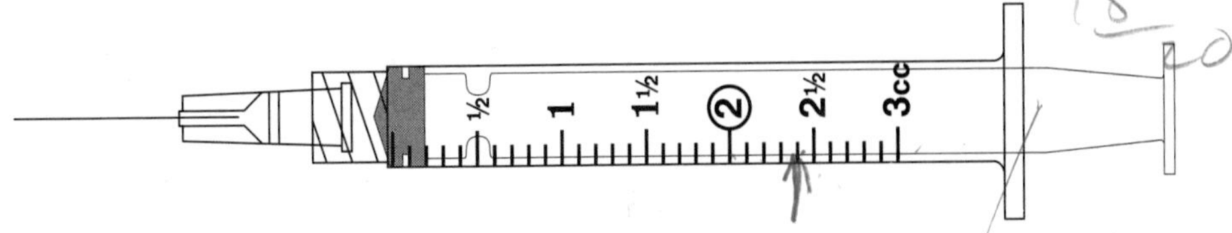

20. Administer 1.1 cc

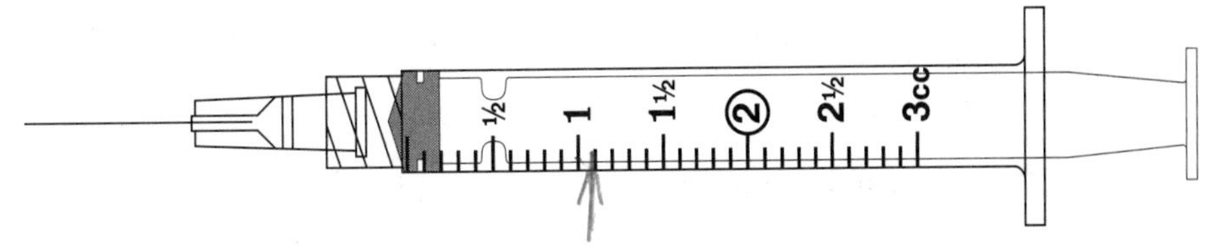

21. Administer 6.2 cc

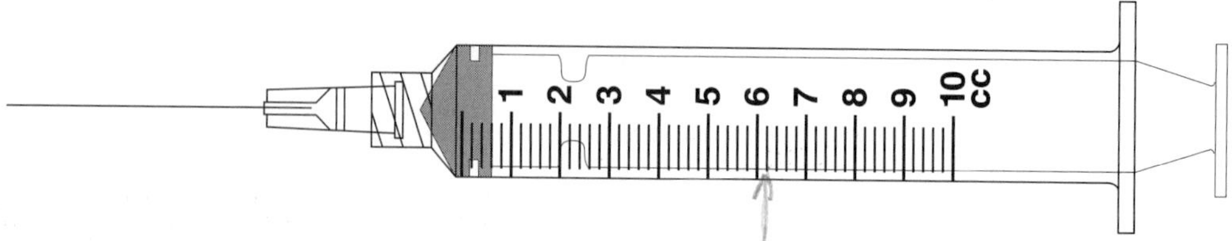

22. Critical Thinking Skill: Describe the strategy that would prevent this medication error.

possible scenario

Suppose a patient with cancer has oral Compazine liquid ordered for nausea. Because the patient has had difficulty taking the medication, the nurse decided to draw up the medication in a syringe without a needle to facilitate giving the medication. The nurse found this to be quite helpful and prepared several doses in syringes without the needle. A nurse from another unit covered for the nurse during lunch, and when the patient complained of nausea, assumed the Compazine prepared in an injection syringe was to be given via injection. The nurse attached a needle and injected the oral medication.

potential outcome

The medication would be absorbed systemically, and the patient could develop an abscess at the site of injection.

prevention

____

____

After completing these problems, see pages 422 and 423 to check your answers.

CHAPTER 7

Interpreting Drug Orders

objectives

Upon mastery of Chapter 7, you will be able to interpret the drug order. To accomplish this you will also be able to:

- Read and write proper medical notation.
- Write the standard medical abbreviation from a list of common terminology.
- Classify the notation that specifies the dosage, route, and frequency of the medication to be administered.
- Interpret physician orders and medication administration records.

The prescription or medication order conveys the therapeutic drug plan for the patient. It is the responsibility of the nurse to:

- interpret the order
- prepare the exact dosage of the prescribed drug
- identify the patient
- administer the proper dosage by the prescribed route, at the prescribed time intervals
- record the administration of the prescribed drug
- monitor the patient's response for desired (therapeutic) or adverse effects

Before you can prepare the proper dosage of the prescribed drug, you must learn to interpret or read the written drug order. For brevity and speed, the health professions have adopted certain standards and common abbreviations for use in notation. You should learn to recognize and interpret the abbreviations from memory. As you practice reading drug orders, you will find that this skill becomes second nature to you.

An example of a typical written drug order is:

9/4/XX Amoxil 500 mg p.o. q.i.d. (p.c. & h.s.)
J. Physician, M.D.

This order means the patient should receive 500 milligrams of an antibiotic named Amoxil (or amoxicillin) orally four times a day (after meals and at bedtime). You can see that the medical notation considerably shortens the written order.

Medical Abbreviations

The following table lists common medical abbreviations used in writing drug orders. The abbreviations are grouped according to those which refer to the route (or method) of administration, the frequency (time interval), and other general terms. Commit these to memory along with the other abbreviations related to systems of measurement presented in Chapter 3.

remember

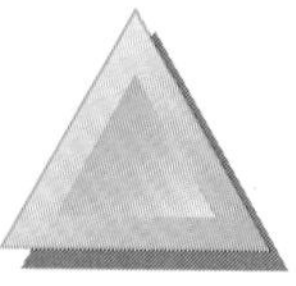

COMMON MEDICAL ABBREVIATIONS

Abbreviation	Interpretation
Route:	
IM	intramuscular
IV	intravenous
IV PB	intravenous piggyback
SC	subcutaneous
SL	sublingual, under the tongue
ID	intradermal
GT	gastrostomy tube
NG	nasogastric tube
NJ	nasojejunal tube
p.o.	by mouth, orally
p.r.	per rectum
O.D.	right eye
O.S.	left eye
O.U.	both eyes
A.D.	right ear
A.S.	left ear
A.U.	both ears
Frequency:	
a.c.	before meals
p.c.	after meals
ad. lib.	as desired, freely
p.r.n.	when necessary
h.s.	hour of sleep, at bed time
stat	immediately, at once
q.d.	once a day, every day
q.o.d.	every other day

Abbreviation	Interpretation
Frequency:	
b.i.d.	twice a day
t.i.d.	three times a day
q.i.d.	four times a day
min	minute
h	hour
q.h	every hour
q.2h	every two hours
q.3h	every three hours
q.4h	every four hours
q.6h	every six hours
q.8h	every eight hours
q.12h	every twelve hours
General:	
$\bar{a}$	before
$\bar{p}$	after
$\bar{c}$	with
$\bar{s}$	without
q	every
aq	water
NPO	nothing by mouth
ss	one-half
gtt	drop
tab	tablet
cap	capsule
et	and
noct	night

The Drug Order

The drug order consists of seven parts:

1. Name of the *patient*
2. Name of the *drug* to be administered
3. *Dosage* of the drug
4. *Route* by which the drug is to be administered
5. *Frequency,* time, and special instructions related to administration

6. *Date and time* when the order was written
7. *Signature* of the person writing the order

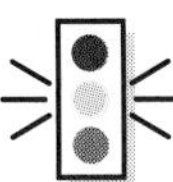

Caution: If any of the seven parts are missing or unclear, the order is considered incomplete and is, therefore, not a legal drug order.

Parts 1 through 5 of the drug order are known as The Five Rights of safe medication administration. They are essential and each one must be faithfully checked every time a medication is prepared and administered.

remember

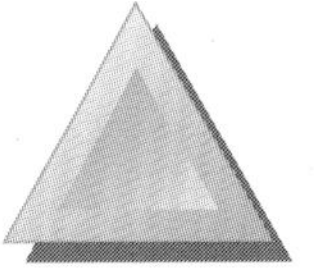

The Five Rights of safe medication administration:

The *right patient* must receive the *right drug* in the *right amount* by the *right route* at the *right time.*

Each drug order should follow a specific sequence. The name of the drug is written first, followed by the dosage, route, and frequency. When correctly written, the brand (or trade) name of the drug begins with a capital or uppercase letter. The generic name begins with a lowercase letter.

Example:

Procan SR 500 mg p.o. q.6h

1. *Procan SR* is the brand name of the drug
2. *500 mg* is the dosage
3. *p.o.* is the route
4. *q.6h* is the frequency

This order means: Give 500 milligrams of Procan SR orally every 6 hours.

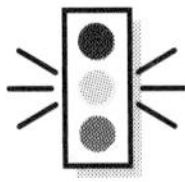

Caution: If the nurse has difficulty understanding and interpreting the drug order, the nurse *must* clarify the order with the writer. Usually this person is the physician or another authorized practitioner, such as an advanced registered nurse practitioner.

Let's practice reading and interpreting drug orders.

Example 1:

Dilantin 100 mg p.o. t.i.d.

Reads: "Give 100 milligrams of Dilantin orally 3 times a day."

Example 2:

procaine penicillin G 400,000 U IM q.6h

Reads: "Give 400,000 units of procaine penicillin G intramuscularly every 6 hours."

Example 3:

Demerol 75 mg IM q.4h p.r.n., pain

Reads: "Give 75 milligrams of Demerol intramuscularly every 4 hours when necessary for pain."

Example 4:

Humulin R U-100 insulin 5 U SC stat

Reads: "Give 5 units of Humulin R U-100 insulin subcutaneously immediately."

Example 5:

Ancef 1 g IV PB q.6h

Reads: "Give one gram of Ancef by intravenous piggyback every 6 hours."

The administration times are designated by hospital policy. For example, t.i.d. administration times may be 0900 or 9 A.M., 1300 or 1 P.M., and 1700 or 5 P.M.

quick review

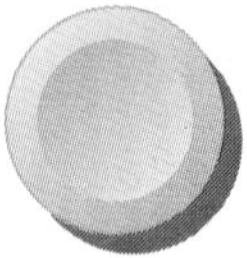

- The *right patient* must receive the *right drug* in the *right amount* by the *right route* at the *right time.*
- Understanding drug orders requires interpreting common medical abbreviations.
- The drug order must contain (in this sequence): drug name, dosage, route, frequency.
- All parts of the drug order must be stated clearly for accurate, exact interpretation.
- If you are ever in doubt as to the meaning of any part of a drug order, ask the writer to clarify before proceeding.

review set 22

Interpret the following medication (drug) orders:

1. *naproxen 250 mg p.o. b.i.d.*
2. *Humulin N NPH U-100 insulin 30 U SC q.d. 30 min ā breakfast*
3. *Ceclor 500 mg p.o. stat, then 250 mg q.8h*
4. *Synthroid 25 mcg p.o. q.d.*
5. *Ativan 10 mg IM q.4h p.r.n., agitation*
6. *furosemide 20 mg IV stat (slowly)*
7. *Gelusil 10 cc p.o. h.s.*

8. atropine sulfate ophthalmic 1% 2 gtt O.D. q. 15 min × 4 ____________________

9. morphine sulfate gr $\frac{1}{4}$ IM q.3–4h p.r.n., pain ____________________

10. Lanoxin 0.25 mg p.o. q.d. ____________________

11. tetracycline 250 mg p.o. q.i.d. ____________________

12. nitroglycerin gr $\frac{1}{400}$ SL stat ____________________

13. Cortisporin otic suspension 2 gtt A.U. t.i.d. et h.s. ____________________

14. Of the preceding medication orders, which are given with the generic name? (Write the numbers of the drug order, e.g., #1, etc.) ____________________

15. Describe your action if no method of administration is written. ____________________

16. Do q.i.d. and q.4h have the same meaning? ________ Explain. ____________________

17. Who determines the medication administration times? ____________________

18. Name the seven parts of a written medication prescription. ____________________

19. Which parts of the written medication prescription/order are included in The Five Rights of medication administration? ____________________

20. State the Five Rights. ____________________

After completing these problems, see pages 423 and 424 to check your answers.

Medication Order and Administration Forms

Hospitals have a special form for recording drug orders. Figure 7-1 shows a sample physician's order form. Find and name each of the seven parts of the drug orders listed. Notice ·· the nurse must verify and initial each order, ensuring that each of the seven parts is ac

ENTERED	FILLED	CHECKED	VERIFIED

NOTE: A NON-PROPRIETARY DRUG OF EQUAL QUALITY MAY BE DISPENSED - IF THIS COLUMN IS NOT CHECKED!

DATE	TIME WRITTEN	PLEASE USE BALL POINT - PRESS FIRMLY	✓	TIME NOTED	NURSES SIGNATURE
11/3/xx	0815	Keflex 250 mg p.o. q.6h	✓	0830	G. Pickar, R.N.
		Humulin N U-100 Insulin 40 U SC ā breakfast	✓		
		Demerol 75 mg IM q. 3–4 h p.r.n. severe pain	✓		
		Codeine 30 mg p.o. q.4h p.r.n. mild–mod pain	✓		
		Tylenol 650 mg p.o. q.4h p.r.n., fever > 101° F	✓		
		Lasix 40 mg p.o. q.d.	✓		
		Slow-K 8 mEq p.o. b.i.d.	✓		
		J. Physician, M.D.			
11/3/xx	2200	Lasix 80 mg IV stat			
		J. Physician, M.D.	✓	2210	M. Smith, R.N.

AUTO STOP ORDERS: UNLESS REORDERED, FOLLOWING WILL BE D/C'D AT 0800 ON:

DATE	ORDER		
		☐ CONT ☐ D/C	PHYSICIAN SIGNATURE
		☐ CONT ☐ D/C	PHYSICIAN SIGNATURE
		☐ CONT ☐ D/C	PHYSICIAN SIGNATURE

CHECK WHEN ANTIBIOTICS ORDERED ☐ Prophylactic ☐ Empiric ☐ Therapeutic

Allergies: None Known

PATIENT DIAGNOSIS: Diabetes

HEIGHT 5'5" WEIGHT 130 lb.

Patient, Mary Q.
#3-11316-7

FORM 069-708 (8-xx) PHYSICIANS ORDER Reynolds + Reynolds LITHO IN U.S.A. K41814 (7-xx) D038060 (1)

FIGURE 7-1 Physician's Order

The drug orders from the physician's order form are transcribed to a medication administration record, Figure 7-2. The nurse uses this record as a guide to:

- check the drug order,
- prepare the correct dosage, and
- record the drug administered.

These three check points help to ensure accurate medication administration.

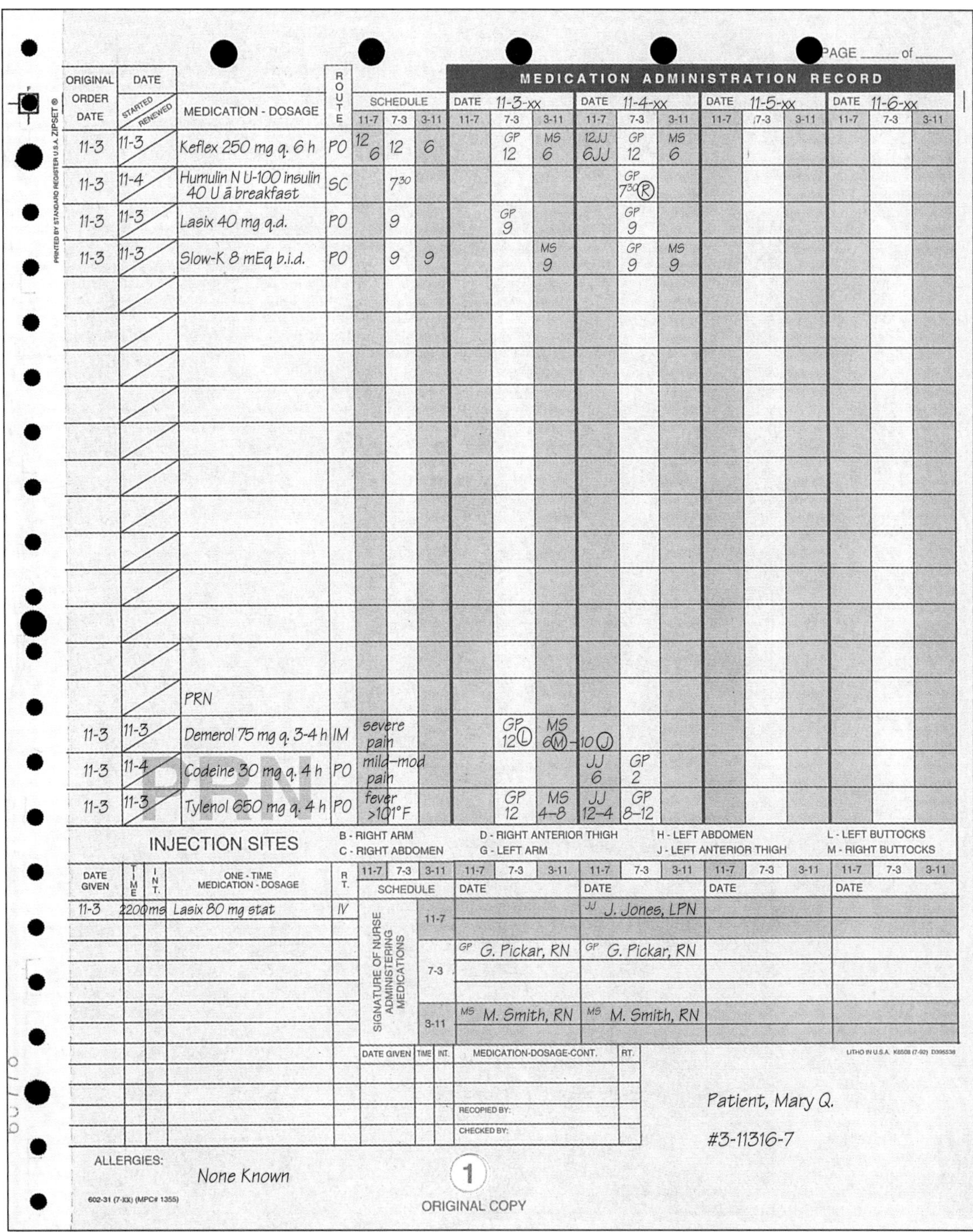

PAGE ____ of ____

MEDICATION ADMINISTRATION RECORD

ORIGINAL ORDER DATE	DATE STARTED / RENEWED	MEDICATION - DOSAGE	ROUTE	SCHEDULE 11-7	7-3	3-11	DATE 11-3-xx 11-7	7-3	3-11	DATE 11-4-xx 11-7	7-3	3-11	DATE 11-5-xx 11-7	7-3	3-11	DATE 11-6-xx 11-7	7-3	3-11
11-3	11-3	Keflex 250 mg q. 6 h	PO	12 6	12	6		GP 12	MS 6	12JJ 6JJ	GP 12	MS 6						
11-3	11-4	Humulin N U-100 insulin 40 U ā breakfast	SC		7^30						GP 7^30 Ⓡ							
11-3	11-3	Lasix 40 mg q.d.	PO		9			GP 9			GP 9							
11-3	11-3	Slow-K 8 mEq b.i.d.	PO		9	9			MS 9		GP 9	MS 9						
		PRN																
11-3	11-3	Demerol 75 mg q. 3-4 h	IM	severe pain				GP 12Ⓛ	MS 6Ⓜ	10Ⓙ								
11-3	11-4	Codeine 30 mg q. 4 h	PO	mild-mod pain						JJ 6	GP 2							
11-3	11-3	Tylenol 650 mg q. 4 h	PO	fever >101°F				GP 12	MS 4-8	JJ 12-4	GP 8-12							

INJECTION SITES: B - RIGHT ARM; C - RIGHT ABDOMEN; D - RIGHT ANTERIOR THIGH; G - LEFT ARM; H - LEFT ABDOMEN; J - LEFT ANTERIOR THIGH; L - LEFT BUTTOCKS; M - RIGHT BUTTOCKS

DATE GIVEN	TIME	INT.	ONE - TIME MEDICATION - DOSAGE	RT.
11-3	2200	ms	Lasix 80 mg stat	IV

SIGNATURE OF NURSE ADMINISTERING MEDICATIONS

SCHEDULE	DATE 11-3	DATE 11-4	DATE	DATE
11-7		JJ J. Jones, LPN		
7-3	GP G. Pickar, RN	GP G. Pickar, RN		
3-11	MS M. Smith, RN	MS M. Smith, RN		

DATE GIVEN | TIME | INT. | MEDICATION-DOSAGE-CONT. | RT.

RECOPIED BY:

CHECKED BY:

Patient, Mary Q.

#3-11316-7

ALLERGIES: None Known

① ORIGINAL COPY

FIGURE 7-2 Medication Administration Record

Computerized Medication Administration Systems

Many health care facilities now use computers for processing drug orders. Drug orders are either electronically transmitted or manually entered into the computer from an order form, such as Figure 7-3. Through the computer, the nurse can transmit the order within seconds to the pharmacy for filling the order. The computer can keep track of drug stock and usage patterns and even notify the business office to post charges to the patient's account. Most importantly, it can scan for information previously entered, such as drug incompatibilities, drug allergies, safe dosage ranges, doses already given, or recommended administration times. The health care

ENTERED	FILLED	CHECKED	VERIFIED

NOTE: A NON-PROPRIETARY DRUG OF EQUAL QUALITY MAY BE DISPENSED - IF THIS COLUMN IS NOT CHECKED!

DATE	TIME WRITTEN	PLEASE USE BALL POINT - PRESS FIRMLY	✓	TIME NOTED	NURSES SIGNATURE
8/31/XX	1500	Procan SR 500 mg p.o. q 6 h	✓		
		J. Physician, M.D.		1515	MS
9/3/XX	0830	Digoxin 0.125 mg p.o. q.o.d.	✓		
		Lasix 40 mg p.o. q.d	✓		
		Reglan 10 mg p.o. stat & a.c. & h.s.	✓		
		K-Lyte 25 mEq p.o. b.i.d.-start 9/4/XX	✓		
		Nitroglycerin gr 1/150 SL p.r.n. chest pain	✓	0845	GF
		Darvocet-N 100 tab. 1 p.o. q. 4-6 h p.r.n. mild-moderate pain	✓		
		Demerol 50 mg IM q. 4 h c̄ } p.r.n. severe pain	✓		
		Phenergan 50 mg IM q. 4h } p.r.n. severe pain	✓		
		J. Physician, M.D.			

AUTO STOP ORDERS: UNLESS REORDERED, FOLLOWING WILL BE D/C^D AT 0800 ON:

DATE	ORDER		
		☐ CONT ☐ D/C	PHYSICIAN SIGNATURE
		☐ CONT ☐ D/C	PHYSICIAN SIGNATURE
		☐ CONT ☐ D/C	PHYSICIAN SIGNATURE

CHECK WHEN ANTIBIOTICS ORDERED ☐ Prophylactic ☐ Empiric ☐ Therapeutic

Allergies: No Known allergies

PATIENT DIAGNOSIS

Patient, John D.
#3-81512-3

HEIGHT WEIGHT

FORM 959-708 (8-XX) PHYSICIANS ORDER Reynolds + Reynolds LITHO IN U.S.A. K41814 (7-XX) D339360

1

FIGURE 7-3 Physician's Order

staff can be readily alerted to potential problems or inconsistencies. The corresponding medication administration record may also be printed directly from the computer, Figure 7-4.

The computerized medication administration record may be viewed at the computer or from a printed copy, Figure 7-4. The nurse may be able to look back at the patient's cumulative medication administration record, document administration times and comments at the computer terminal, and then keep a printed copy of the information obtained and entered. The data

PHARMACY MAR

START	STOP	MEDICATION	SCHEDULED TIMES	OK'D BY	0001 HRS. TO 1200 HRS.	1201 HRS. TO 2400 HRS.
08/31/xx 1800 SCH		PROCAN SR 500 MG TAB-SR 500 MG Q6H PO	0600 1200 1800 2400	JD	0600GP 1200 GP	1800 MS 2400 JD
09/03/xx 0900 SCH		DIGOXIN (LANOXIN) 0.125 MG TAB 1 TAB QOD PO ODD DAYS-SEPT	0900	JD	0900 GP	
09/03/xx 0900 SCH		FUROSEMIDE (LASIX) 40 MG TAB 1 TAB QD PO	0900	JD	0900 GP	
09/03/xx 0845 SCH		REGLAN 10 MG TAB 10 MG AC&HS PO GIVE ONE NOW!!	0730 1130 1630 2100	JD	0730 GP 1130 GP	1630 MS 2100 MS
09/04/xx 0900 SCH		K-LYTE 25 MEQ EFFERVESCENT TAB 1 EFF. TAB BID PO DISSOLVE AS DIR START 9-4	0900 1700	JD	0900 GP	1700 GP
09/03/xx 1507 PRN		NITROGLYCERIN 1/50 GR 0.4 MG TAB-SL 1 TABLET PRN* SL PRN CHEST PAIN		JD		
09/03/xx 1700 PRN		DARVOCET-N 100* 1 TAB Q4-6H PO PRN MILD–MODERATE PAIN		JD		
09/03/xx 2100 PRN		MEPERIDINE* (DEMEROL) INJ 50 MG Q4H IM PRN SEVERE PAIN W PHENERGAN		JD		2200 Ⓗ MS
09/03/xx 2100 PRN		PROMETHAZINE (PHENERGAN) INJ 50 MG Q4H IM PRN SEVERE PAIN W DEMEROL		JD		2200 Ⓗ MS

Gluteus	Thigh
A. Right	H. Right
B. Left	I. Left
Ventro Gluteal	
C. Right	J. Right
D. Left	K. Left
E. Abdomen 1 | 2 / 3 | 4	

730-13 (12/xx)

	NURSE'S SIGNATURE	INITIAL
7–3	G. Pickar, R.N.	GP
3–11	M. Smith, R.N.	MS
11–7	J. Doe, R.N.	JD

ALLERGIES: NKA

DIAGNOSIS: CHF

Patient: Patient, John D.
Patient # 3-81512-3
Admitted: 08/31/xx
Physician: J. Physician, MD
Room: PCU-14 PCU

FIGURE 7-4 Computerized Medication Administration Record

analysis, storage, and retrieval abilities of computers are making them essential tools for safe and accurate medication administration.

quick review

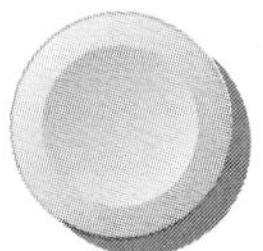

- Drug orders are prescribed on the Physician's Order form.
- The person who administers a drug records it on the Medication Administration Record (MAR). This record may be manual or computerized.
- All parts of the drug order must be stated clearly for accurate, exact interpretation. If you are ever in doubt as to the meaning of any part of a drug order, ask the writer to clarify.

review set 23

Refer to the Computerized Pharmacy MAR (Figure 7-4) on page 121 to answer items 1 through 10.

Convert the scheduled international time to traditional A.M./P.M. time.

1. Scheduled times for administering Procan SR. ______
2. Scheduled times for administering Lanoxin and Lasix. ______
3. Scheduled times for administering Reglan. ______
4. Scheduled times for administering K-Lyte. ______
5. How often can the Demerol be given? ______
6. If the Lanoxin was last given on 9/5/xx at 0900, when is the next time and date it will be given? ______
7. What is the ordered route of administration for the nitroglycerin? ______
8. How many times a day is furosemide ordered? ______
9. The equivalent dosage of Lanoxin is ______ mcg.
10. Which drugs are ordered to be administered "as necessary?" ______

Refer to the Medication Administration Record (Figure 7-2) on page 119 to answer items 11 through 20.

11. What is the route of administration for the insulin? ______
12. How many times in a 24-hour period will Lasix be administered? ______
13. What is the only medication ordered to be given routinely at noon? ______
14. What time of day is the insulin to be administered? ______
15. A dosage of 8 mEq of Slow-K is ordered. What does mEq mean? ______
16. You work 3 to 11 P.M. on November 5. Which routine medications will you administer to Mary Q. Patient during your shift? ______
17. Mary Q. Patient has a fever of 101.4°F. What medication should you administer? ______
18. How many times in a 24-hour period will Slow-K be administered? ______
19. What is the equivalent of the scheduled administration time(s) for the Slow-K as converted to international time? ______
20. What is the equivalent of the scheduled administration time(s) for the Keflex as converted to international time? ______
21. Identify the place on the MAR where the stat IV Lasix was charted. ______

After completing these problems, see page 424 to check your answers.

critical thinking skills

It is the responsibility of the nurse to clarify any drug order that is incomplete; that is, an order that does not contain the essential seven parts discussed in this chapter. Let's look at an example in which this error occurred.

error

Failing to clarify incomplete orders.

possible scenario

Suppose a physician ordered *Pepcid tablet p.o. h.s.* for a patient with an active duodenal ulcer. You will note there is no dosage listed.

The nurse thought the dosage came in only one strength, added 20 mg to the order, and sent it to the pharmacy. The pharmacist prepared the dosage written on the physician's order sheet. Two days later, during rounds, the physician noted that the patient had not responded well to the Pepcid. When asked about the Pepcid, the nurse explained that the patient had received 20 mg at bedtime. The physician informed the nurse that the patient should have received the 40-mg tablet.

potential outcome

Potentially, the delay in correct dose could result in gastrointestinal bleeding or delayed healing of the ulcer.

prevention

This medication error could have been avoided simply by the physician writing the strength of the medication. When this was omitted, the nurse should have checked the dosage before sending the order to the pharmacy. When you fill in an incomplete order, you are essentially practicing medicine without a license, which is illegal and potentially dangerous.

practice problems—chapter 7

Interpret the following abbreviations and symbols without consulting another source.

1. ℥ ______
2. p.r. ______
3. a.c. ______
4. $\bar{p}$ ______
5. t.i.d. ______
6. q.4h ______
7. p.r.n. ______
8. p.o. ______
9. q.d. ______
10. O.D. ______
11. stat ______
12. ad.lib. ______
13. h.s. ______
14. IM ______
15. $\bar{s}$ ______

Give the abbreviation or symbol for the following terms without consulting another source.

16. one-half ______
17. drop ______
18. milliliter ______
19. grain ______
20. gram ______
21. four times a day ______
22. both eyes ______
23. subcutaneous ______
24. teaspoon ______
25. twice daily ______
26. every 3 hours ______
27. after meals ______
28. before ______
29. kilogram ______

Interpret the following physician's drug orders without consulting another source.

30. *Toradol 60 mg IM stat et q.6h* ____________________
31. *procaine penicillin G 300,000 U IM q.i.d.* ____________________
32. *Mylanta 5 mL p.o. 1 h a.c., 1 h p.c., h.s., et q.2h p.r.n. @ noct* ____________________
33. *Librium 25 mg p.o. q.6h p.r.n., agitation* ____________________
34. *heparin 5,000 U SC stat* ____________________
35. *Demerol 50 mg IM q.3–4h p.r.n., pain* ____________________

PAGE 1 of 1

MEDICATION ADMINISTRATION RECORD

ORIGINAL ORDER DATE	DATE STARTED / RENEWED	MEDICATION - DOSAGE	ROUTE	SCHEDULE 11-7	SCHEDULE 7-3	SCHEDULE 3-11	DATE 11-3-xx 11-7	7-3	3-11	DATE 11-4-xx 11-7	7-3	3-11	DATE 11-5-xx 11-7	7-3	3-11	DATE 11-6-xx 11-7	7-3	3-11
11-3	11-3	Heparin lock Central line flush (10U/cc solution) 2cc	IV bid		1000	2200												
11-3	11-3	Isosorbide SR 40 mg q.8h	PO	2400	0800	1600												
11-3	11-3	Cipro 500 mg. q. 12h	PO		1000	2200												
11-3	11-3	Humulin N U-100insulin 15U q. am	SC	0700														
11-3	11-3	Humulin R U-100 insulin 30 min. ac and hs	SC		0730 1130	1730 2200												
		per sliding scale: Blood glucose																
		0-150 3U 151-250 8U																
		251-350 13U 351-400 18U																
		>400 call Dr.																
		PRN																
11-3	11-3	Tylenol tabs 2 q.3-4 h prn headache	PO															

PRN

INJECTION SITES: B - RIGHT ARM; C - RIGHT ABDOMEN; D - RIGHT ANTERIOR THIGH; G - LEFT ARM; H - LEFT ABDOMEN; J - LEFT ANTERIOR THIGH; L - LEFT BUTTOCKS; M - RIGHT BUTTOCKS

DATE GIVEN	TIME	INT.	ONE - TIME MEDICATION - DOSAGE	RT.

SCHEDULE 11-7, 7-3, 3-11 — DATE — SIGNATURE OF NURSE ADMINISTERING MEDICATIONS (11-7 / 7-3 / 3-11)

DATE GIVEN	TIME	INT.	MEDICATION-DOSAGE-CONT.	RT.

RECOPIED BY:

CHECKED BY:

Patient, Pat H.
#6-33725-4

ALLERGIES: None Known

602-31 (7-XX) (MPC# 1355)

PRINTED BY STANDARD REGISTER U.S.A. ZIPSET ®

LITHO IN U.S.A. K6508 (7-92) D39S536

1 ORIGINAL COPY

FIGURE 7-5 Medication Administration Record for Chapter 7 Practice Problems (Questions 40–44)

36. *digoxin 0.25 mg p.o. q.d.* __________

37. *Neo-Synephrine ophthalmic 10% 2 gtt O.S. q. 30 min × 2* __________

38. *Lasix 40 mg IM stat* __________

39. *Decadron 4 mg IV b.i.d.* __________

Refer to the Medication Administration Record (Figure 7-5) to answer items 40 through 44.

40. Convert the scheduled times for Isosorbide SR to traditional A.M./P.M. time.

__________ __________ __________

41. How many units of heparin will the patient receive at 2200? __________

42. What route is ordered for the Humulin R insulin? __________

43. Interpret the order for Cipro. __________

44. If the administration times for the sliding scale insulin are accurate (30 minutes before meals), what times will meals be served? (Use traditional A.M./P.M. time.) __________

Refer to the Computerized Pharmacy MAR (Figure 7-6) on page 126 to answer items 45 through 49.

45. The physician visited about 5:00 P.M. on 8/8/xx. What order did the physician write?

____

46. Using the time, as a clue, interpret the symbol "w/" in the Zantac order and give the proper medical abbreviation. __________

47. Interpret the order for ranitidine. __________

48. Which of the routine medications is(are) ordered for 6:00 P.M.? __________

49. How many hours are between the scheduled administration times for Megace? __________

50. Critical Thinking Skill: Describe the strategy that would prevent this medication error.

possible scenario

Suppose a physician wrote an order for gentamicin 100 mg to be given IV q.8h to a patient hospitalized with meningitis. The unit secretary transcribed the order as:

Gentamicin 100 mg IV q.8h

(12 am–6 am–12 pm–6 pm)

The medication nurse checked the order without noticing the discrepancy in the administration times. Suppose the patient received the medication every six hours for three days before the error was noticed.

potential outcome

The patient would have received one extra dose each day, which is equivalent to one-third more medication daily. Most likely, the physician would be notified of the error, and the medication would be discontinued with serum gentamicin levels drawn. The levels would likely be in the toxic range, and the patient's gentamicin levels would be monitored until the levels returned to normal. This patient would be at risk of developing ototoxicity or nephrotoxicity from the overdose of gentamicin.

prevention

____

____

After completing these problems, see page 424 to check your answers.

PHARMACY MAR

START	STOP	MEDICATION	SCHEDULED TIMES	OK'D BY	0701 TO 1500	1501 TO 2300	2301 TO 0700
21:00 8/17/xx SCH		MEGESTROL ACETATE (MEGACE) 40 MG TAB 2 TABS PO BID	0900 2100				
12:00 8/17/xx SCH		VANCOMYCIN 250 MG CAP 1 CAPSULE PO QID	0800 1200 1800 2200				
9:00 8/13/xx SCH		FLUCONAZOLE (DIFLUCAN) 100 MG TAB 100 MG PO QD	0900				
21:00 8/11/xx SCH		PERIDEX ORAL RINSE 480 ML 30 ML ORAL RINSE BID SWISH & SPIT	0900 2100				
17:00 8/10/xx SCH		RANITIDINE (ZANTAC) 150 MG TAB 1 TABLET PO BID W/BREAK.&SUPPER	0800 1700				
17:00 8/08/xx SCH		DIGOXIN (LANOXIN) 0.125 MG TAB 1 TAB PO QD1700	1700				
0:01 8/27/xx PRN		LIDOCAINE 5% OINT 35 GM TUBE APPLY TOPICAL PRN* TO RECTAL AREA					
14:00 8/22/xx PRN		SODIUM CHLORIDE INJ 10 ML AS DIR IV TID DILUENT FOR ATIVAN IV					
14:00 8/22/xx PRN		LORAZEPAM (ATIVAN)*2 MG INJ 1 MG IV TID PRN ANXIETY					
9:30 8/21/xx PRN		TUCKS 40 PADS APPLY APPLY TOPICAL Q4-6H TO RECTUM PRN					
9:30 8/21/xx PRN		ANUSOL SUPP 1 SUPP 1 SUPP PR Q4-6H					
16:00 8/18/xx PRN		MEPERIDINE* (DEMEROL) INJ 25 MG 10 MG IV Q1H PRN PAIN IN ADDITION TO PCA					

Gluteus	Thigh
A. Right	H. Right
B. Left	I. Left
Ventro Gluteal	Deltoid
C. Right	J. Right
D. Left	K. Left
E. Abdomen 1 2 / 3 4	QD

Page 1 of 2

STANDARD TIMES
QD = 0900
BID = Q12H = 0900 & 2100
TID = 0800, 1400, 2200
Q8H = 0800, 1600, 2400
QID = 0800, 1200, 1800, 2200
Q6H = 0600, 1200, 1800, 2400
Q4H = 0400, 0800, 1200. . .
QD DIGOXIN = 1700
QD WARFARIN = 1600

NURSE'S SIGNATURE INITIAL
0701-1500 ______
1501-2300 ______
2301-0700 ______
Ok'd by ______

ALLERGIES: NAFCILLIN, BACTRIM, SULFA, TRIMETHOPRIM, CIPROFLOXACIN HCL

Patient: Smith, John
Patient #: 3-90301-4
Physician: J. Physician, M.D.
Room: 407-4 South

FROM: 08/30/xx 0701 TO: 08/31/xx 0700

FIGURE 7-6 Computerized Pharmacy MAR for Chapter 7 Practice Problems (Questions 45–49)

CHAPTER

8

Understanding Drug Labels

objectives

Upon mastery of Chapter 8, you will be able to read and understand the labels of the medications you have available. To accomplish this you will also be able to:

- Find and differentiate the brand and generic names of drugs.
- Determine the dosage strength.
- Determine the form in which the drug is supplied.
- Determine the supply dosage or concentration.
- Identify the total volume of the drug container.
- Differentiate the total volume of the container from the supply dosage.
- Find the directions for mixing or preparing the supply dosage of drugs as needed.
- Recognize and follow drug alerts.
- Identify the administration route.
- Check the expiration date.
- Identify the lot number, National Drug Code, and bar code symbols.
- Recognize the manufacturer's name.
- Differentiate labels for multi-dose containers from unit dose packets.
- Identify combination drugs.

The drug order prescribes how much of a drug the patient is to receive. The nurse must prepare the order from the drugs on hand. The drug label tells how the available drug is supplied.

Look at the following common drug labels and learn to recognize pertinent information about the drugs supplied.

Brand and generic names of the drug: The brand, trade, or proprietary name is the manufacturer's name for a drug. Notice that the brand name is usually the most prominent word on the drug label—large type and boldly visible to promote the product. It is followed by the sign ® meaning that both the name and formulation are registered. The generic or established, nonproprietary name appears directly under the brand name in lowercase letters. Sometimes the generic name is also placed inside parentheses. By law, the generic name must be identified on all drug labels.

Generic equivalents of many brand name drugs are ordered as substitutes by physician preference or pharmacy policy. Because only the generic name appears on these labels, nurses need to carefully cross check all medications. Failure to do so could cause inaccurate drug identification.

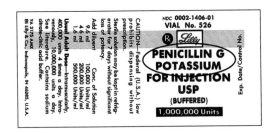

Generic Name (penicillin G potassium)

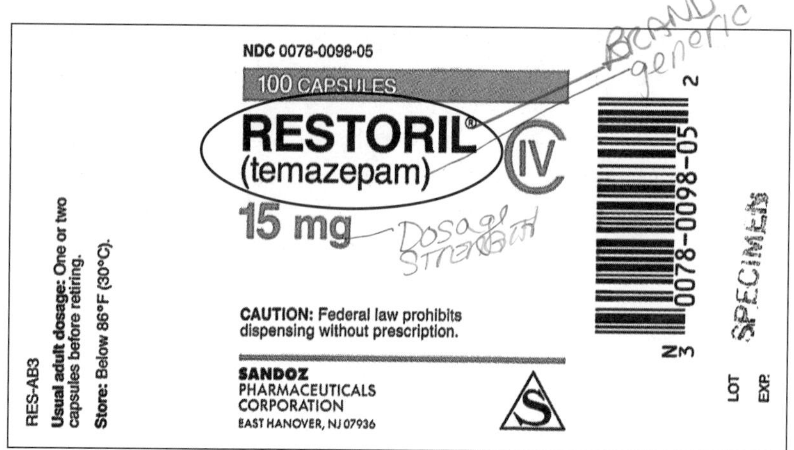

Brand Name (Restoril) and Generic Name (temazepam)

Dosage strength: This refers to the dosage *weight* or amount of drug provided in a specific unit of measurement. The dosage strength of Amoxil capsules is 250 milligrams (the weight and specific unit of measurement) per capsule. Some drugs, like V-cillin K, have two different but equivalent dosage strengths. V-cillin K has a dosage strength of 250 milligrams per tablet or 400,000 units per tablet. This allows physicians to order the drug using either unit of measurement.

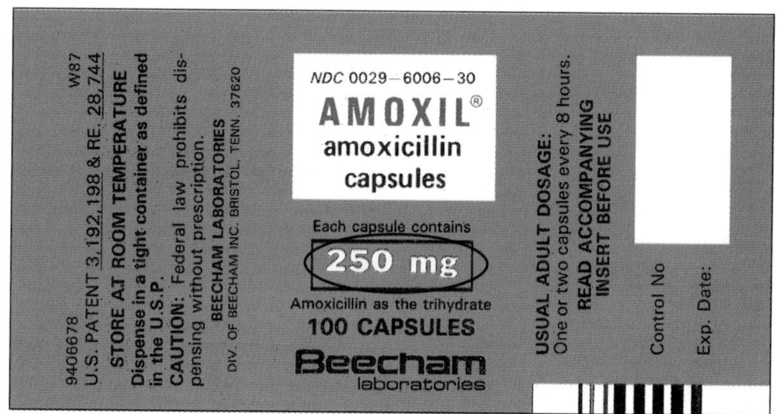

250 mg

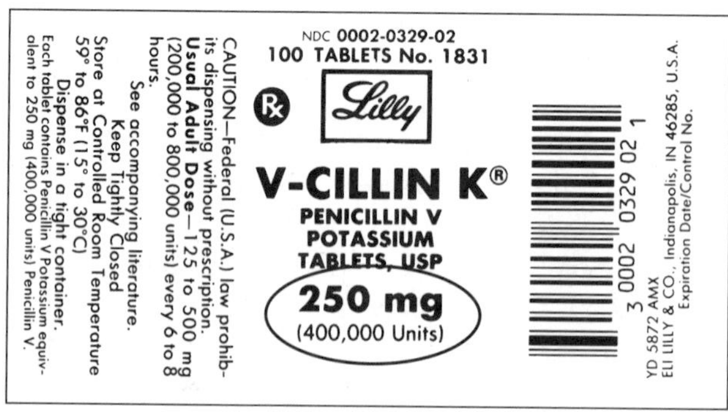

250 mg (400,000 units)

Form: This identifies the *structure and composition* of the drug. Solid dosage forms for oral use include tablets and capsules. Some powdered or granular medications, not manufactured in tablet or capsule form, can be directly combined with food or beverages and administered. Others must be reconstituted (liquefied) and measured in a precise liquid volume, such as milliliters, drops, or ounces. They may be a crystaloid (clear solution) or a suspension (solid particles in liquid that separate when held in a container).

Injectable medications may be supplied in solution or dry powdered form to be reconstituted. Once reconstituted they are measured in milliliters or cubic centimeters.

Medications are also supplied in a variety of other forms, such as suppositories, creams, and patches.

Otic Sterile Suspension Drops

Fiber Granular Drug Added to Beverage

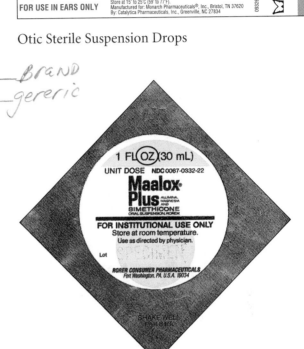

Ounces

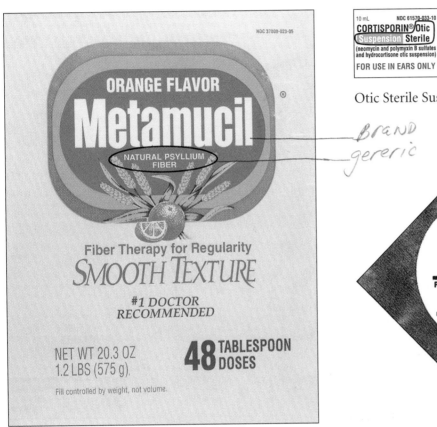

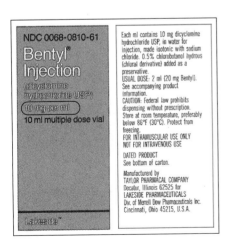

Milliliters

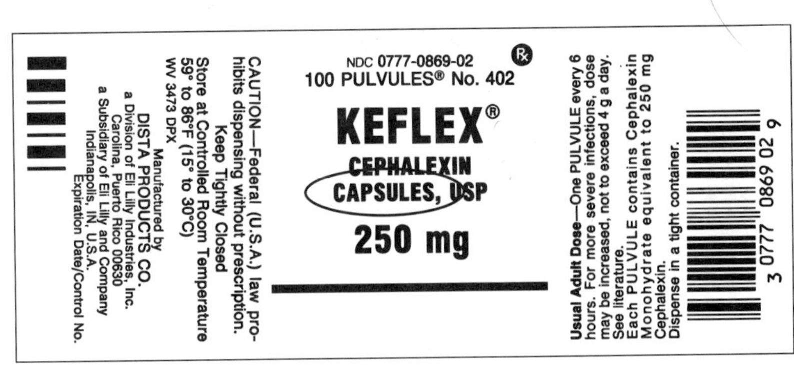

Capsules

Supply dosage: This refers to both *dosage strength* and *form*. It is read "X measured units per some quantity." For solid form medications, such as tablets, the supply dosage is X measured units per tablet. For liquid medications, the supply dosage is the same as the medication's concentration, such as X measured units per milliliter. Take a minute to read the supply dosage printed on the following labels.

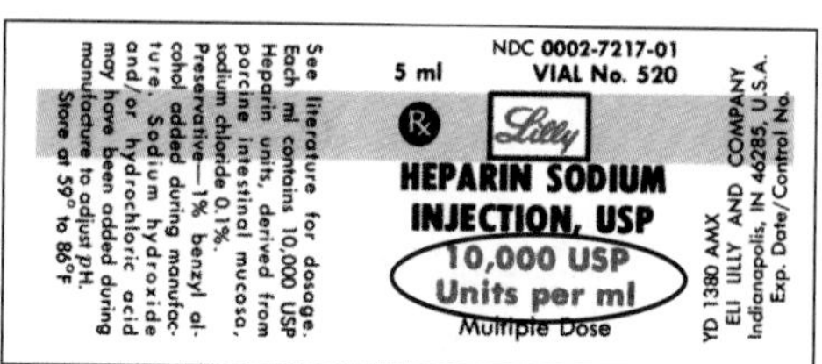

10,000 units per milliliter

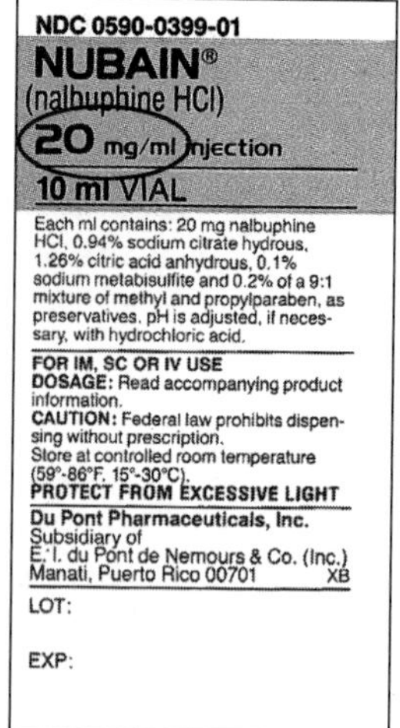

20 milligrams per milliliter

Total volume: This refers to the *full quantity* contained in a package, bottle, or vial. For tablets and other solid medications, it is the total number of individual items. For liquids, it is the total fluid volume.

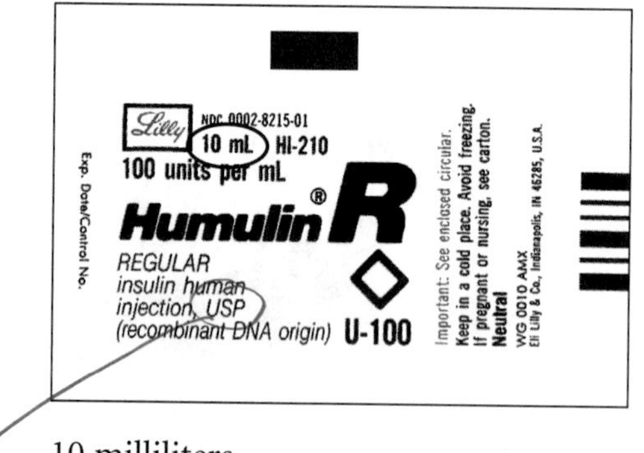

10 milliliters

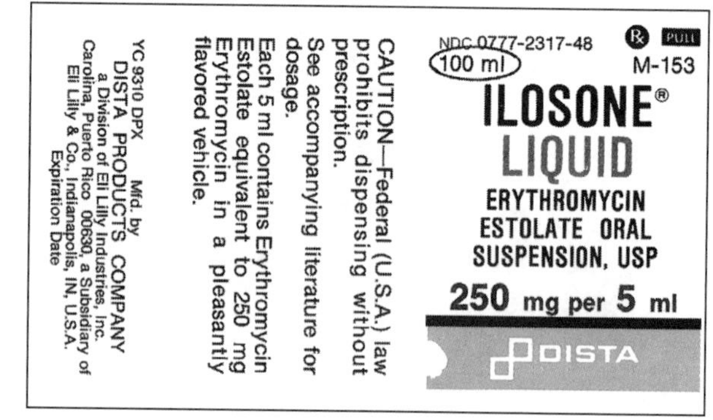

100 milliliters

Administration route: This refers to the *site* of the body or *method of drug delivery* into the patient. Examples of routes of administration include oral, enteral (into the gastrointestinal tract through a tube), sublingual, injection (IV, IM), otic, optic, topical, rectal, vaginal, and others. Unless specified otherwise, tablets, capsules, and caplets are intended for oral use.

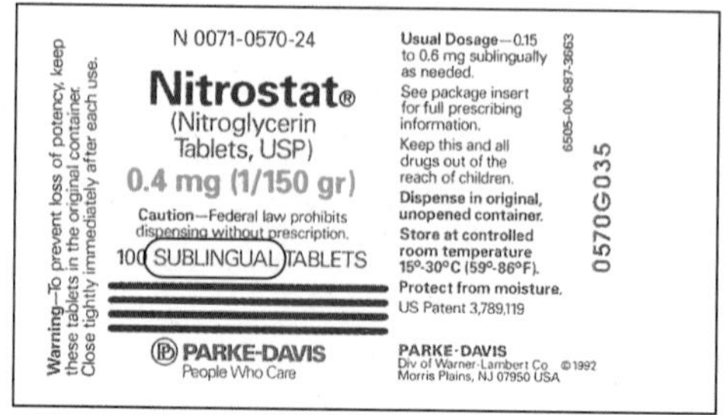

Sublingual

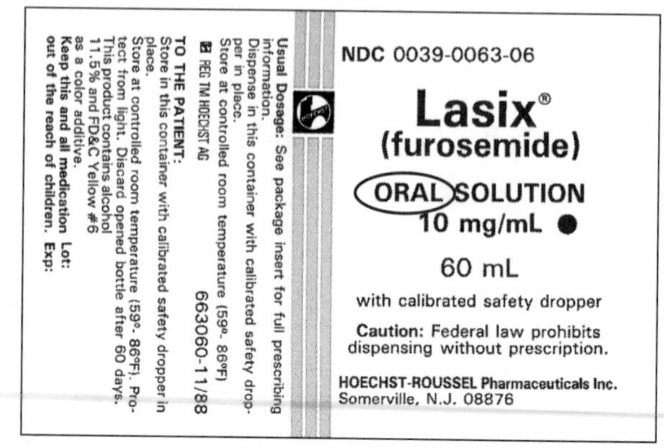

Oral

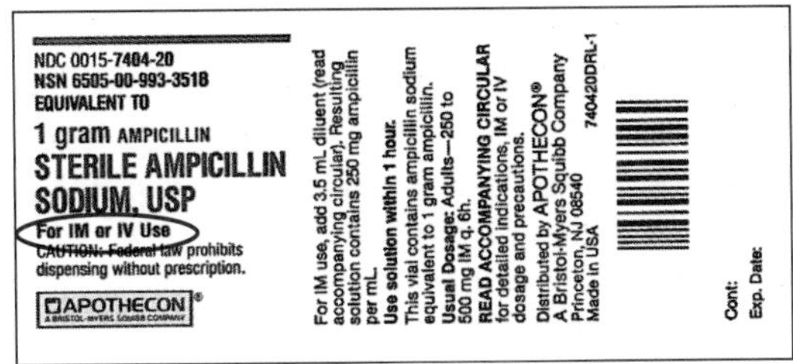

Intramuscular (IM) or Intravenous (IV)

Directions for mixing or reconstituting: This refers to drugs that are dispensed in *powder form* and must be *reconstituted for use.* (Reconstitution is discussed further in Chapters 9, 10, and 13.)

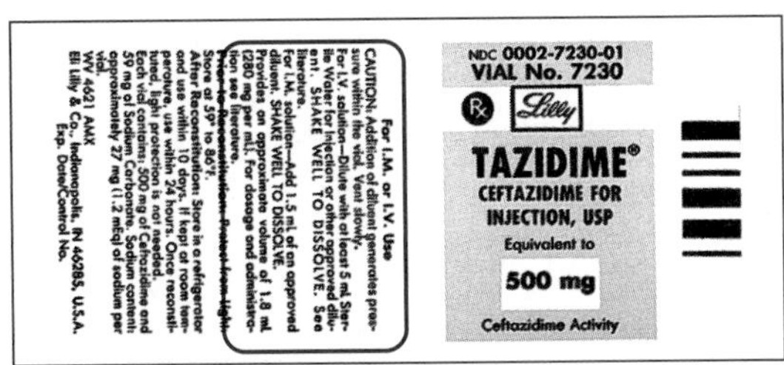

See Directions

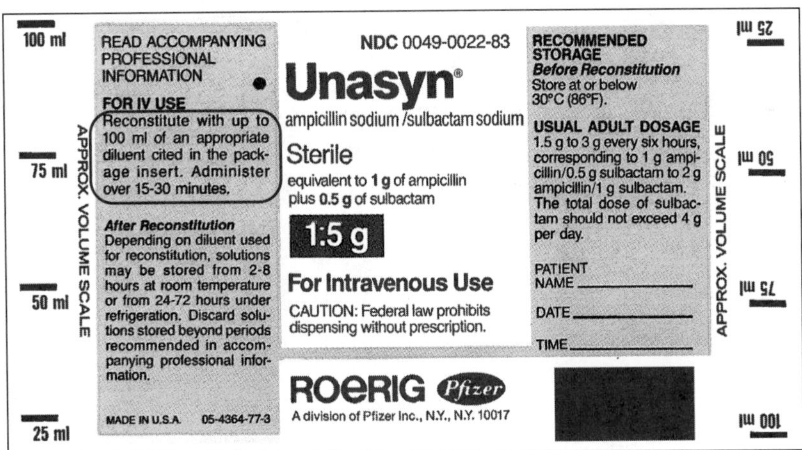

See Directions

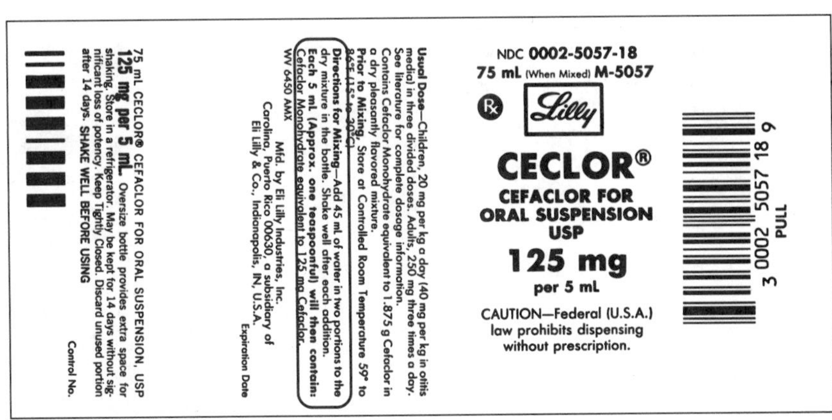

See Directions

Label alerts: Manufacturers may print warnings on the packaging or special alerts may be added by the pharmacy before dispensing. Look for special storage alerts such as "refrigerate at all times," "keep in a dry place," "replace cap and close tightly before storing," or "protect from light." Reconstituted suspensions may be dispensed already prepared for use, and directions may instruct the nurse to "shake well before using" as a reminder to remix the components. Read and follow all label instructions carefully.

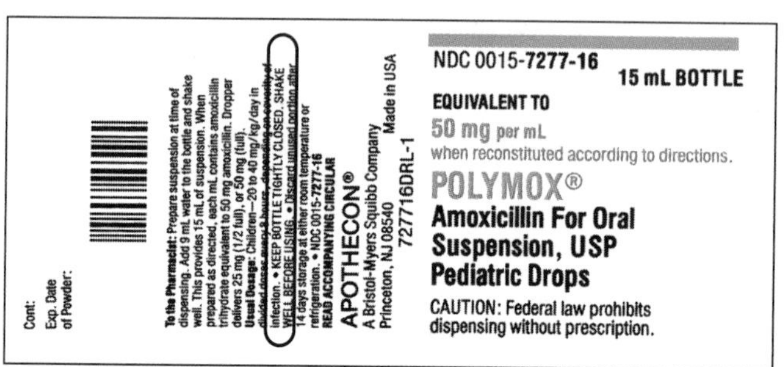

See Alert

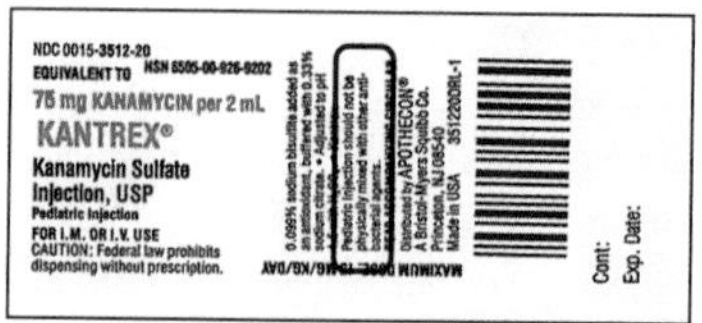

See Alert

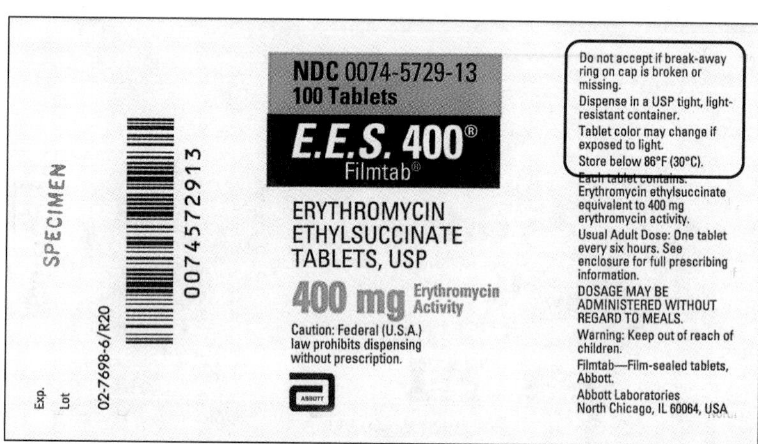

See Alert

Name of the manufacturer: Manufacturer is circled on the following labels.

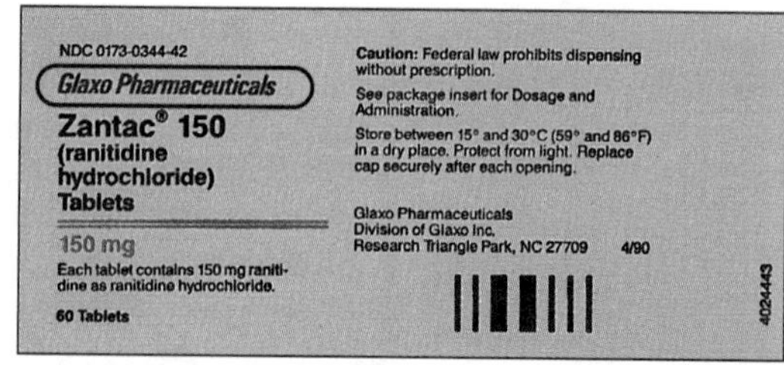

Glaxo Pharmaceuticals

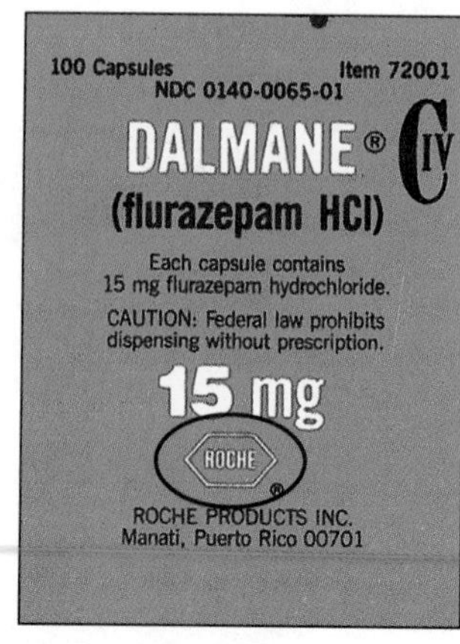

Roche Products, Inc.

Expiration date: The medication should be used, discarded, or returned to the pharmacy by this date. Further, note the special expiration instructions given on labels for reconstituted medications. Refer to the Tazidime and Unasyn labels on page 000.

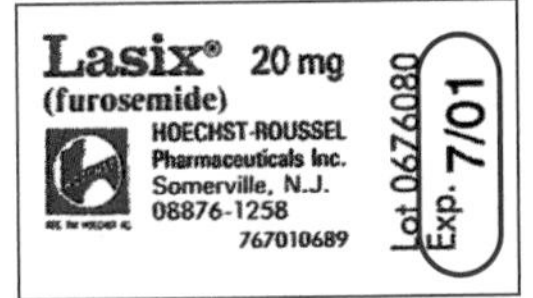

7/01

Lot or control numbers: Federal law requires all medication packages to be identified with a lot or control number. If a drug is recalled, for reasons such as damage or tampering, the lot number quickly identifies the particular group of medication packages to be removed from shelves. Recently this has been invaluable in relation to vaccine and over-the-counter medication recalls.

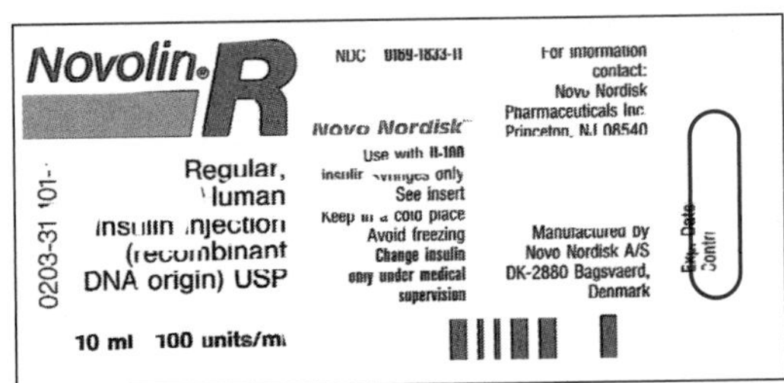

Control Number

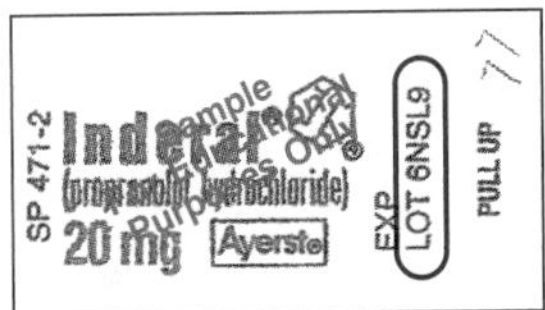

Lot Number

National Drug Code (NDC): Federal law requires that every prescription medication has a unique identifying number, much like every U.S. citizen has a unique Social Security number. This number must appear on every manufacturer's label and is printed as "NDC-*XXXX-XXXX-XX*" with the NDC followed by three groups of discrete numbers.

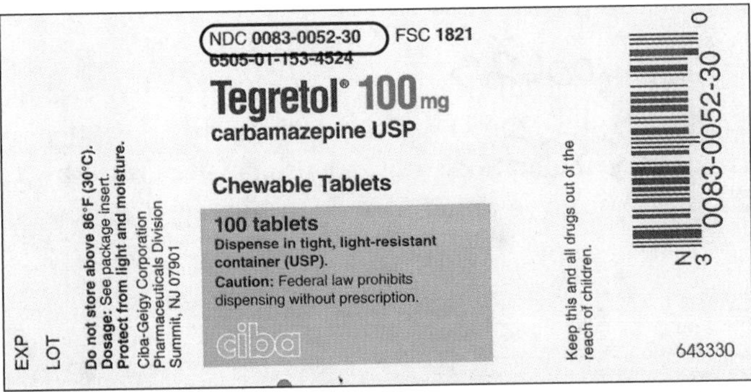

NDC

Bar code symbols: Bar code symbols are commonly used in retail sales. Bar code symbols serve to document drug dosing for recordkeeping and stock reorder, and may soon automate medication documentation right at the patient's bedside. The horizontal ones look like "picket fences" and the vertical ones look like "ladders."

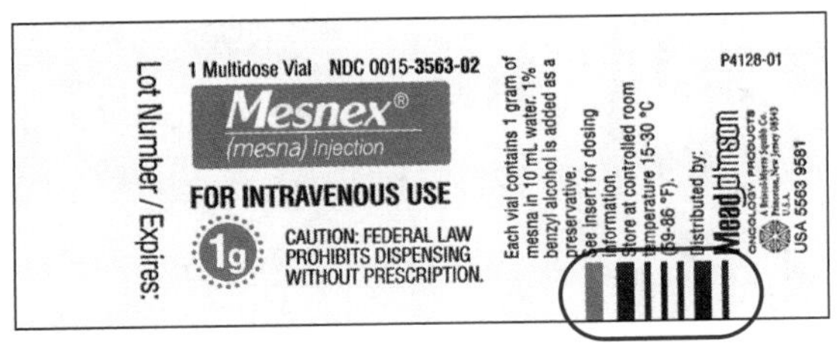

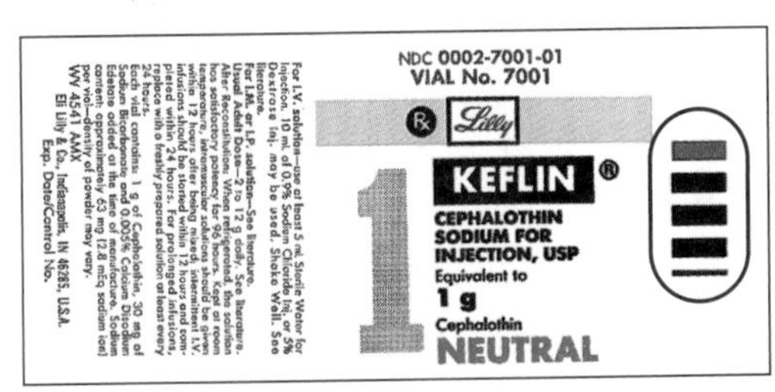

Bar Codes

United States Pharmacopeia (USP) and National Formulary (NF): These codes are found on many manufacturer-printed medication labels. The USP and the NF are the two official national lists of approved drugs. Each manufacturer follows special guidelines that determine when to include these initials on a label. These initials are placed after the generic drug name. Be careful not to mistake these abbreviations for other initials that designate specific characteristics of a drug, such as *SR*, which means "sustained release."

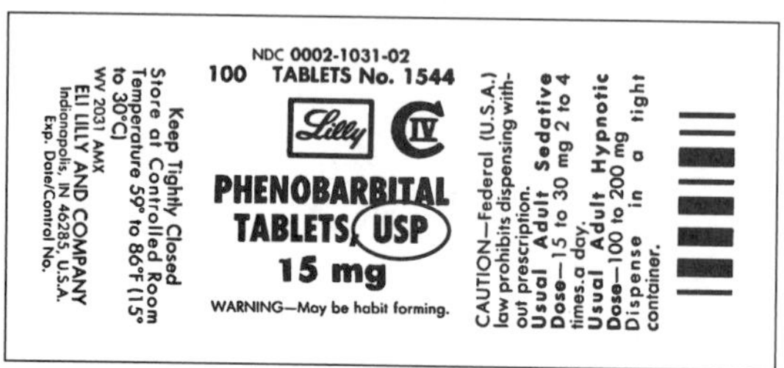

USP

Unit dose labels: Most oral medications administered in the hospital setting are available in unit dosage, in which a single capsule or tablet is packaged separately in a typical blister pack. The pharmacy provides a 24-hour supply of each drug for the patient. Notice that the only major difference in this form of labeling is that the total volume of the container is omitted, because the volume is *one* tablet or capsule. Likewise, the dosage strength is understood as *per one.*

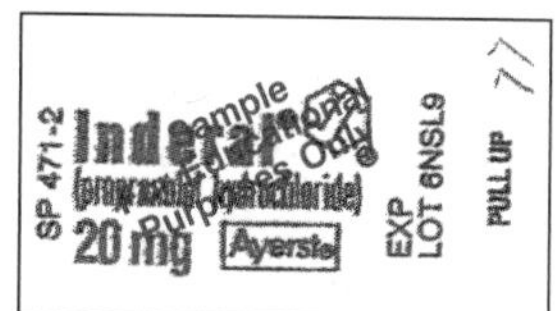

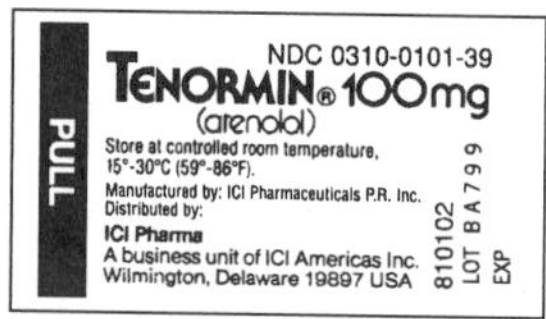

Unit Dose Labels

Combination drugs: Some medications are a combination of two or more drugs in one form. Read the labels for Claritin-D and Darvocet-N and notice the different substances that are combined in each tablet. Combination drugs are usually prescribed by the number of tablets, capsules, or milliliters to be given rather than by the dosage strength.

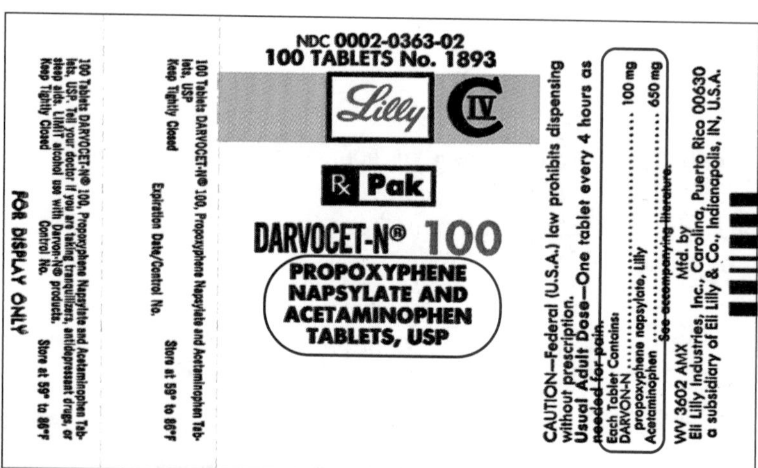

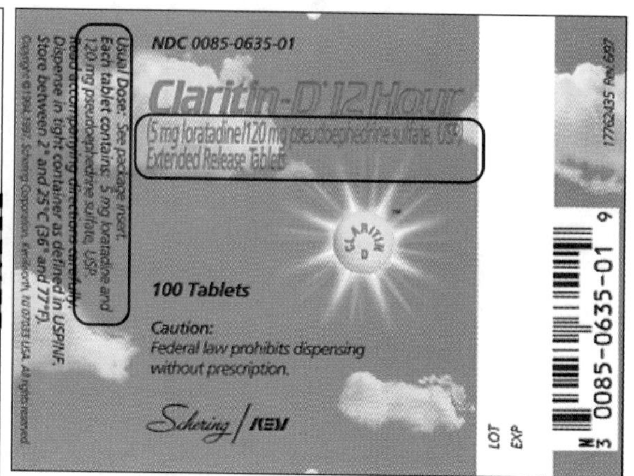

(Reproduced with permission of Schering Corporation. All rights reserved.)

Combination Drug labels

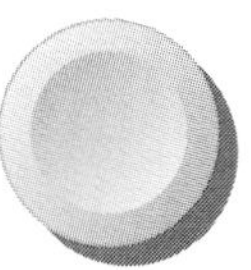

quick review

Read labels carefully to:

- identify the drug and the manufacturer.
- differentiate between dosage strength, form, supply dosage, total container volume, and administration route.
- recognize that the drug's supply dosage similarly refers to a drug's weight per unit of measure or *concentration*.
- find the directions for reconstitution, as needed.
- note expiration date.
- describe lot or control number.

review set 24

Use labels A through G which follow, to find the information requested in Questions 1–13. Indicate your answer by letter (A through G).

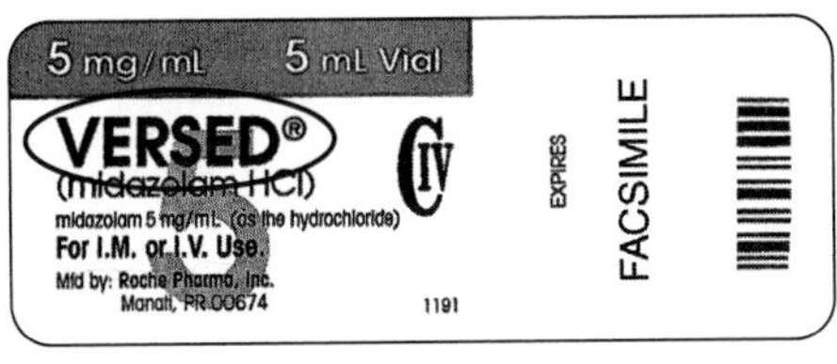

A

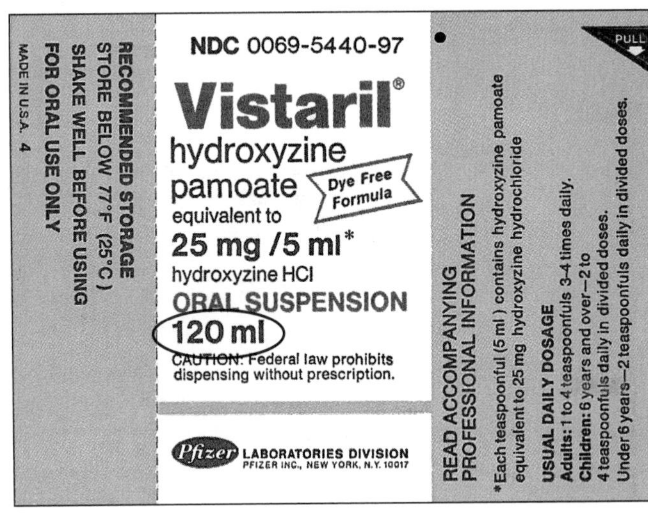

B

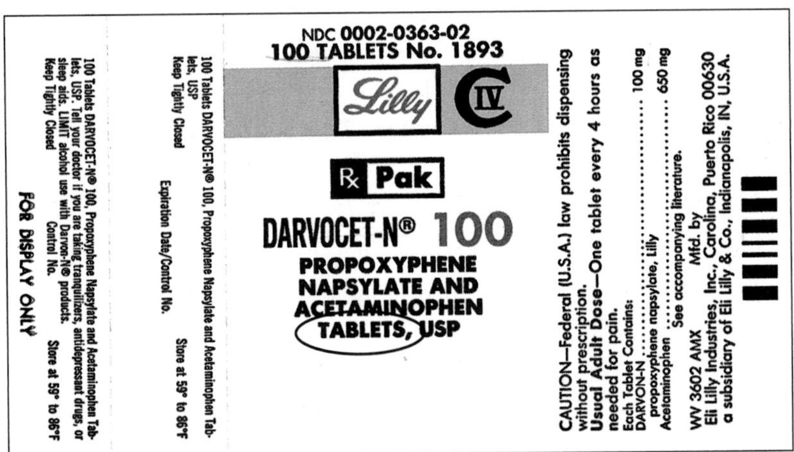

C

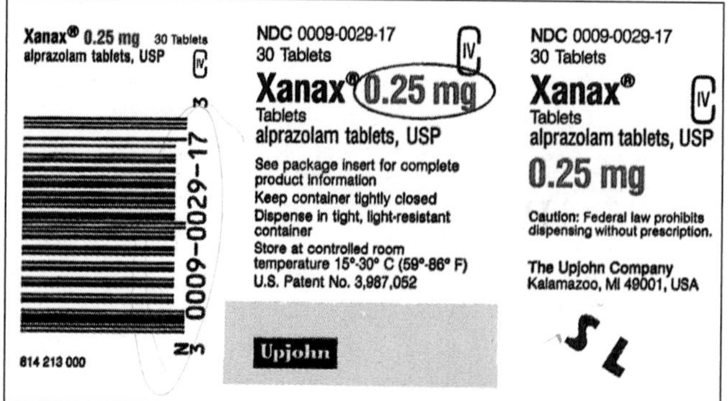

D

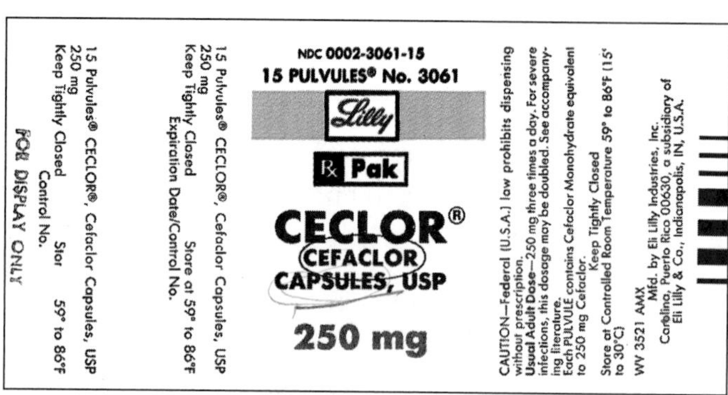

E

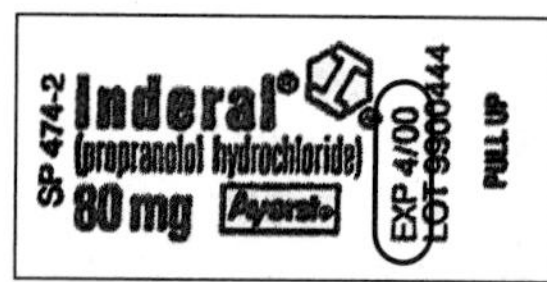

F

NDC 0310-0101-39
TENORMIN® 100mg
(atenolol)
Store at controlled room temperature, 15°-30°C (59°-86°F).
Manufactured by: ICI Pharmaceuticals P.R. Inc.
Distributed by:
ICI Pharma
A business unit of ICI Americas Inc.
Wilmington, Delaware 19897 USA
PULL
LOT BA799

G

1. The total volume of the liquid container is circled. ________
2. The dosage strength is circled. ________
3. The form of the drug is circled. ________
4. The brand name of the drug is circled. ________
5. The generic name of the drug is circled. ________
6. The expiration date is circled. ________
7. The lot number is circled. ________
8. Look at label E and determine how much of the supply drug you will administer to the patient per dose for the order *Ceclor 250 mg p.o. q.8h p.r.n.* ________
9. Look at label A and determine the route of administration. ________
10. Indicate which labels have an imprinted bar code symbol. ________
11. Look at label C. What does the number *100*, printed next to Darvocet-N, represent on this label? ________
12. Look at label B, and determine the supply dosage per 1 mL. ________
13. Look at label G, and determine how much of the supply drug you will administer to the patient per dose for the order *Tenormin 50 mg po q.d. hs.* ________

Refer to the following label to identify the specific drug information described in Questions 14–20.

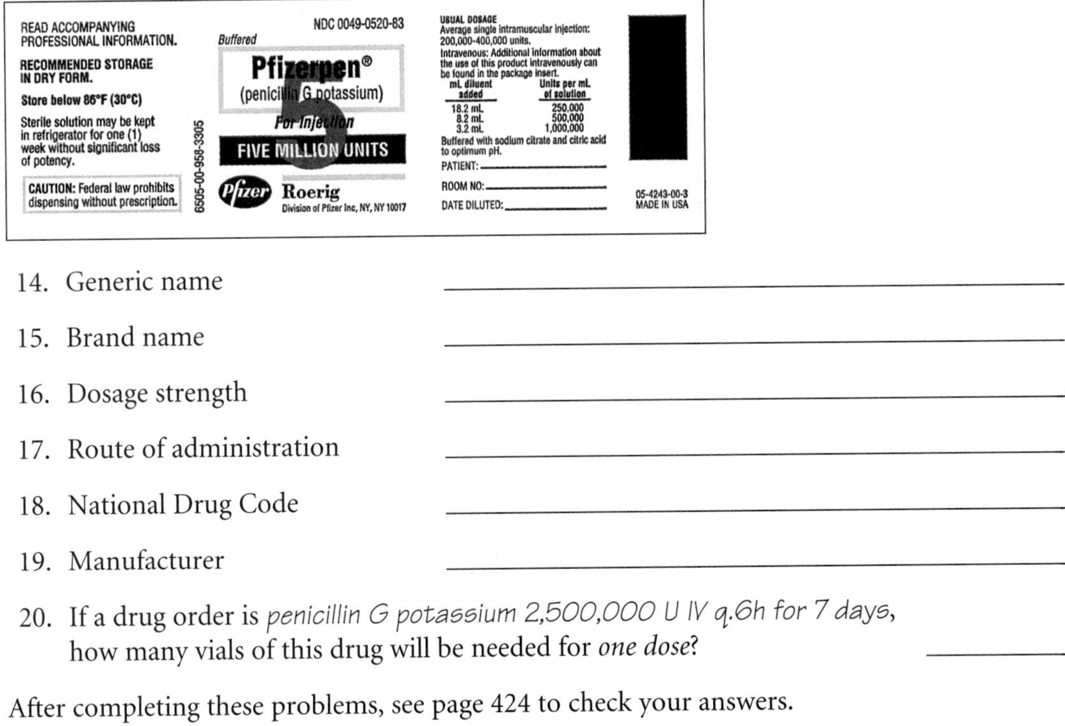

14. Generic name ______________________
15. Brand name ______________________
16. Dosage strength ______________________
17. Route of administration ______________________
18. National Drug Code ______________________
19. Manufacturer ______________________
20. If a drug order is *penicillin G potassium 2,500,000 U IV q.6h for 7 days*, how many vials of this drug will be needed for *one dose*? __________

After completing these problems, see page 424 to check your answers.

critical thinking skills

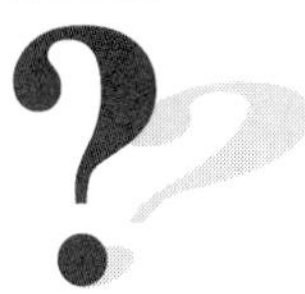

Reading the labels of medications is critical. Make sure that the drug you want is what you have on hand before you prepare it. Let's look at an example of a medication error related to reading the label incorrectly.

error

Not checking the label for correct dosage.

possible scenario

A nurse flushed a triple central venous catheter (an IV with three ports). According to hospital policy, the nurse was to flush each port with 10 mL of normal saline followed by 2 mL of heparin flush solution in the concentration of 100 units/mL. The nurse mistakenly picked up a vial of heparin containing heparin 10,000 units/mL. Without checking the label, she prepared the solution for all three ports. The patient received 60,000 units of heparin instead of 600 units.

potential outcome

The patient in this case would be at great risk for hemorrhage, leading to shock and death. Protamine sulfate would likely be ordered to counteract the action of the heparin, but a successful outcome is questionable.

prevention

There is no substitute for checking the label before administering a medication. The nurse in this case had three opportunities to catch the error, having drawn three different syringes of medication for the three ports.

practice problems—chapter 8

Look at labels A through G, and identify the information requested.

Label A:

1. The supply dosage of the drug in milliequivalents is ______________________.
2. The National Drug Code is ______________________.
3. The supply dosage of the drug in milligrams is ______________________.

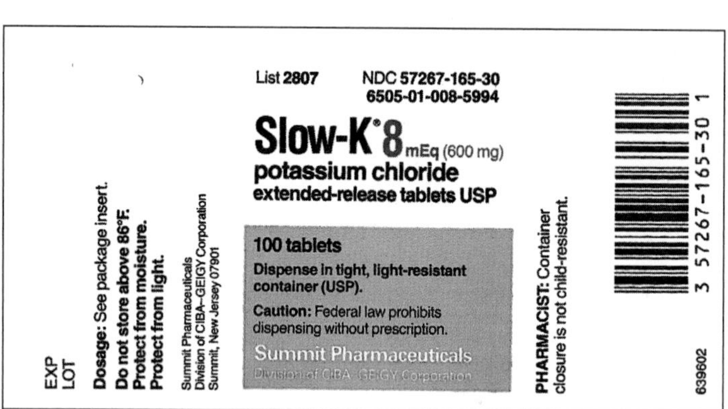

A

Label B:

4. The generic name of the drug is ______________________.
5. The reconstitution instruction to mix a supply dosage of 1.5 g per 100 mL for intravenous use is ______________________.
6. The manufacturer of the drug is ______________________.

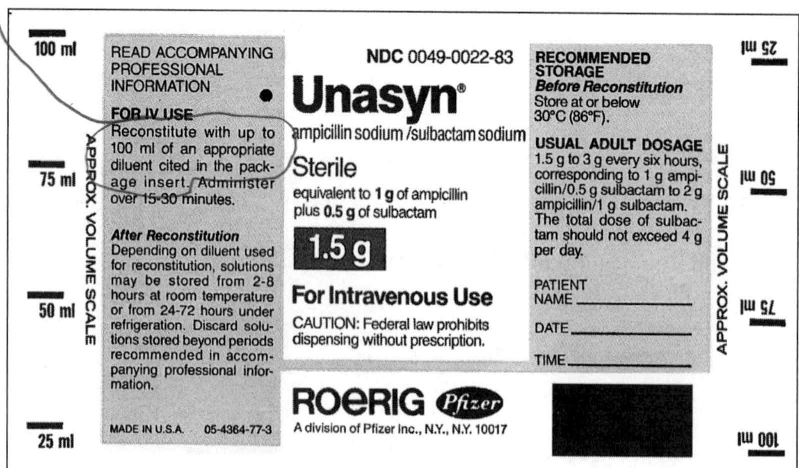

B

Label C:

7. The total volume of the medication container is 10 ml .
8. The supply dosage is 25 mg/ml .
9. How much will you administer to the patient per dose for the order *Methotrexate 25 mg IV stat?* 1 ml .

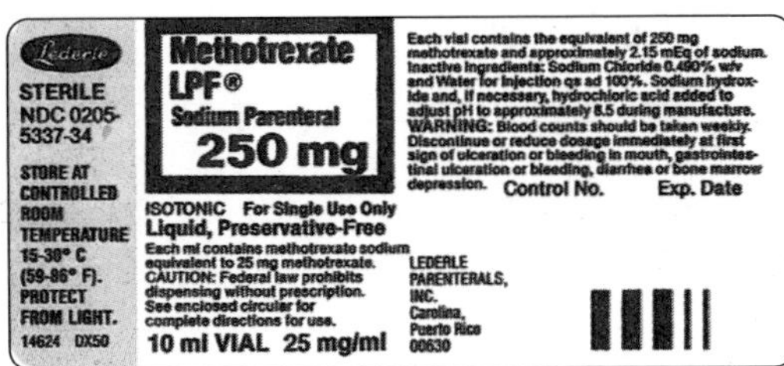

C

Label D:

10. The brand name of the drug is Keflin .
11. The generic name is CEPHALOTHIN SODIUM .
12. The National Drug Code of the drug is NDC0002-7001-01 .

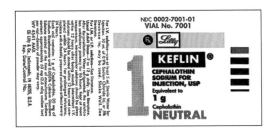

D

Label E:

13. The form of the drug is SOLUTION .
14. The total volume of the drug container is 10 ml .
15. The administration route is IM .

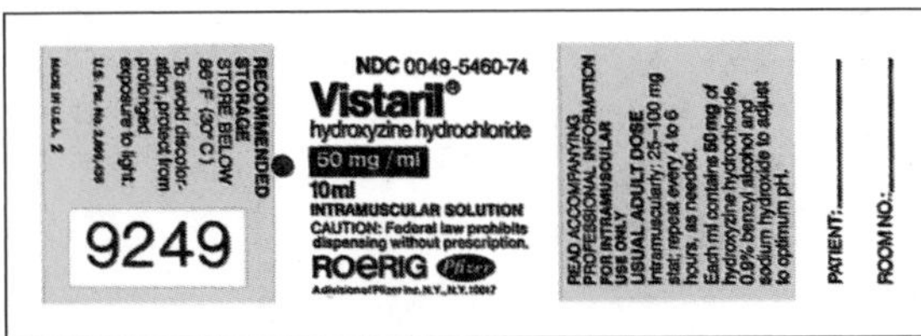

E

Label F:

16. The name of the drug manufacturer is Roche.
17. The form of the drug is CAPSULE.
18. The appropriate range of temperatures for storage of this drug is 59°–86°F.

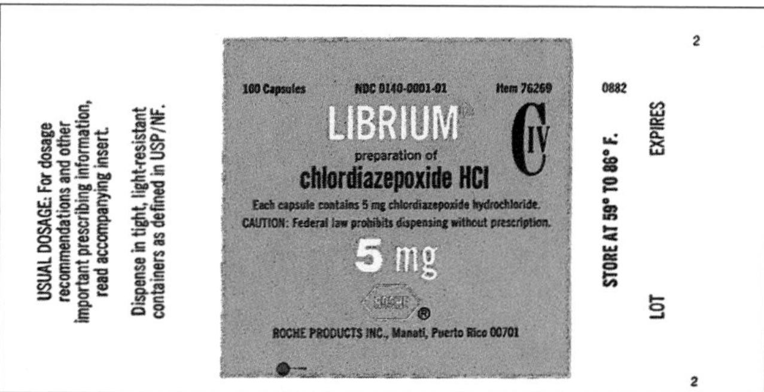

F

Label G:

19. The expiration date of the drug is 4/00.
20. The dosage strength of the drug is 80 mg.

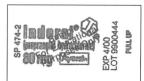

G

Match label H or I with the correct descriptive statement.

21. This label represents a unit dose drug. I
22. This label represents a combination drug. H
23. This label represents a drug usually ordered by the number of tablets or capsules to be administered rather than the dosage strength. H
24. The administration route for the drug labeled H is orally.
25. The lot number for the drug labeled I is 0666060.

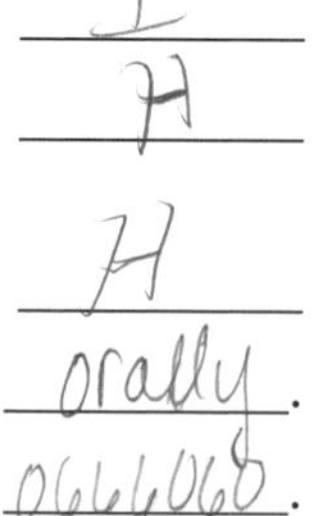

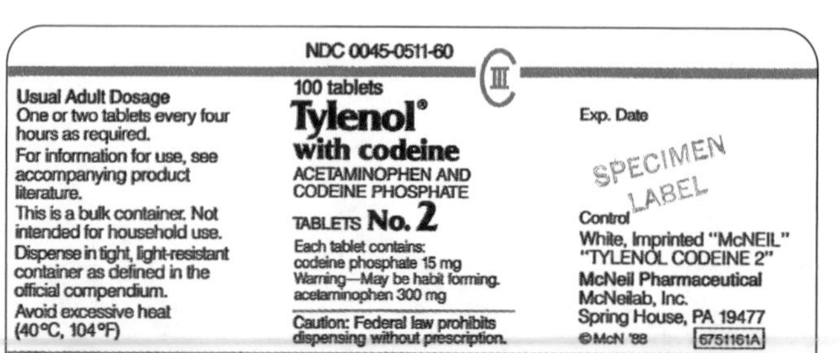

H

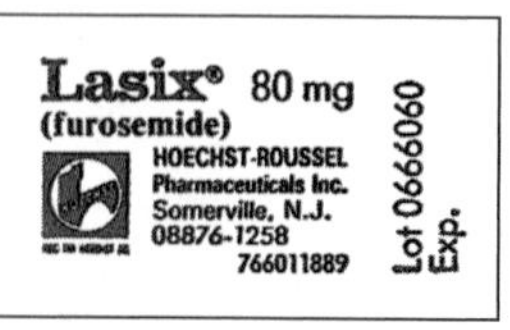

I

26. Critical Thinking Skill: Describe the strategy you would implement to prevent this medication error.

possible scenario

Suppose a physician ordered an antibiotic *Principen .5 g p.o. q.6h.* The writing was not clear on the order, and Prinivil (an antihypertensive medication) 5 mg was sent up by the pharmacy. However, the order was correctly transcribed to the medication administration record (MAR). In preparing the medication, the nurse did not read the MAR or label carefully and administered Prinivil, the wrong medication.

potential outcome

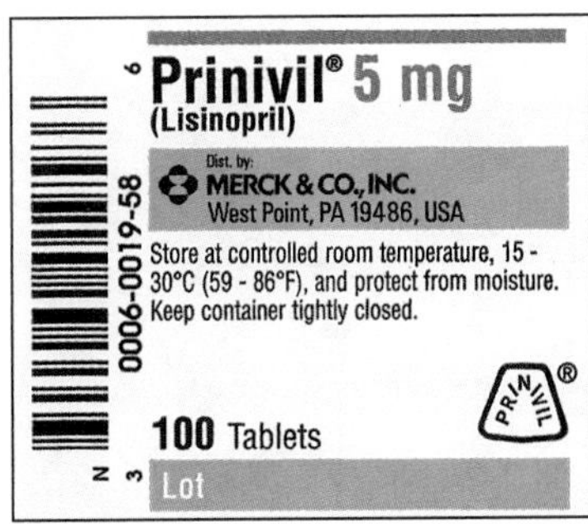

(Used with permission from Merck & Co., Inc.)

A medication error occurred because the wrong medication was given. The patient's infection treatment would be delayed. Furthermore, the erroneous blood pressure drug could have harmful effects.

prevention

Always double check the label against the MAR.

____

After completing these problems, see page 424 to check your answers.

Section 2 Self-Evaluation

Directions:

1. Round decimal answers to two decimal places. Round temperatures to one decimal place.
2. Express fractions in lowest terms.

Chapter 3: Systems of Measurement

Express the following amounts in proper medical notation.

1. two-thirds grain ______
2. four teaspoons ______
3. one three-hundredths grain ______
4. one-half milliliter ______
5. one-half ounce ______

Interpret the following notations.

6. 4 gtt ______
7. 450 mg ______
8. gr $\frac{1}{100}$ ______
9. gr viiss ______
10. 0.25 L ______

Chapters 4 and 5: Conversions

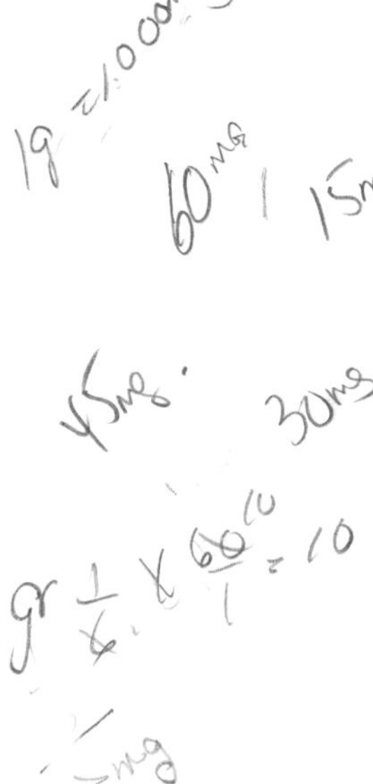

Fill in the missing decimal numbers next to each metric unit as indicated.

11.	7.13	kg	=	______	g	=	______	mg	=	______	mcg
12.	______	kg	=	______	g	=	______	mg	=	925	mcg
13.	______	kg	=	______	g	=	125	mg	=	______	mcg
14.	______	kg	=	16.4	g	=	______	mg	=	______	mcg

Convert each of the following to the equivalent units indicated.

15. gr $\frac{1}{6}$ = 10 mg = 0.01 g
16. 20 mg = 0.02 g = gr ______
17. 4 T = ______ t = ______ mL
18. qt ix = ______ L = ______ mL
19. 15 in = ______ cm = ______ mm
20. 56.2 mm = ______ cm = ______ in
21. 198 lb = ______ kg = ______ g
22. 11.59 kg = ______ g = ______ lb
23. A patient is told to take 180 mg of a medication. What is the equivalent dosage in grains? ______
24. A patient is being treated for chronic pain with gr $\frac{3}{4}$ of morphine sulphate every 3 hours. How many milligrams will he receive in 24 hours? ______
25. Your patient uses nitroglycerin for chest pain. The prescription is for gr $\frac{1}{300}$ of nitroglycerin. What is the equivalent dosage in milligrams? ______

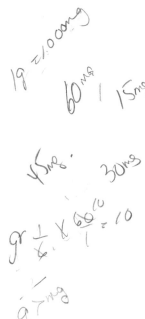

26. Most adults have about 6000 mL of circulating blood volume. This is equivalent to __________ L or qt __________ of blood volume.

27. Your patient drinks the following for breakfast: 3 ounces orange juice, 8 ounces coffee with 1 teaspoon cream, and 4 ounces of water. The total intake is __________ mL.

Convert the following times as indicated. Denote AM or PM where needed.

	Traditional Time	*International Time*
28.	11:35 PM	__________
29.	__________	1844
30.	4:17 AM	__________
31.	__________	0803

Convert the following temperatures as indicated.

	°C	*°F*
32.	38°C	_______ °F
33.	_______ °C	101.5°F
34.	37.2°C	_______ °F

Chapter 6: Equipment Used in Dosage Measurement

Draw an arrow to demonstrate the correct measurement of the doses given.

35. 1.5 mL

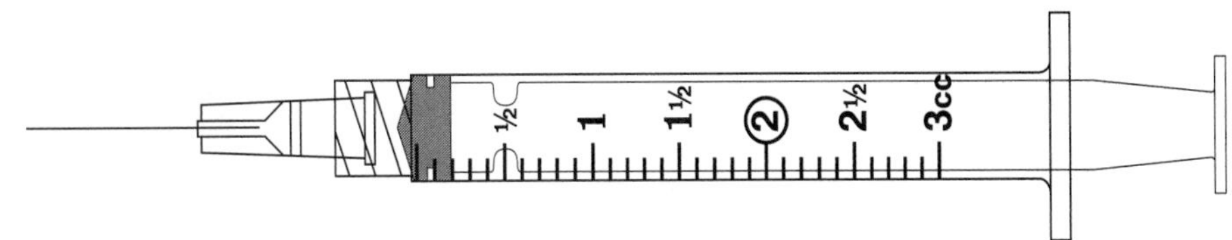

36. 0.33 mL

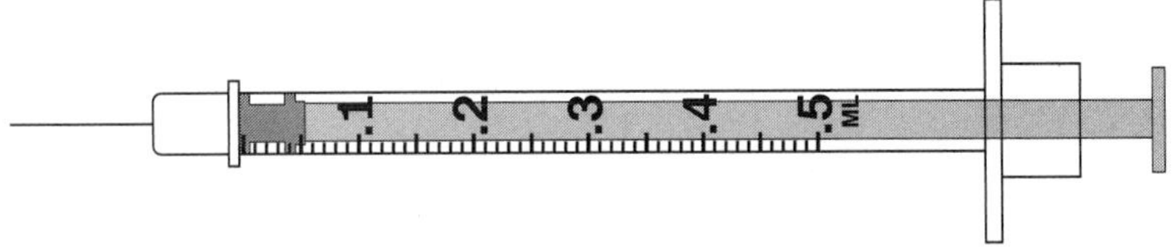

37. 44 U NPH U-100 insulin

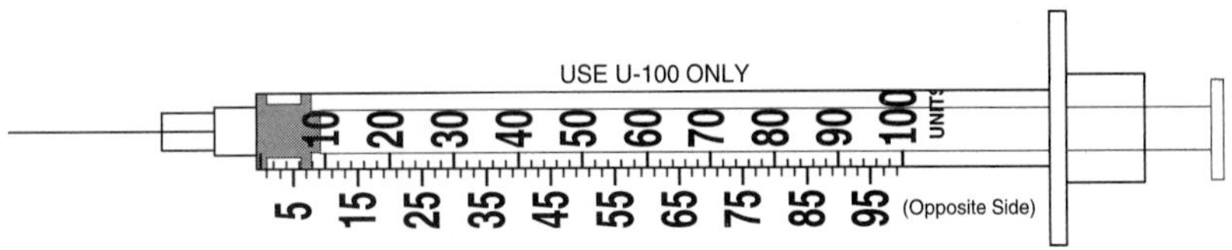

38. 37 U NPH U-100 insulin

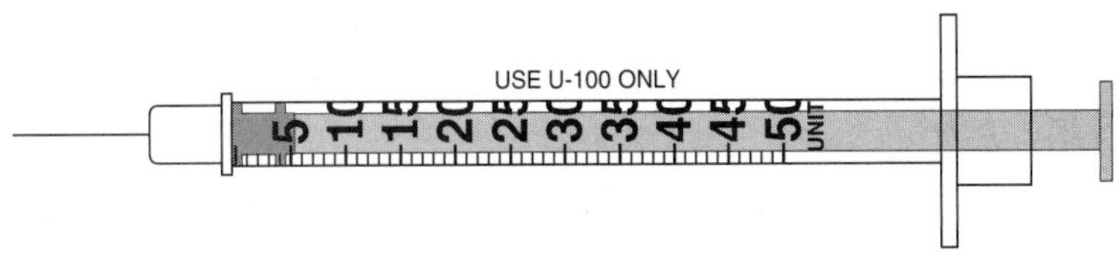

39. $1\frac{1}{2}$ t

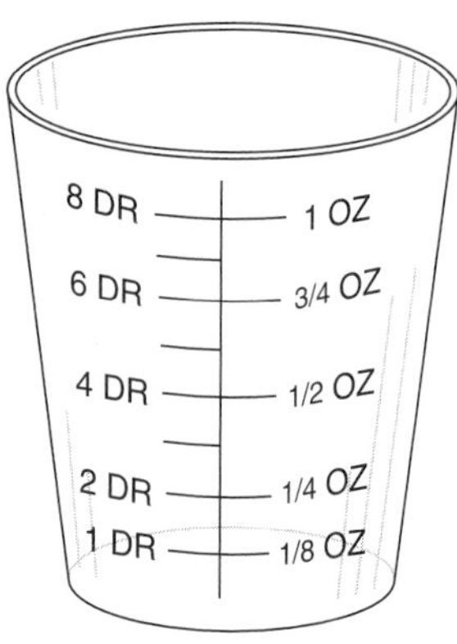

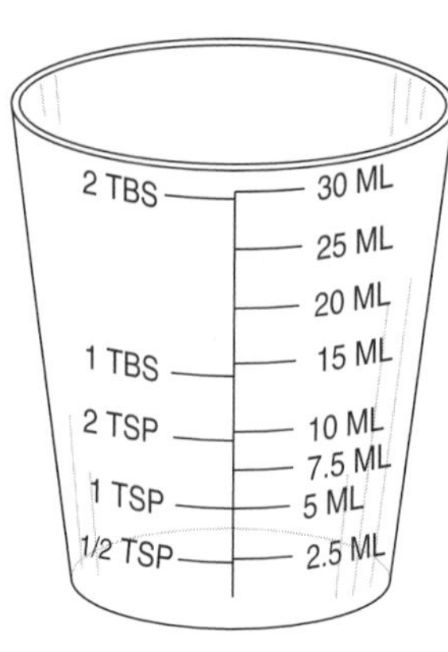

Chapter 7 and 8: Interpreting Drug Orders and Understanding Drug Labels

Use label A to identify the information requested.

40. The generic name is __________.
41. This drug is an otic solution and is intended for __________.
42. The total volume of this container is __________.
43. Interpret: *Cortisporin Otic Solution 2 gtt A.U. q.15 min × 3*

10 mL NDC 61570-034-10
CORTISPORIN® Otic Solution Sterile
(neomycin and polymyxin B sulfates and hydrocortisone otic solution)
FOR USE IN EARS ONLY

Each mL contains: neomycin sulfate equivalent to 3.5 mg neomycin base, polymyxin B sulfate equivalent to 10,000 polymyxin B units, hydrocortisone 10 mg (1%), and potassium metabisulfite 0.1% (added as a preservative). Vehicle contains the inactive ingredients cupric sulfate, glycerin, hydrochloric acid, propylene glycol, and Water for Injection.
USUAL DOSAGE: Four drops in the affected ear.
For indications, dosage, precautions, etc., see accompanying package insert.
CAUTION: Federal law prohibits dispensing without prescription.
Store at 15° to 25°C (59° to 77°F).
Manufactured for: Monarch Pharmaceuticals®, Inc., Bristol, TN 37620
By: Catalytica Pharmaceuticals, Inc., Greenville, NC 27834

Rev. 8/97
0932674
Monarch Pharmaceuticals®
unvarnished

A

Use label B to identify the information requested.

44. The supply dosage is __________.
45. The National Drug Code is __________.
46. Interpret: *heparin 3,750 U SC q.8h*

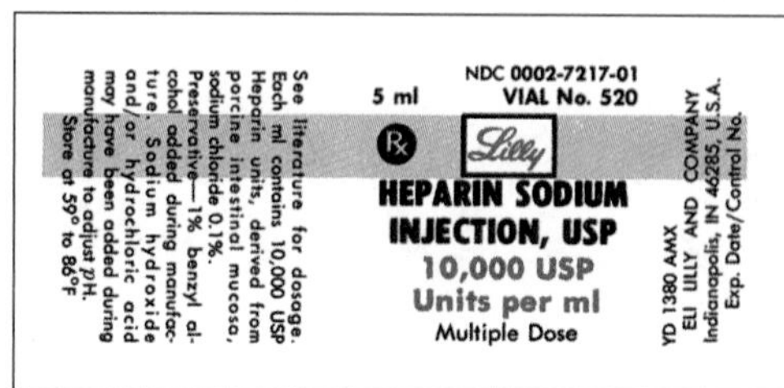

B

Use label C to identify the information requested.

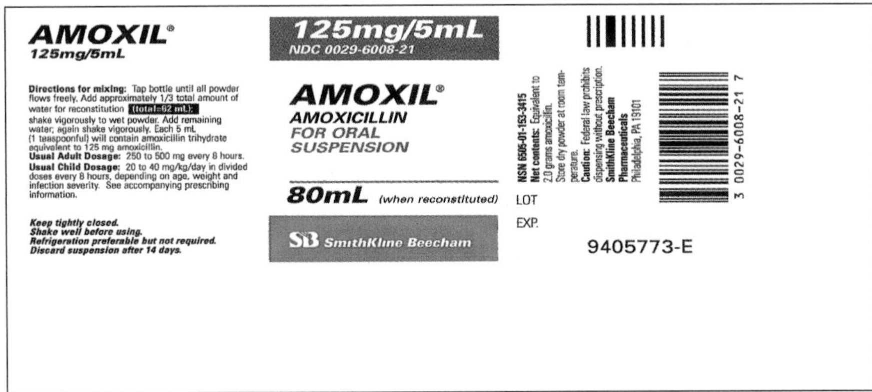

C

47. The trade name is ______________________________.
48. The supply dosage, when reconstituted, is ____________.
49. What amount would be given for one dose if the drug order is *Amoxil 125 mg p.o. stat*?
 a. ____________ mL or b. ____________ t
 c. Draw an arrow on the medicine cup to demonstrate the dose volume.

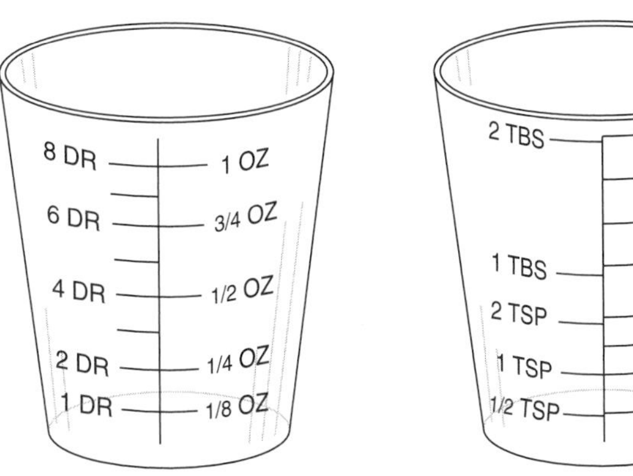

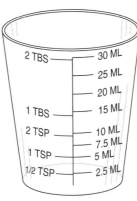

50. Interpret: *Amoxil 250 mg p.o. t.i.d.* ______________________________.

After completing these problems, see pages 424–426 to check your answers.

Perfect score = 100

Minimum mastery score = 86% (43 correct) My score = ______________

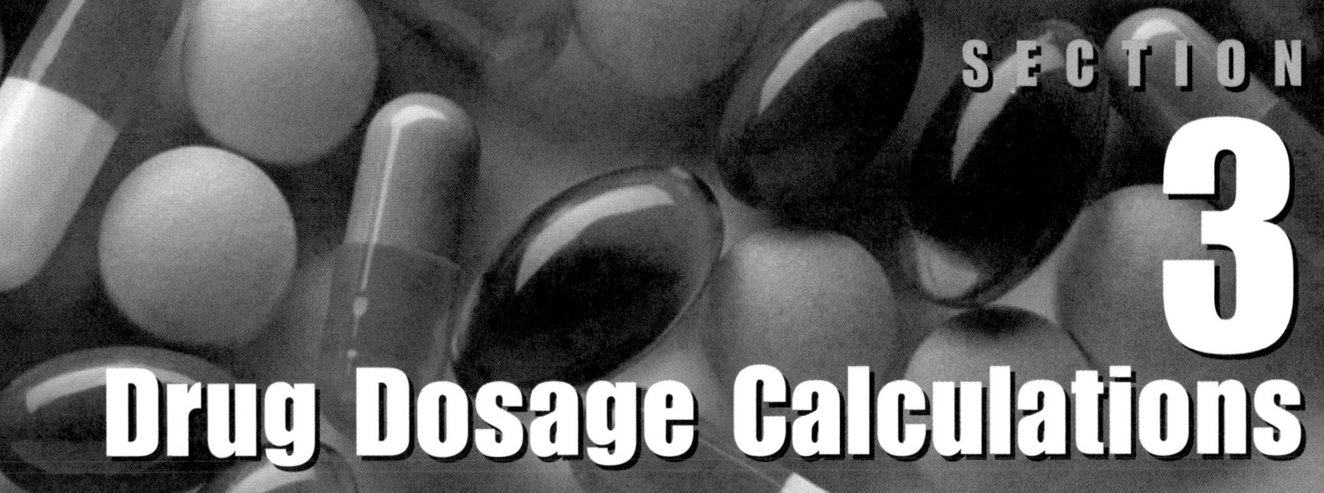

SECTION 3
Drug Dosage Calculations

CHAPTER 9

Oral Dosage of Drugs

objectives

Upon mastery of Chapter 9, you will be able to calculate oral dosages of drugs. To accomplish this you will also be able to:

- Convert all units of measurement to the same system and same size units.
- Estimate the reasonable amount of the drug to be administered.
- Use the formula $\frac{D}{H} \times Q = X$ to calculate drug dosage.
- Calculate the number of tablets or capsules that are contained in prescribed dosages.
- Calculate the volume of liquid per dose when the prescribed dosage is in solution form.

Medications for oral administration are supplied in a variety of forms such as tablets, capsules, and liquids. They are usually ordered to be administered by mouth, or *p.o.*, which is an abbreviation for the Latin phrase, "*per os.*"

When a liquid form of a drug is unavailable, children and many elderly patients may need to have a tablet crushed or a capsule opened and prepared in a small volume of food or fluid to enable them to swallow the medication. Many of these crushed medications and oral liquids also may be ordered to be given enterally, or into the gastrointestinal tract via a specially placed tube. Such tubes and their associated enteral routes include the *nasogastric* (NG) tube from nares to stomach; the *nasojejunal* (NJ) tube from nares to jejunum; and the *gastrostomy* tube (GT) placed directly through the abdomen into the stomach.

It is important to recognize that some solid form medications are intended to be given whole to achieve a specific effect in the body. For example, enteric-coated medications protect the stomach by dissolving in the duodenum. Sustained-release capsules allow for gradual release of medication over time and should be swallowed whole. Consult a drug reference or the pharmacist if you are in doubt about the safety of crushing tablets or opening capsules.

Tablets and Capsules

Medications prepared in tablet and capsule form are supplied in the strengths or dosages in which they are commonly prescribed (Figure 9-1). It is desirable to obtain the drug in the same strength as the dosage ordered or in multiples of that dosage. When necessary, scored tablets (those marked for division) can be divided into halves or quarters. Only scored tablets are intended to be divided.

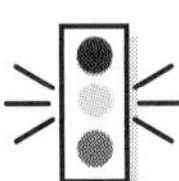

Caution: It is safest and most accurate to give the fewest number of whole, undivided tablets possible.

Example 1:

The doctor's order reads: *Tylenol (acetaminophen) 500 mg p.o. q.3–4h p.r.n. for mild pain.*

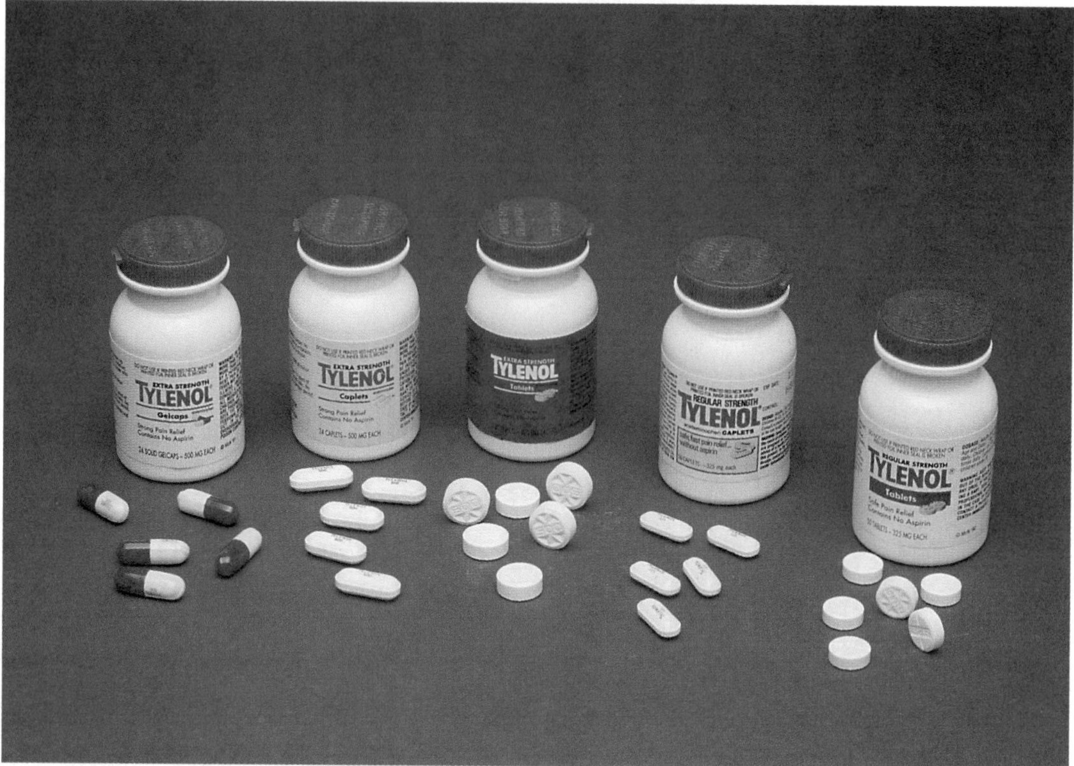

FIGURE 9-1 Tablets, Caplets, and Gelcaps

Tylenol comes in strengths of 325 milligrams per tablet or caplet and 500 milligrams per tablet, caplet, or gelcap. When both strengths are available, the nurse should select the 500-milligram strength, and give one whole tablet for each dose.

Example 2:

The doctor's order reads: *Codeine 45 mg p.o. stat.*

Codeine comes in strengths of 15 mg, 30 mg, and 60 mg scored tablets. When the three strengths are available, the nurse should select one 15 mg tablet and one 30 mg tablet (15 mg + 30 mg = 45 mg). This provides the ordered dose of 45 mg and is the least amount of tablets (2 tablets total) for the patient to swallow.

You might want to halve the 60 mg tablet to obtain two 30 mg parts and pair one-half with a 15 mg tablet. This would also equal 45 mg and give you $1\frac{1}{2}$ tablets. But, cutting any scored tablet in half may produce slightly unequal halves. Your patient may not get the ordered dose as a result. It is preferable to give whole, undivided tablets, when they are available.

Three-Step Approach to Dosage Calculations

Now you are ready to learn to solve dosage problems. The following simple three-step method has been proven to reduce anxiety about calculations and ensure that your results are accurate. Take notice that you will be asked to think or estimate before you apply a formula. Learn and commit this simple three-step approach to memory and use it for every dosage calculation every time.

remember

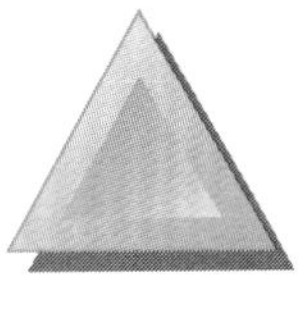

Simple Three-Step Approach to Dosage Calculations

STEP 1	**CONVERT**	Ensure all measurements are in the same system of measurement and the same size unit of measurement. If not, convert before proceeding.
STEP 2	**THINK**	Estimate what is a *reasonable amount* of the drug to be administered.
STEP 3	**CALCULATE**	Apply the formula: $\frac{D}{H} \times Q = X$ $\frac{\text{D (desired)}}{\text{H (have)}} \times \text{Q (quantity)} = \text{X (amount)}$

Let's carefully examine each of the three steps as essential consecutive rules of accurate dosage calculation.

rule

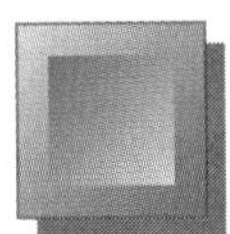

STEP 1	**CONVERT**	Be sure that all measurements are in the same system and all units are in the same size, converting when necessary.

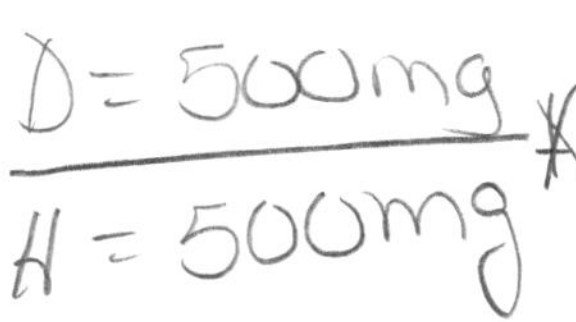

Many medications are both ordered and supplied in the same system of measurement and the same size unit of measurement. This makes dosage calculation very easy, because no conversion is necessary. When this is not the case, then you must convert to the same system or the same size units. Let's look at two examples where conversion is a necessary first step in dosage calculation.

Example 1:

The drug order reads: *Keflex 0.5 g p.o. q.6h.* The supply dosage (what is available on hand) is labeled "*Keflex 500 mg per capsule.*" This is an example of a medication order written and supplied in the same system (metric), but in different size units (g and mg). A drug order written in grams but supplied in milligrams will need to be converted to the same size unit.

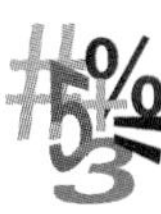

math tip: In most cases, it is more practical to change to the smaller unit (such as g to mg). This requires multiplication and usually eliminates the decimal or fraction, keeping the calculation in whole numbers.

To continue with Example 1, you should convert 0.5 gram to milligrams. Notice that milligrams is the smaller unit and converting eliminates the decimal fraction.

Equivalent: 1 g = 1000 mg

Remember: You are converting from a larger to a smaller unit. Therefore, you will multiply by the conversion factor of 1000 or move the decimal point three places to the right.

0.5 g = 0.5 × 1000 = 0.500. = 500 mg

Order: Keflex 500 mg

Supply: Keflex 500 mg per capsule

You would give the patient 1 Keflex 500 mg capsule.

math tip: Convert apothecary and household measurements to their metric equivalents. This will be helpful for your calculations even if the conversion is to a larger unit. The metric system is the predominant system of measurement for drugs.

Example 2:

The drug order reads: *Phenobarbital gr ss p.o. q.12h.* The supply dosage (what you have available on hand) is labeled *phenobarbital 15 mg per tablet.* This is an example of the medication ordered in one system but supplied in a different system. The medication order is written in the apothecary system, and the medication is supplied in the metric system. You must recall the approximate equivalents and convert both amounts to the same system. You should convert the apothecary measure to metric.

Approximate equivalent: gr i = 60 mg

Remember: You are converting from a larger to a smaller unit; therefore, you will multiply by the conversion factor of 60.

gr ss $= \frac{1}{2} \times 60 = \frac{60}{2} = 30$ mg

Now the problem looks like this:

Order: phenobarbital 30 mg

Supply: phenobarbital 15 mg per tablet

Now you can probably solve this problem in your head. That's what step 2 is about.

rule

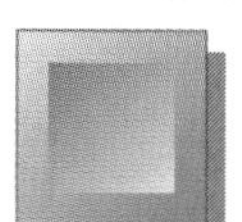

STEP 2 **THINK** Carefully consider what is the reasonable amount of the drug that should be administered.

Once you have converted all units to the same system and size, step 2 asks you to logically conclude what amount should be given. Before you go on to step 3, you may be able to picture in your mind a reasonable amount of medication to be administered, such as demonstrated in the previous two examples. At least you should be able to estimate a very close approximation, such as more or less than one tablet (capsule or milliliter). Basically step 2 asks you to *stop and think before you go any farther.*

In the phenobarbital example, you estimate that the patient should receive more than one tablet. In fact, you realize that you would administer two of the 15 mg tablets to complete the order for gr ss or 30 mg.

rule

STEP 3 **CALCULATE** Apply the dosage calculation formula: $\frac{D}{H} \times Q = X$

Always doublecheck your estimated amount from step 2 with the simple formula $\frac{D}{H} \times Q = X$.

In this formula, *D* represents the *desired* dosage or the dosage ordered. *H* represents the dosage you have on *hand* per a *quantity, Q.*

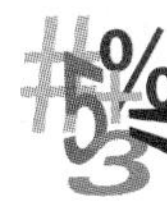

math tip: When solving dosage problems for drugs supplied in tablets or capsules, Q (quantity) is always 1, because the supply dosage is per one tablet or capsule.

Therefore, Q = 1 tablet or capsule.

Let's use the $\frac{D}{H} \times Q = X$ formula to doublecheck our thinking, and calculate the dosages for the previous phenobarbital example.

Order: *Phenobarbital gr ss p.o. q.12h,* convert to phenobarbital 30 mg

Supply: *phenobarbital 15 mg per tablet*

D = desired = 30 mg

H = have = 15 mg

Q = quantity = 1 tablet

$$\frac{D}{H} \times Q = \frac{30 \text{ mg}}{15 \text{ mg}} \times 1 \text{ tablet}$$

$$\frac{\overset{2}{\cancel{30}}\ \cancel{\text{mg}}}{\underset{1}{\cancel{15}}\ \cancel{\text{mg}}} \times 1 \text{ tablet} = 2 \times 1 \text{ tablet} = 2 \text{ tablets}$$ (Notice that mg cancel out.)

Give two of the 15 mg phenobarbital tablets. The calculations verify your estimate from step 2.

Notice that the formula is set up with *D (desired dosage)* as the numerator and *H* (dosage you *have* on hand) as the denominator of a fraction. You are calculating for some portion of Q (*quantity* you have on hand). You can see that setting up a dosage calculation like this makes sense. Let's look at two more examples to reinforce this concept.

Example 3:

Order: *Lasix 10 mg p.o. b.i.d.*

Supply: *Lasix 20 mg per tablet*

$$\frac{D}{H} \times Q = \frac{10 \text{ mg}}{20 \text{ mg}} \times 1 \text{ tablet}$$

$$\frac{\overset{1}{\cancel{10}}\ \cancel{\text{mg}}}{\underset{2}{\cancel{20}}\ \cancel{\text{mg}}} \times 1 \text{ tablet} = \frac{1}{2} \times 1 \text{ tablet} = \frac{1}{2} \text{ tablet}$$

Notice that you want to give $\frac{1}{2}$ of the Q (quantity of the supply dosage you have on hand, which in this case is 1 tablet). Therefore, you want to give $\frac{1}{2}$ tablet.

Example 4:

Order: *Tylenol 1000 mg p.o. q.3–4h p.r.n., headache*

Supply: *Tylenol 500 mg per tablet*

$$\frac{D}{H} \times Q = \frac{1000 \text{ mg}}{500 \text{ mg}} \times 1 \text{ tablet}$$

$$\frac{\overset{2}{\cancel{1000}}\ \cancel{\text{mg}}}{\underset{1}{\cancel{500}}\ \cancel{\text{mg}}} \times 1 \text{ tablet} = \frac{2}{1} \times 1 \text{ tablet} = 2 \text{ tablets}$$

Notice that you want to give 2 times the amount of Q or you want to give 2 tablets.

Now you are ready to apply all three steps of this logical approach to dosage calculations. The same three steps will be used to solve both oral and parenteral dosage calculation problems. It is most important that you develop the ability to reason for the answer or estimate before you apply the $\frac{D}{H} \times Q = X$ formula.

Note to Learner

Errors are often made unknowingly because nurses rely solely on a formula rather than first asking themselves what the answer should be. As a nurse or allied health professional, you are expected to be able to reason sensibly, problem solve, and justify your judgments rationally. With these same skills you gain admission to your educational program and to your profession. While you sharpen your math skills, your ability to think and estimate are your best resources to ensure that you avoid errors. Use the formula as a calculation tool to validate the dose amount you anticipate should be given, rather than the reverse. If your reasoning is sound, you will find the dosages you compute make sense and are accurate. For example, if your calculations result in directing you to administer 15 tablets of any medication, you would question this.

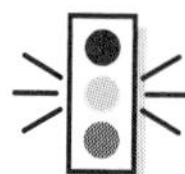

Caution: The maximum number of tablets or capsules for a single dose is *usually* three. Recheck your calculation if a single dose requires more.

Let's examine more examples of oral dosages supplied in capsules and tablets to reinforce the three basic steps. Then you will be ready to solve problems like these on your own.

Example 1:

The drug order is *Lopressor 100 mg p.o. b.i.d.* The medicine container is labeled *Lopressor 50 mg per tablet.* Calculate one dose.

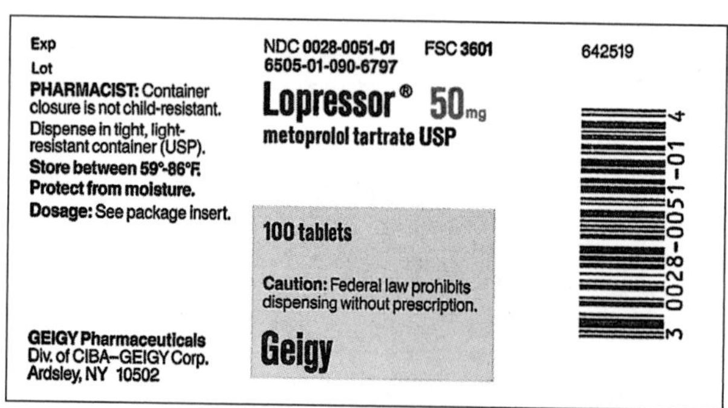

STEP 1 CONVERT No conversion is necessary. The units are in the same system (metric) and the same size (mg).

STEP 2 THINK You want to administer 100 milligrams, and you have 50 milligrams in each tablet. You want to give twice the equivalent of each tablet, or you want to administer 2 tablets per dose.

STEP 3 CALCULATE $\frac{D}{H} \times Q = \frac{100 \text{ mg}}{50 \text{ mg}} \times 1 \text{ tablet}$

$\frac{\overset{2}{\cancel{100 \text{ mg}}}}{\underset{1}{\cancel{50 \text{ mg}}}} \times 1 \text{ tablet} = 2 \times 1 \text{ tablet} = 2$ tablets; given orally twice daily

Doublecheck to be sure your calculated dosage matches your *reasonable* dosage from step 2. If for example, you had calculated to give more or less than 2 tablets of Lopressor, you would suspect a calculation error.

Example 2:

The physician prescribes *Ampicillin 0.5 g p.o. q.i.d.* The dosage available is *Ampicillin 250 mg per capsule.* How many capsules should the nurse give to the patient per dose?

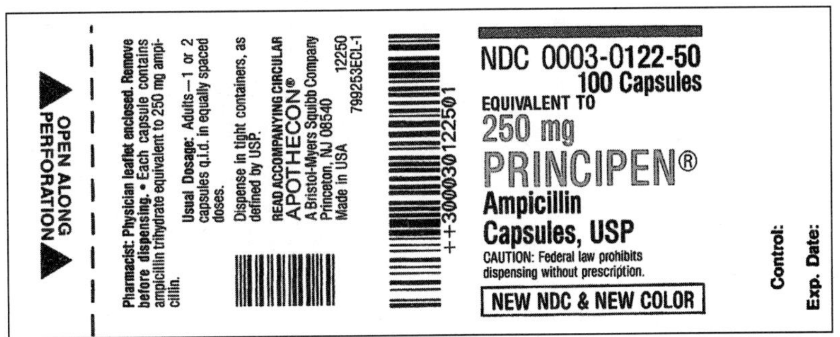

STEP 1 CONVERT

To the same size units. Convert 0.5 g to mg. Remember the math tip: Convert larger unit (g) to the smaller unit (mg).

Equivalent: 1 g = 1000 mg. Conversion factor is 1000.

Larger → Smaller: (×)

$0.5 \text{ g} = 0.5 \times 1000 = 0.500. = 500 \text{ mg}$

Cross out 0.5 g in the order, and write the equivalent of 500 mg above it.

Order: Ampicillin ~~0.5 g~~ 500 mg

Supply: Ampicillin 250 mg capsules

By now you probably can do conversions like this from memory.

STEP 2 THINK

500 mg is twice as much as 250 milligrams. You want to give 2 capsules.

STEP 3 CALCULATE

$$\frac{D}{H} \times Q = \frac{500 \text{ mg}}{250 \text{ mg}} \times 1 \text{ capsule}$$

$$\frac{\overset{2}{\cancel{500 \text{ mg}}}}{\underset{1}{\cancel{250 \text{ mg}}}} \times 1 \text{ capsule} = 2 \times 1 \text{ capsule} = 2 \text{ capsules; given orally 4 times daily.}$$

Example 3:

The drug order reads *Codeine sulfate gr $\frac{3}{4}$ p.o. q.4h p.r.n., pain.* The drug supplied is *Codeine sulfate 30 mg per tablet.* Calculate one dose.

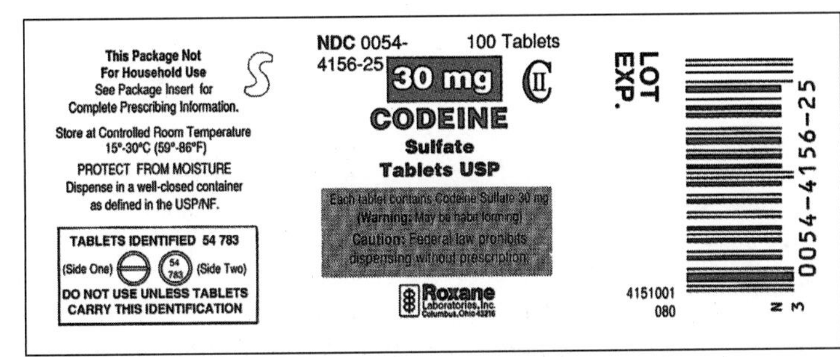

STEP 1 CONVERT

To equivalent units in the same system of measurement. Convert gr to mg. Approximate equivalent: gr i = 60 mg. Conversion factor is 60. Larger → Smaller: (×).

$$\text{gr } \frac{3}{4} = \frac{3}{\cancel{4}_{1}} \times \cancel{60}^{15} = 45 \text{ mg}$$

Order: Codeine ~~gr 3/4~~ 45 mg

Supply: Codeine 30 mg tablets

STEP 2 THINK

You estimate that you want to give more than one tablet but less than two tablets.

STEP 3 CALCULATE

$$\frac{D}{H} \times Q = \frac{45 \text{ mg}}{30 \text{ mg}} \times 1 \text{ tablet}$$

$$\frac{\cancel{45 \text{ mg}}^{3}}{\cancel{30 \text{ mg}}_{2}} \times 1 \text{ tablet} = \frac{3}{2} \text{ tablets} = 1\frac{1}{2} \text{ tablets; given every 3 to 4 hours as needed for pain}$$

Now you can see that a dosage problem that may have seemed difficult on first reading is actually very simple. Approach every dosage calculation just like this: one step at a time.

Example 4:

Halcion 0.25 mg tablets are available.

The order is *Halcion 125 mcg p.o. h.s.* How many tablets will you give?

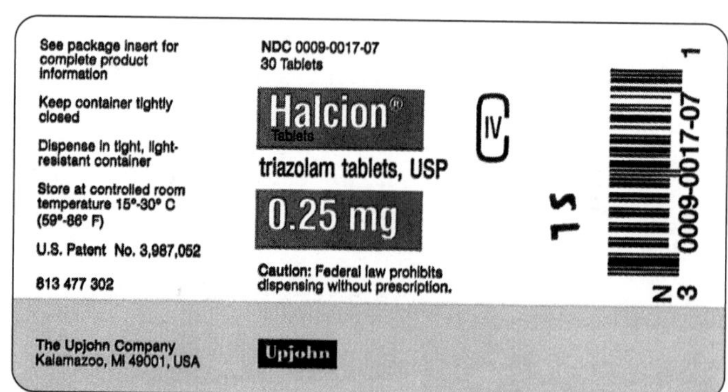

STEP 1 CONVERT

To same size units. Remember the math tip: Convert larger unit (mg) to smaller unit (mcg).

Approximate equivalent: 1 mg = 1000 mcg. Conversion factor is 1000.

Larger → Smaller: (×)

0.25 mg = 0.25 × 1000 = 0.250. = 250 mcg

Order: Halcion 125 mcg

Supply: Halcion ~~0.25 mg~~ 250 mcg tablets

STEP 2 THINK

As soon as you convert the supply dosage of Halcion 0.25 mg to Halcion 250 mcg, you realize that to give the ordered dosage of 125 mcg, you want to give less than 1 tablet for each dose. In fact, you want to give $\frac{1}{2}$ of the supply dosage, which is the same as $\frac{1}{2}$ tablet.

Avoid getting confused by the way the original problem is presented. Be sure that you recognize which is the dosage ordered (D—desired) and which is the supply dosage (H—have on hand) per the quantity on hand (Q). A common error is to misread the information and mix up the calculations in step 3. This demonstrates the importance of thinking (step 2) before you calculate.

STEP 3 CALCULATE

$$\frac{D}{H} \times Q = \frac{125\text{ mg}}{250\text{ mg}} \times 1\text{ tablet}$$

$$\frac{\overset{1}{\cancel{125\text{ mg}}}}{\underset{2}{\cancel{250\text{ mg}}}} \times 1\text{ tablet} = \frac{1}{2} \times 1\text{ tablet} = \frac{1}{2}\text{ tablet; given at bedtime}$$

Example 5:

Your client is to receive *Nitrostat gr $\frac{1}{400}$ SL p.r.n. for angina pain.* The label on the available Nitrostat bottle tells you that each tablet provides 0.3 mg (gr $\frac{1}{200}$). How much will you give your client?

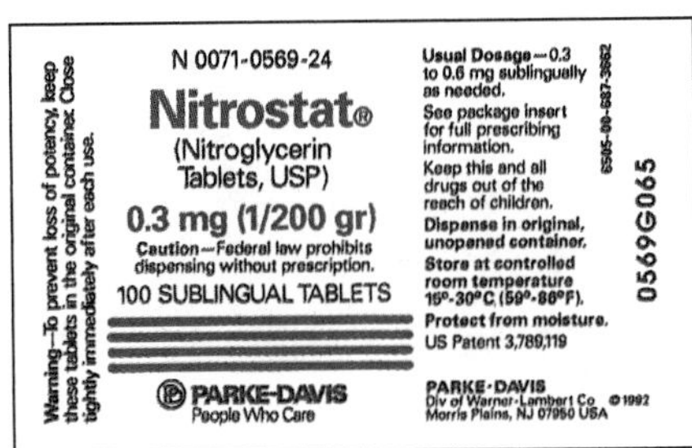

STEP 1 CONVERT

To equivalent units in the same system of measurement. Remember the math tip: Convert apothecary measurement to metric units. Convert the order in grains to milligrams. Approximate equivalent: gr i = 60 mg. Conversion factor is 60. Larger → Smaller: (×).

$$\text{gr } \frac{1}{400} = \frac{1}{\underset{20}{\cancel{400}}} \times \overset{3}{\cancel{60}} = \frac{3}{20} = 0.15\text{ mg}$$

Order: Nitrostat ~~gr 1/400~~ 0.15 mg

Supply: Nitrostat 0.3 mg tablets

STEP 2 THINK

Look at the supply dosage and add a zero at the end of the decimal number: 0.3 mg = 0.30 mg. Now you can compare the ordered dosage of 0.15 mg with the supply dosage of 0.30 mg per tablet. You can reason that you want to give less than 1 tablet. Further, you can see that 0.15 is $\frac{1}{2}$ of 0.30, and you know that you want to give $\frac{1}{2}$ tablet. Check your reasoning in step 3.

STEP 3 **CALCULATE** $\frac{D}{H} \times Q = \frac{0.15 \text{ mg}}{0.30 \text{ mg}} \times 1 \text{ tablet}$

$$\frac{\overset{1}{\cancel{0.15 \text{ mg}}}}{\underset{2}{\cancel{0.30 \text{ mg}}}} \times 1 \text{ tablet} = \frac{1}{2} \times 1 \text{ tablet} = \frac{1}{2} \text{ tablet; given sublingually for angina pain}$$

quick review

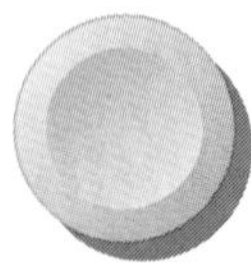

Simple Three-Step Approach to Dosage Calculations

STEP 1 **CONVERT** To units of the same system and the same size.

STEP 2 **THINK** Estimate for a reasonable amount to give.

STEP 3 **CALCULATE** $\frac{D}{H} \times Q = X$

$$\frac{\text{D (desired)}}{\text{H (have)}} \times \text{Q (quantity)} = \text{X (amount)}$$

- For most dosage calculation problems:
  - convert to smaller size unit. Example: g → mg
  - convert from the apothecary or household system to the metric system. Example: gr → mg
- Consider the reasonableness of the calculated amount to give. Example: You would question giving 10 tablets or capsules per dose for oral administration.

review set 25

Calculate the correct number of tablets or capsules to be administered per dose. Tablets are scored.

1. The physician writes an order for *Diabinese 0.1 g p.o. q.d.* The drug container label reads Diabinese 100 mg tablets.

   Give: ________ tablet(s)

2. Duricef 500 mg tablets available. The order is for *Duricef 0.5 g p.o. b.i.d.*

   Give: ________ tablet(s)

3. Urecholine 10 mg tablets available. Order: *Urecholine 15 mg p.o. t.i.d.*

   Give: ________ tablet(s)

4. Order: *Hydrochlorothiazide 12.5 mg p.o. t.i.d.* 25 mg tablets available.

   Give: ________ tablet(s)

5. Order: *Lanoxin 0.125 mg p.o. q.d.*

   Supply: Lanoxin 0.25 mg tablets

   Give: ________ tablet(s)

6. Order: *Motrin 600 mg p.o. b.i.d.*

   Supply: Motrin 300 mg tablets

   Give: ________ tablet(s)

7. Order: *Slow-K 16 mEq p.o. stat*

   Supply: Slow-K 8 mEq tablets

   Give: __________ tablet(s)

8. Cytoxan 25 mg tablets available. Order: *Cytoxan 50 mg p.o. q.d.*

   Give: __________ tablet(s)

9. Zaroxolyn 5 mg tablets available. Order: *Zaroxolyn 7.5 mg p.o. b.i.d.*

   Give: __________ tablet(s)

10. *Coumadin 5 mg p.o. q.d.* ordered. Coumadine 2.5 mg tablets available.

    Give: __________ tablet(s)

11. Drug "X" is available in 0.5 g tablets. Ordered dose is *Drug "X" 1.5 g p.o. q.i.d.* How many tablets are needed for each dose? __________ tablet(s)

    How many grams will the patient receive per day? __________ g

12. Order: *Trandate 150 mg p.o. b.i.d.*

    Supply: Trandate 300 mg tablets

    Give: __________ tablet(s)

13. Order: *Duricef 1 g p.o. q.i.d. a.c.*

    Supply: Duricef 500 mg capsules

    Give: __________ capsule(s)

14. Synthroid 50 mcg tablets available. Order: *Synthroid 0.1 mg p.o. q.d.*

    Give: __________ tablet(s)

15. *Tranxene 7.5 mg p.o. q.i.d.* is ordered and you have 3.75 mg Tranxene capsules available.

    Give: __________ capsule(s)

16. Order: *Inderal 15 mg p.o. t.i.d.*

    Supply: Inderal 10 mg tablets

    Give: __________ tablet(s)

17. The doctor orders *Loniten gr $\frac{1}{6}$ p.o. stat* and you have available Loniten 10 mg and 2.5 mg scored tablets. Select __________ mg tablets and give __________ tablet(s).

18. Order: *Peritrate gr ss p.o. 1 h a.c. et h.s.* You have available Peritrate 10 mg, 20 mg, and 40 mg scored tablets. Select __________ mg tablets and give __________ tablet(s). How many doses of Peritrate will the patient receive in 24 hours? __________ dose(s)

19. Order: *Phenobarbital gr $\frac{1}{4}$ p.o. q.d.*

    Supply: Phenobarbital 15 mg, 30 mg, 60 mg scored tablets.

    Select __________ mg tablets and give __________ tablet(s).

20. Order: *Tylenol $\bar{c}$ codeine gr i p.o..q.4h p.r.n. pain*

    Supply: Tylenol with codeine 7.5 mg, 15 mg, 30 mg, and 60 mg tablets.

    Select __________ mg tablets and give __________ tablet(s).

Calculate one dose for each of the medication orders 21 through 30. The labels lettered A through J are the drugs you have available. Indicate the letter corresponding to the label you select.

21. Order: *Dilatrate-SR 80 mg p.o. b.i.d.*
    Select: ________
    Give: ________
22. Order: *Carbamazepine 0.2 g p.o. t.i.d.*
    Select: ________
    Give: ________
23. Order: *Lopressor 50 mg p.o. b.i.d.*
    Select: ________
    Give: ________
24. Order: *Potassium chloride 16 mEq p.o. q.d.*
    Select: ________
    Give: ________
25. Order: *Procan SR 1 g p.o. q.6h*
    Select: ________
    Give: ________
26. Order: *Cephalexin 0.5 g q.i.d.*
    Select: ________
    Give: ________
27. Order: *Danazol 0.4 g p.o. b.i.d.*
    Select: ________
    Give: ________
28. Order: *Digoxin 0.5 mg p.o. q.d.*
    Select: ________
    Give: ________
29. Order: *Meclofenamate sodium 0.1 g p.o. t.i.d.*
    Select: ________
    Give: ________
30. Order: *Procainamide hydrochloride 1000 mg q.6h*
    Select: ________
    Give: ________

After completing these problems, see page 426 to check your answers.

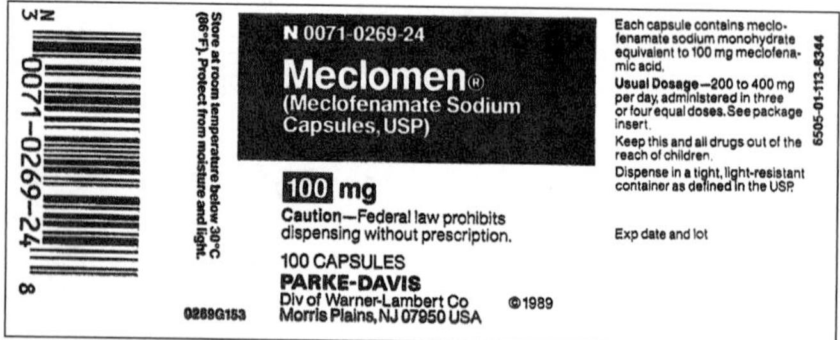

A

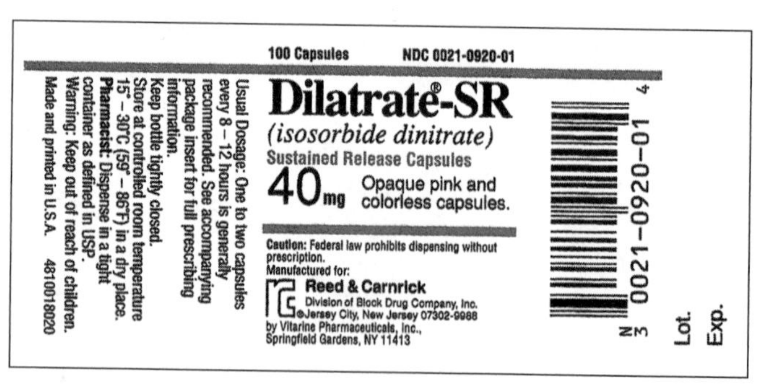

B

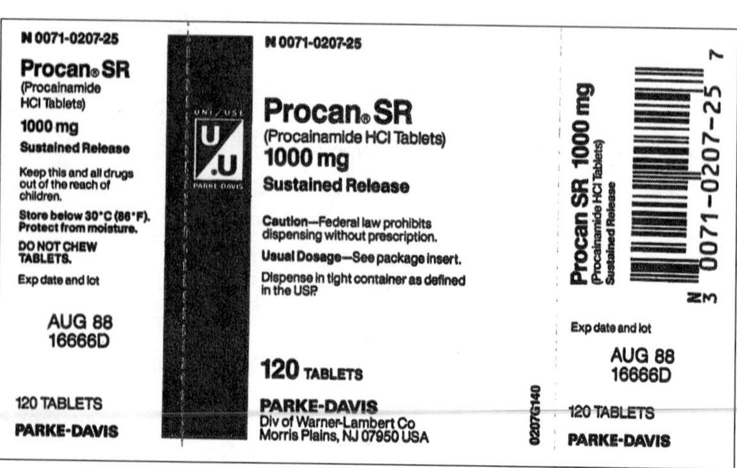

C

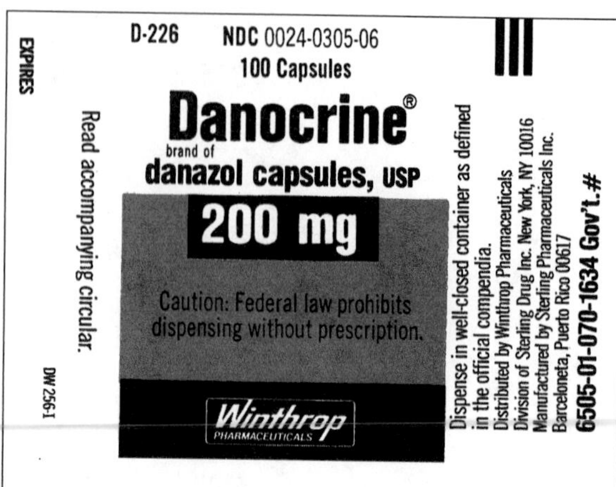

D

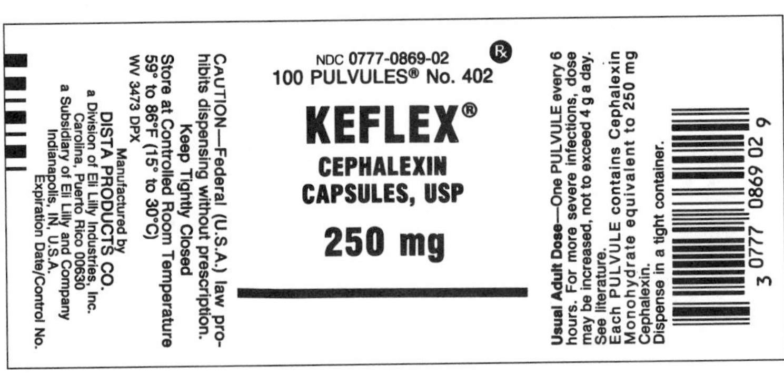
NDC 0777-0869-02
100 PULVULES® No. 402
KEFLEX®
CEPHALEXIN
CAPSULES, USP
250 mg
CAUTION—Federal (U.S.A.) law prohibits dispensing without prescription.
Keep Tightly Closed
Store at Controlled Room Temperature 59° to 86°F (15° to 30°C)
WV 3473 DPX
Manufactured by
DISTA PRODUCTS CO.
a Division of Eli Lilly Industries, Inc.
Carolina, Puerto Rico 00630
a Subsidiary of Eli Lilly and Company
Indianapolis, IN, U.S.A.
Expiration Date/Control No.
Usual Adult Dose—One PULVULE every 6 hours. For more severe infections, dose may be increased, not to exceed 4 g a day. See literature.
Each PULVULE contains Cephalexin Monohydrate equivalent to 250 mg Cephalexin.
Dispense in a tight container.
3 0777 0869 02 9

E

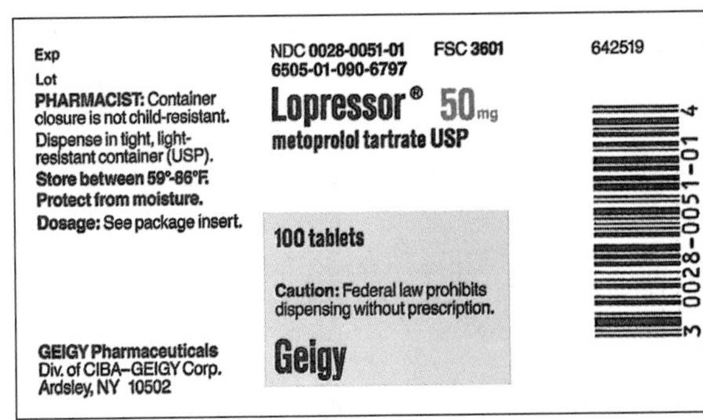
Exp
Lot
PHARMACIST: Container closure is not child-resistant.
Dispense in tight, light-resistant container (USP).
Store between 59°-86°F.
Protect from moisture.
Dosage: See package insert.
GEIGY Pharmaceuticals
Div. of CIBA-GEIGY Corp.
Ardsley, NY 10502
NDC 0028-0051-01 FSC 3601
6505-01-090-6797
Lopressor® 50 mg
metoprolol tartrate USP
100 tablets
Caution: Federal law prohibits dispensing without prescription.
Geigy
642519
3 0028-0051-01 4

F

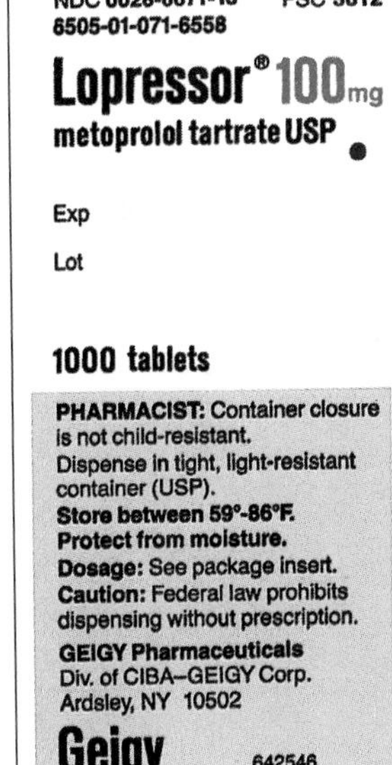
NDC 0028-0071-10 FSC 3612
6505-01-071-6558
Lopressor® 100 mg
metoprolol tartrate USP
Exp
Lot
1000 tablets
PHARMACIST: Container closure is not child-resistant.
Dispense in tight, light-resistant container (USP).
Store between 59°-86°F.
Protect from moisture.
Dosage: See package insert.
Caution: Federal law prohibits dispensing without prescription.
GEIGY Pharmaceuticals
Div. of CIBA-GEIGY Corp.
Ardsley, NY 10502
Geigy
642546

G

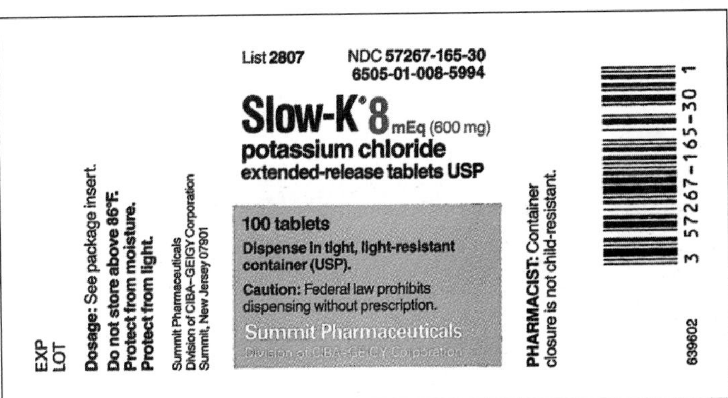
For indications, dosage, precautions, etc., see accompanying package insert.
Made in U.S.A.
100 Tablets
Professional Package Not To Be Sold
LANOXIN®
(DIGOXIN)
Each scored tablet contains
250 μg (0.25 mg)
Store at 15°-30°C (59°-86°F) in a dry place.
CAUTION: Federal law prohibits dispensing without prescription.
BURROUGHS WELLCOME CO.
Research Triangle Park, NC 27709
Sample for Educational Use Only

H

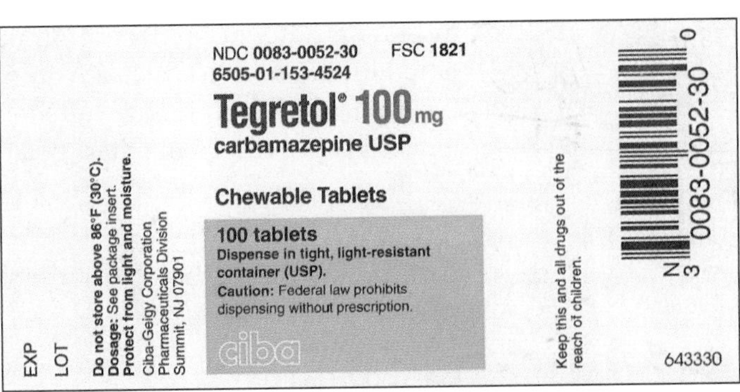
List 2807
NDC 57267-165-30
6505-01-008-5994
Slow-K® 8 mEq (600 mg)
potassium chloride
extended-release tablets USP
EXP
LOT
Dosage: See package insert.
Do not store above 86°F.
Protect from moisture.
Protect from light.
Summit Pharmaceuticals
Division of CIBA-GEIGY Corporation
Summit, New Jersey 07901
100 tablets
Dispense in tight, light-resistant container (USP).
Caution: Federal law prohibits dispensing without prescription.
Summit Pharmaceuticals
Division of CIBA-GEIGY Corporation
PHARMACIST: Container closure is not child-resistant.
3 57267-165-30 1
639602

I

NDC 0083-0052-30 FSC 1821
6505-01-153-4524
Tegretol® 100 mg
carbamazepine USP
Chewable Tablets
100 tablets
Dispense in tight, light-resistant container (USP).
Caution: Federal law prohibits dispensing without prescription.
ciba
EXP
LOT
Do not store above 86°F (30°C).
Dosage: See package insert.
Protect from light and moisture.
Ciba-Geigy Corporation
Pharmaceuticals Division
Summit, NJ 07901
Keep this and all drugs out of the reach of children.
N 3 0083-0052-30 0
643330

J

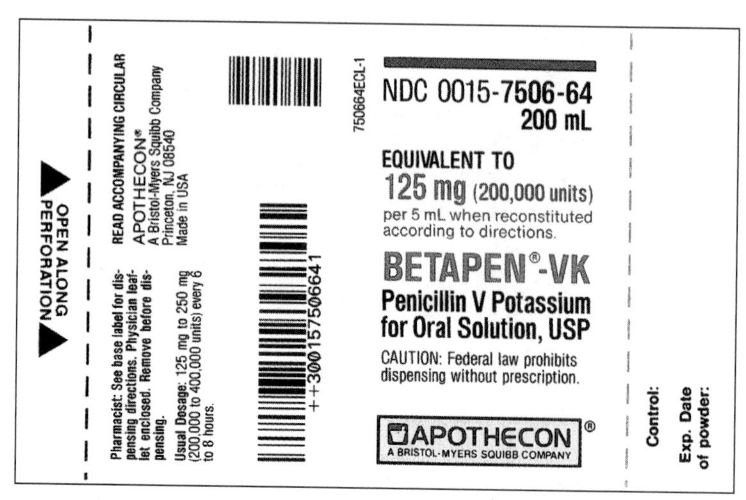

FIGURE 9-2 (a) Oral Liquid: Betapen-VK 125 mg per 5 mL

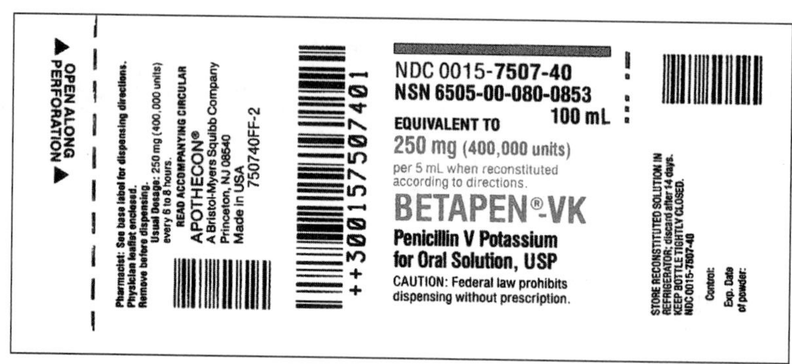

FIGURE 9-2 (b) Oral Liquid: Betapen-VK 250 mg per 5 mL

Oral Liquids

Oral liquids are supplied in solution form and contain a specific amount of drug in a given amount of solution as stated on the label (Figures 9-2a and 9-2b).

In solving dosage problems when the drug is supplied in solid form, you calculated the number of tablets or capsules that contained the prescribed dosage. The supply container label indicates the amount of medication per one tablet or one capsule. For medications supplied in liquid form, you must calculate the volume of the liquid that contains the prescribed dosage of the drug. The supply dosage noted on the label may indicate the amount of drug per one milliliter or per multiple milliliters of solution, such as 10 mg per 2 mL, 125 mg per 5 mL, or 1.2 g per 30 mL.

Steps 1, 2, and 3 can be used to solve liquid oral dosage calculations in the same way that solid form oral dosages were calculated. Let's apply the three steps to dosage calculations in a few examples.

Example 1:

The doctor orders *Betapen-VK 100 mg p.o. q.i.d.* Look at the labels of Betapen-VK available in Figure 9-2a and 9-2b. You choose *Betapen-VK 125 mg per 5 mL.* Follow the three steps to dosage calculations.

STEP 1 CONVERT No conversion is necessary, because the order and supply dosage are both in the same units.

STEP 2 THINK You want to give less than 125 mg, so you want to give less than 5 mL. Doublecheck your thinking with the $\frac{D}{H} \times Q = X$ formula.

STEP 3 CALCULATE $\frac{D}{H} \times Q = \frac{100 \text{ mg}}{125 \text{ mg}} \times 5 \text{ mL} = X$

$$\frac{\overset{4}{\cancel{100}\ \cancel{\text{mg}}}}{\underset{5}{\cancel{125}\ \cancel{\text{mg}}}} \times 5 \text{ mL} = \frac{20}{5} \text{ mL} = 4 \text{ mL}$$

You will give 4 mL of the Betapen-VK with the dosage strength of 125 mg per 5 mL. Doublecheck to be sure your calculated dosage is consistent with your *reasonable* dosage from step 2. If, for instance, you calculate to give *more* than 5 mL, then you should suspect an error.

Example 2:

Suppose, using the same drug order in Example 1, *Betapen-VK 100 mg p.o. q.i.d.*, you choose the other oral solution, *Betapen-VK 250 mg per 5 mL*. Follow the three steps to dosage calculations.

STEP 1 CONVERT No conversion is necessary, because the order and supply dosage are both in the same units and system.

STEP 2 THINK You want to give 100 mg, and you have 250 mg per 5 mL so you will give less than half of 5 mL. Doublecheck your thinking with the $\frac{D}{H} \times Q = X$ formula.

STEP 3 CALCULATE $\frac{D}{H} \times Q = \frac{100 \text{ mg}}{250 \text{ mg}} \times 5 \text{ mL}$

$$\frac{\overset{2}{\cancel{100}\ \cancel{\text{mg}}}}{\underset{5}{\cancel{250}\ \cancel{\text{mg}}}} \times 5 \text{ mL} = \frac{10}{5} = 2 \text{ mL}$$

Notice that in both Example 1 and Example 2, the supply quantity is the same (5 mL), but the dosage strength (weight) of medication is different (125 mg per 5 mL vs. 250 mg per 5 mL). This results in the calculated dose volume (amount to give) being different (4 mL vs. 2 mL). This difference is the result of each liquid's *concentration*. *Betapen-VK 125 mg per 5 mL* is half as concentrated as *Betapen-VK 250 mg per 5 mL*. In other words, there is half as much drug in 5 mL of the *125 mg per 5 mL* supply as there is in 5 mL of the *250 mg per 5 mL* supply. Likewise, *Betapen-VK 250 mg per 5 mL* is twice as concentrated as *Betapen-VK 125 mg per 5 mL*. The more concentrated solution allows you to give the patient less volume per dose for the same dosage. This is significant when administering medication to infants and small children when a smaller quantity is needed. Think about this carefully until it is clear.

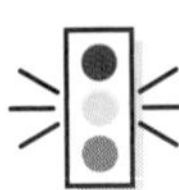

Caution: Think before you calculate. It is important to estimate before you apply any formula. In this way, if you make a careless error in math or if you set up the problem incorrectly, your thinking will alert you to *try again*.

Example 3:

The doctor orders *potassium chloride 40 mEq p.o. q.d.* The label on the package reads *potassium chloride 20 mEq per 15 mL.* How many mL should you administer?

NDC 0054-8714
DELIVERS 15 ml
POTASSIUM CHLORIDE
20 mEq per 15 ml (10%)
Oral Solution USP
SUGAR FREE Alcohol 5%
Dilute Before Using
Caution: Federal law prohibits dispensing without prescription.
See Package Insert
Roxane Laboratories, Inc.
Columbus, Ohio 43216
PEEL
012

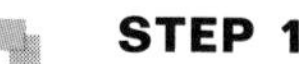

STEP 1 CONVERT No conversion is necessary.

STEP 2 THINK You want to give more than 15 mL. In fact, you want to give exactly twice as much as 15 mL. You know this is true because 40 mEq is twice as much as 20 mEq; therefore, it will take 2 × 15 or 30 mL to give 40 mEq. Continue to step 3 to doublecheck your thinking.

STEP 3 CALCULATE $\frac{D}{H} \times Q = \frac{\overset{2}{\cancel{40}\text{ mEq}}}{\underset{1}{\cancel{20}\text{ mEq}}} \times 15 \text{ mL} = 30 \text{ mL}$

quick review

Look again at Steps 1 through 3 as a valuable dosage calculation checklist.

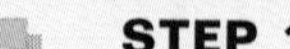

STEP 1 CONVERT Be sure that all measurements are in the same system, and all units are in the same size.

STEP 2 THINK Carefully estimate the reasonable amount of the drug that should be administered.

STEP 3 CALCULATE $\frac{D}{H} \times Q = X$ $\frac{D \text{ (desired)}}{H \text{ (have)}} \times Q \text{ (quantity)} = X \text{ (amount)}$

review set 26

Calculate one dose of the drugs ordered.

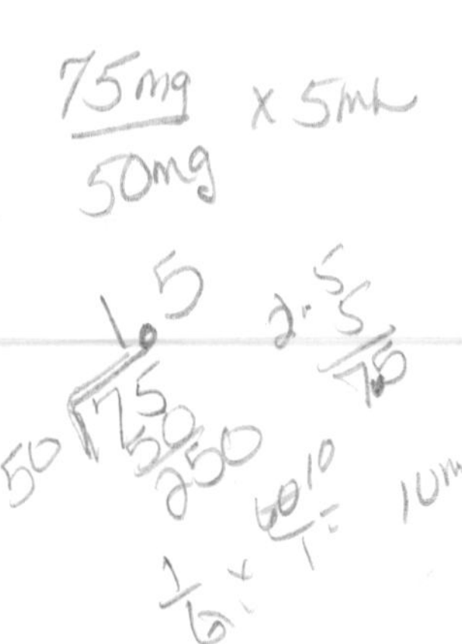

1. Order: *Demerol syrup 75 mg p.o. q.4h p.r.n. pain*

   Supply: Demerol syrup 50 mg per 5 mL

   Give: ________ mL

2. Order: *Phenergan c̄ codeine gr $\frac{1}{6}$ p.o. q.4–6h p.r.n. cough*

   Supply: Phenergan c̄ codeine solution 10 mg per 5 mL

   Give: ________ mL

3. Order: *Pen-Vee K 1 g p.o. 1h pre-op dental surgery*

   Supply: Pen-Vee K oral suspension 250 mg (400,000 U) per 5 mL

   Give: ________ mL

4. Order: *Amoxicillin 100 mg p.o. q.i.d.*

   Supply: 80 mL bottle of Amoxil (amoxicillin) oral pediatric suspension 125 mg per 5 mL

   Give: ________ mL

5. Order: *Tylenol 0.5 g p.o. q.4h p.r.n. pain*

   Supply: Tylenol 500 mg in 5 mL

   Give: __________ t

6. Order: *Promethazine HCl 25 mg p.o. h.s. pre-op*

   Supply: Phenergan Plain (promethazine HCl) 6.25 mg per teaspoon

   Give: __________ mL

7. Order: *Pathocil 125 mg p.o. q.6h a.c.*

   Supply: Pathocil suspension 62.5 mg per 5 mL

   Give: __________ t

8. Order: *Erythromycin suspension 600 mg p.o. q.6h*

   Supply: Erythromycin 400 mg/5 mL

   Give: __________ mL

9. Order: *Ceclor suspension 225 mg p.o. b.i.d.*

   Supply: Celcor suspension 375 mg per 5 mL

   Give: __________ mL

10. Order: *Septra-DS suspension 200 mg p.o. b.i.d.*

    Supply: Septra-DS suspension 400 mg per 5 mL

    Give: __________ mL

11. Order: *Elixophyllin liquid 0.24 g p.o. stat*

    Supply: Elixophyllin liquid 80 mg/7.5 mL

    Give: __________ mL

12. Order: *Trilisate liquid 750 mg p.o. t.i.d.*

    Supply: Trilisate liquid 250 mg/2.5 mL

    Give: __________ mL

13. Order: *Esidrix solution 100 mg p.o. b.i.d.*

    Supply: Esidrix solution 50 mg/5 mL

    Give: __________ t

14. Order: *Pepcid 20 mg p.o. q.i.d.*

    Supply: Pepcid 80 mg/10 mL

    Give: __________ mL

15. Order: *Digoxin elixir 0.25 mg p.o. q.d.*

    Supply: Digoxin elixir 50 mcg/mL

    Give: __________ mL

16. Order: *Nafcillin sodium 0.75 g p.o. q.6h*

    Supply: Nafcillin sodium 250 mg/5 mL

    Give: __________

17. Order: *cephalexin 375 mg p.o. t.i.d.*

    Supply: cephalexin 250 mg/5 mL

    Give: __________ t

18. Order: *Maalox 0.4 g p.o. q.6h p.r.n.*

    Supply: Maalox 400 mg/10 mL

    Give: __________ t

19. Order: *erythromycin 1.2 g p.o. q.8h*

    Supply: erythromycin 400 mg/5 mL

    Give: __________ mL

20. Order: *oxacillin sodium 0.25 g p.o. q.8h*

    Supply: oxacillin sodium 125 mg/2.5 mL

    Give: __________ t

21. Order: *amoxicillin suspension 100 mg p.o. q.6h*

    Supply: amoxicillin suspension 250 mg/5 mL

    Give: __________ mL

Use the labels A, B, and C on page 166 to calculate one dose of the following orders (22, 23, and 24). Indicate the letter corresponding to the label you select.

22. Order: *Erythromycin 125 mg p.o. t.i.d.*

    Select: __________

    Give: __________

23. Order: *Keflex 50 mg p.o. q.6h*

    Select: __________

    Give: __________

24. Order: *Vistaril 10 mg p.o. q.i.d.*

    Select: __________

    Give: __________

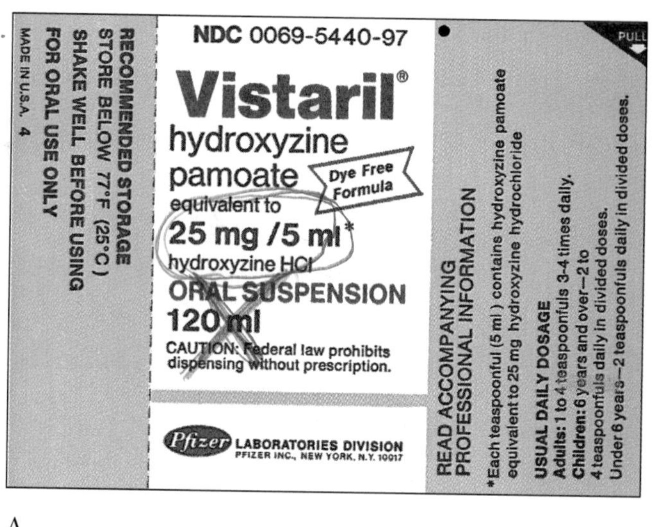

A

NDC 0777-2317-48 ℞ PULL
100 ml
M-153
ILOSONE®
LIQUID
ERYTHROMYCIN ESTOLATE ORAL SUSPENSION, USP
250 mg per 5 ml
DISTA

CAUTION—Federal (U.S.A.) law prohibits dispensing without prescription.
See accompanying literature for dosage.
Each 5 ml contains Erythromycin Estolate equivalent to 250 mg Erythromycin in a pleasantly flavored vehicle.

YC 9310 DPX
Mfd. by
DISTA PRODUCTS COMPANY
a Division of Eli Lilly Industries, Inc.
Carolina, Puerto Rico 00630, a Subsidiary of Eli Lilly & Co., Indianapolis, IN, U.S.A.
Expiration Date

B

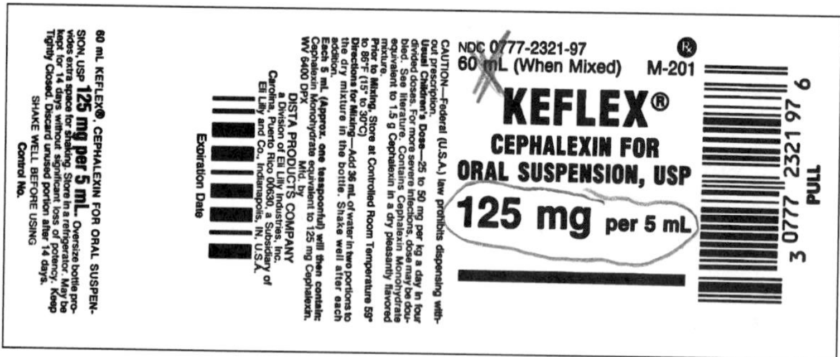

NDC 0777-2321-97 ℞
60 mL (When Mixed)
M-201
KEFLEX®
CEPHALEXIN FOR ORAL SUSPENSION, USP
125 mg per 5 mL
PULL
3 0777 2321 97 6
Expiration Date
60 mL KEFLEX® CEPHALEXIN FOR ORAL SUSPENSION, USP 125 mg per 5 mL
SHAKE WELL BEFORE USING
Control No.

C

Calculate the information requested based on the drugs ordered. The labels provided are the drugs available.

25. Order: *Lanoxin elixir 0.25 mg p.o. q.d.*

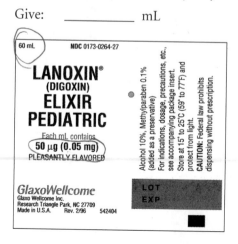

Give: __________ mL

60 mL NDC 0173-0264-27
LANOXIN®
(DIGOXIN)
ELIXIR
PEDIATRIC
Each mL contains
50 μg (0.05 mg)
PLEASANTLY FLAVORED

Alcohol 10%, Methylparaben 0.1% (added as a preservative)
For indications, dosage, precautions, etc., see accompanying package insert.
Store at 15° to 25°C (59° to 77°F) and protect from light.
CAUTION: Federal law prohibits dispensing without prescription.

GlaxoWellcome
Glaxo Wellcome Inc.
Research Triangle Park, NC 27709
Made in U.S.A. Rev. 2/96 542404
LOT
EXP

26. Order: *Lactulose 20 g via gastric tube b.i.d. today*

Give: ℥ __________

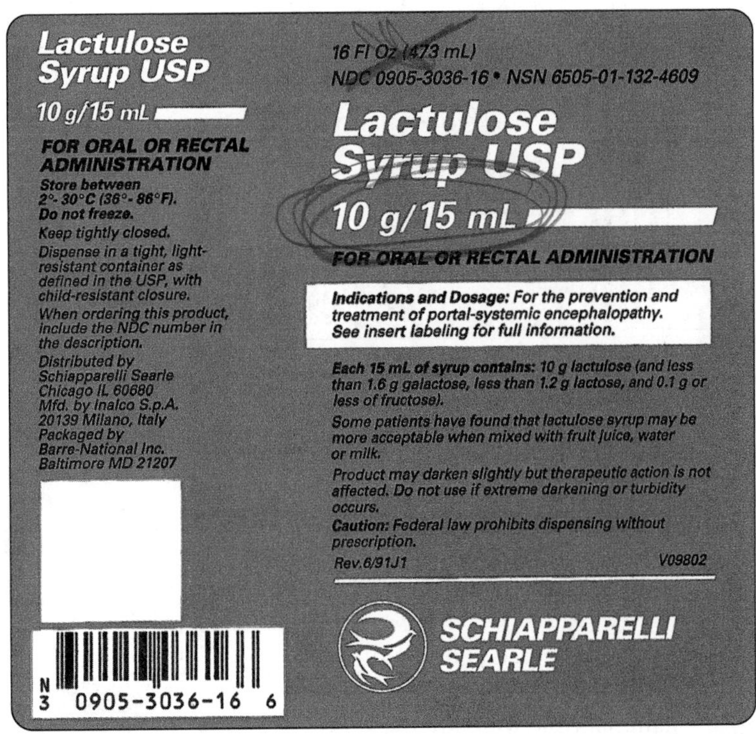

27. Order: *Tussi-Organidin DM 10 mL p.o. q.4h p.r.n. cough*

How many full doses are available in this bottle? __________ full doses

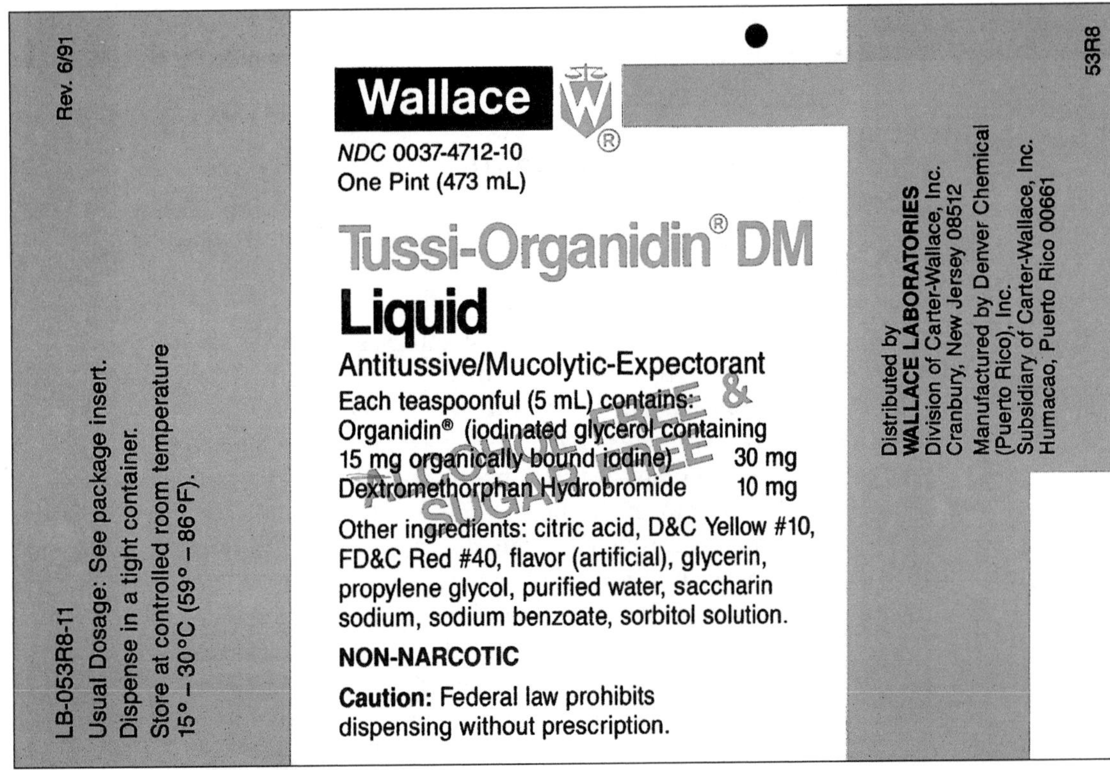

28. Order: *Lomotil 2.5 mg p.o. q.8h p.r.n.*

    Give: __________ mL

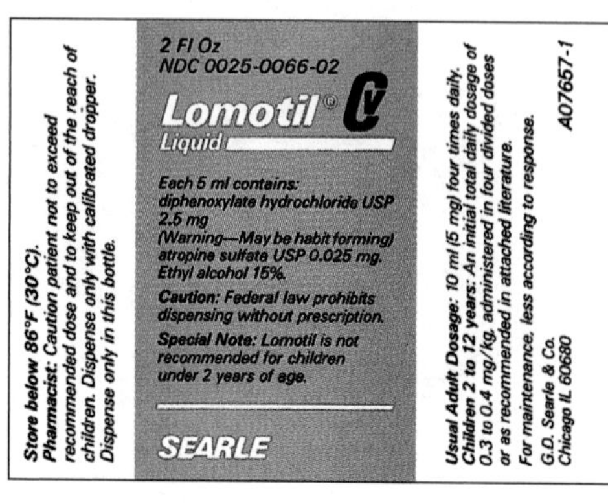

29. Order: *Maalox Plus 30 mL p.o. 30 min. p.c. and h.s.*

    How many containers will be needed for a 24-hour period? __________ containers

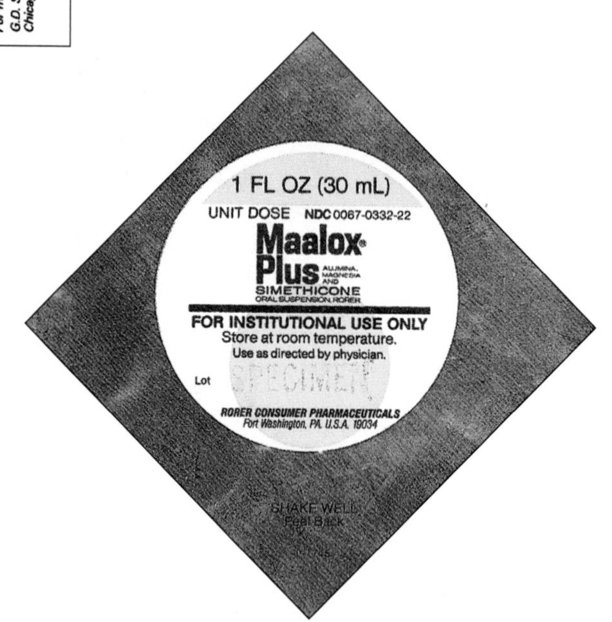

30. Meals are served at 8 AM, 12 noon, and 6 PM. Using international time what are the administration times for the 30 min p.c. dosages? (Allow 30 minutes for each meal to be eaten.) __________

After completing these problems, see page 427 to check your answers.

Summary

Let's examine where you are in mastering the skill of dosage calculations. You have learned to convert equivalent units within systems of measurements and from one system to another. You have also applied this conversion skill to the calculation of oral dosages—both solid and liquid forms. By now, you know that solving dosage problems requires that all units of measurement first be expressed in the same system and same size.

Next, you learned to think through the dosage ordered and dosage supplied to estimate the amount to be given. *To minimize medication errors, it is essential that you consider the reasonableness of the amount before applying a calculation method or formula.*

Finally, you have learned the formula method $\frac{D}{H} \times Q = X$ (desired over have times quantity = amount to give). This method is so simple and easy to recall that you will find that it will stick with you throughout your career.

Review the Critical Thinking Skills and work the practice problems for Chapter 9. If you are having difficulty, get help from an instructor before proceeding to Chapter 10. Continue to concentrate on accuracy. Keep in mind that one error can be a serious mistake when you are calculating the dosages of medicines. Medication administration is a *legal responsibility*. Remember, when you give a medication, you are legally responsible for your action.

critical thinking skills

Inaccuracy in dosage calculation is often attributed to errors in calculating the dosage. By first asking the question, "What is the reasonable amount to give?" many medication errors can often be avoided.

error

Incorrect calculation and not assessing the reasonableness of the calculation before administering the medication.

possible scenario

The physician ordered *phenobarbital 60 mg p.o. b.i.d.* for a patient with seizures. The pharmacy supplied phenobarbital 30 mg per tablet. The nurse did not use step 2 to think about the reasonable dosage, and calculated the dosage this way:

$$\frac{\text{DESIRED}}{\text{HAVE}} \times \text{QUANTITY} = \text{AMOUNT}$$

$$\frac{60\text{ mg}}{30\text{ mg}} \times 1\text{ tab} = 20\text{ tab (Incorrect)}$$

Suppose the nurse then gave the patient 20 tablets of the 30 mg per tablet of phenobarbital. The patient would have received 600 mg of phenobarbital, or 10 times the correct dosage. This is a very serious error.

potential outcome

The patient would likely develop signs of phenobarbital toxicity such as nystagmus (rapid eye movement), ataxia (lack of coordination), central nervous system depression, respiratory depression, hypothermia, and hypotension. When the error was caught and the physician notified, the patient would likely be given doses of charcoal to hasten elimination of the drug. Depending on the severity of the symptoms, the patient would likely be moved to the intensive care unit for monitoring of respiratory and neurological status.

prevention

This medication error could have been prevented if the nurse used the three-step method and estimated for the reasonable dosage of the drug to give. The order is for 60 mg of phenobarbital and the available drug has 30 mg per tablet, so the nurse should give 2 tablets. Such a large amount of tablets to give per dose should have alerted the nurse to a possible error. The formula $\frac{D}{H} \times Q = X$ should be used to verify thinking about the *reasonable* dosage. Further, the nurse should double check the math to find the error.

$$\frac{60\text{ mg}}{30\text{ mg}} \times 1\text{ tablet} = \frac{\overset{2}{\cancel{60}}\ \cancel{\text{mg}}}{\underset{1}{\cancel{30}}\ \cancel{\text{mg}}} \times 1\text{ tablet} = 2\text{ tablets, not 20 tablets}$$

practice problems—chapter 9

Calculate one dose of the following drug orders. The tablets are scored in half.

1. Order: *Orinase 250 mg p.o. b.i.d.*
   Supply: Orinase 0.5 g tablets
   Give: __________ tablet(s)
2. Order: *Codeine gr ss p.o. q.4h p.r.n., pain*
   Supply: Codeine 15 mg tablets
   Give: __________ tablet(s)
3. Order: *Synthroid 0.075 mg p.o. q.d.*
   Supply: Synthroid 150 mcg tablets
   Give: __________ tablet(s)
4. Order: *Phenobarbital gr$\frac{1}{6}$ p.o. t.i.d.*
   Supply: Phenobarbital elixir 20 mg/5 mL
   Give: __________ mL

5. Order: *Keflex 500 mg p.o. q.i.d.*

   Supply: Keflex, 250 mg/5 mL

   Give: __________ mL

6. Order: *Inderal 20 mg p.o. q.i.d.*

   Supply: Inderal 10 mg tablets

   Give: __________ tablet(s)

7. Order: *Amoxil 400 mg p.o. q.6h*

   Supply: Amoxil 250 mg per 5 mL

   Give: __________ mL

8. Order: *Diabenese 150 mg p.o. b.i.d.*

   Supply: Diabenese 0.1 g tablets

   Give: __________ tablet(s)

9. Order: *Phenobarbital gr $\frac{3}{4}$ p.o. q.i.d.*

   Supply: Phenobarbital 30 mg tablets

   Give: __________ tablet(s)

10. Order: *Codeine gr $\frac{1}{4}$ p.o. q.d.*

    Supply: Codeine 30 mg tablets

    Give: __________ tablet(s)

11. Order: *Inderal 30 mg p.o. q.i.d. p.c.*

    Supply: Inderal 20 mg tablets

    Give: __________ tablet(s)

12. Order: *Synthroid 300 mcg p.o. q.d.*

    Supply: Synthroid 0.3 mg tablets

    Give: __________ tablet(s)

13. Order: *Lasix 60 mg p.o. q.d.*

    Supply: Lasix 40 mg tablets

    Give: __________ tablet(s)

14. Order: *Tylenol $\bar{c}$ codeine gr $\frac{1}{8}$ p.o. q.d.*

    Supply: Tylenol with 7.5 mg codeine tablets

    Give: __________ tablet(s)

15. Order: *Penicillin G 400,000 U p.o. q.i.d.*

    Supply: Pentids (Penicillin G) 250 mg = 400,000 U tablets

    Give: __________ tablet(s)

16. Order: *Vasotec 7.5 mg p.o. q.d.*

    Supply: Vasotec 5 mg and 10 mg tablets

    Select: __________ mg tablets

    and give __________ tablet(s)

17. Order: *V-Cillin K 300,000 U p.o. q.i.d.*

    Supply: V-Cillin K 200,000 U/5 mL

    Give: __________ mL

18. Order: *Neomycin 0.75 g p.o. b.i.d.*

    Supply: Neomycin 500 mg tablets

    Give: __________ tablet(s)

19. Order: *Halcion 0.25 mg p.o. h.s.*

    Supply: Halcion 0.125 mg tablets

    Give: __________ tablet(s)

20. Order: *Dilantin gr i p.o. t.i.d.*

    Supply: Dilantin 30 mg capsules

    Give: __________ capsule(s)

21. Order: *Decadron 750 mcg p.o. b.i.d.*

    Supply: Decadron 0.75 mg and 1.5 mg tablets

    Select: __________ mg tablets

    Give: __________ tablet(s)

22. Order: *Edecrin 12.5 mg p.o. b.i.d.*

    Supply: Edecrin 25 mg tablets

    Give: __________ tablet(s)

23. Order: *Urecholine 50 mg p.o. t.i.d.*

    Supply: Urecholine 25 mg tablets

    Give: __________ tablet(s)

24. Order: *Robaxin 1.5 g p.o. stat*

    Supply: Robaxin 750 mg tablets

    Give: __________ tablet(s)

25. Order: *Robaxin 1 g p.o. q.i.d.*

    Supply: Robaxin 500 mg tablets

    Give: __________ tablet(s)

26. Order: *Tranxene 7.5 mg p.o. q.AM*

    Supply: Tranxene 3.75 mg capsules

    Give: __________ capsules

27. Order: *Phenobarbitol gr $\frac{3}{4}$ p.o. q.d.*

    Supply: Phenobarbital 15 mg, 30 mg, and 60 mg scored tablets

    Which strength of tablet(s) would you select, and how much would you give?

    Select: __________ mg tablets

    Give: __________ tablet(s)

28. Order: *Acetaminophen 240 mg p.o. q.4–6h p.r.n., pain or T>102*

    Supply: Acetaminophen drops 80 mg per 0.8 mL

    Give: __________ mL

29. Order: *Acetaminophen 160 mg p.o. q.4–6h p.r.n., pain or T>102*

    Supply: Acetaminophen liquid 80 mg per $\frac{1}{2}$ t

    Give: __________ mL

30. Order: *Coumadin gr $\frac{1}{6}$ p.o. q.d.*

    Supply: Coumadin 5 mg tablets

    Give: __________ tablet(s)

See the three medication administration records and accompanying labels on the following pages for problems 31 through 49.

Calculate one dose of each of the drugs prescribed. Labels A–O provided on pages 174–176 are the drugs you have available. Indicate the letter corresponding to the label you select.

PRINTED BY STANDARD REGISTER U.S.A. ZIPSET ®

PAGE ____ of ____

MEDICATION ADMINISTRATION RECORD

	ORIGINAL ORDER DATE	DATE STARTED / RENEWED	MEDICATION - DOSAGE	ROUTE	SCHEDULE 11-7	SCHEDULE 7-3	SCHEDULE 3-11	DATE 1/5/xx 11-7	7-3	3-11	DATE 11-7	7-3	3-11	DATE 11-7	7-3	3-11	DATE 11-7	7-3	3-11
31.	1/5/xx	1/5	*Tegretol 200 mg bid*	*PO*		*9*	*9*		*9 GP*	*9 MS*									
32.	1/5/xx	1/5	*Allegra 60 mg bid*	*PO*		*9*	*9*		*9 GP*	*9 MS*									
33.	1/5/xx	1/5	*Halcion 125 mcg hs*	*PO*			*10*			*10 MS*									
34.	1/5/xx	1/5	*Ludiomil 150 mg qd*	*PO*	*9*				*9 GP*										

PRN

INJECTION SITES: B - RIGHT ARM; C - RIGHT ABDOMEN; D - RIGHT ANTERIOR THIGH; G - LEFT ARM; H - LEFT ABDOMEN; J - LEFT ANTERIOR THIGH; L - LEFT BUTTOCKS; M - RIGHT BUTTOCKS

DATE GIVEN	TIME	INT.	ONE - TIME MEDICATION - DOSAGE	RT.	SCHEDULE 11-7	7-3	3-11	DATE *1/5/xx* 11-7	7-3	3-11	DATE 11-7	7-3	3-11	DATE 11-7	7-3	3-11	DATE 11-7	7-3	3-11

SIGNATURE OF NURSE ADMINISTERING MEDICATIONS

	1/5/xx
11-7	
7-3	*GP G. Pickar, RN*
3-11	*MS M. Smith, R.N.*

DATE GIVEN	TIME	INT.	MEDICATION-DOSAGE-CONT.	RT.

RECOPIED BY:

CHECKED BY:

LITHO IN U.S.A. K6508 (7-92) D095538

Patient, Mary Q.

ALLERGIES: *NKA*

602-31 (7-XX) (MPC# 1355)

1 ORIGINAL COPY

31. Select: __________

    Give: __________

32. Select: __________

    Give: __________

33. Select: __________

    Give: __________

34. Select: __________

    Give: __________

PAGE ______ of ______

MEDICATION ADMINISTRATION RECORD

PRINTED BY STANDARD REGISTER U.S.A. ZIPSET ®

	ORIGINAL ORDER DATE	DATE STARTED / RENEWED	MEDICATION - DOSAGE	ROUTE	SCHEDULE 11-7	SCHEDULE 7-3	SCHEDULE 3-11	DATE 1/5/xx 11-7	7-3	3-11	DATE 11-7	7-3	3-11	DATE 11-7	7-3	3-11	DATE 11-7	7-3	3-11
35.	1/5/xx	1/5	Synthroid 0.2 mg qd	PO		9			GP 9										
36.	1/5/xx	1/5	Micronase 10 mg qd	PO		9			GP 9										
37.	1/5/xx	1/5	Ilosone 250 mg q6h	PO	12 6	12	6		GP 12	MS 6									
38.	1/5/xx	1/5	Phenobarbital 30 mg bid	PO		9	9		GP 9	MS 9									
39.	1/5/xx	1/5	Potassium Chloride 40 mEq in ʒiv juice bid	PO		9	9		GP 9	MS 9									
			PRN																

INJECTION SITES
B - RIGHT ARM
C - RIGHT ABDOMEN
D - RIGHT ANTERIOR THIGH
G - LEFT ARM
H - LEFT ABDOMEN
J - LEFT ANTERIOR THIGH
L - LEFT BUTTOCKS
M - RIGHT BUTTOCKS

DATE GIVEN	TIME	INT.	ONE - TIME MEDICATION - DOSAGE	RT.

SIGNATURE OF NURSE ADMINISTERING MEDICATIONS	SCHEDULE	DATE 1/5/xx	DATE	DATE	DATE
	11-7				
	7-3	GP G. Pickar, RN			
	3-11	MS M. Smith, R.N.			

DATE GIVEN	TIME	INT.	MEDICATION-DOSAGE-CONT.	RT.
			RECOPIED BY:	
			CHECKED BY:	

LITHO IN U.S.A. K6508 (7-92) D395538

Patient, John Q.

ALLERGIES:

602-31 (7-XX) (MPC# 1355)

1 ORIGINAL COPY

35. Select: __________

    Give: __________

36. Select: __________

    Give: __________

37. Select: __________

    Give: __________

38. Select: __________

    Give: __________

39. Select: __________

    Give: __________

PAGE ____ of ____

MEDICATION ADMINISTRATION RECORD

	ORIGINAL ORDER DATE	DATE STARTED / RENEWED	MEDICATION - DOSAGE	ROUTE	SCHEDULE 11-7	SCHEDULE 7-3	SCHEDULE 3-11	DATE 1/5/xx 11-7	7-3	3-11
40.	1/5/xx	1/5	Nitroglycerin 5 mg q8h	PO	6	2	10		2 GP	10 MS
41.	1/5/xx	1/5	Potassium Chloride gr x tid	PO		8 2	8		8 GP 2 GP	8 MS
42.	1/5/xx	1/5	Lopid 0.6 g bid ac	PO		7^30	4^30		7^30 GP	4^30 MS
43.	1/5/xx	1/5	Furosemide 40 mg qd	PO		9			9 GP	
44.	1/5/xx	1/5	Lopressor 100 mg bid	PO		9	9		9 GP	9 MS
			PRN							
45.	1/5/xx	1/5	Darvocet-N 100 1 tab q4h prn headache	PO					7^30 GP 11^30 GP	

PRN

INJECTION SITES: B - RIGHT ARM; C - RIGHT ABDOMEN; D - RIGHT ANTERIOR THIGH; G - LEFT ARM; H - LEFT ABDOMEN; J - LEFT ANTERIOR THIGH; L - LEFT BUTTOCKS; M - RIGHT BUTTOCKS

DATE GIVEN	TIME	INT.	ONE - TIME MEDICATION - DOSAGE	RT.

SIGNATURE OF NURSE ADMINISTERING MEDICATIONS

SCHEDULE	DATE 1/5/xx	DATE	DATE	DATE
11-7				
7-3	GP G. Pickar RN			
3-11	MS M. Smith, R.N.			

DATE GIVEN	TIME	INT.	MEDICATION-DOSAGE-CONT.	RT.

RECOPIED BY:

CHECKED BY:

Doe, Jane Q.

ALLERGIES: NKA

1 ORIGINAL COPY

602-31 (7-xx) (MPC# 1355)

40. Select: __________
    Give: __________

41. Select: __________
    Give: __________

42. Select: __________
    Give: __________

43. Select: __________
    Give: __________

44. Select: __________
    Give: __________

45. Select: __________
    Give: __________

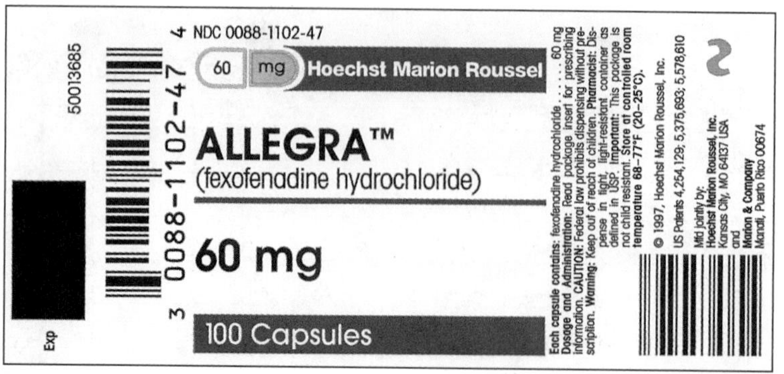

A

List 1730 NDC 0083-0135-30

Ludiomil® 75 mg
maprotiline HCl USP

100 tablets CIBA

Dispense in tight container (USP).

Caution: Federal law prohibits dispensing without prescription.

EXP
LOT

Dosage: See package insert.

Do not store above 86°F.

CIBA Pharmaceutical Company
Division of CIBA-GEIGY Corporation
Summit, New Jersey 07901

PHARMACIST: Container closure is not child-resistant.

3 0083-0135-30 0

637183

B

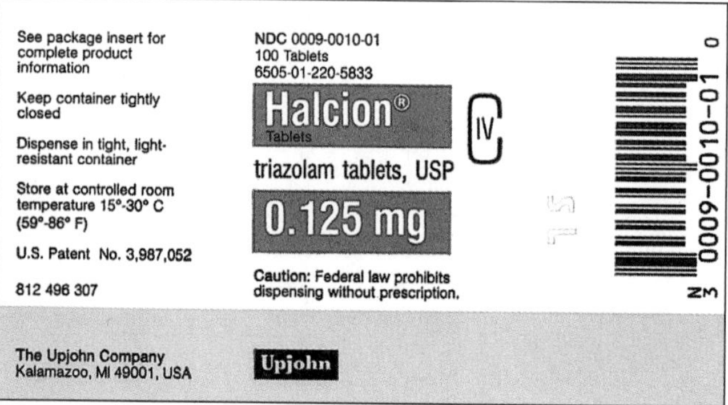

C

NDC 0083-0052-30 FSC 1821
6505-01-153-4524

Tegretol® 100 mg
carbamazepine USP

Chewable Tablets

100 tablets
Dispense in tight, light-resistant container (USP).
Caution: Federal law prohibits dispensing without prescription.
ciba

EXP
LOT

Do not store above 86°F (30°C).
Dosage: See package insert.
Protect from light and moisture.
Ciba-Geigy Corporation
Pharmaceuticals Division
Summit, NJ 07901

Keep this and all drugs out of the reach of children.

N 3 0083-0052-30 0

643330

D

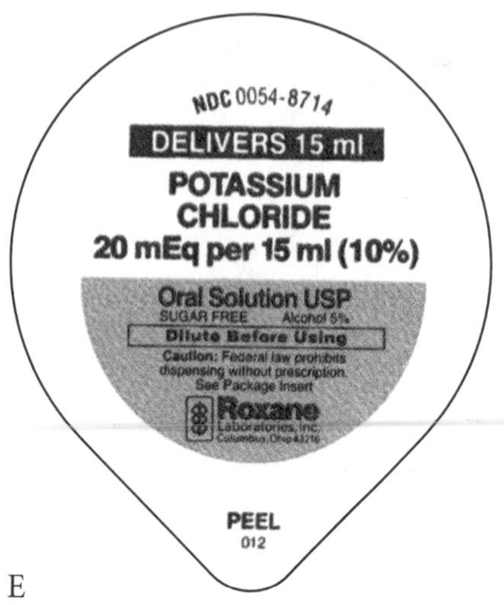

NDC 0054-8714
DELIVERS 15 ml
POTASSIUM
CHLORIDE
20 mEq per 15 ml (10%)
Oral Solution USP
SUGAR FREE Alcohol 5%
Dilute Before Using
Caution: Federal law prohibits dispensing without prescription.
See Package Insert
Roxane
Laboratories, Inc.
PEEL
012

E

NDC 0777-2317-48
100 ml
M-153
℞ PULL

ILOSONE®
LIQUID
ERYTHROMYCIN
ESTOLATE ORAL
SUSPENSION, USP
250 mg per 5 ml
DISTA

CAUTION—Federal (U.S.A.) law prohibits dispensing without prescription.
See accompanying literature for dosage.
Each 5 ml contains Erythromycin Estolate equivalent to 250 mg Erythromycin in a pleasantly flavored vehicle.

YC 9310 DPX Mfd. by
DISTA PRODUCTS COMPANY
a Division of Eli Lilly Industries, Inc.
Carolina, Puerto Rico 00630, a Subsidiary of
Eli Lilly & Co., Indianapolis, IN, U.S.A.
Expiration Date

F

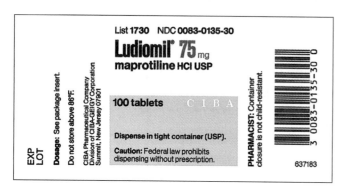

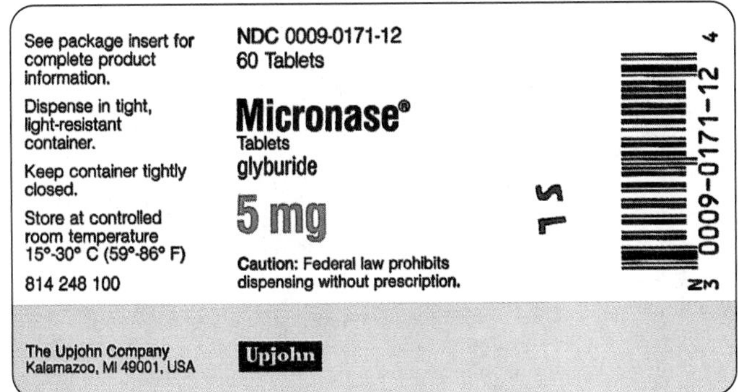
See package insert for complete product information.
Dispense in tight, light-resistant container.
Keep container tightly closed.
Store at controlled room temperature 15°-30° C (59°-86° F)
814 248 100
NDC 0009-0171-12
60 Tablets
Micronase®
Tablets
glyburide
5 mg
Caution: Federal law prohibits dispensing without prescription.
The Upjohn Company
Kalamazoo, MI 49001, USA
Upjohn

G

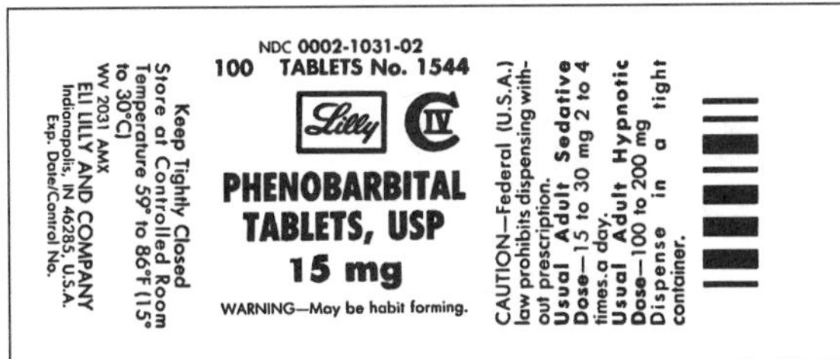
NDC 0002-1031-02
100 TABLETS No. 1544
PHENOBARBITAL TABLETS, USP
15 mg
WARNING—May be habit forming.

H

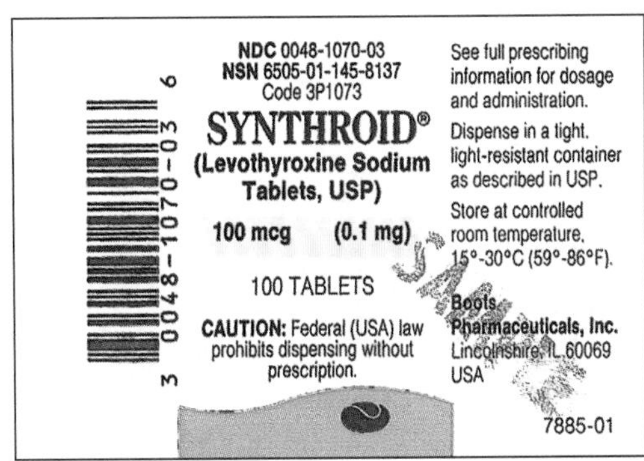
NDC 0048-1070-03
NSN 6505-01-145-8137
Code 3P1073
SYNTHROID®
(Levothyroxine Sodium Tablets, USP)
100 mcg (0.1 mg)
100 TABLETS
CAUTION: Federal (USA) law prohibits dispensing without prescription.
See full prescribing information for dosage and administration.
Dispense in a tight, light-resistant container as described in USP.
Store at controlled room temperature, 15°-30°C (59°-86°F).
Boots Pharmaceuticals, Inc.
Lincolnshire, IL 60069
USA
7885-01

I

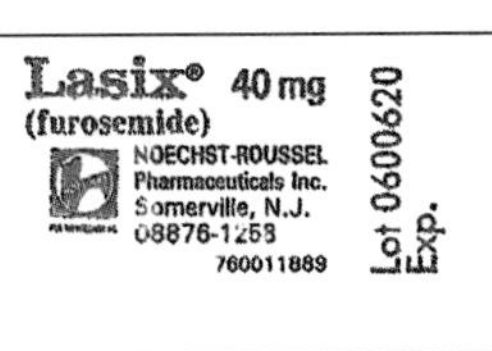
Lasix® 40 mg
(furosemide)
HOECHST-ROUSSEL
Pharmaceuticals Inc.
Somerville, N.J.
08876-1258
760011889

J

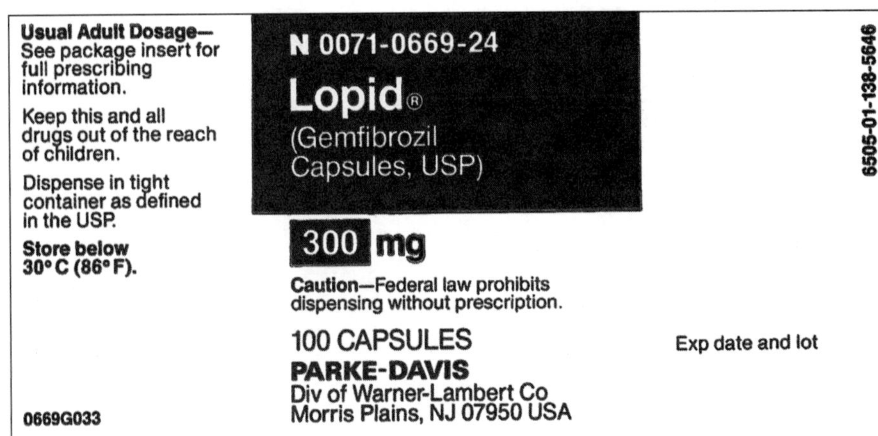
Usual Adult Dosage—See package insert for full prescribing information.
Keep this and all drugs out of the reach of children.
Dispense in tight container as defined in the USP.
Store below 30°C (86°F).
0669G033
N 0071-0669-24
Lopid®
(Gemfibrozil Capsules, USP)
300 mg
Caution—Federal law prohibits dispensing without prescription.
100 CAPSULES
PARKE-DAVIS
Div of Warner-Lambert Co
Morris Plains, NJ 07950 USA
Exp date and lot
6505-01-138-5646

K

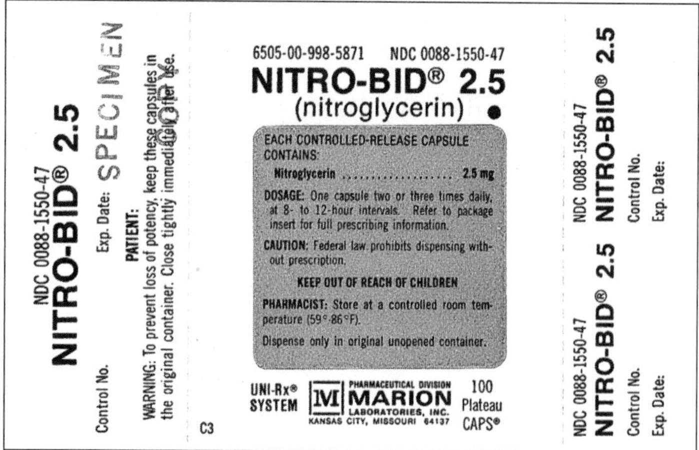
6505-00-998-5871 NDC 0088-1550-47
NITRO-BID® 2.5
(nitroglycerin)
EACH CONTROLLED-RELEASE CAPSULE CONTAINS:
Nitroglycerin .... 2.5 mg
DOSAGE: One capsule two or three times daily, at 8- to 12-hour intervals. Refer to package insert for full prescribing information.
CAUTION: Federal law prohibits dispensing without prescription.
KEEP OUT OF REACH OF CHILDREN
PHARMACIST: Store at a controlled room temperature (59°-86°F).
Dispense only in original unopened container.
UNI-Rx® SYSTEM
MARION LABORATORIES, INC. KANSAS CITY, MISSOURI 64137
100 Plateau CAPS®
NDC 0088-1550-47
NITRO-BID® 2.5
Control No.
Exp. Date: SPECIMEN
PATIENT:
WARNING: To prevent loss of potency, keep these capsules in the original container. Close tightly immediately after use.
C3

L

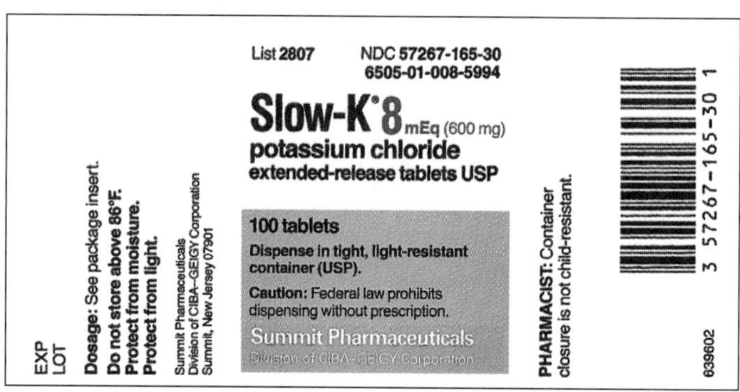
List 2807 NDC 57267-165-30
6505-01-008-5994
Slow-K® 8 mEq (600 mg)
potassium chloride
extended-release tablets USP
100 tablets
Dispense in tight, light-resistant container (USP).
Caution: Federal law prohibits dispensing without prescription.
Summit Pharmaceuticals
Division of CIBA-GEIGY Corporation
EXP
LOT
Dosage: See package insert.
Do not store above 86°F.
Protect from moisture.
Protect from light.
Summit Pharmaceuticals
Division of CIBA-GEIGY Corporation
Summit, New Jersey 07901
PHARMACIST: Container closure is not child-resistant.
3 57267-165-30 1
639602

M

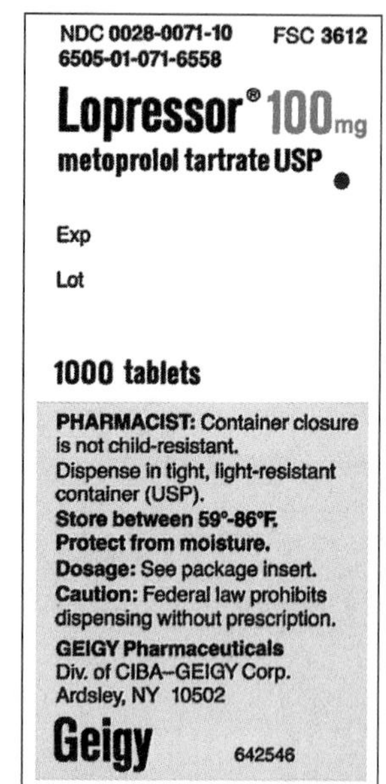
NDC 0028-0071-10 FSC 3612
6505-01-071-6558
Lopressor® 100 mg
metoprolol tartrate USP
Exp
Lot
1000 tablets
PHARMACIST: Container closure is not child-resistant.
Dispense in tight, light-resistant container (USP).
Store between 59°-86°F.
Protect from moisture.
Dosage: See package insert.
Caution: Federal law prohibits dispensing without prescription.
GEIGY Pharmaceuticals
Div. of CIBA-GEIGY Corp.
Ardsley, NY 10502
Geigy
642546

N

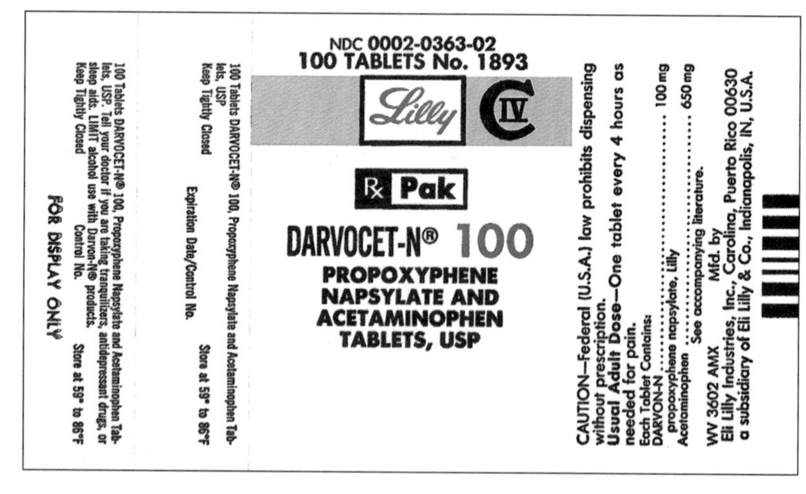
NDC 0002-0363-02
100 TABLETS No. 1893
Lilly
C IV
Rx Pak
DARVOCET-N® 100
PROPOXYPHENE NAPSYLATE AND ACETAMINOPHEN TABLETS, USP
CAUTION—Federal (U.S.A.) law prohibits dispensing without prescription.
Usual Adult Dose—One tablet every 4 hours as needed for pain.
Each Tablet Contains:
DARVON-N propoxyphene napsylate, Lilly ...... 100 mg
Acetaminophen ...... 650 mg
See accompanying literature.
WV 3602 AMX Mfd. by
Eli Lilly Industries, Inc., Carolina, Puerto Rico 00630
a subsidiary of Eli Lilly & Co., Indianapolis, IN, U.S.A.
FOR DISPLAY ONLY

O

Calculate one dose of the medications indicated on the MAR. Labels P–T provided on pages 178 and 179 are the drugs available. Indicate the letter corresponding to the label you select, as requested.

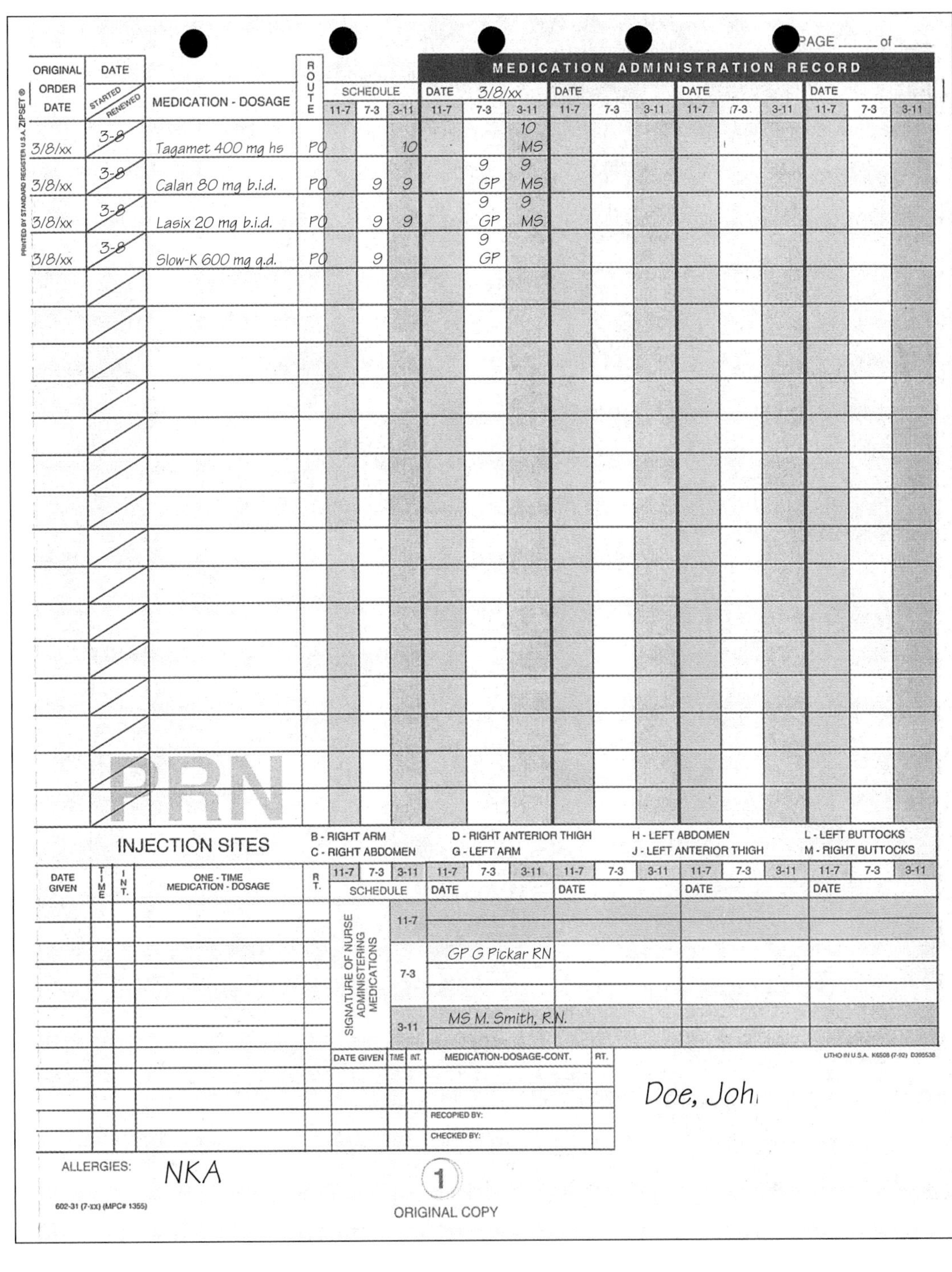

PAGE ____ of ____

MEDICATION ADMINISTRATION RECORD

	ORIGINAL ORDER DATE	DATE STARTED/RENEWED	MEDICATION - DOSAGE	ROUTE	SCHEDULE 11-7	SCHEDULE 7-3	SCHEDULE 3-11	DATE 3/8/xx 11-7	7-3	3-11
46.	3/8/xx	3-8	Tagamet 400 mg hs	PO			10			10 MS
47.	3/8/xx	3-8	Calan 80 mg b.i.d.	PO		9	9		9 GP	9 MS
48.	3/8/xx	3-8	Lasix 20 mg b.i.d.	PO		9	9		9 GP	9 MS
49.	3/8/xx	3-8	Slow-K 600 mg q.d.	PO		9			9 GP	

PRN

INJECTION SITES: B - RIGHT ARM, C - RIGHT ABDOMEN, D - RIGHT ANTERIOR THIGH, G - LEFT ARM, H - LEFT ABDOMEN, J - LEFT ANTERIOR THIGH, L - LEFT BUTTOCKS, M - RIGHT BUTTOCKS

DATE GIVEN | TIME | INT. | ONE - TIME MEDICATION - DOSAGE | RT. | SCHEDULE 11-7 7-3 3-11

SIGNATURE OF NURSE ADMINISTERING MEDICATIONS:
11-7:
7-3: GP G Pickar RN
3-11: MS M. Smith, R.N.

DATE GIVEN | TIME | INT. | MEDICATION-DOSAGE-CONT. | RT.

RECOPIED BY:
CHECKED BY:

Doe, John

ALLERGIES: NKA

602-31 (7-xx) (MPC# 1355)

1 ORIGINAL COPY

46. Select: __________

Give: __________

47. Select: __________

Give: __________

48. Select: __________

Give: __________

49. Select: __________

Give: __________

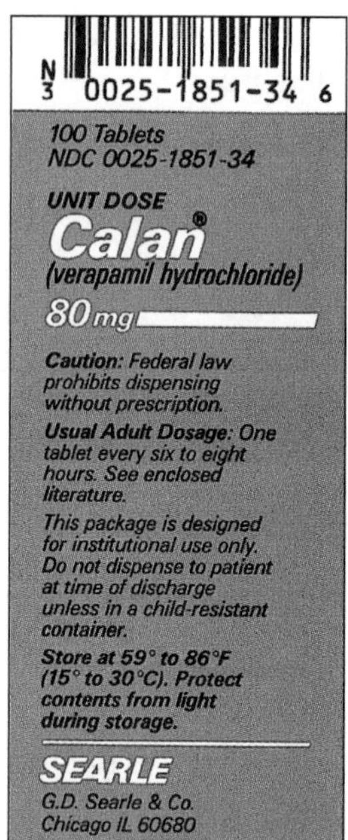
N 3 0025-1851-34 6
100 Tablets
NDC 0025-1851-34
UNIT DOSE
Calan®
(verapamil hydrochloride)
80 mg
Caution: Federal law prohibits dispensing without prescription.
Usual Adult Dosage: One tablet every six to eight hours. See enclosed literature.
This package is designed for institutional use only. Do not dispense to patient at time of discharge unless in a child-resistant container.
Store at 59° to 86°F (15° to 30°C). Protect contents from light during storage.
SEARLE
G.D. Searle & Co.
Chicago IL 60680

P

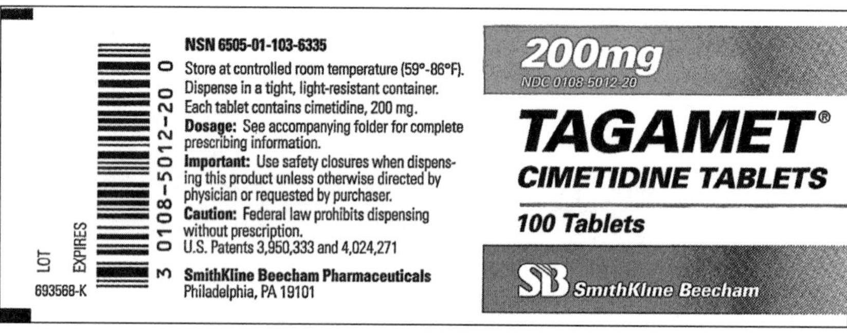
LOT
EXPIRES
693568-K
3 0108-5012-20 0
NSN 6505-01-103-6335
Store at controlled room temperature (59°-86°F).
Dispense in a tight, light-resistant container.
Each tablet contains cimetidine, 200 mg.
Dosage: See accompanying folder for complete prescribing information.
Important: Use safety closures when dispensing this product unless otherwise directed by physician or requested by purchaser.
Caution: Federal law prohibits dispensing without prescription.
U.S. Patents 3,950,333 and 4,024,271
SmithKline Beecham Pharmaceuticals
Philadelphia, PA 19101
200mg
NDC 0108-5012-20
TAGAMET®
CIMETIDINE TABLETS
100 Tablets
SB SmithKline Beecham

Q

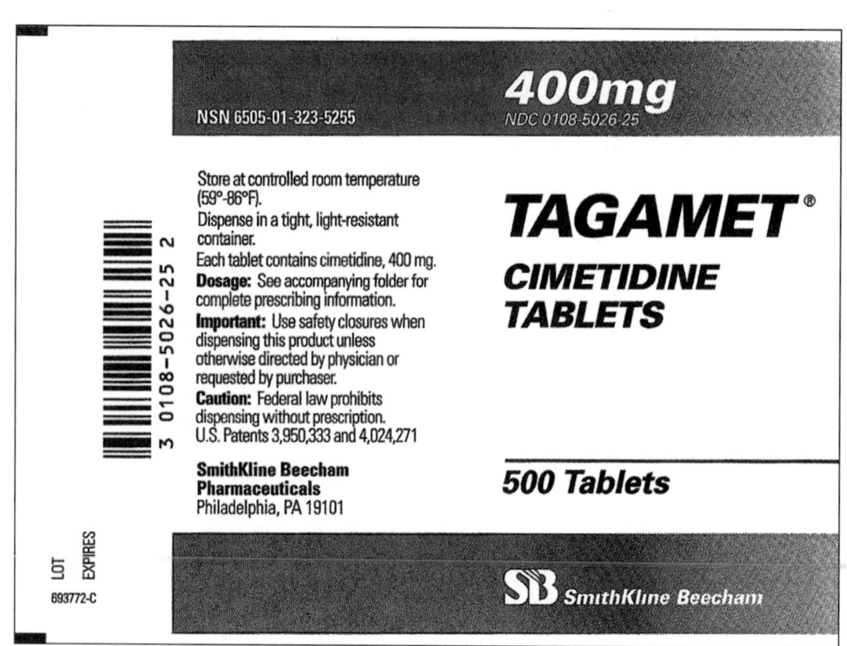
NSN 6505-01-323-5255
400mg
NDC 0108-5026-25
Store at controlled room temperature (59°-86°F).
Dispense in a tight, light-resistant container.
Each tablet contains cimetidine, 400 mg.
Dosage: See accompanying folder for complete prescribing information.
Important: Use safety closures when dispensing this product unless otherwise directed by physician or requested by purchaser.
Caution: Federal law prohibits dispensing without prescription.
U.S. Patents 3,950,333 and 4,024,271
SmithKline Beecham Pharmaceuticals
Philadelphia, PA 19101
3 0108-5026-25 2
TAGAMET®
CIMETIDINE TABLETS
500 Tablets
LOT
EXPIRES
693772-C
SB SmithKline Beecham

R

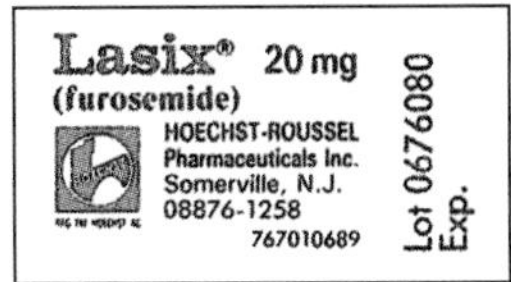

S

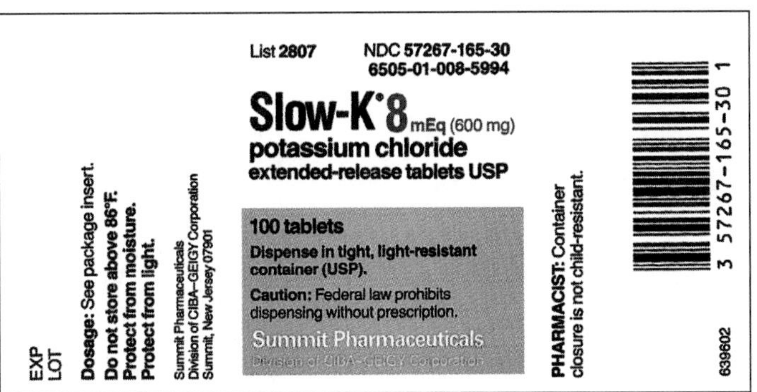

T

50. Critical Thinking Skill: Describe the strategy to prevent this medication error.

possible scenario 4XD

Suppose the physician ordered *Betapen VK 5 mL (250 mg) p.o. q.i.d.* for a patient with an upper respiratory tract infection. The pharmacy supplied *Betapen VK 125 mg per 5 mL*. In a rush to administer the medication on time, the nurse read the order as "Betapen VK 5 mL," checked the label for Betapen VK and poured that amount and administered the drug. In a hurry, the nurse failed to recognize that 5 mL of the supply dose of 125 mg/5 mL did not provide the ordered dose of 250 mg and underdosed the patient.

potential outcome

The patient received one-half of the ordered dose of antibiotic needed to treat the respiratory infection. If this error was not caught, the patient's infection would not be halted. This would add to the patient's illness time and might lead to a more severe infection and additional tests to determine why the patient was not responding to the medication.

prevention

always check the label against the order MAR

After completing these problems, see pages 427 and 428 to check your answers.

CHAPTER

10

Parenteral Dosage of Drugs

objectives

Upon mastery of Chapter 10, you will be able to calculate the parenteral dosages of drugs. To accomplish this you will also be able to:

- Apply the three steps for dosage calculations: convert, think, and calculate.
- Use the formula $\frac{D}{H} \times Q = X$ to calculate the amount to give.
- Reconstitute and label medications supplied in powder or dry form.
- Differentiate between varying directions for reconstitution and select the correct set to prepare the dosage ordered.
- Measure insulin in a matching insulin syringe.
- Convert insulin units to milliliters.
- Calculate parenteral dosages when the supply dosage is given in ratio or percent.

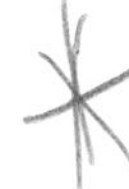

The term *parenteral* is used to designate routes of administration other than gastrointestinal, such as the injection routes of IM, SC, ID, and IV. In this chapter intramuscular (IM) and subcutaneous (SC) injection will be emphasized. Intravenous (IV) drug calculations are discussed in Chapters 14–16. Intramuscular indicates an injection given into a muscle, such as Demerol given IM for pain. Subcutaneous means an injection given into the subcutaneous tissue, such as an insulin injection for the management of diabetes given SC. Intradermal (ID) means an injection given under the skin, such as an allergy test or tuberculin skin test.

Injectable Solutions

Most parenteral medications are prepared in liquid or solution form, and packaged in dosage vials, ampules, or prefilled syringes (Figure 10-1). Injectable drugs are measured in syringes.

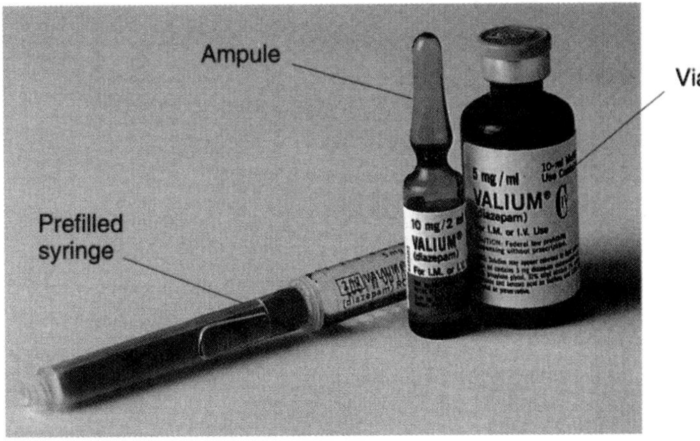

FIGURE 10-1 Parenteral Solutions

rule

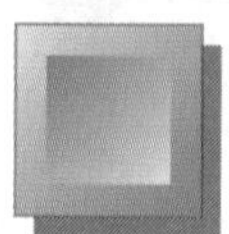

The maximum dosage volume to be administered per intramuscular injection site for:

1. An average 150-lb adult = 3 mL
2. Children age 6 to 12 years = 2 mL
3. Children birth to age 5 years = 1 mL

For example, if you must give an adult patient 4 milliliters of a drug, divide the dose into two injections of 2 milliliters each. The condition of the patient must be considered when applying this rule. *Adults or children who have decreased muscle or subcutaneous tissue mass or poor circulation may not be able to tolerate the maximum dosage volumes.*

To solve parenteral dosage problems, apply the same steps used for the calculation of oral dosages.

remember

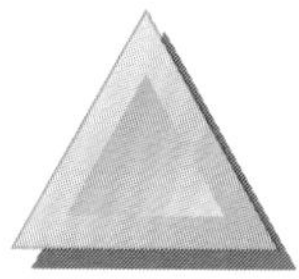

STEP 1	**CONVERT**	All units of measurement to the same system, and all units to the same size.
STEP 2	**THINK**	Estimate the logical amount.
STEP 3	**CALCULATE**	$\frac{\text{D (desired)}}{\text{H (have)}} \times \text{Q (quantity)} = \text{X (amount)}$

Use the following rules to help you decide which size syringe to select to administer parenteral dosages.

rule

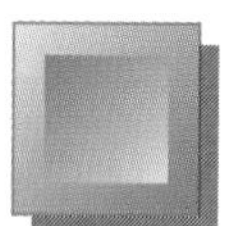

As you calculate parenteral dosages:

1. Round X (amount to be administered) to tenths if the amount is greater than 1 mL and measure it in a 3 cc syringe.
2. Measure amounts of less than 1 mL rounded to hundredths in a tuberculin syringe.
3. Amounts of 0.5 to 1 mL, rounded to tenths, can be accurately measured in either a tuberculin or 3 cc syringe.

Let's look at some examples of appropriate syringe selections for the dosages to be measured and how to read the calibrations. Refer to Chapter 6, *Equipment Used in Dosage Measurement*, regarding how to measure medication in a syringe. To review, the top black ring should align with the desired calibration, not the raised mid-section and not the bottom ring. Look carefully at the illustrations that follow.

Example 1:

Measure 0.33 mL in a 0.5 mL tuberculin syringe.

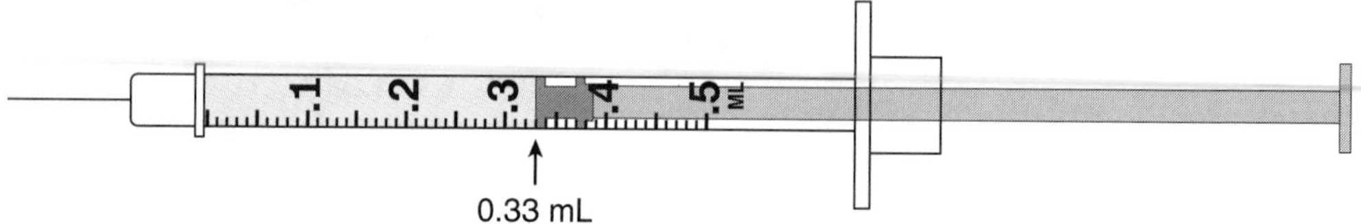

Example 2:

Round 1.33 mL to 1.3 mL, and measure in a 3 cc syringe.

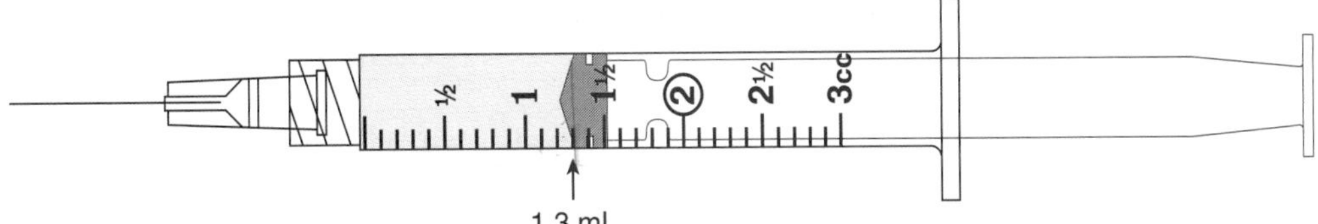

Example 3:

Measure 0.6 mL in either a 1 mL tuberculin or 3 cc syringe. (Notice that the amount is measured in tenths.)

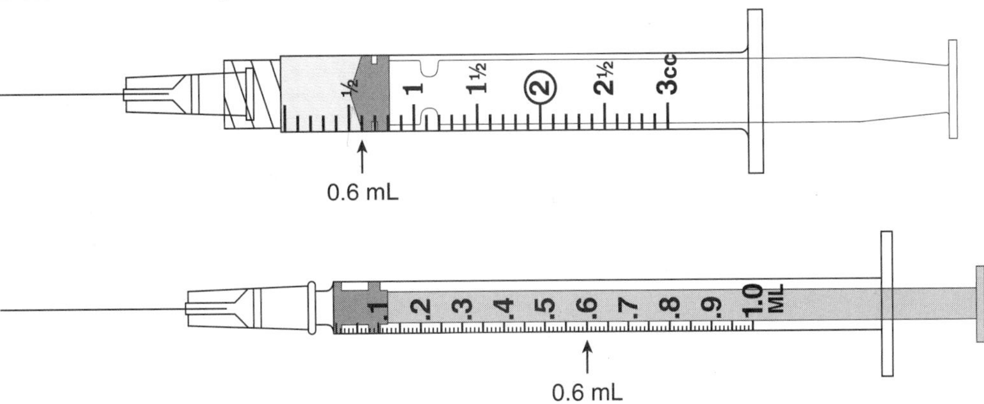

Example 4:

Measure 0.65 mL in a 1 mL tuberculin syringe. (Notice that the amount is measured in hundredths and is less than 1 mL.)

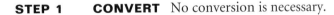

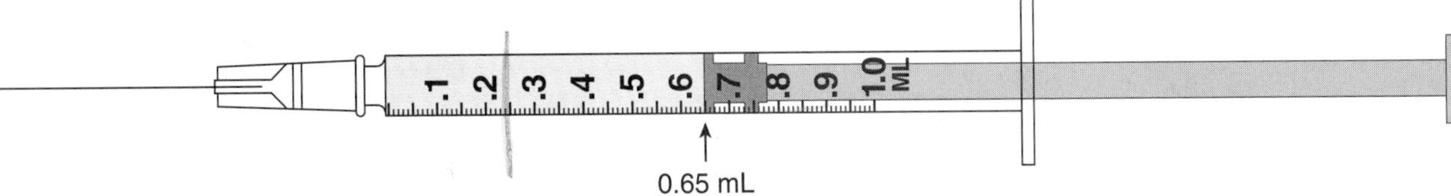

An amber color has been added to selected syringe drawings throughout the text *to simulate a specific amount of medication*, as indicated in the example or problem. Because the color used may not correspond to the actual color of the medications named, **it must not be used as a reference for identifying medications.**

Let's look at some examples of parenteral dosage calculations.

Example 1:

The drug order reads *Bentyl 20 mg IM q.i.d.* Available is *Bentyl injection 10 mg per mL* in a 10 mL multiple dose vial. How many milliliters should be administered to the patient?

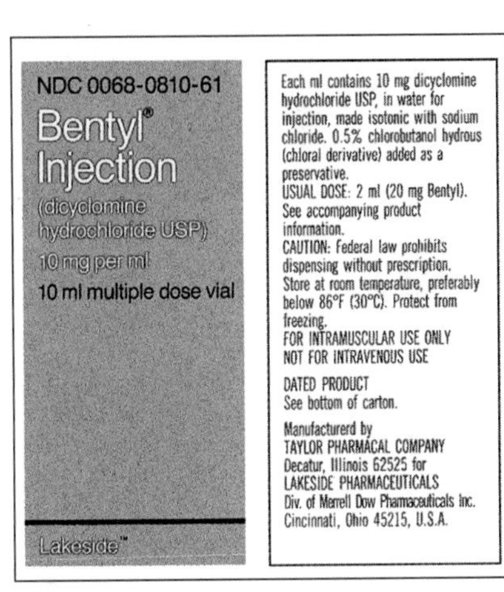

NDC 0068-0810-61
Bentyl®
Injection
(dicyclomine
hydrochloride USP)
10 mg per ml
10 ml multiple dose vial
Lakeside™
Each ml contains 10 mg dicyclomine hydrochloride USP, in water for injection, made isotonic with sodium chloride. 0.5% chlorobutanol hydrous (chloral derivative) added as a preservative.
USUAL DOSE: 2 ml (20 mg Bentyl).
See accompanying product information.
CAUTION: Federal law prohibits dispensing without prescription.
Store at room temperature, preferably below 86°F (30°C). Protect from freezing.
FOR INTRAMUSCULAR USE ONLY
NOT FOR INTRAVENOUS USE
DATED PRODUCT
See bottom of carton.
Manufacturerd by
TAYLOR PHARMACAL COMPANY
Decatur, Illinois 62525 for
LAKESIDE PHARMACEUTICALS
Div. of Merrell Dow Phamaceuticals Inc.
Cincinnati, Ohio 45215, U.S.A.

STEP 1 **CONVERT** No conversion is necessary.

STEP 2 **THINK** You want to give more than 1 mL. In fact, you want to give twice as much, because 20 mg is twice as much as 10 mg.

STEP 3 **CALCULATE** $\frac{D}{H} \times Q = \frac{\overset{2}{\cancel{20}}\ \cancel{\text{mg}}}{\underset{1}{\cancel{10}}\ \cancel{\text{mg}}} \times 1\ \text{mL} = 2\ \text{mL}$

given intramuscularly four times daily

Select a *3 cc syringe and measure 2 mL* of Bentyl 10 mg per mL. Look carefully at the illustration to clearly identify the part of the black rubber stopper that measures the exact dosage.

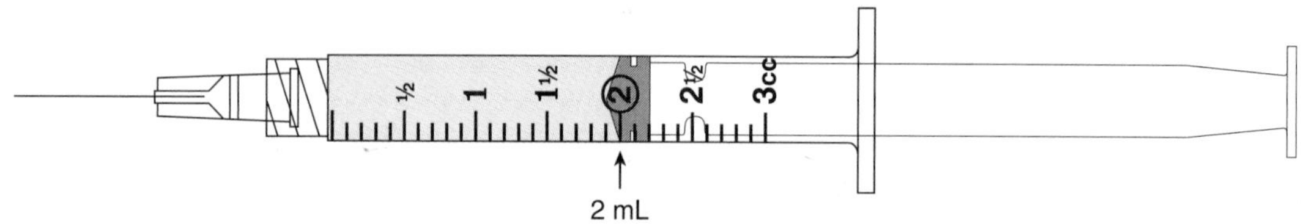

Example 2:

The drug order reads *Bricanyl 0.25 mg SC bid.* The ampule is labeled *1 mg per mL.*

NDC 0068-0702-20
Bricanyl®
(terbutaline sulfate)
1 mg per ml
A STERILE AQUEOUS SOLUTION FOR SUBCUTANEOUS INJECTION
10 ampuls 1 ml each
TO BE SOLD ONLY AS AN UNBROKEN PACKAGE
Lakeside™

STEP 1 **CONVERT** No conversion necessary.

STEP 2 **THINK** You want to give less than 1 mL. Actually you want to give 0.25 of a mL.

STEP 3 **CALCULATE** $\frac{D}{H} \times Q = \frac{0.25\ \cancel{\text{mg}}}{\cancel{1}\ \cancel{\text{mg}}} \times \cancel{1}\ \text{mL} = 0.25\ \text{mL}$

given subcutaneously twice daily

remember

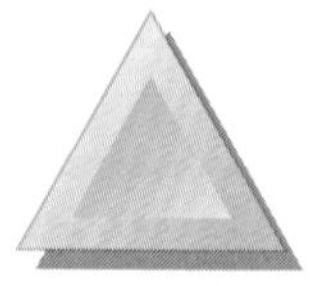

Dosages measured in hundredths (such as 0.25 mL) and all amounts less than 0.5 mL should be prepared in a tuberculin syringe, which is calibrated in hundredths.

Select a *0.5 mL tuberculin syringe and measure 0.25 mL* of Bricanyl 1 mg per mL. Look carefully at the illustration to clearly identify the part of the black rubber stopper that measures the exact dosage.

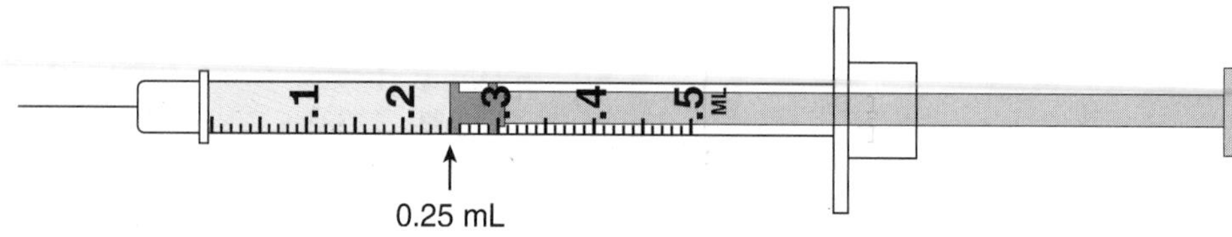

Example 3:

Drug order: *Demerol (meperidine hydrochloride) 35 mg IM q.3–4h p.r.n., pain*

Tubex on hand: *Meperidine HCl 50 mg per mL*

1/2 mL 1 mL 1-1/2 mL 2 mL
MEPERIDINE 50 MG/ML
HCL INJECTION, USP
WARNING—MAY BE HABIT-FORMING
FOR IM OR SC USE
FOR IV USE SEE DIRECTIONS
(1 ML FILL IN 2 ML SIZE)
LOT EXP
TUBEX® Wyeth® PHILA. TL 87-4

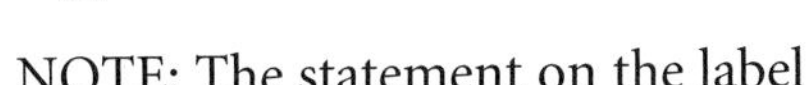

NOTE: The statement on the label "(1 ML FILL IN 2 ML SIZE)" means that the total capacity of the Tubex syringe is 2 mL, but it is filled with 1 mL of meperidine.

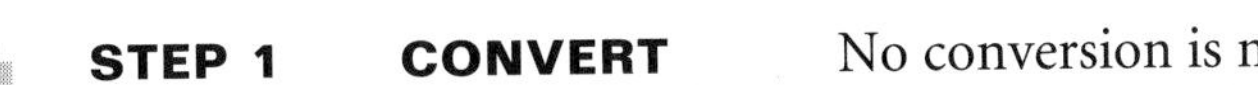

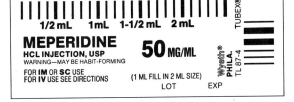

STEP 1 **CONVERT** No conversion is necessary.

STEP 2 **THINK** You want to give less than 1 mL but more than 0.5 mL.

STEP 3 **CALCULATE** $\frac{D}{H} \times Q = \frac{\overset{7}{\cancel{35}}\ \cancel{\text{mg}}}{\underset{10}{\cancel{50}}\ \cancel{\text{mg}}} \times 1 \text{ mL} = \frac{7}{10} \text{ mL} = 0.7 \text{ mL}$

given intramuscularly every 3 to 4 hours as needed for pain

Select the *2 mL-Tubex and discard 0.3 mL to administer 0.7 mL* of meperidine (Demerol) 50 mg/mL. You must discard the 0.3 mL in the presence of another nurse because meperidine is a controlled substance.

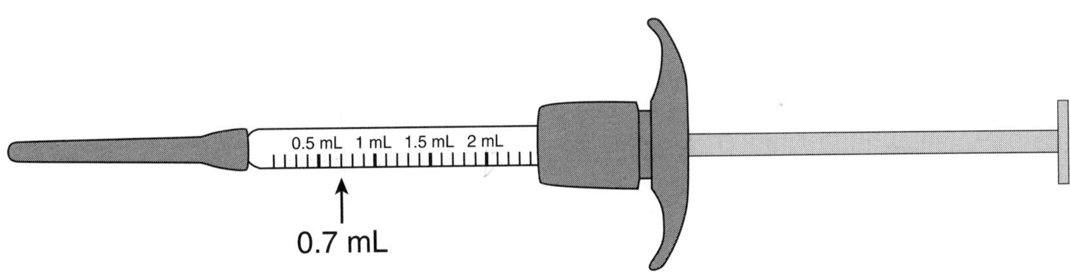

Example 4:

Order: *Heparin 8,000 U SC b.i.d.*

Available: A vial of *heparin sodium injection 10,000 U per mL*

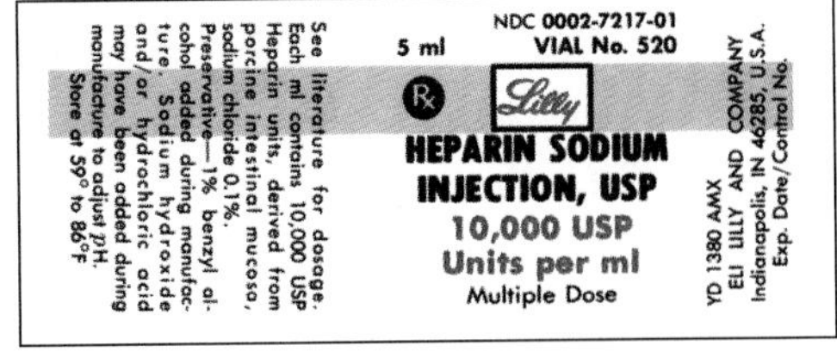

STEP 1 **CONVERT** No conversion is necessary.

STEP 2 **THINK** You want to give less than 1 mL but more than 0.5 mL

STEP 3 **CALCULATE** $\frac{D}{H} \times Q = \frac{8{,}\cancel{000}\ \cancel{U}}{10{,}\cancel{000}\ \cancel{U}} \times 1 \text{ mL} = \frac{8}{10} \text{ mL} = 0.8 \text{ mL}$

given subcutaneously twice daily

Select a *1 mL* or a *3 cc syringe and measure 0.8 mL* of heparin 10,000 U/mL.

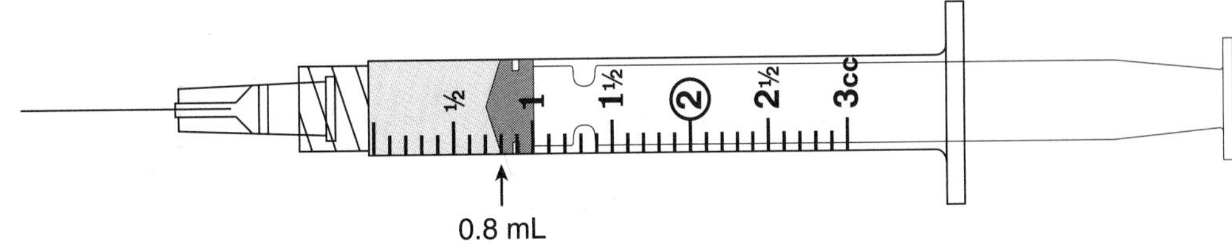

Example 5:

Order: *Cleocin 150 mg IM q.12h*

Available: *Cleocin (clindamycin phosphate) 300 mg per 2 mL*

LOT
EXP
NDC 0009-0870-21
2 ml Vial
Cleocin Phosphate®
Sterile Solution
clindamycin phosphate injection, USP
300 mg
Equivalent to 300 mg clindamycin
Single Dose Container
See package insert for complete product information.
Store at controlled room temperature 15°-30°C (59°-86°F)
812 728 103
The Upjohn Company
Kalamazoo, MI 49001, USA

STEP 1 CONVERT No conversion is necessary.

STEP 2 THINK You want to give less than 2 mL. Actually, you want to give 150 mg which is $\frac{1}{2}$ of 300 mg and $\frac{1}{2}$ of 2 mL, or 1 mL. Calculate to doublecheck your estimate.

STEP 3 CALCULATE $\frac{D}{H} \times Q = \frac{\overset{1}{\cancel{150}}\ \cancel{mg}}{\underset{2}{\cancel{300}}\ \cancel{mg}} \times 2\text{ mL} = \frac{\overset{1}{\cancel{2}}}{\underset{1}{\cancel{2}}}\text{ mL} = 1\text{ mL}$

given intramuscularly every 12 hours

Select a *3 cc syringe, and measure 1 mL* of Cleocin 300 mg/2 mL.

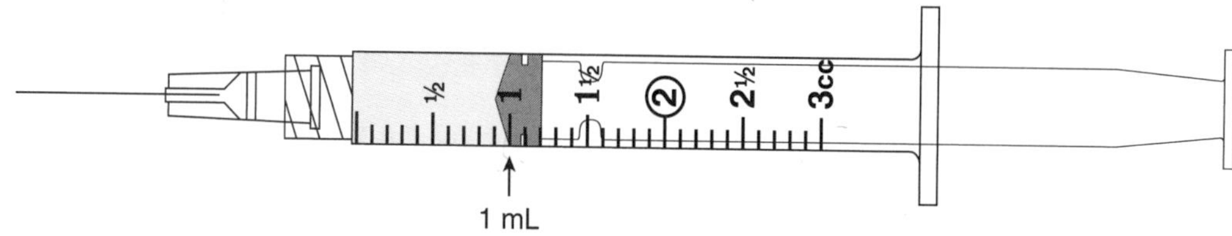

Example 6:

Order: (pediatric dose) *Atropine sulfate 0.15 mg SC stat*

Supply: *Atropine sulfate 0.4 mg per mL*

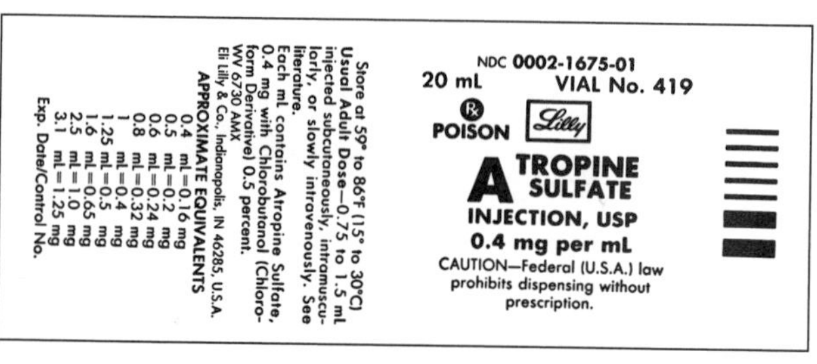

STEP 1 CONVERT No conversion necessary.

STEP 2 THINK You want to give less than 1 mL. Be careful with the decimals. Don't be fooled into thinking 0.15 is more than 0.4. Add a zero to 0.4, and you can see that 0.15 is *much less:* $0.15 < 0.40$.

STEP 3 CALCULATE $\frac{D}{H} \times Q = \frac{\overset{3}{\cancel{0.15}}\ \cancel{mg}}{\underset{8}{\cancel{0.40}}\ \cancel{mg}} \times 1\text{ mL} = \frac{3}{8}\text{ mL} = 0.375\text{ mL}$

given subcutaneously immediately

This is a small pediatric dosage, so round to hundredths: $0.375 = 0.38$ mL.

Select a *0.5 mL tuberculin syringe, and measure 0.38 mL* of atropine sulfate 0.4 mg/mL.

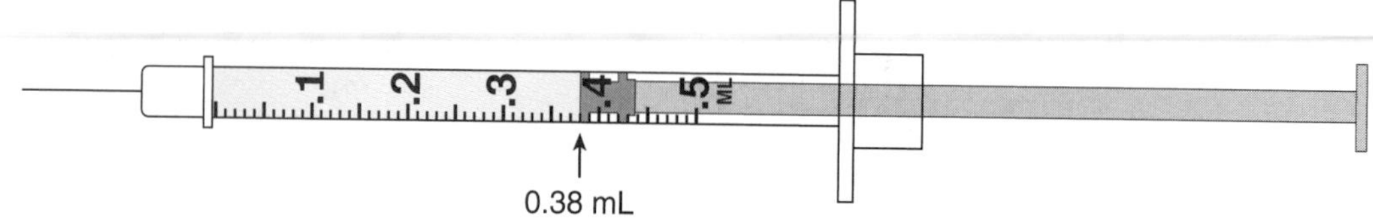

Example 7:

The drug order reads *Morphine sulfate gr$\frac{1}{6}$ IM q.3–4h p.r.n.*, and the label on the Tubex syringe states *Morphine sulfate 15 mg per mL.*

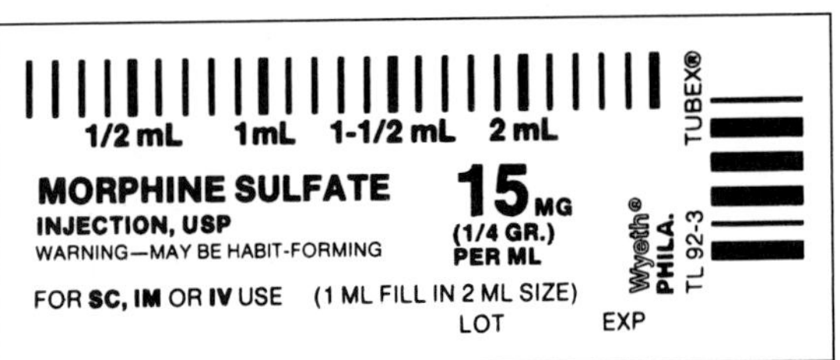

1/2 mL 1 mL 1-1/2 mL 2 mL
MORPHINE SULFATE
INJECTION, USP
WARNING—MAY BE HABIT-FORMING
15 MG
(1/4 GR.)
PER ML
FOR SC, IM OR IV USE (1 ML FILL IN 2 ML SIZE)
LOT
EXP
Wyeth®
PHILA.
TL 92-3
TUBEX®

STEP 1 CONVERT

Order: *Morphine sulfate* ~~gr 1/6~~ *10 mg*

Equivalent: gr i = 60 mg

$$\text{gr}\,\frac{1}{6} = \frac{1}{\cancel{6}_{1}} \times \frac{\cancel{60}^{10}}{1} = 10 \text{ mg}$$

Supply: Morphine sulfate 15 mg/mL

STEP 2 THINK

You want to give less than 1 mL but more than 0.5 mL.

STEP 3 CALCULATE

$$\frac{D}{H} \times Q = \frac{\cancel{10\text{ mg}}^{2}}{\cancel{15\text{ mg}}_{3}} \times 1 \text{ mL} = \frac{2}{3} \text{ mL} = 0.67 \text{ mL} = 0.7 \text{ mL};$$

given intramuscularly every 3 to 4 hours as needed for pain

NOTE: This dose is rounded to tenths because the medication is supplied in a Tubex syringe, which is calibrated in tenths.

Select the *2 mL Tubex syringe, and first discard 0.3 mL of the prefilled amount (1 mL)*. Then give 0.7 mL of morphine sulfate 15 mg/mL. You must discard 0.3 mL in the presence of another nurse, because this is a controlled substance.

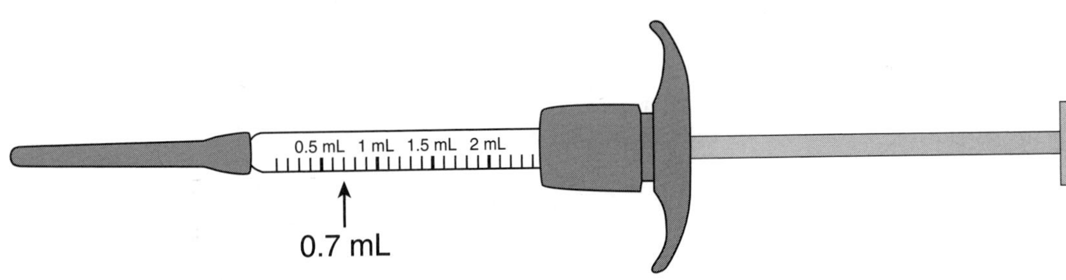

quick review

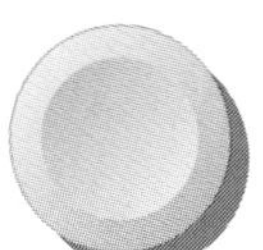

- To solve parenteral dosage problems, apply the three steps to dosage calculations:

  STEP 1 CONVERT

  STEP 2 THINK

  STEP 3 CALCULATE $\frac{\text{D (desired)}}{\text{H (have)}} \times \text{Q (quantity)} = \text{X (amount)}$

- Prepare a maximum of 3 mL per intramuscular injection site for an average size adult, 2 mL per site for children ages 6 through 12 and 0.5 to 1 mL for children under age 6.
- Calculate dose volumes and prepare injectable fractional doses in a syringe using these guidelines:
  - Standard doses over 1 mL: Round to *tenths* and measure in a 3 cc syringe. The 3 cc syringe is calibrated to 0.1 cc increments. Example: 1.53 mL is rounded to 1.5 mL and drawn up in a 3 cc syringe.

- Small (less than 0.5 mL), critical care, or children's doses: Round to *hundredths* and measure in a tuberculin (0.5 or 1 mL) syringe. The tuberculin syringe is calibrated in 0.01 mL increments. Example: 0.257 mL is rounded to 0.26 mL and drawn up in a tuberculin syringe.
- Measure amounts of 0.5–1 mL in either a tuberculin or 3cc syringe.

review set 27

Calculate the amount you will prepare for each dose. Draw an arrow to the syringe calibration that corresponds to the amount you will administer. Indicate dosages that need to be divided.

1. Order: *Codeine gr $\frac{1}{4}$ SC q.4h p.r.n., pain*

   Supply: 20 mL vial codeine labeled 30 mg per mL

   Give: ___Ø.5___ mL

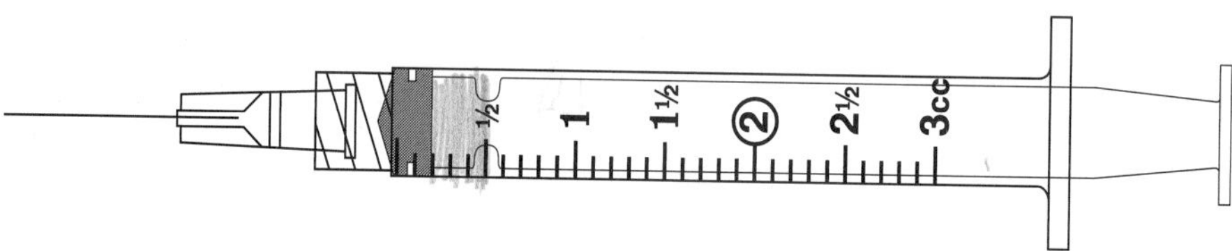

2. Order: *Bicillin 2,400,000 U IM stat*

   Supply: 10 mL vial of Bicillin containing 600,000 U per mL

   Give: ___4___ mL

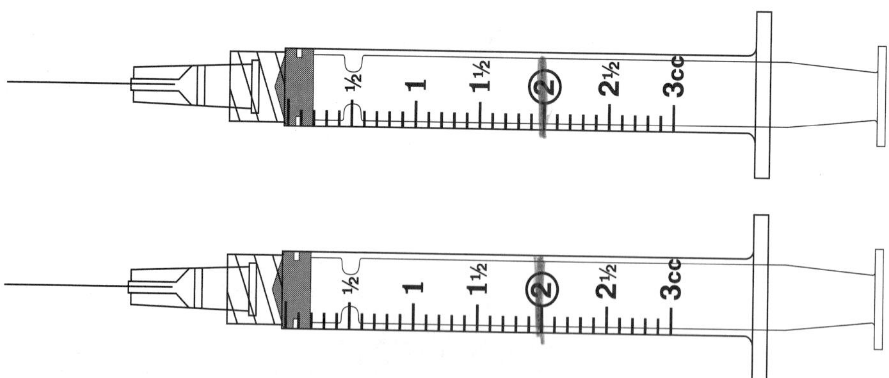

3. Order: *Digoxin 600 mcg IV stat*

   Supply: See label

   Give: ___2.4___ mL

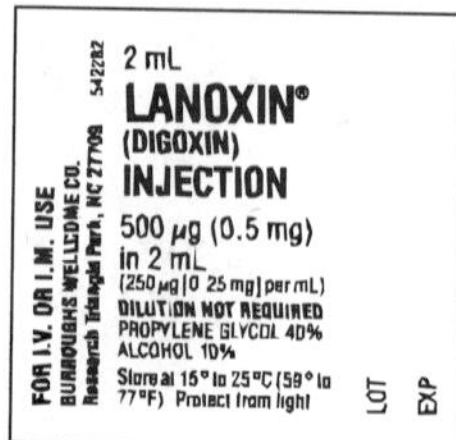

2 mL
LANOXIN®
(DIGOXIN)
INJECTION
500 µg (0.5 mg)
in 2 mL
(250 µg [0.25 mg] per mL)
DILUTION NOT REQUIRED
PROPYLENE GLYCOL 40%
ALCOHOL 10%
Store at 15° to 25°C (59° to 77°F) Protect from light
FOR I.V. OR I.M. USE
BURROUGHS WELLCOME CO.
Research Triangle Park, NC 27709
LOT
EXP

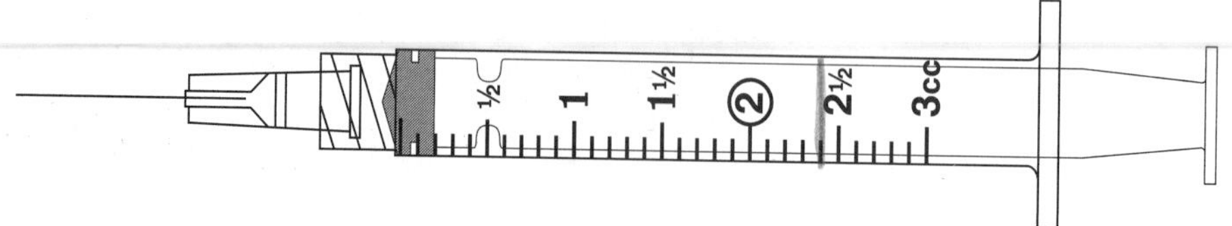

4. Order: *Procaine penicillin G 2.4 million U IM stat*

Supply: Wycillin (Procaine penicillin G) disposable, single-dose syringe containing 2,400,000 U/2 mL

Give: ________ mL

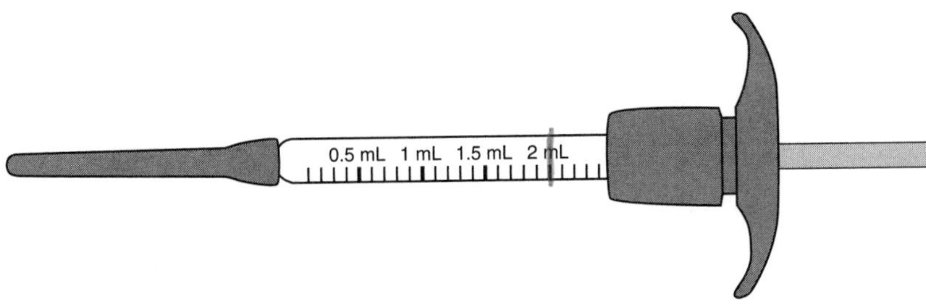

5. Order: *Tigan 200 mg IM stat, then 100 mg q.6h p.r.n. nausea*

Supply: 2 mL ampule Tigan containing 100 mg per mL

Give: ________ mL stat and ________ mL q.6h

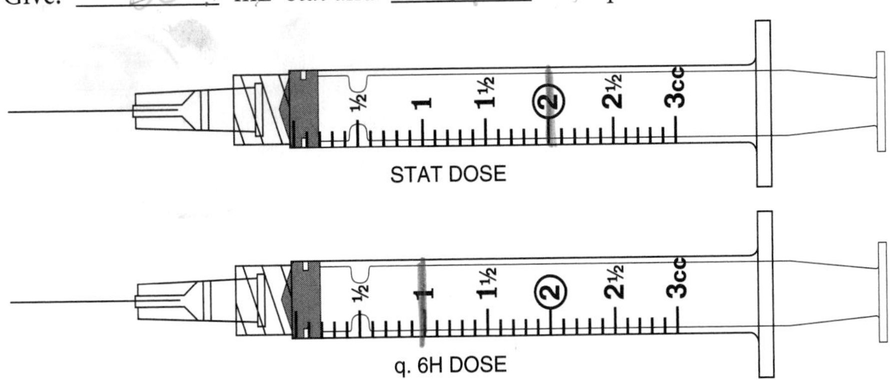

6. Order: *Heparin 8000 U SC q.8h*

Supply: See label

Give: ________ mL

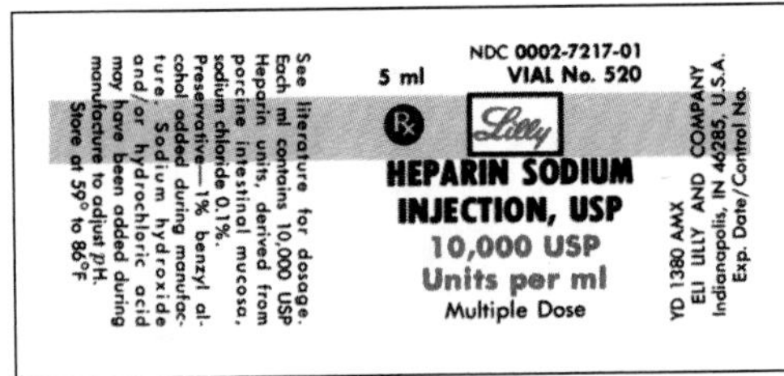

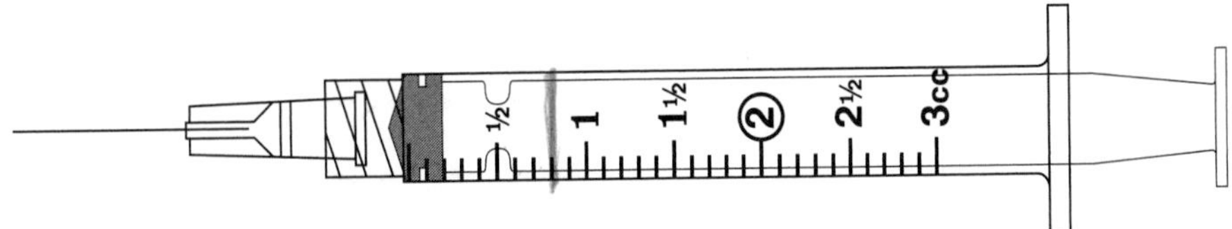

7. Order: *Potassium chloride 15 mEq added to each 1000 mL IV fluid container*

Supply: Potassium chloride 30 mL vial containing 2 mEq/mL

Give: ________ mL

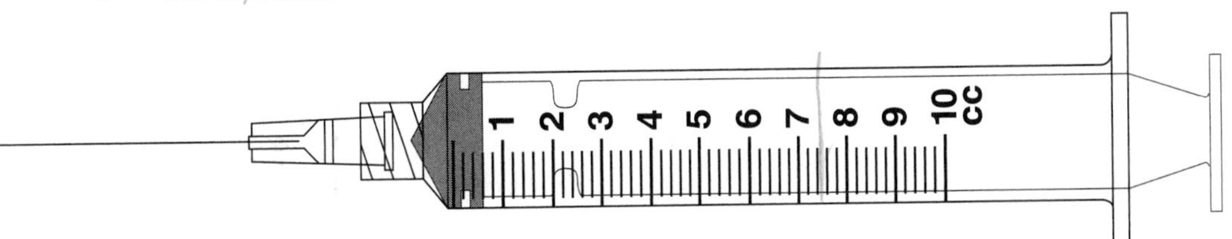

8. Order: *Demerol 60 mg IM q.4h p.r.n., pain*

   Supply: Demerol 75 mg per 1.5 mL

   Give: 1.2 mL

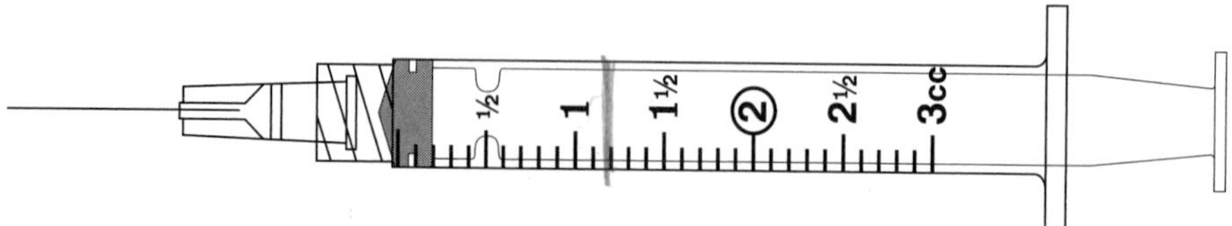

9. Order: *Atropine gr $\frac{1}{100}$ IM on call preoperatively*

   Supply: See label

   Give: 1.5 mL

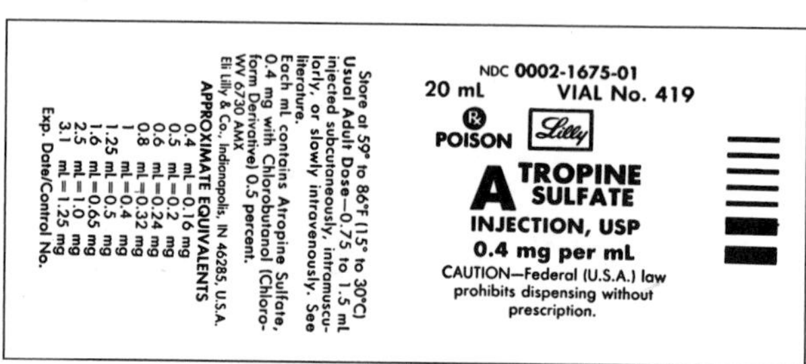

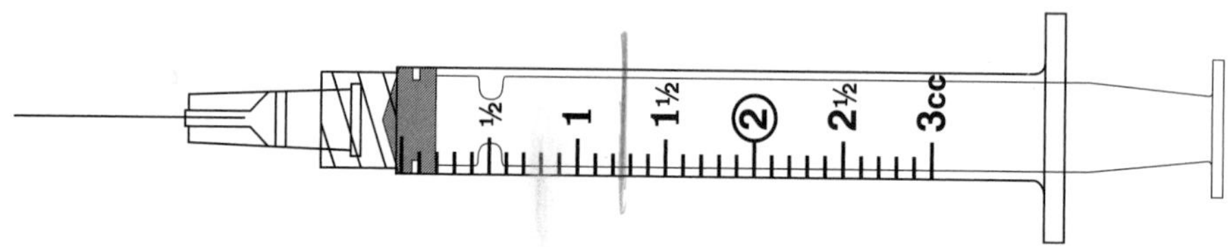

10. Order: *Morphine sulfate gr $\frac{1}{6}$ IM q.3–4h p.r.n.*

    Supply: Morphine sulfate 10 mg per mL

    Give: 1 mL

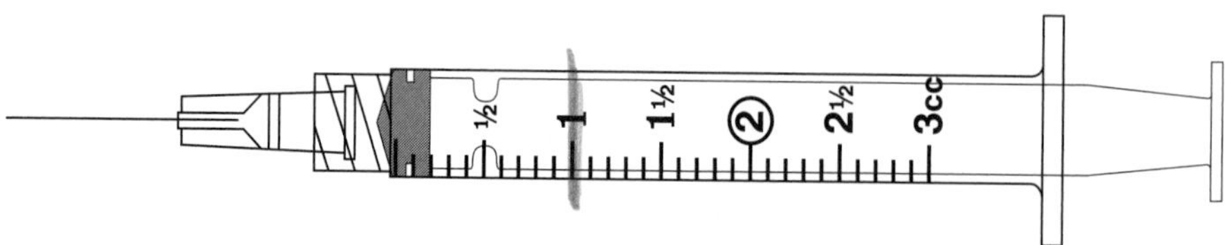

11. Order: *Procaine penicillin G 400,000 U IM t.i.d.*

    Supply: see label

    Give: 1.3 mL

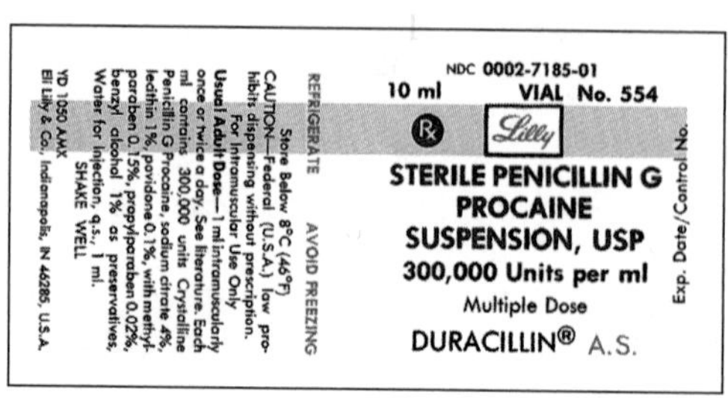

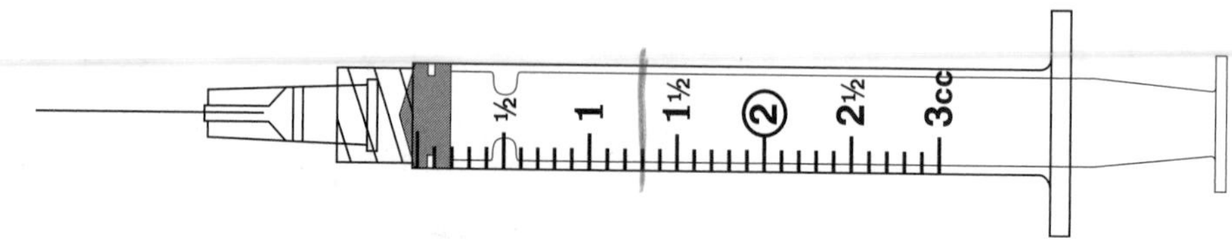

12. Order: *Heparin 4500 U SC q.d.*

    Supply: See label

    Give: __________ mL

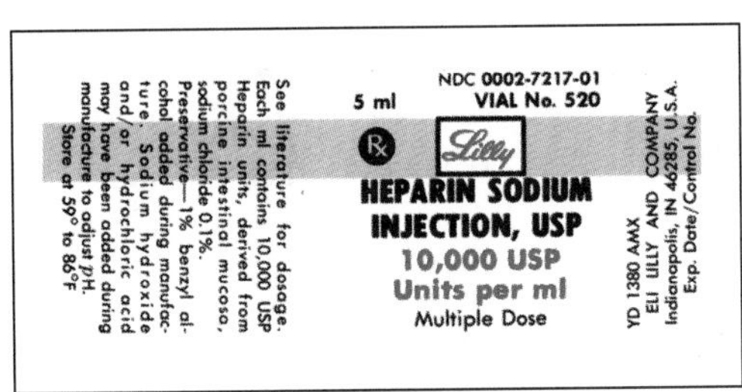

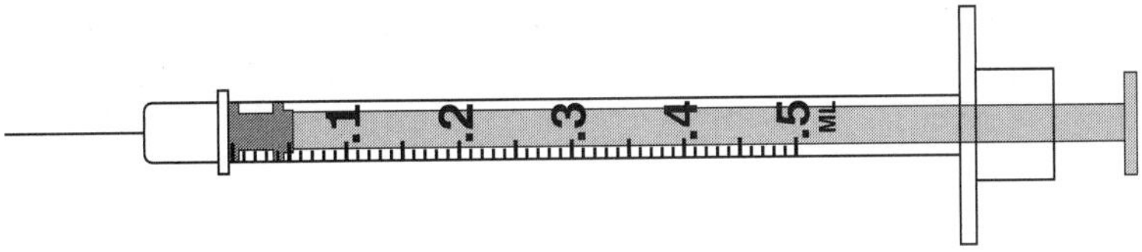

13. Order: *Compazine 7.5 mg IM q.3–4h p.r.n. nausea and vomiting*

    Supply: 10 mL vial Compazine containing 5 mg per mL

    Give: __________ mL

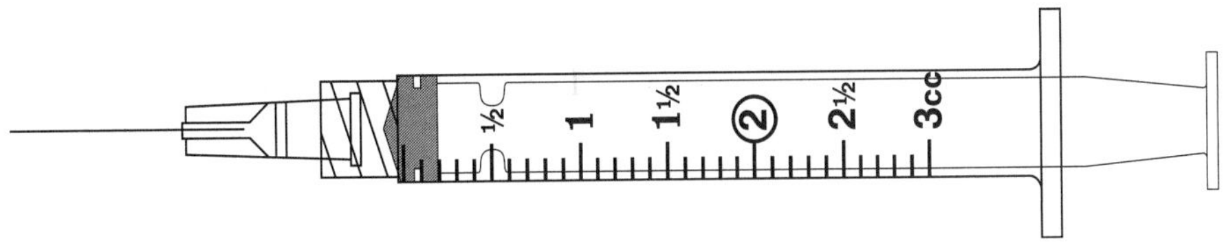

14. Order: *Vistaril 20 mg IM q.4h p.r.n. nausea*

    Supply: 10 mL vial of Vistaril 25 mg/mL

    Give: __________ mL

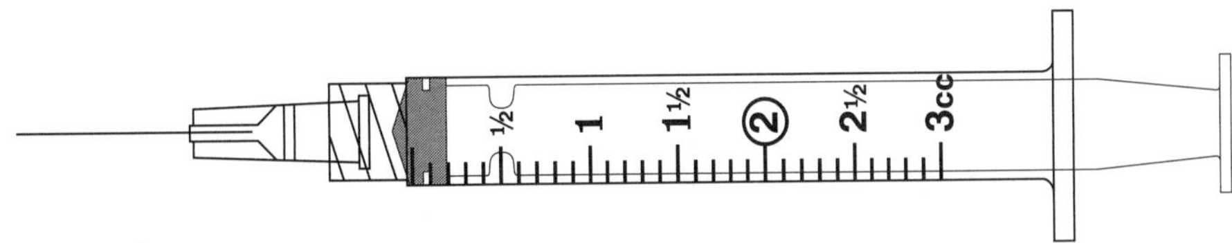

15. Order: *Gentamicin sulfate 60 mg IM b.i.d.*

    Supply: 2 mL vial Garamycin (gentamicin sulfate) 40 mg/mL

    Give: __________ mL

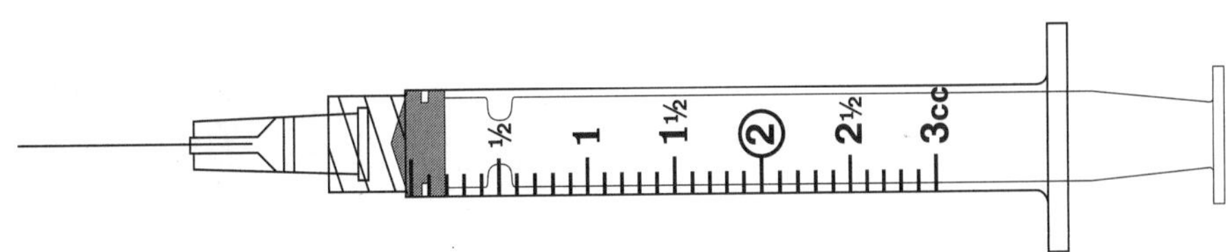

16. Order: *Ativan 3 mg IM on-call pre-operatively*

    Supply: 10 mL vial of Ativan 2 mg per mL

    Give: __________ mL

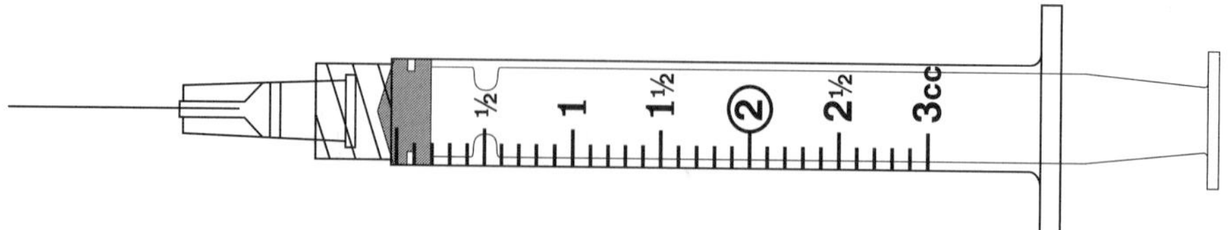

17. Order: *Vitamin B_{12} 0.5 mg IM once/week*

    Supply: See label

    Give: __________ mL

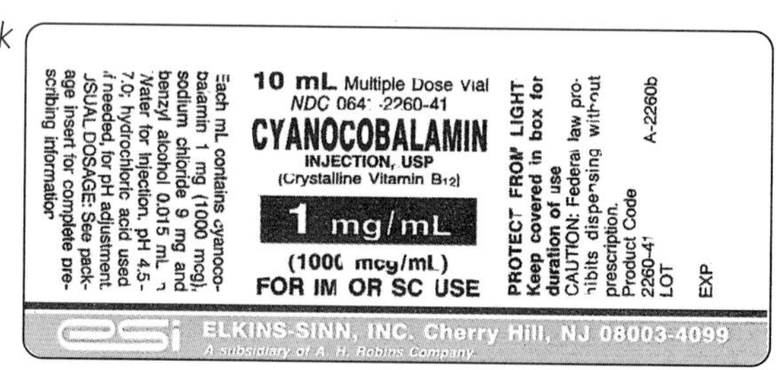

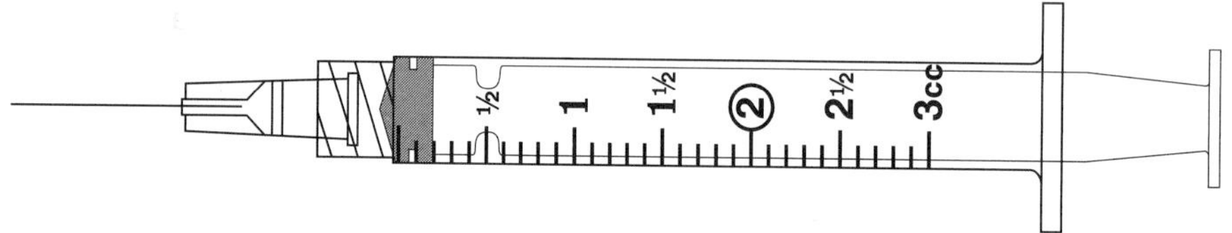

18. Order: *Zantac 20 mg IM q.6h*

    Supply: See label

    Give: __________ mL

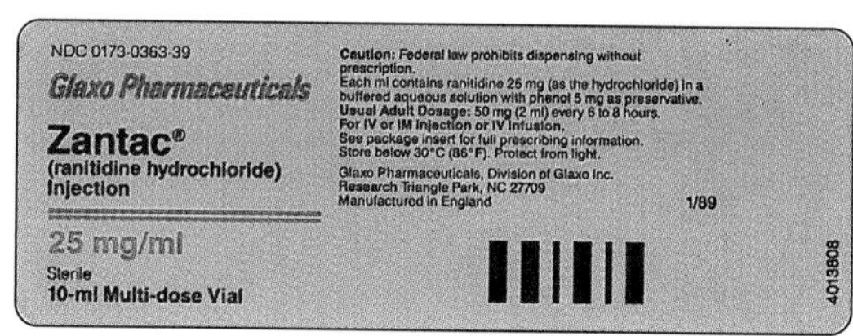

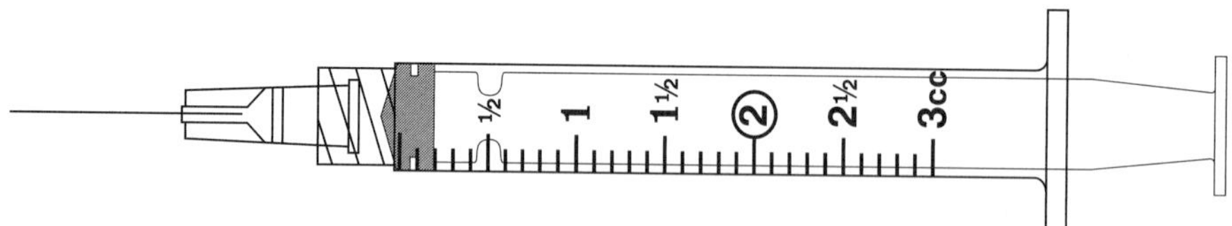

19. Order: *Phenergan 12.5 mg IM stat*

    Supply: See label

    Give: __________ mL

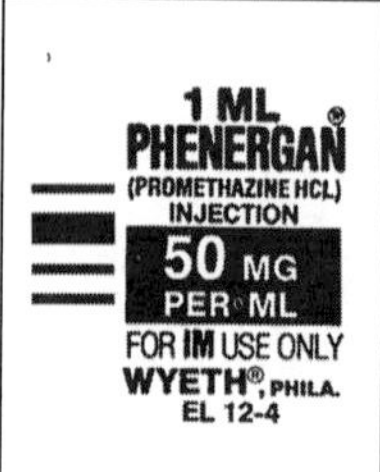

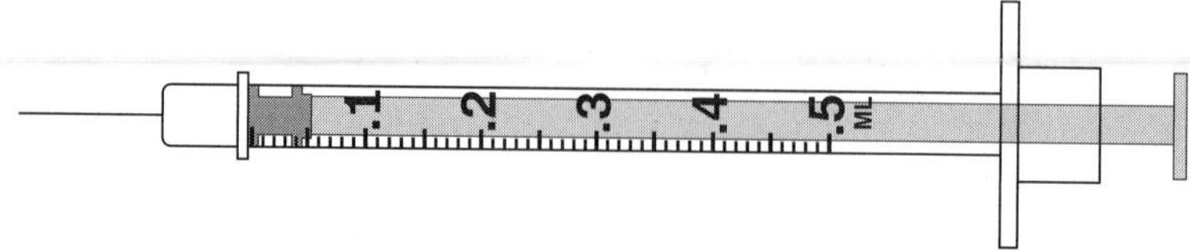

20. Order: *Valium 8 mg IM stat*

 Supply: Valium 10 mg per 2 mL

 Give: __________

After completing these problems, see pages 428–431 to check your answers.

Injectable Medications in Powder Form

Some medications are unstable when stored in solution or liquid form. Thus they are packaged in powdered form and must be dissolved by a liquid called a solvent or *diluent*. This dissolving procedure is referred to as *reconstitution*. Reconstitution is a necessary step in medication preparation to create a measurable and usable dosage form. The pharmacist often does this before dispensing most liquid medications for oral as well as parenteral routes. However, nurses need to understand reconstitution and know how to accomplish this. Some medications must be liquefied by the nurse just prior to administration.

The reconstitution process is easily compared to the preparation of a familiar liquid, such as hot chocolate from a powder mix. By adding the correct amount of water (the solvent or diluent) to the package of powdered, hot chocolate mix (solute) the resulting hot chocolate drink (solution) is in a properly mixed form.

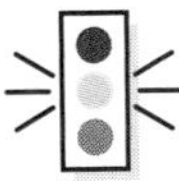

Caution: Before reconstituting injectable drugs, read and follow the label or package insert directions carefully. Consult a pharmacist with *any* questions.

Let's look at the rules of reconstitution of injectable medications from powder to liquid form. Follow these rules carefully to ensure that the patient receives the intended solution.

rule

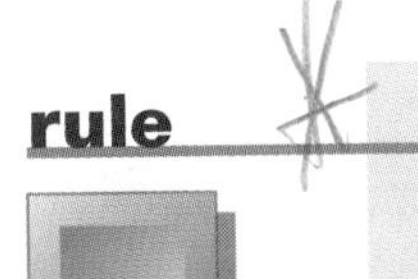

When reconstituting injectable medications, you must determine both the *type* and *amount* of diluent to be used.

Some powdered medications are packaged by the manufacturer with special solutions for reconstitution. Sterile water and 0.9% sodium chloride (normal saline) are most commonly used as diluents in parenteral medications. Both sterile water (Figure 10-2) and normal saline are available *preservative-free* when intended for single-use only, as well as in *bacteriostatic* form with preservative when intended for more than one use. Carefully check the instructions and vial label for the appropriate diluent.

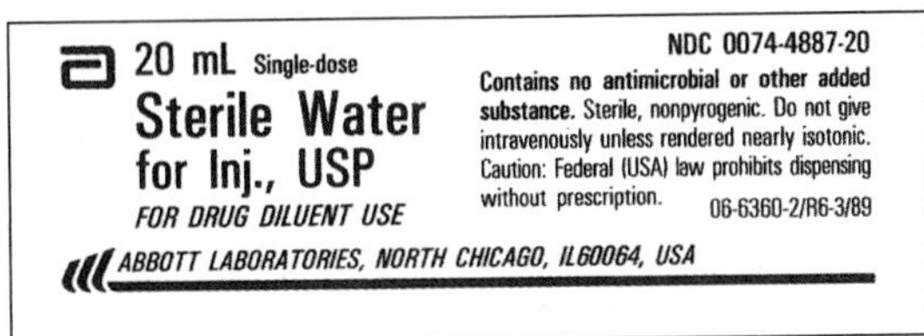

20 mL Single-dose
Sterile Water
for Inj., USP
FOR DRUG DILUENT USE
NDC 0074-4887-20
Contains no antimicrobial or other added substance. Sterile, nonpyrogenic. Do not give intravenously unless rendered nearly isotonic. Caution: Federal (USA) law prohibits dispensing without prescription.
06-6360-2/R6-3/89
ABBOTT LABORATORIES, NORTH CHICAGO, IL60064, USA

FIGURE 10-2 Reconstitution Diluent for Parenteral Powdered Drugs

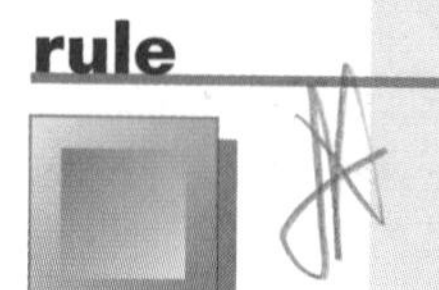

rule

When reconstituting injectable medications, you must determine the *volume in mL* of diluent to be used, then reconstitute the drug and *note the resulting supply dosage* on the vial.

Because many reconstituted medications can be administered either intramuscularly (IM) or intravenously (IV), it is essential to verify the route of administration before reconstituting the medication. Remember that the intramuscular volume of 3 mL or less per injection site is determined by the patient's age and condition and the intramuscular site selected. The directions take this into account by stating the minimal volume or quantity of diluent that should

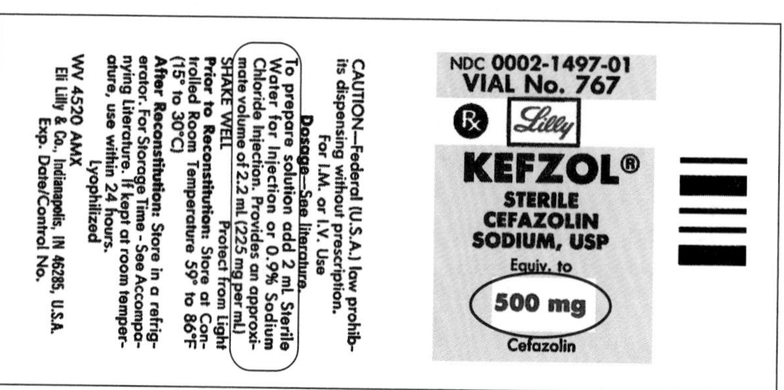

DOSAGE AND ADMINISTRATION

Kefzol may be administered intramuscularly or intravenously after reconstitution. Total daily dosages are the same for either route of administration.

Intramuscular Administration—Reconstitute as directed by Table 3 with 0.9% Sodium Chloride Injection, Sterile Water for Injection, or Bacteriostatic Water for Injection. Shake well until dissolved. Kefzol should be injected into a large muscle mass. Pain on injection is infrequent with Kefzol.

TABLE 3. DILUTION TABLE

Vial Size	Diluent to Be Added	Approximate Available Volume	Approximate Average Concentration
250 mg	2 mL	2 mL	125 mg/mL
500 mg	2 mL	2.2 mL	225 mg/mL
1 g*	2.5 mL	3 mL	330 mg/mL

*The 1-g vial should be reconstituted only with Sterile Water for Injection or Bacteriostatic Water for Injection.

Intravenous Administration—Kefzol may be administered by intravenous injection or by continuous or intermittent infusion.

Intermittent intravenous infusion: Kefzol can be administered along with primary intravenous fluid management programs in a volume control set or in a separate, secondary IV bottle. Reconstituted 500 mg or 1 g of Kefzol may be diluted in 50 to 100 mL of 1 of the following intravenous solutions: 0.9% Sodium Chloride Injection, 5% or 10% Dextrose Injection, 5% Dextrose in Lactated Ringer's Injection, 5% Dextrose and 0.9% Sodium Chloride Injection (also may be used with 5% Dextrose and 0.45% or 0.2% Sodium Chloride Injection), Lactated Ringer's Injection, 5% or 10% Invert Sugar in Sterile Water for Injection, Ringer's Injection, Normosol®-M in D5-W, Ionosol® B with Dextrose 5%, or Plasma-Lyte® with 5% Dextrose.

ADD-Vantage Vials of Kefzol are to be reconstituted *only* with 0.9% Sodium Chloride Injection or 5% Dextrose Injection in the 50-mL or 100-mL Flexible Diluent Containers.

Intravenous injection (Administer solution directly into vein or through tubing): Dilute the reconstituted 500 mg or 1 g of Kefzol in a minimum of 10 mL of Sterile Water for Injection. Inject solution slowly over 3 to 5 minutes. Do not inject in less than 3 minutes. (NOTE: ADD-VANTAGE VIALS ARE NOT TO BE USED IN THIS MANNER.)

Dosage—The usual adult dosages are given in Table 4.

TABLE 4. USUAL ADULT DOSAGE

Type of Infection	Dose	Frequency
Pneumococcal pneumonia	500 mg	q12h
Mild infections caused by susceptible gram-positive cocci	250 to 500 mg	q8h
Acute uncomplicated urinary tract infections	1 g	q12h
Moderate to severe infections	500 mg to 1 g	q6 to 8h
Severe, life-threatening infections (eg, endocarditis, and septicemia)*	1 g to 1.5 g	q6h

*In rare instances, doses up to 12 g of cefazolin per day have been used.

FIGURE 10-3 Kefzol Label with Portion of the Accompanying Package Insert

be added to the powdered drug for IM use. Often the powdered drug itself *adds* volume to the solution. The powder displaces the liquid as it dissolves and increases the total resulting volume. The resulting volume of the reconstituted drug is usually given on the label. This resulting volume determines the liquid's concentration or *supply dosage*. Figure 10-3 shows the reconstitution directions for the drug Kefzol as printed on the vial label with additional instructions as seen in the package insert.

NOTE: Figure 10-3 and subsequent reproductions of package inserts represent only the portion of the information relative to the specific problem under study.

Look at the directions on the Kefzol label. They state, "To prepare solution add 2 mL Sterile Water for Injection or 0.9% Sodium Chloride Injection. Provides an approximate volume of 2.2 mL (225 mg per mL)." Notice that when 2 mL of diluent is added, the 500 mg of powdered drug displaces an additional 0.2 mL for a total solution volume of 2.2 mL. Then the supply dosage available after reconstitution is *225 mg of Kefzol per mL of solution.* Figure 10-4 demonstrates the reconstitution procedure for Kefzol 500 mg.

Single-dose vials contain only enough medication for one dose, and the resulting contents are administered after the powder is diluted. But in some cases the nurse also may dilute a powdered medication in a multiple-dose vial that will result in more than one dose. When this

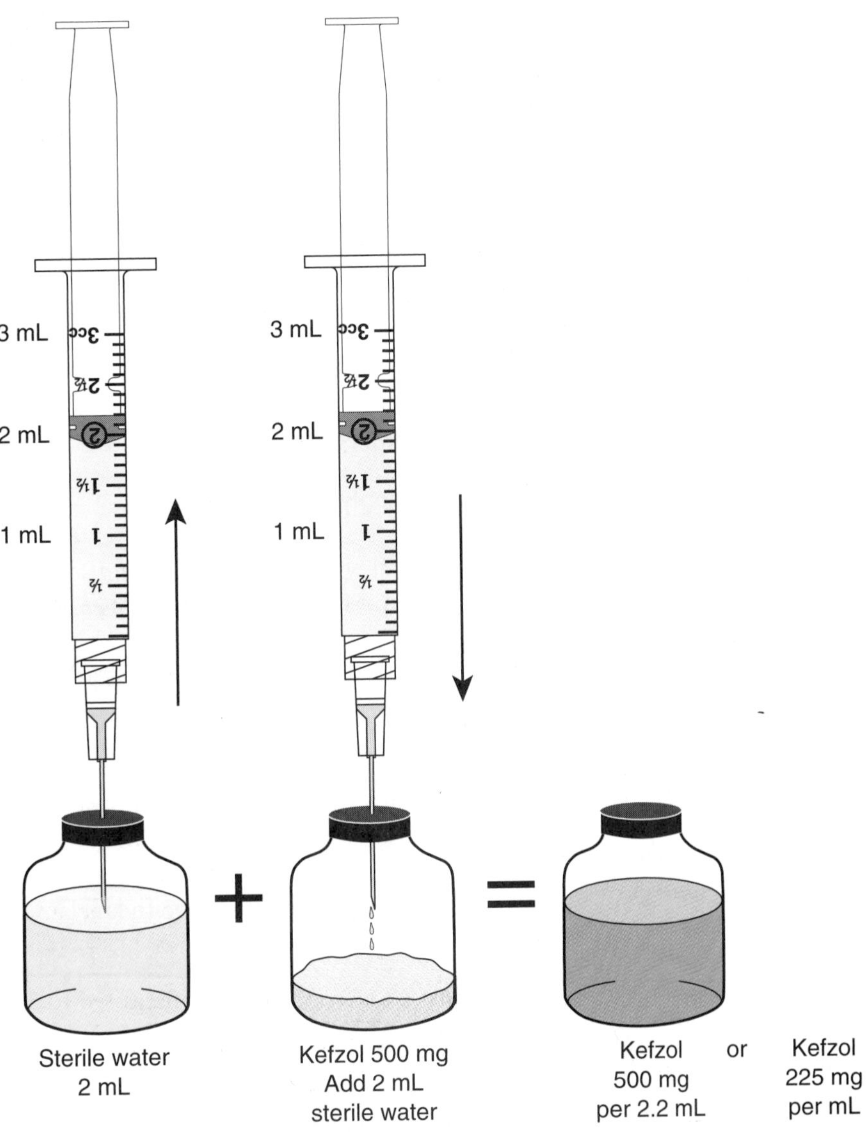

FIGURE 10-4 Kefzol Reconstitution Procedure

is the case, it is important to clearly label the vial after reconstitution. Labeling will be discussed in the next section.

There are two types of reconstituted parenteral solutions: single strength and multiple strength. The simplest type to dilute is a *single strength* solution. This type usually has the recommended dilution directions and resulting supply dosage printed on the label, such as the Kefzol 500 mg label at the top of Figure 10-3 (p. 194).

Some medications have several directions for dilution that allow the nurse to select the best supply dosage. This is called a *multiple strength* solution and requires even more careful reading of the instructions. Often these directions for reconstitution will not fit on the vial label. The package insert or other printed instructions are then consulted to ensure accurate dilution of the parenteral medication.

Let's look at some examples of powdered medications to clarify what the nurse needs to do to correctly reconstitute parenteral medications from powder to liquid form.

Example 1:

Single-strength solution/single-dose vial

Order: *Ancef 750 mg IM q.8h*

Supply: *1 g vial of powdered Ancef* with directions on the right side of the label as follows: "For IM use, add 2.5 mL Sterile Water . . . Provides an approximate volume of 3.0 mL (330 mg/mL)."

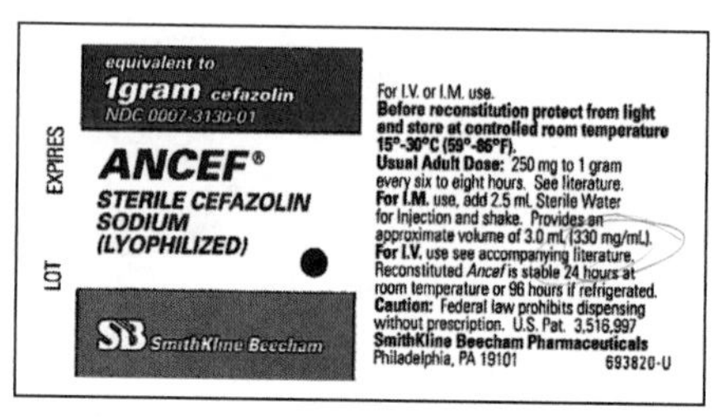

This means you have available a vial of 1 gram of *Ancef* to which you will add 2.5 milliliters of diluent (sterile water). The powdered drug displaces 0.5 mL. Then each 3 milliliters contains 1 g of the drug, and there are 330 mg in each 1 mL.

STEP 1 CONVERT No conversion is necessary.

Order: *Ancef 750 mg*

Supply: 330 mg/1 mL

STEP 2 THINK You want to give more than 1 mL. In fact you want to give more than twice as much as 330 mg or more than 2 mL.

STEP 3 CALCULATE $\frac{D}{H} \times Q = \frac{75\not{0} \text{ mg}}{33\not{0} \text{ mg}} \times 1 \text{ mL} = \frac{75}{33} \text{ mL} = 2.27 \text{ mL}$; rounded to 2.3 mL

Give 2.3 mL of Ancef intramuscularly every 8 hours.

The vial of Ancef contains only one full ordered dose of reconstituted drug. Any remaining medication is usually discarded. Because this Ancef vial provides only one dose, the nurse will not have to label and store any of the reconstituted drug.

Select a *3 cc syringe, and measure 2.3 mL* of Ancef reconstituted to 330 mg/mL.

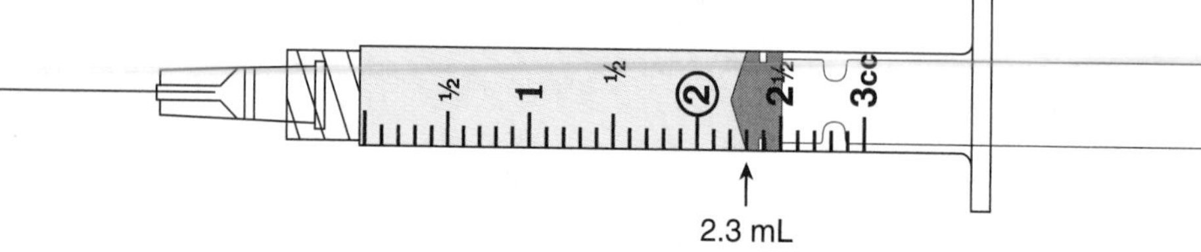

Example 2:

Single-strength solution/multiple-dose vial

Suppose the drug order reads *Ancef 330 mg IM q.8h.* Using the same size vial of Ancef and the same dilution instructions as in Example 1, you would now have 3 full doses of Ancef, making this a multiple-dose vial.

Select a 3 cc syringe, and measure 1 mL of Ancef reconstituted to 330 mg/mL.

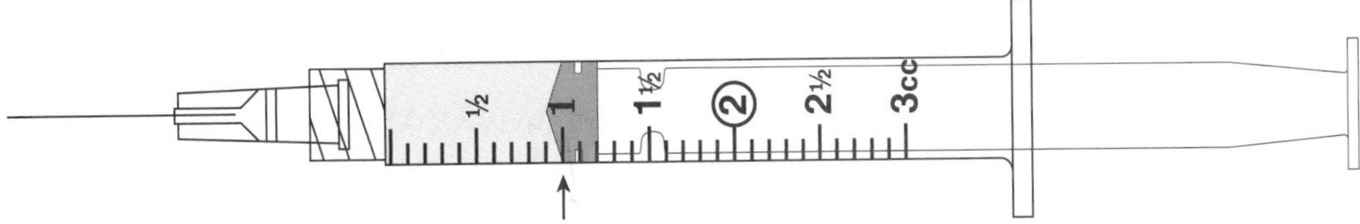

rule

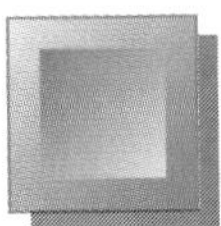

When reconstituting multiple-dose injectable medications, verify the length of drug potency. Store the reconstituted drug appropriately with the label attached.

If multiple doses result from the reconstitution of a powdered drug, the solution must be used in a timely manner. Because the drug potency (or stability) may be several hours to several days, check the drug label, package information sheet, or *Hospital Formulary* for how long the drug may be used after reconstitution. Store the drug appropriately at room temperature or refrigerate per the manufacturer's instructions. Notice the directions provided on the Ancef label that state, "Reconstituted Ancef is stable 24 hours at room temperature or 96 hours if refrigerated."

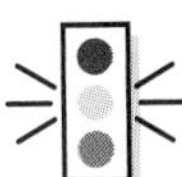

Caution: The length of potency is different from the expiration date. The expiration date is provided by the manufacturer on the label. It indicates the *last* date the drug may be reconstituted and used.

When you reconstitute or mix a multiple-dose vial of medication in powdered form, it is important that it be *clearly labeled* with the *date* and *time* of preparation, the strength or *supply dosage* you prepared, *length of potency, storage directions*, and your *initials*. Because the medication becomes unstable after storage for long periods, the date and time are especially important. Figure 10-5 demonstrates the proper label for the Ancef reconstituted to 330 mg/mL. Because there are only 3 doses of reconstituted Ancef in this vial, and 3 doses will be administered within 16 hours (now at 0800, then again at 1600 and 2400), this drug can be safely stored at room temperature.

1/30/xx, 0800, reconstituted as 330 mg/mL. Expires 1/31/xx, 0800 at room temperature.
G.D.P.

FIGURE 10-5 Reconstitution Label for Ancef

Example 3:

Multiple-strength solution/multiple-dose vial

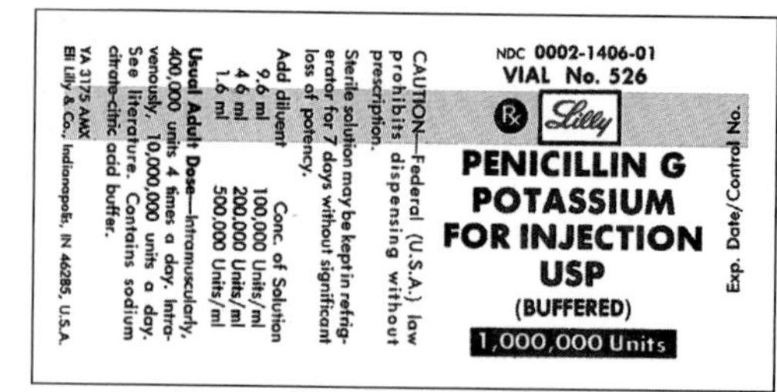

Some parenteral powdered medications allow the nurse to select a particular dosage strength. This results in a reasonable amount to be given to a particular patient.

Order: *Penicillin G potassium 300,000 U IM q.i.d.*

Supply: *Penicillin G potassium 1,000,000 U vial*

This vial contains a total of 1,000,000 U of penicillin. The reconstitution instructions are shown on the left side of the label. The instructions detail three different intramuscular solution strengths or concentrations that are determined by the added diluent volume. Let's look at each of the three instructions. Notice how these reconstituted strengths differ and when they might be selected.

Refer to the first directions, which state "Add diluent *9.6 mL* (for a) Conc(entration) of Solution *100,000 Units/mL*." This means when you add 9.6 milliliters of sterile diluent to this vial of powdered penicillin, the result is 1,000,000 units of penicillin in 10 milliliters of solution. The diluent is 9.6 milliliters; the powder displaces 0.4 more milliliter for a total of 1,000,000 units in 10 milliliters, resulting in a reconstituted solution strength of *100,000 U per mL.*

STEP 1 **CONVERT** No conversion is necessary.

STEP 2 **THINK** Estimate that you want to give 3 times 100,000 U or 3 times 1 mL, which is 3 mL.

STEP 3 **CALCULATE** $\frac{D}{H} \times Q = \frac{\overset{3}{\cancel{300,000\text{ U}}}}{\underset{1}{\cancel{100,000\text{ U}}}} \times 1\text{ mL} = 3\text{ mL};$

given intramuscularly four times daily

Because each dose is 3 mL and the total volume is 10 mL, you still have enough for 2 additional full doses. As an IM dose, 3 mL is the maximum volume for a large, adult muscle.

Select a *3 cc syringe, and measure 3 mL* of penicillin reconstituted to 100,000 units/mL.

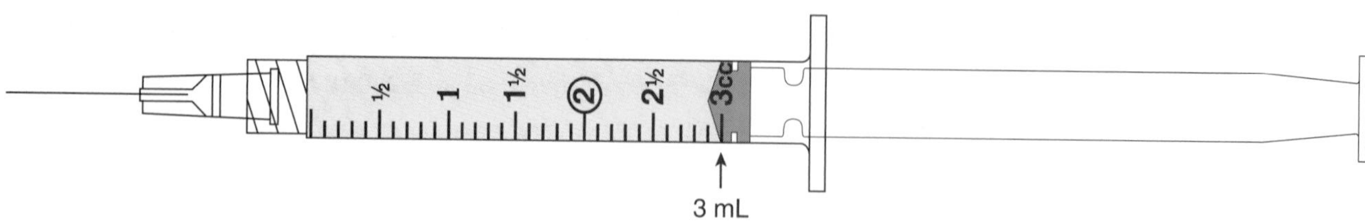

Caution: The supply dosage of a reconstituted drug is an essential detail that the nurse must write on a multiple-dose vial label. Once reconstituted, there is no way to verify how much diluent was actually added without proper labeling.

Be sure to add a label to the reconstituted penicillin G 100,000 U/mL vial, Figure 10-6.

> 1/30/xx, 0800, reconstituted as
> 100,000 U/mL. Expires 2/06/xx, 0800,
> keep refrigerated. G.D.P.

FIGURE 10-6 Reconstitution Label for Penicillin G Potassium, 1 g, Reconstituted with 9.2 mL Diluent

Next, refer to the second set of directions on the penicillin label which state, "Add diluent *4.6 mL* (for a) Conc(entration) of Solution *200,000 Units/mL*. This means when you add 4.6 mL of sterile diluent to the vial of powdered penicillin, the result is 1,000,000 U of penicillin in 5 mL of solution. The diluent is 4.6 mL. The powder displaces 0.4 mL more, for a total of 1,000,000 U in 5 mL and a solution strength of 200,000 U per mL.

STEP 1 **CONVERT** No conversion is necessary.

STEP 2 **THINK** Estimate that you want to give more than 1 mL but less than 2 mL.

STEP 3 **CALCULATE** $\frac{D}{H} \times Q = \frac{\overset{3}{\cancel{300,000\ U}}}{\underset{2}{\cancel{200,000\ U}}} \times 1\ mL = \frac{3}{2}\ mL = 1.5\ mL;$

given intramuscularly four times daily.

Because each dose is 1.5 mL and the total volume is 5 mL, you still have enough for 2 more full doses. As an IM dose, 1.5 mL is a more reasonable volume than 3 mL, and 1.5 mL would be appropriate for a variety of ages and muscle sizes.

Select a *3 cc syringe, and measure 1.5 mL* of penicillin reconstituted to 200,000 units/mL.

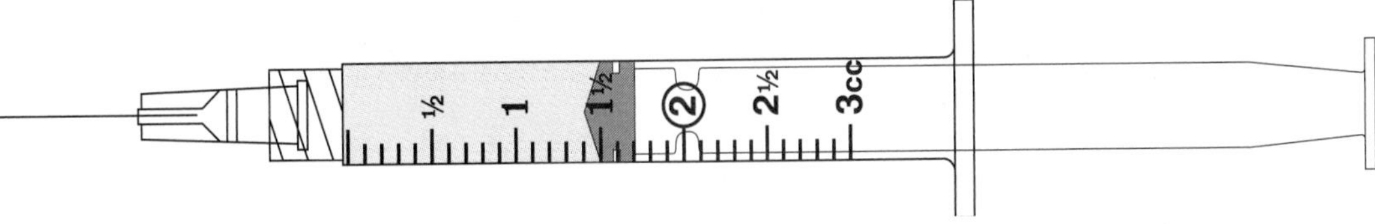

Now add the label to the reconstituted penicillin G 200,000 U/mL vial, Figure 10-7.

> 1/30/xx, 0800, reconstituted as
> 200,000 U/mL. Expires 2/06/xx,
> 0800, keep refrigerated. G.D.P.

FIGURE 10-7 Reconstitution Label for Penicillin G Potassium, 1 g, Reconstituted with 4.6 mL Diluent

You could also reconstitute this drug to a solution strength of 500,000 U/mL by following the third set of instructions and adding 1.6 mL to the vial for a total volume of 2 mL.

STEP 1 **CONVERT** No conversion is necessary.

STEP 2 **THINK** Estimate that you want to give less than 1 mL but more than 0.5 mL.

STEP 3 **CALCULATE** $\frac{D}{H} \times Q = \frac{\overset{3}{\cancel{300{,}000\ U}}}{\underset{5}{\cancel{500{,}000\ U}}} \times 1\ mL = \frac{3}{5}\ mL = 0.6\ mL$; given intramuscularly four times daily

Each dose is 0.6 mL, and the total volume is 2 mL. You still have enough for 2 more full doses. As an IM dose, 0.6 mL is the most concentrated and smallest volume that could be utilized for a parenteral dose. It would be ideal for an infant, small child, or anyone with wasted muscle mass.

Select a *3 cc syringe, and measure 0.6 mL* of penicillin reconstituted to 500,000 units/mL.

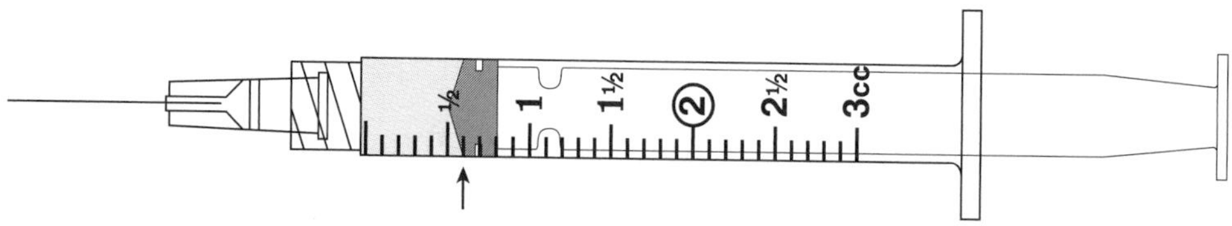

Finally, add the label to the reconstituted penicillin G 500,000 U/mL vial, Figure 10-8.

1/30/xx, 0800, reconstituted as
500,000 U/mL. Expires 2/06/xx, 0800
keep refrigerated. G.D.P.

FIGURE 10-8 Reconstitution Label for Penicillin G Potassium, 1 g, Reconstituted with 1.6 mL Diluent

As you can see from these three possible reconstituted strengths, there are three full doses available from this multiple-dose vial in each case. The added diluent volume is the key factor that determines the resulting concentration. It is the *supply dosage* that ultimately determines the *injectable volume per dose.*

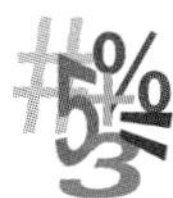

math tip: When multiple directions for diluting are given, the *smaller* the amount of diluent added, the *greater* the resulting solution concentration will be.

quick review

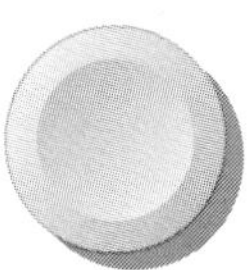

It is important that you remember the following points when reconstituting drugs:

- If any medicine remains for future use after reconstitution, clearly label:
  1. date and time of preparation
  2. strength or concentration per volume
  3. potency expiration
  4. recommended storage
  5. your initials
- Read all instructions carefully. If no instructions accompany the vial, confer with the pharmacist before proceeding.
- When reconstituting multiple strength parenteral powders, select the dosage strength that is appropriate for the patient's age, size, and condition.

review set 28

Calculate the amount you will prepare for each dose. The labels provided are the drugs available. Draw an arrow to the syringe calibration that corresponds with the amount you will draw up.

1. Order: *Ceftazidime 250 mg IM q.i.d.*

   Reconstitute with __________ mL diluent and give __________ mL.

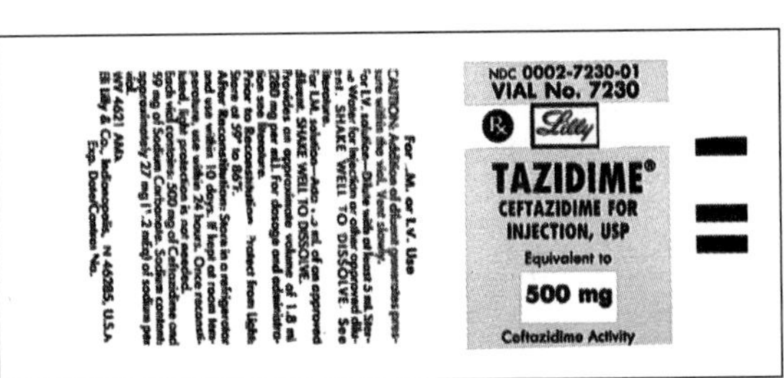

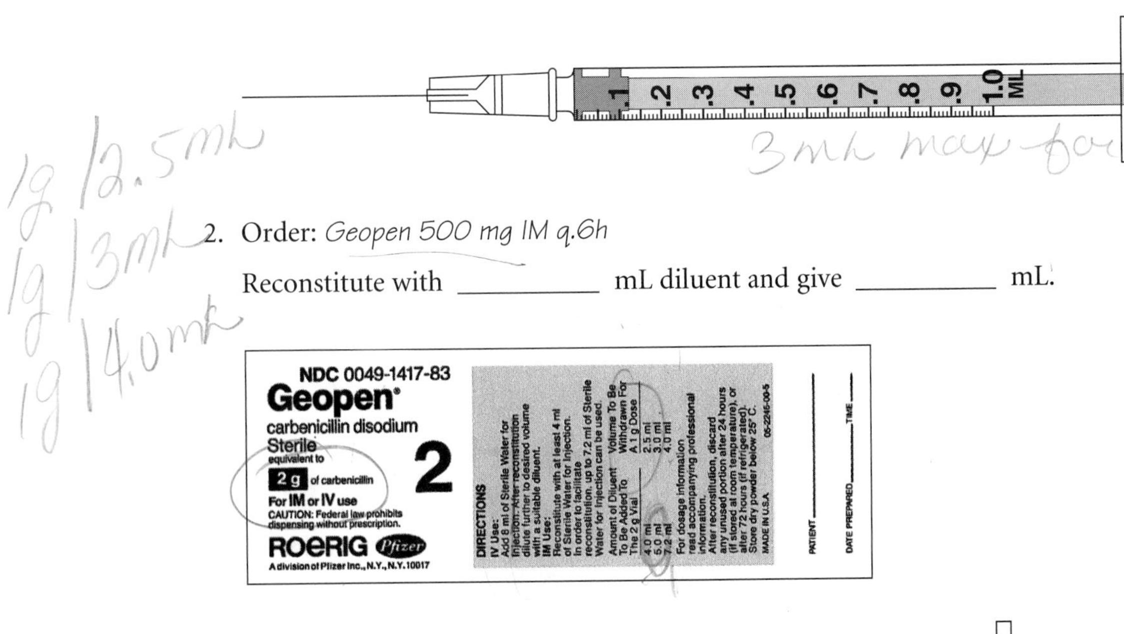

2. Order: *Geopen 500 mg IM q.6h*

   Reconstitute with __________ mL diluent and give __________ mL.

3. Order: *Librium 25 mg IM q.6h p.r.n.*

Directions: Add 2 mL Special Diluent to yield 100 mg per 2 mL. Reconstitute with __2__ mL diluent and give __0.5__ mL.

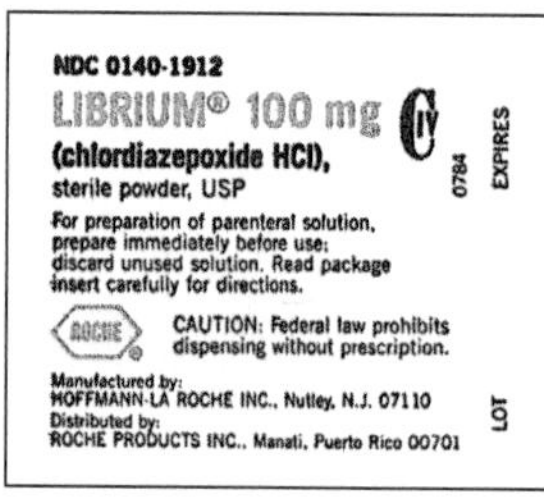

2 ml SIZE Special Intramuscular Diluent
For use with LIBRIUM® (chlordiazepoxide HCl) sterile powder.
FOR INTRAMUSCULAR USE ONLY, NOT FOR INTRAVENOUS USE.
DO NOT USE IF OPALESCENT OR HAZY.
Mfd. by: HOFFMANN-LA ROCHE INC. Nutley, N.J. 07110
Distr. by: ROCHE PRODUCTS INC. Manati, Puerto Rico 00701
0784 Expires

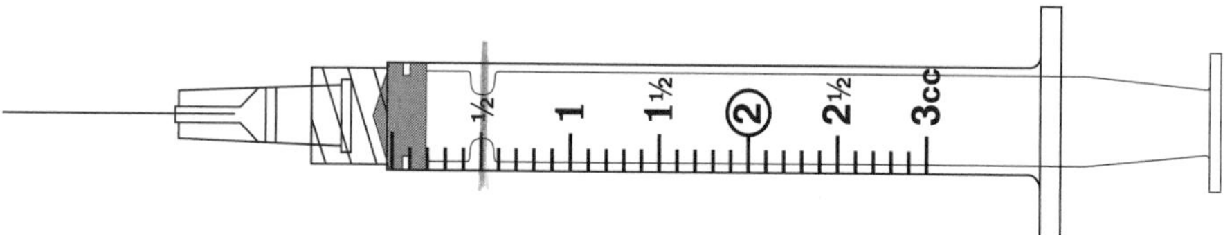

4. Order: *Cytoxan 250 mg IV q.d. × 5 days*

Reconstitute with __50__ mL diluent and give __12.5__ mL.

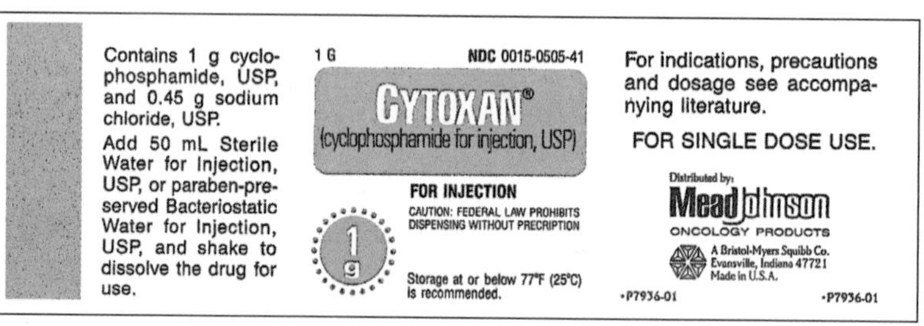

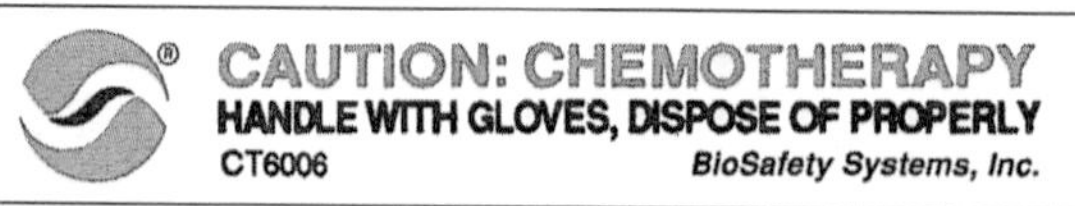

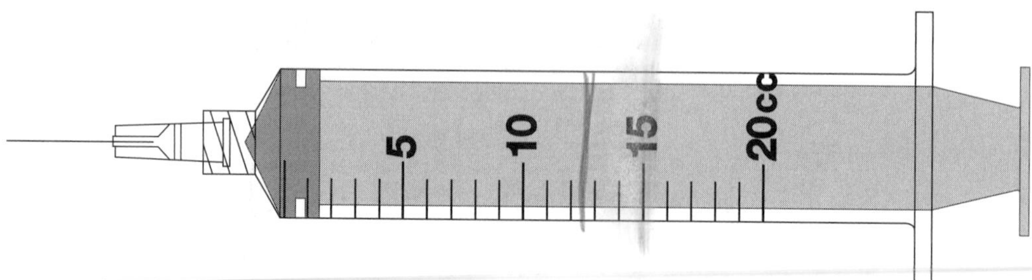

5. Order: *Polycillin-N 300 mg IV PB q.6h in 50 mL D_5W*

Reconstitute with __50__ mL diluent and give __15__ mL.

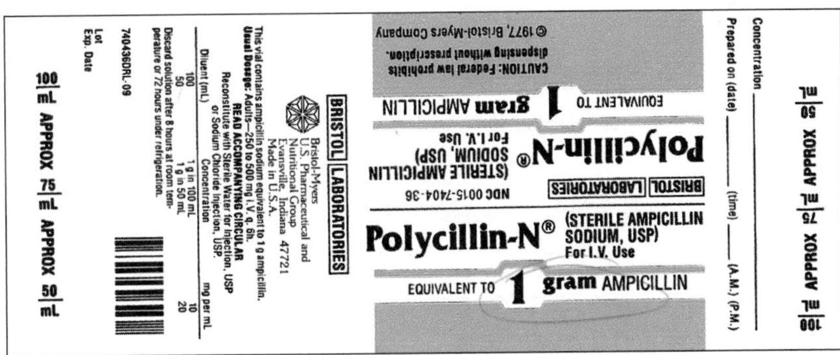

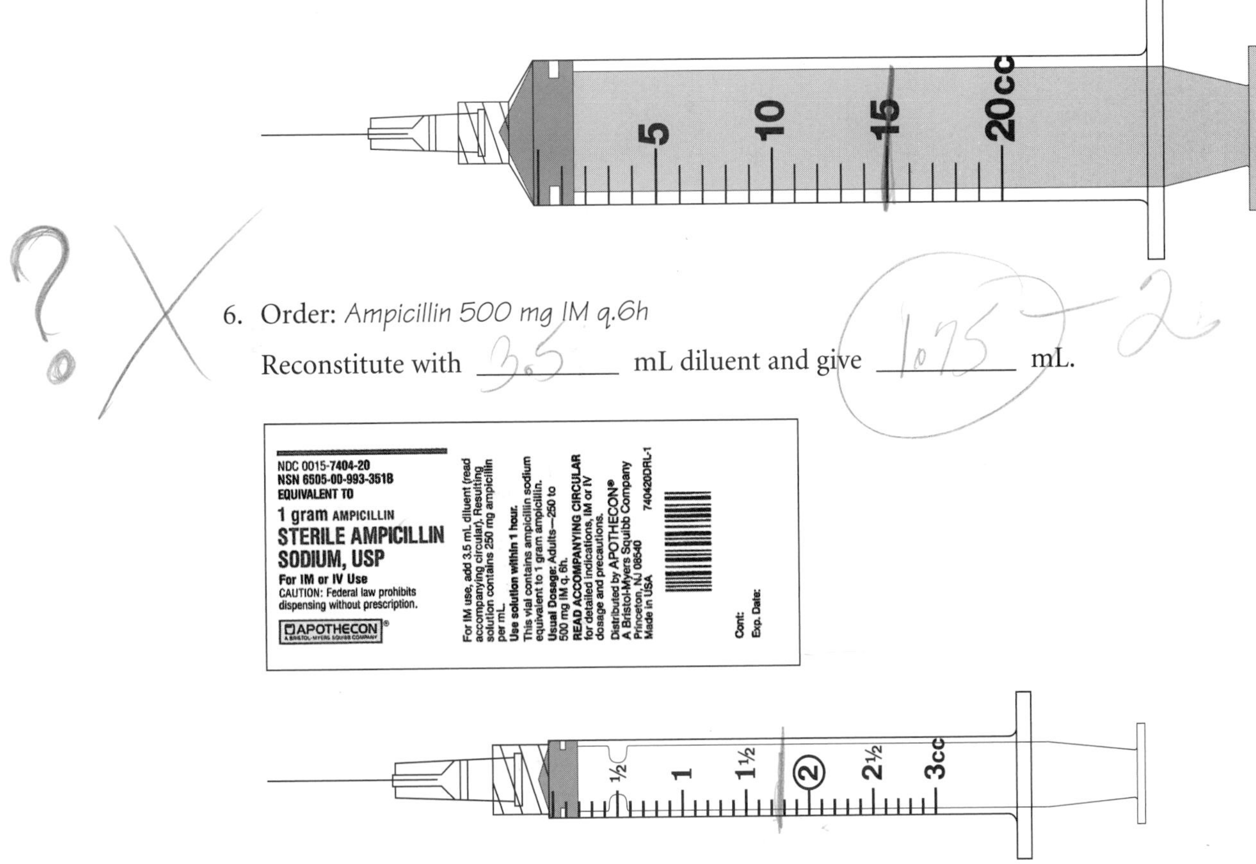

6. Order: *Ampicillin 500 mg IM q.6h*

Reconstitute with ________ mL diluent and give ________ mL.

7. Order: *Solu-Medrol 175 mg IM q.d.*

Reconstitute with ________ mL diluent and give ________ mL.

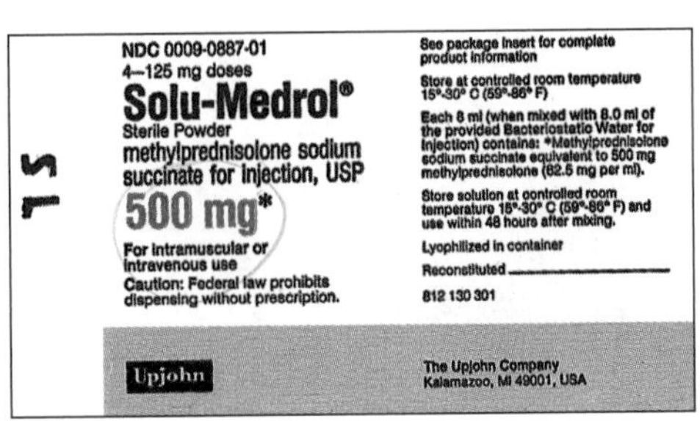

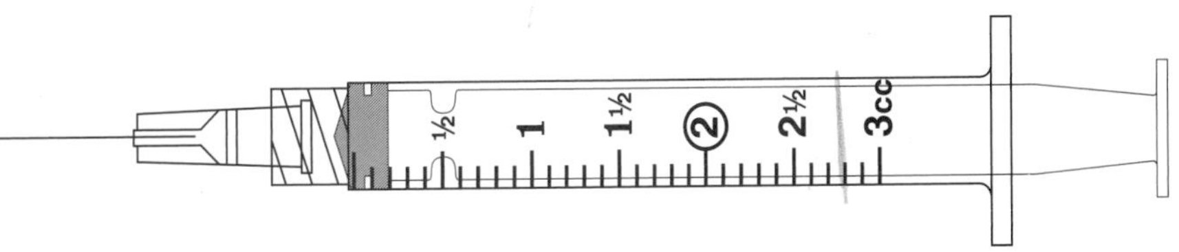

8. Order: *Pipracil 200 mg IM q.6h*

   Directions: Adding 4 cc diluent yields 1 g per 2.5 mL

   Reconstitute with ________ mL diluent and give ________ mL.

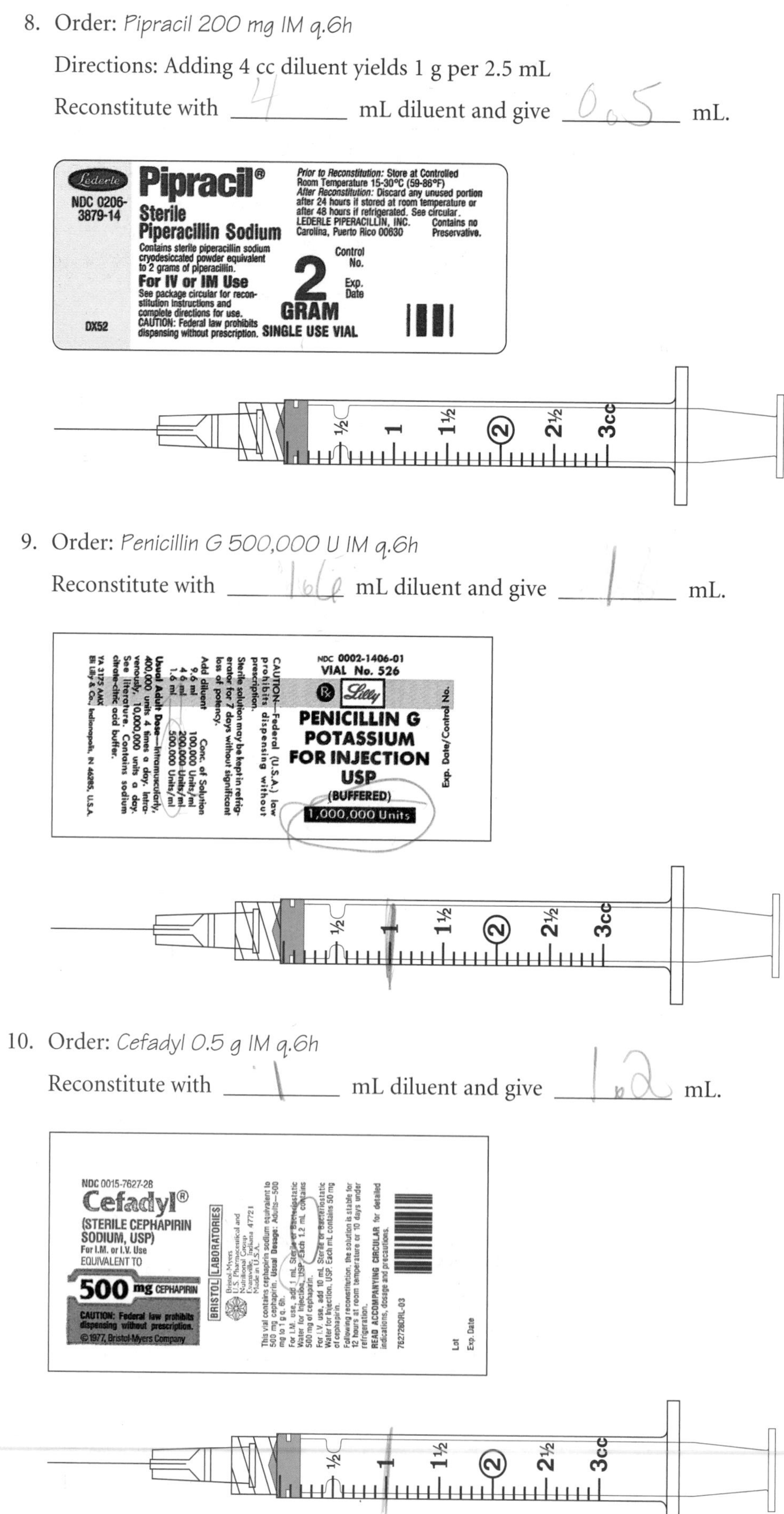

9. Order: *Penicillin G 500,000 U IM q.6h*

   Reconstitute with ________ mL diluent and give ________ mL.

10. Order: *Cefadyl 0.5 g IM q.6h*

    Reconstitute with ________ mL diluent and give ________ mL.

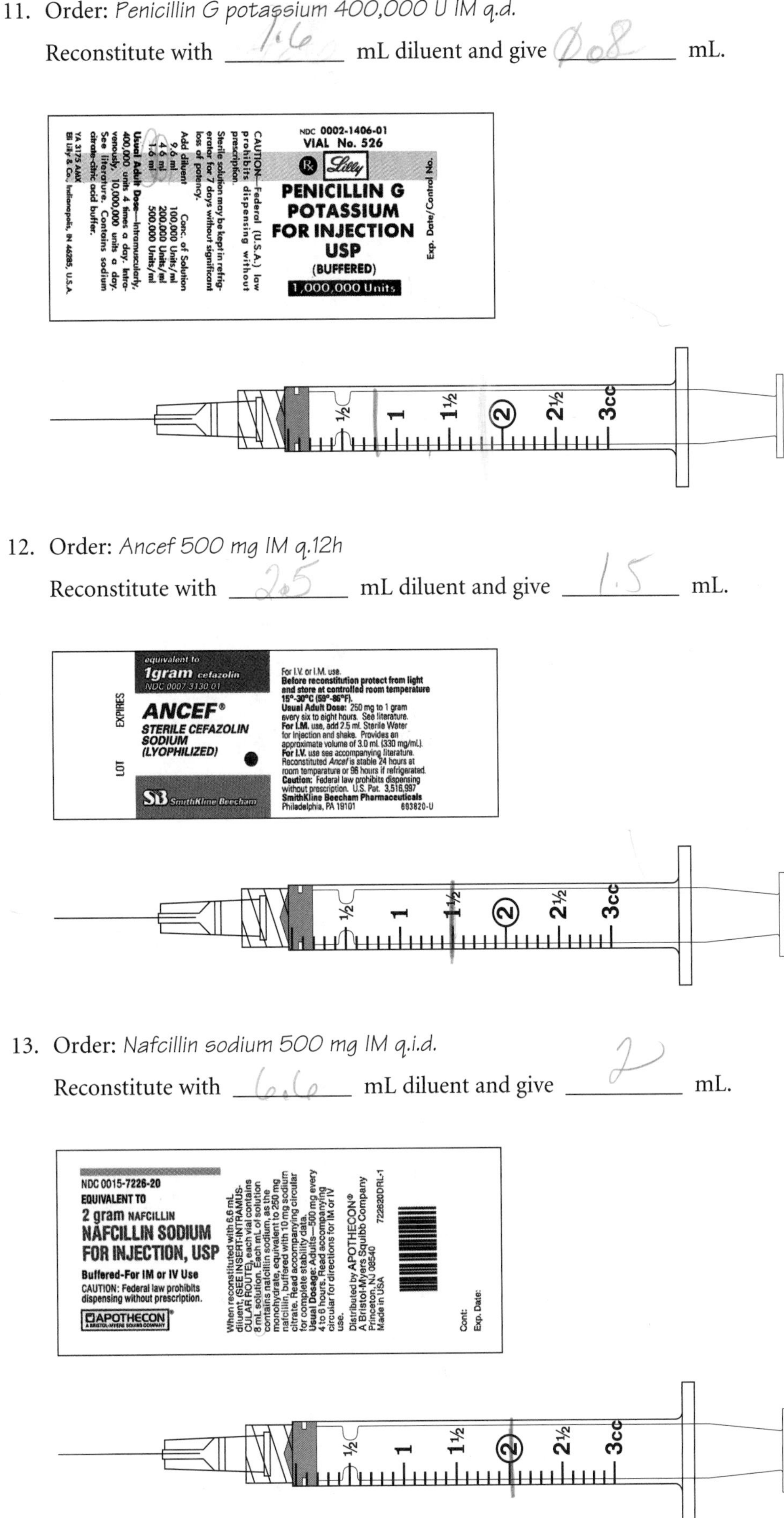

11. Order: *Penicillin G potassium 400,000 U IM q.d.*

Reconstitute with ________ mL diluent and give ________ mL.

12. Order: *Ancef 500 mg IM q.12h*

Reconstitute with ________ mL diluent and give ________ mL.

13. Order: *Nafcillin sodium 500 mg IM q.i.d.*

Reconstitute with ________ mL diluent and give ________ mL.

14. Order: *Wydase 75 U SC stat*

    Directions in package insert: Add 10 mL of diluent to provide a solution containing 150 U/mL

    Reconstitute with ___10___ mL diluent and give ___0.5___ mL.

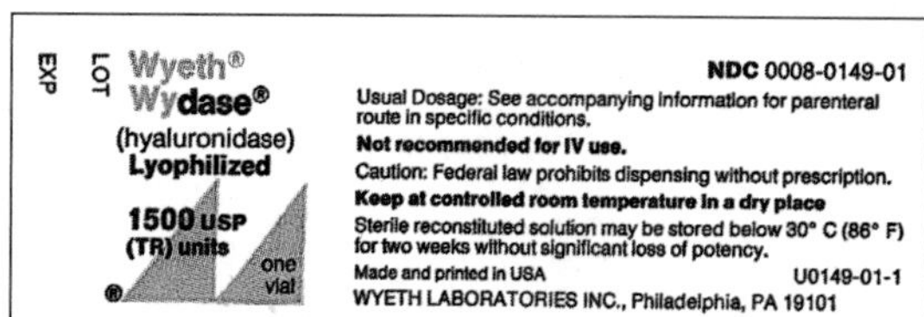

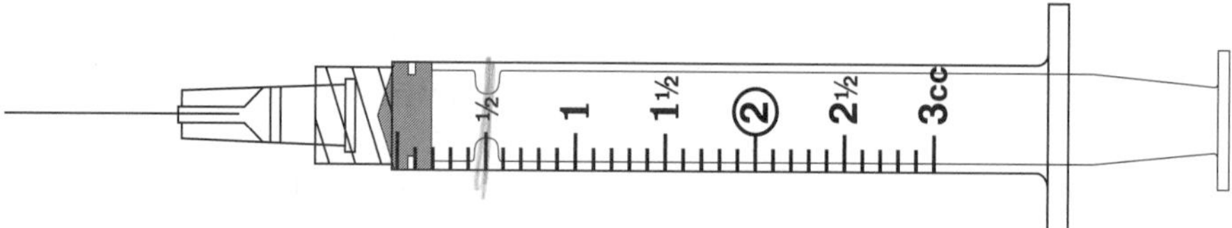

15. Order: *Kefzol 250 mg IM q.6h*

    Reconstitute with ___2mL___ mL diluent and give ___1.1___ mL.

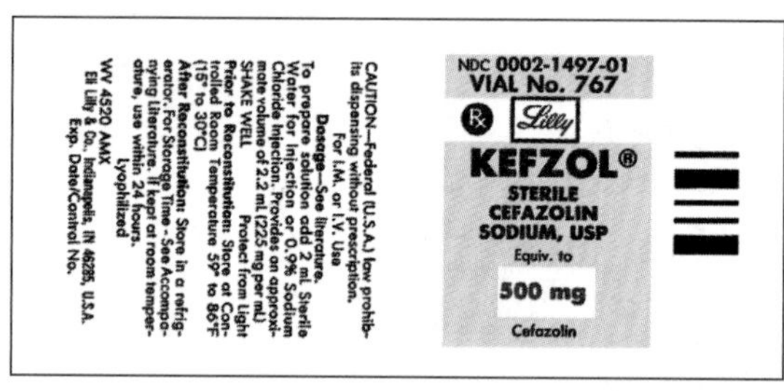

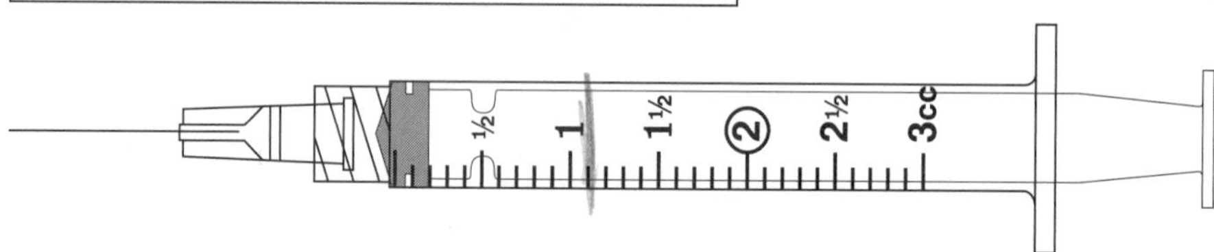

After completing these problems, see pages 432–434 to check your answers.

Insulin

Insulin, a hormone made in the pancreas, is necessary for the metabolism of glucose, proteins, and fats. Patients who are deficient in insulin (insulin-dependent diabetics) are required to take insulin by injection daily. Insulin is a ready-to-use solution that is measured in units (U). The most common supply dosage is *100 U per mL.*

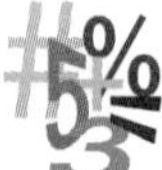

math tip: The supply dosage of insulin is **100 U per mL**, which is abbreviated on the label as **U-100**. Think: U-100 = 100 U per mL.

Insulin is also available as 500 U per mL (or U-500). This supply dosage is only used under special circumstances and is not commercially dispensed.

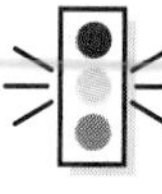

Caution: Accuracy in insulin preparation and administration is critical. Inaccuracy is potentially life threatening. It is essential for nurses to *understand the information on the insulin label*, to correctly *interpret the insulin order*, and to *select the correct syringe* to measure insulin for administration.

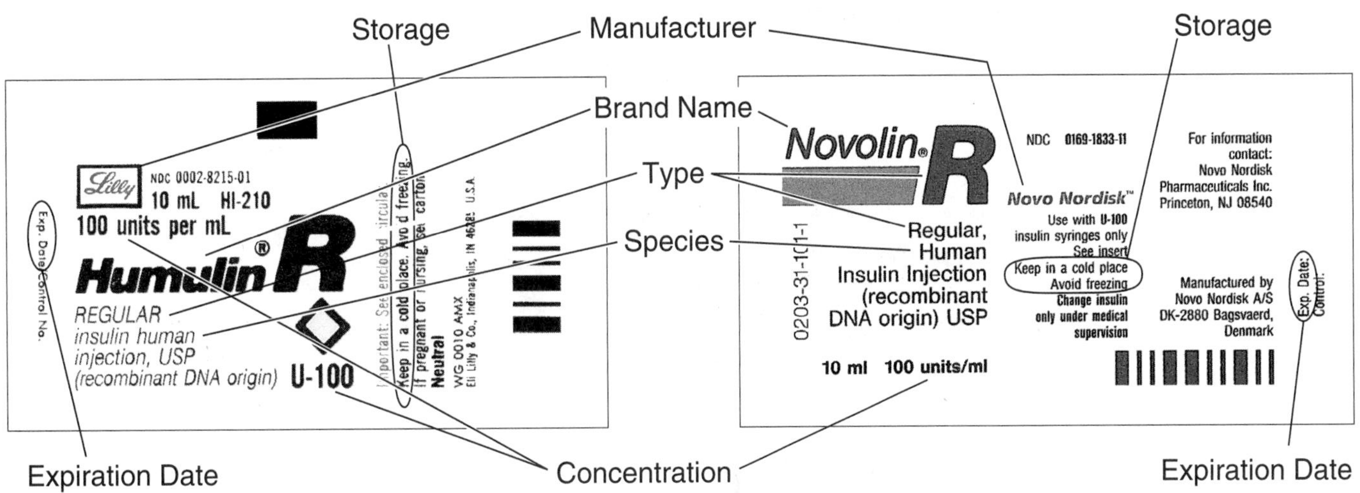

FIGURE 10-9 Insulin Labels

Insulin Label

Figure 10-9 identifies the essential components of insulin labels. These similar products are distributed by Eli Lilly & Company and Novo Nordisk, the two major U.S. insulin manufacturers. The insulin label specifies pertinent information. The *brand and generic names*, the *concentration*, and the *storage* instructions are details commonly found on most parenteral drug labels. Chapter 8 explains these and other typical drug label components. Notice that Eli Lilly & Company also includes unique international symbols on its human insulin-type labels for worldwide identification. Let's look closely at different insulin types classified by the insulin *action times* and insulin *species*, which are critical identifiers of this important hormone supplement.

Insulin Action Times

Figure 10-10 shows a sampling of labels arranged by the three action times: rapid-acting (Regular, Lispro), intermediate-acting (Lente, NPH or *N*eutral *P*rotamine *H*agedorn), and long-acting (Ultralente). Regular and NPH insulin are the two types of insulin used most often. Notice the uppercase, bold letters on each insulin label: **R** for Regular insulin; **L** for Lente insulin; **N** for NPH insulin; **P** for Protamine Zinc insulin; and **U** for Ultralente insulin. These letters are important visual identifiers when selecting the insulin type.

Species of Insulin

Insulin comes from various sources:

- beef insulin—from the pancreas of cattle
- pork insulin—from the pancreas of pigs
- beef-pork mixture—a combination of beef and pork insulin
- human insulin
  a. bio-synthetic—bacteria genetically altered to create human insulin.
  b. semi-synthetic—pork insulin chemically altered to produce human insulin.

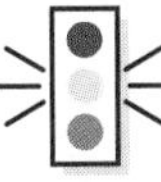

Caution: Avoid a potentially life-threatening medication error. Carefully read the label, and compare it to the drug order to ensure that you select the correct action time and species of insulin.

Rapid Acting

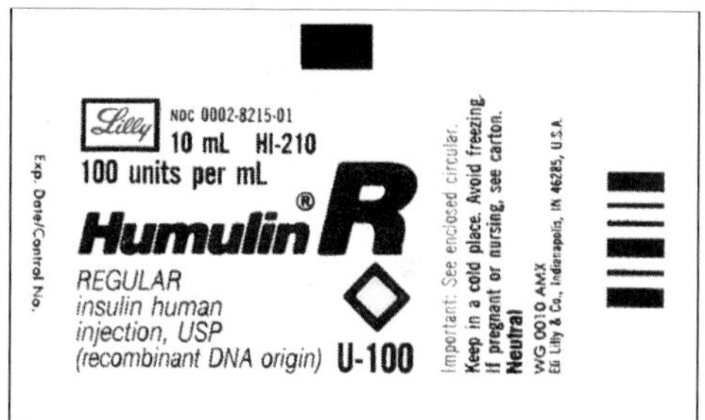

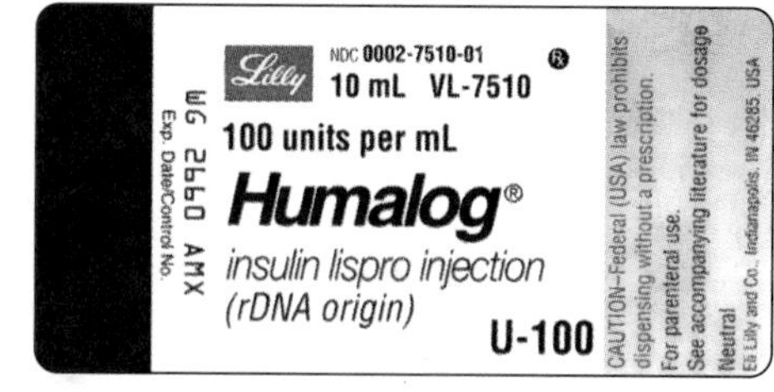

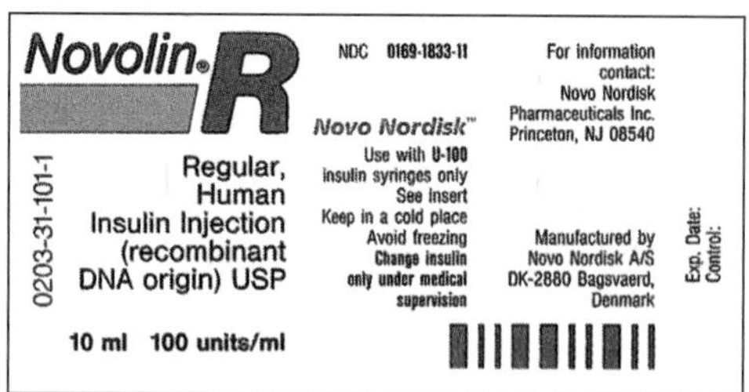

Intermediate Acting

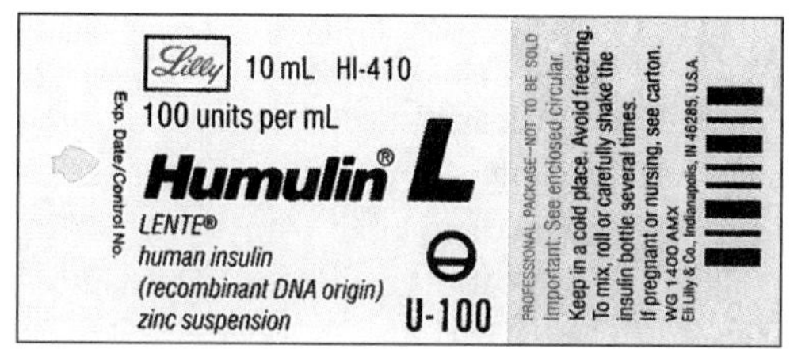

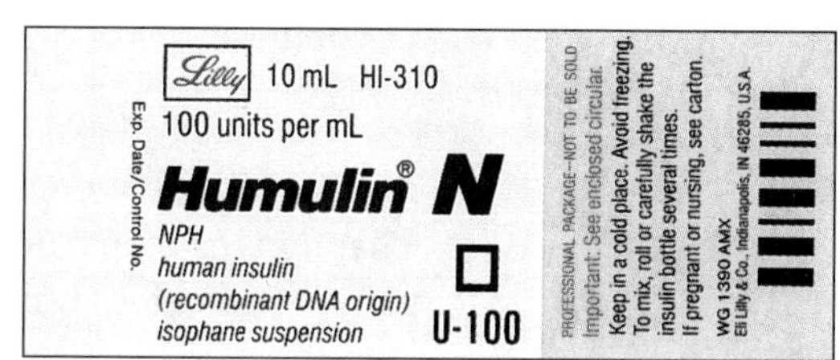

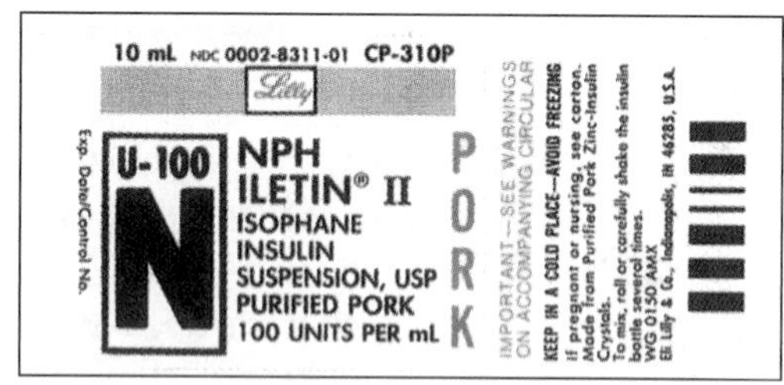

Long Acting

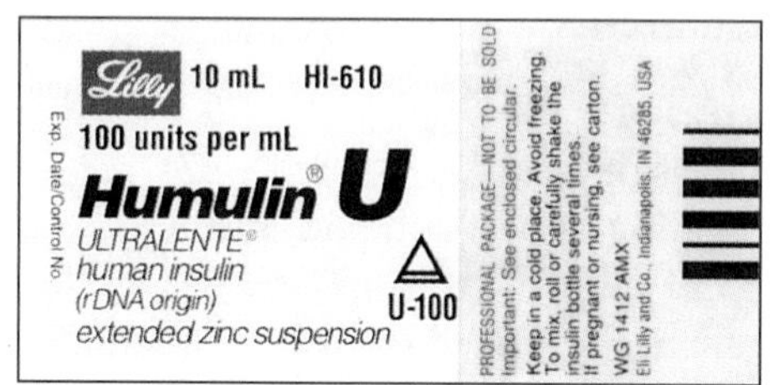

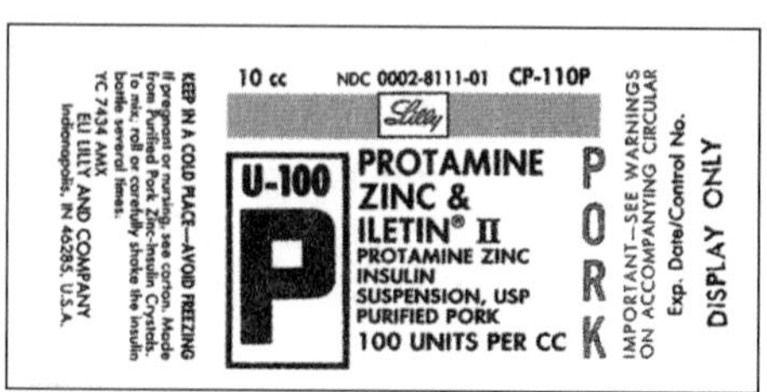

FIGURE 10-10 Insulin Types Grouped by Action Times

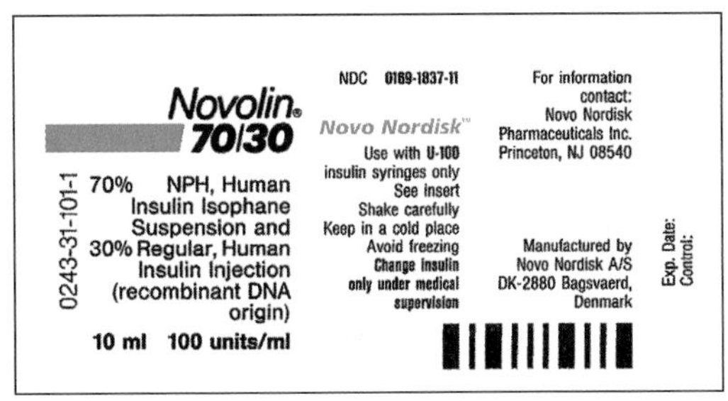

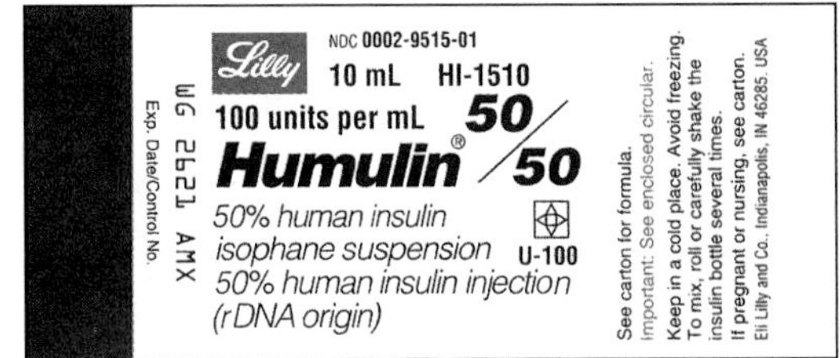

FIGURE 10-11 Premixed, Combination Insulins

Premixed, Combination Insulin

Two pre-mixed insulin combinations that are commercially available are 70/30 U-100 insulin and 50/50 U-100 insulin (Figure 10-11). The 70/30 insulin concentration means there is 70% NPH insulin and 30% Regular insulin in each unit. Therefore, if the physician orders 10 units of 70/30 insulin, the patient would receive 7 units of NPH insulin (70% or 0.7 × 10 U = 7 U) and 3 units of Regular insulin (30% or 0.3 × 10 U = 3 U) in the 70/30 concentration. If the physician orders 20 units of 70/30 insulin, the patient would receive 14 units (0.7 × 20 = 14) of NPH and 6 units (0.3 × 20 = 6) of Regular insulin.

The 50/50 insulin concentration means there is 50% NPH insulin and 50% Regular insulin in each unit. Therefore, if the physician orders 12 units of 50/50 insulin, the patient would receive 6 units of NPH insulin (50% or 0.5 × 12 U = 6 U) and 6 units of Regular insulin (50% or 0.5 × 12 U = 6 U).

Interpreting the Insulin Order

Insulin orders must be written clearly and contain specific information to ensure correct administration and prevent errors. An insulin order should contain:

1. The *brand name, including the species and action time.* Patients are instructed to stay with the same manufacturer's brand name insulin and species. Slight variations between brands can affect an individual's response. Verify both the usual brand name used and the actual insulin supplied with the patient before administration. Most brand names imply the species, such as Humulin (human origin) and Iletin (animal origin). Different species of insulin may cause allergy-like symptoms in some patients, so check carefully. Look for one of the three action times: rapid-acting (*R*egular, *S*emilente), intermediate-acting (*L*ente, *N*PH), and long-acting (*U*ltralente).
2. The *supply dosage and number of units* to be given; such as, U-100 40U
3. The *route* of administration and *time or frequency.* All insulin may be administered subcutaneously (SC), and regular insulin may additionally be administered intravenously (IV).

Examples:

Humulin R Regular U-100 14 U SC stat

Iletin II NPH U-100 24 U SC $\frac{1}{2}$ hour ā breakfast

Insulin Coverage—the "Sliding Scale"

A special insulin order is sometimes needed to "cover" a patient's increasing blood sugar level that is not yet regulated. Regular insulin will be used because of its rapid-acting time. The physician will specify the amount of insulin in units, which "slide up or down" based on a specific blood sugar level range. Sliding scales are individualized for each patient. Here's an example of a sliding scale order:

Example:

Order: *Humulin R Regular U-100 SC based on glucose reading at 1600:*

Insulin Dose	Glucose Reading*
No coverage	Glucose < 160
2 U	160–220
4 U	221–280
6 U	281–340
8 U	341–400

*Glucose > 400: Hold insulin; call MD stat.

Measuring Insulin in an Insulin Syringe

The insulin syringe and measurement of insulin were introduced in Chapter 6. This critical skill warrants your attention again. Once you understand how insulin is packaged and how to use the insulin syringe, you will find insulin dosage simple.

rules

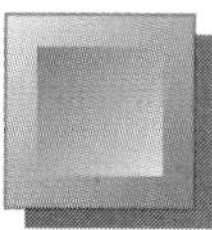

- Measure insulin in an insulin syringe only. Do not use a 3 cc or tuberculin syringe to measure insulin.
- Use U-100 insulin syringes to measure U-100 insulin only. Do not measure other drugs supplied in units in an insulin syringe.

Measuring insulin with the insulin syringe is very simple. The insulin syringe makes it possible to obtain a correct dosage without mathematical calculation. Let's look at three different insulin syringes. They are the *standard* (100 unit) capacity and the *lo-dose* 50 unit and 30 unit capacity.

Standard U-100 Insulin Syringes

Example 1:

The standard U-100 insulin syringe in Figure 10-12 is a dual-scale syringe with 100 U/mL capacity. It is calibrated on one side in *even*-numbered, 2-unit increments (2, 4, 6...) with every 10 units labeled (10, 20, 30...). It is calibrated on the reverse side in odd-numbered, 2-unit increments (1, 3, 5...) with every 10 units labeled (5, 15, 25...). The measurement of 73 units of U-100 insulin is illustrated in Figure 10-12.

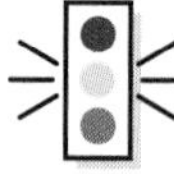

Caution: Look carefully at the increments on the dual scale. The volume from one mark to the next (on either side) is 2 units. You are probably comfortable counting by 2s for even numbers. Pay close attention when counting by 2s with odd numbers.

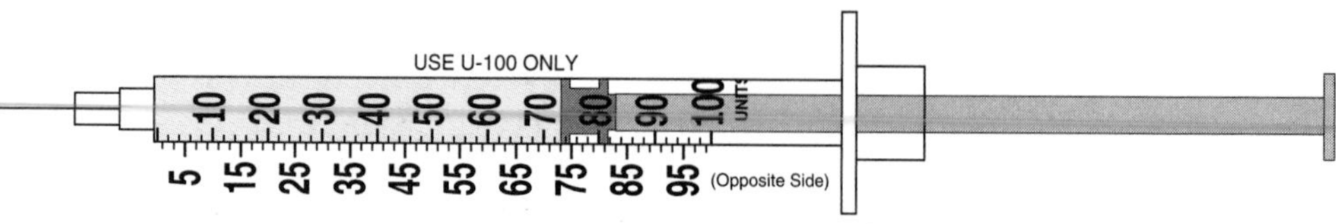

FIGURE 10-12 Standard U-100 Insulin Syringe Measuring 73 U

Lo Dose U-100 Insulin Syringes

Example 2:

The Lo-Dose U-100 insulin syringe in Figure 10-13 is a single-scale syringe with 50 U/0.5 mL capacity. It is calibrated in 1-unit increments with every five units (5, 10, 15, ...) labeled up to 50 units. The enlarged 50 unit calibration makes this syringe easy to read and to measure low dosages of insulin. To measure 32 units, withdraw U-100 insulin to the 32 unit mark.

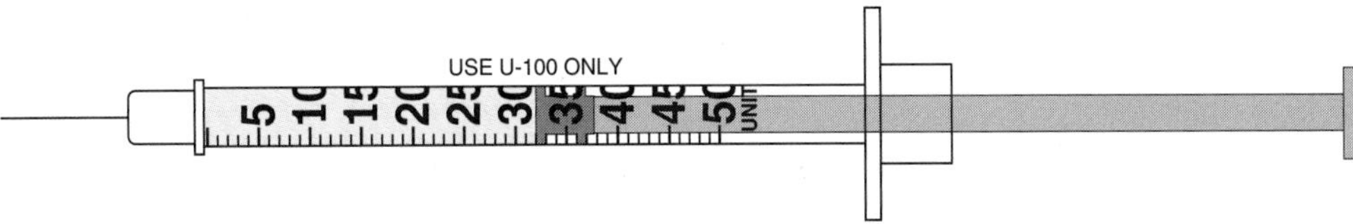

FIGURE 10-13 50-U Lo-Dose U-100 Insulin Syringe Measuring 32 U

Example 3:

The Lo-Dose U-100 insulin syringe in Figure 10-14 is a single-scale syringe with 30 U/0.3 mL capacity. It is calibrated in 1 unit increments with every five units (5, 10, 15, ...) labeled up to 30 units. The enlarged 30 unit calibration accurately measures very small amounts of insulin, such as for children. To measure 12 units, withdraw U-100 insulin to the 12 unit mark.

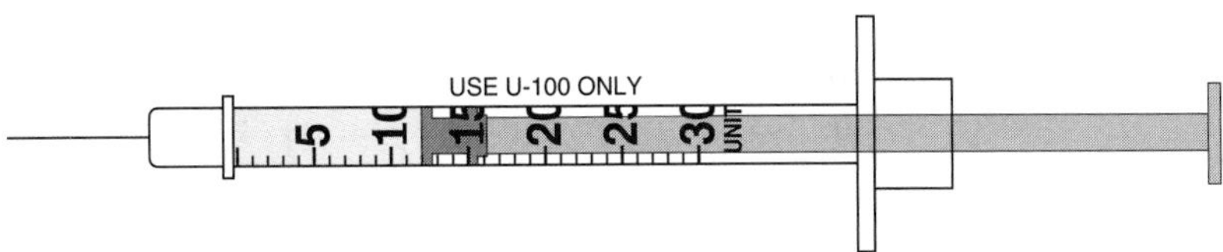

FIGURE 10-14 30-U Lo-Dose U-100 Insulin Syringe Measuring 12 U

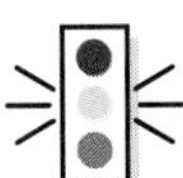

Caution: Always choose the *smallest* capacity insulin syringe available for accurate insulin measurement. Use Standard and Lo-Dose U-100 syringes to measure U-100 insulin *only*. Although the Lo-Dose U-100 insulin syringes only measure a maximum of 30 or 50 units, they are still intended for the measurement of U-100 insulin only.

Combination Insulin Dosage

The patient may have two types of insulin prescribed to be administered at the same time. To avoid injecting the patient twice, it is common practice to draw up both insulins in the same syringe.

rule

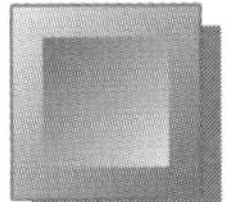

Draw up *clear insulin first,* then draw up cloudy insulin.
Regular insulin is clear. NPH insulin is cloudy.
Think: *First clear, then cloudy.* **Think:** *First Regular, then NPH.*

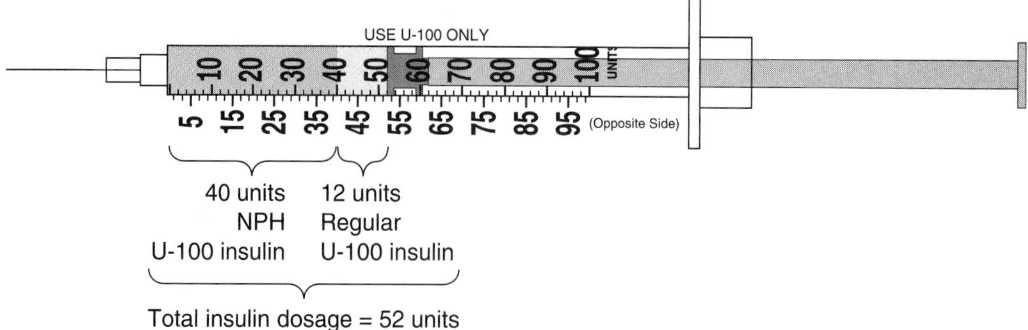

FIGURE 10-15 Combination Insulin Dosage

Example 1:

Order: *Novolin R Regular U-100 insulin 12 U with Novolin N NPH U-100 insulin 40 U SC ā breakfast.*

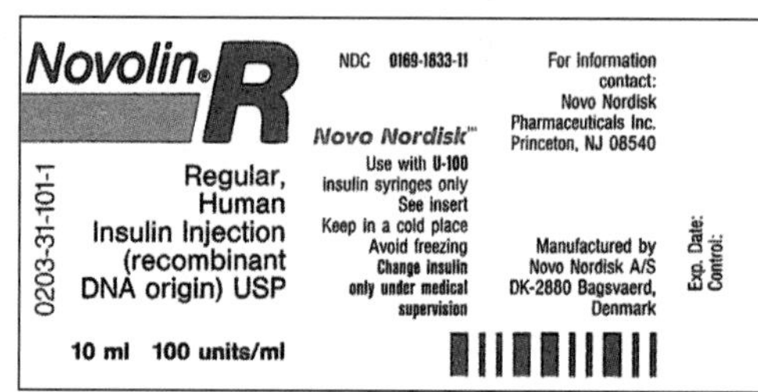

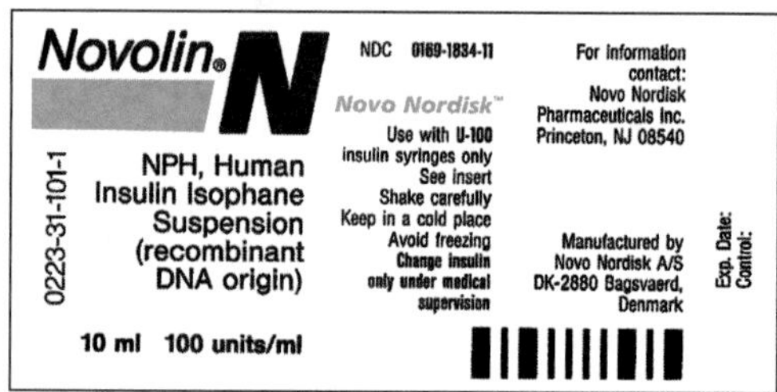

To accurately withdraw both insulins into the same syringe you will need to know the total units of both insulins: 12 + 40 = 52 units. Withdraw 12 units of the Regular U-100 insulin (clear) and then withdraw 40 more units of the NPH U-100 insulin (cloudy) up to the 52 unit mark, Figure 10-15. In this case, the smallest capacity syringe you can use is the standard U-100 syringe. Notice that the NPH insulin is drawn up last and is closest to the needle.

The second example gives step-by-step directions for this procedure.

Look closely at Figures 10-16 and 10-17 to demonstrate the procedure as you study Example 2.

Example 2:

The physician orders *Novolin R Regular U-100 insulin 10 U with Novolin N NPH U-100 insulin 30 U SC $\frac{1}{2}$ hour ā dinner.*

1. Draw back and inject 30 units of air into the NPH insulin vial (cloudy liquid). Remove needle.
2. Draw back and inject 10 units of air into the Regular insulin vial (clear liquid) and leave the needle in the vial.
3. Turn the vial of Regular insulin upside down, and draw out the insulin to the 10-unit mark on the syringe. Make sure all air bubbles are removed.
4. Roll the vial of the NPH insulin in your hands to mix; do not shake it. Insert the needle into the NPH insulin vial, turn the vial upside down and draw back to the 40-unit mark. 10 units of Regular + 30 units of NPH = 40 units of insulin total, Figure 10-17.

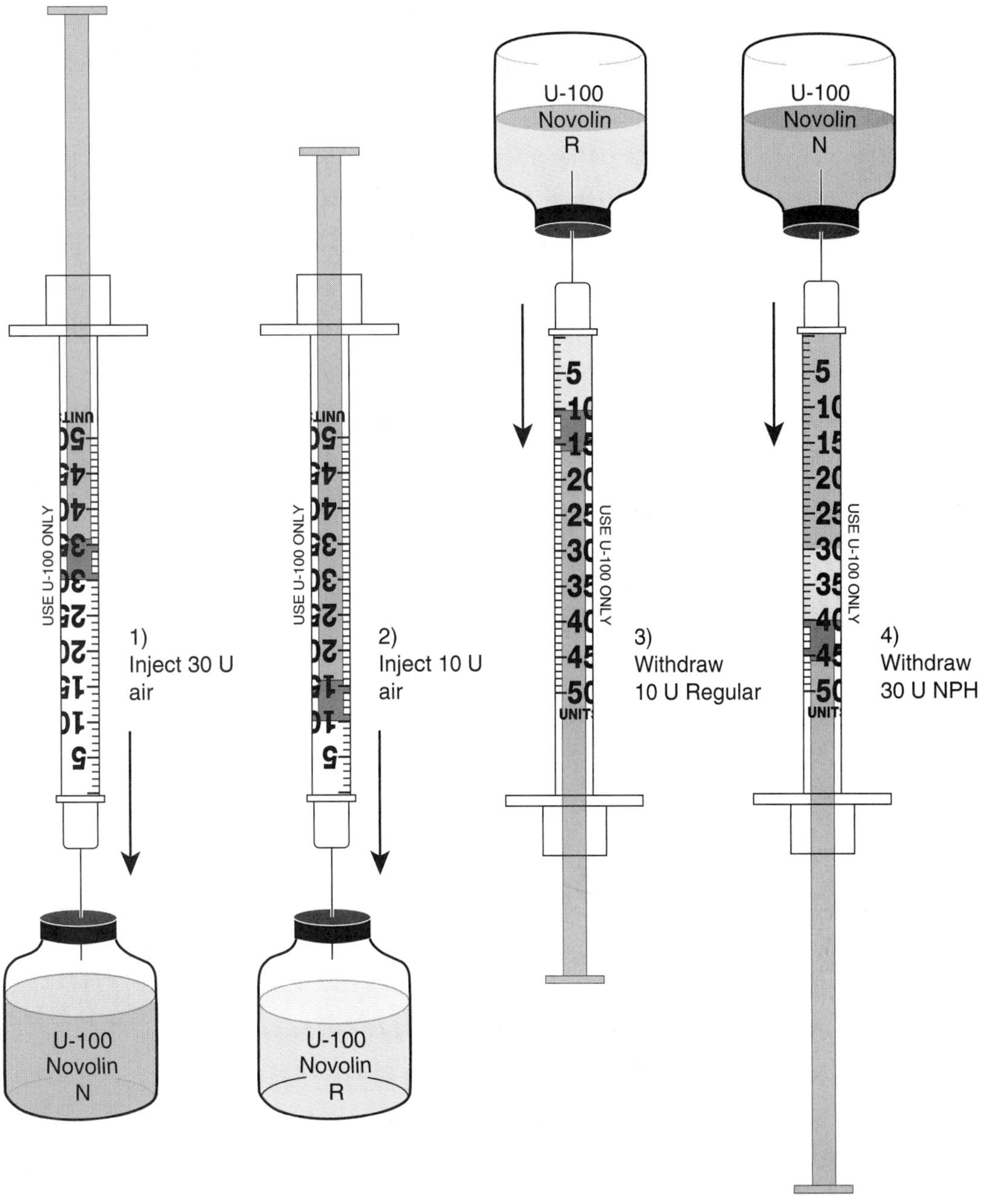

U-100
Novolin
R
U-100
Novolin
N
1)
Inject 30 U
air
2)
Inject 10 U
air
3)
Withdraw
10 U Regular
4)
Withdraw
30 U NPH
USE U-100 ONLY
U-100
Novolin
N
U-100
Novolin
R

FIGURE 10-16 Procedure for Drawing Up Combination Insulin Dosage: 10 U Regular U-100 Insulin with 30 U NPH U-100 Insulin

USE U-100 ONLY
30 units
NPH
U-100 Insulin
10 units
Regular
U-100 Insulin
Total insulin dosage = 40 units

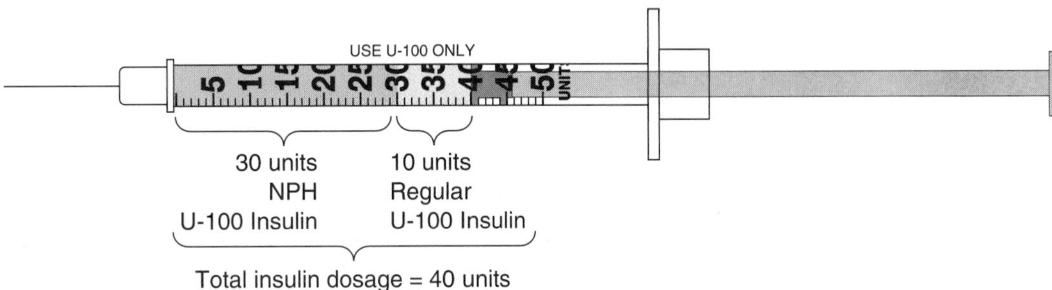

FIGURE 10-17 Combination Insulin Dosage

Avoiding Insulin Dosage Errors

Insulin dosage errors are very costly and unfortunately too common. They can be avoided by following two important rules.

rules

- Insulin dosages must be checked by two nurses.
- When combination dosages are prepared, two nurses must verify each step of the process.

quick review

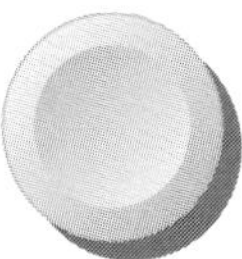

- Carefully read the physician's order, and match the supply dosage for type and species of insulin.
- Always measure insulin in an insulin syringe.
- An insulin syringe is used to measure insulin *only.* Insulin syringes must not be used to measure other medications measured in units.
- Use the smallest capacity insulin syringe possible to most accurately measure insulin doses.
- When drawing up combination insulin doses, think *clear first, then cloudy.*
- Avoid insulin dosage errors. The insulin dosage should be checked by two nurses.
- There are 100 units per mL for U-100 insulin.

review set 29

Read the following labels. Identify the insulin trade name, its action time (fast acting, intermediate acting, or long acting), and its species.

1. Insulin trade name ____________
   Action time ____________
   Species ____________

Lilly NDC 0002-8215-01
10 mL HI-210
100 units per mL
Humulin® R
REGULAR
insulin human
injection, USP
(recombinant DNA origin) U-100
Exp. Date/Control No.
Important: See enclosed circular.
Keep in a cold place. Avoid freezing.
If pregnant or nursing, see carton.
Neutral
WG 0010 AMX
Eli Lilly & Co., Indianapolis, IN 46285, U.S.A.

2. Insulin trade name ____________
   Action time ____________
   Species ____________

10 mL NDC 0002-8311-01 CP-310P
Lilly
U-100
N
NPH
ILETIN® II
ISOPHANE
INSULIN
SUSPENSION, USP
PURIFIED PORK
100 UNITS PER mL
PORK
Exp. Date/Control No.
IMPORTANT—SEE WARNINGS ON ACCOMPANYING CIRCULAR
KEEP IN A COLD PLACE—AVOID FREEZING
If pregnant or nursing, see carton.
Made from Purified Pork Zinc-Insulin Crystals.
To mix, roll or carefully shake the insulin bottle several times.
WG 0150 AMX
Eli Lilly & Co., Indianapolis, IN 46285, U.S.A.

3. Insulin trade name ____________
   Action time ____________
   Species ____________

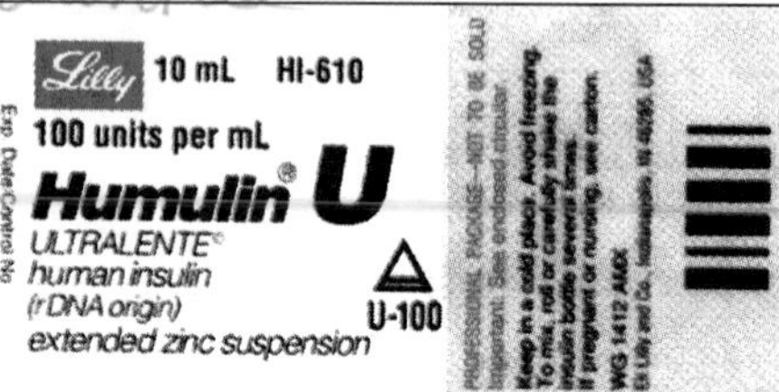

4. Insulin trade name ______________
   Action time ______________
   Species ______________

10 cc NDC 0002-8111-01 CP-110P
Lilly
U-100 P
PROTAMINE ZINC & ILETIN® II
PROTAMINE ZINC INSULIN SUSPENSION, USP
PURIFIED PORK
100 UNITS PER CC
PORK
KEEP IN A COLD PLACE—AVOID FREEZING
IMPORTANT—SEE WARNINGS ON ACCOMPANYING CIRCULAR
Exp. Date/Control No.
DISPLAY ONLY
ELI LILLY AND COMPANY Indianapolis, IN 46285, U.S.A.

5. Insulin trade name ______________
   Action time ______________
   Species ______________

Lilly 10 mL HI-410
100 units per mL
Humulin® L
LENTE®
human insulin
(recombinant DNA origin)
zinc suspension
U-100
Exp. Date/Control No.
PROFESSIONAL PACKAGE—NOT TO BE SOLD
Important: See enclosed circular.
Keep in a cold place. Avoid freezing.
To mix, roll or carefully shake the insulin bottle several times.
If pregnant or nursing, see carton.
WG 1400 AMX
Eli Lilly & Co., Indianapolis, IN 46285, U.S.A.

6. Describe the three syringes available to measure U-100 insulin. ______________

7. What would be your preferred syringe choice to measure 24 units of U-100 insulin? ______________

8. What would be your preferred syringe choice to measure 35 units of U-100 insulin? ______________

9. There are 60 units of U-100 insulin per ______ mL.

10. There are 25 units of U-100 insulin per ______ mL.

11. 65 units of U-100 insulin should be measured in a(an) ______ syringe.

12. The 50 unit Lo-Dose U-100 insulin syringe is intended to measure U-50 insulin only.
    ______ (True) (False)

Identify the U-100 insulin dosage indicated by the colored area of the syringe.

13. ______ U

USE U-100 ONLY
10 20 30 40 50 60 70 80 90 100 UNITS
5 15 25 35 45 55 65 75 85 95 (Opposite Side)

14. ______ U

USE U-100 ONLY
5 10 15 20 25 30 UNITS

15. ______ U

USE U-100 ONLY
5 10 15 20 25 30 35 40 45 50 UNITS

16. __________ U

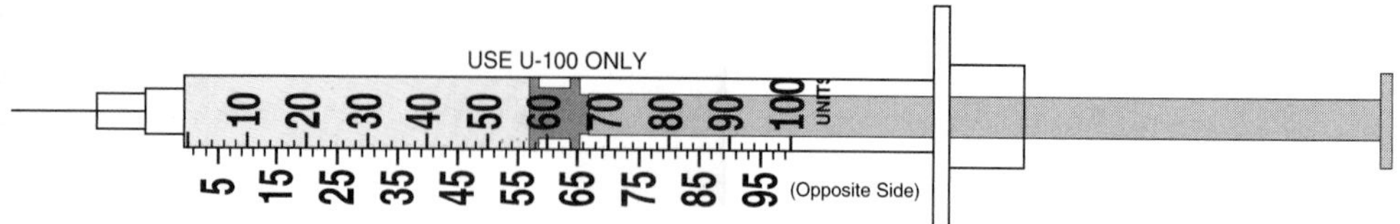

Draw an arrow on the syringe to identify the given dosages.

17. 80 units U-100 insulin

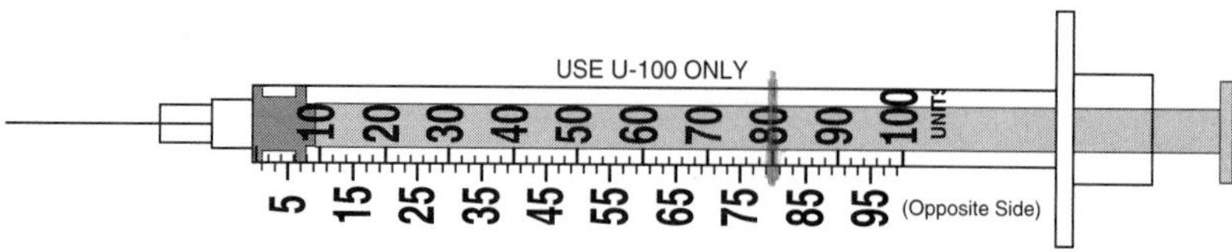

18. 15 units U-100 insulin

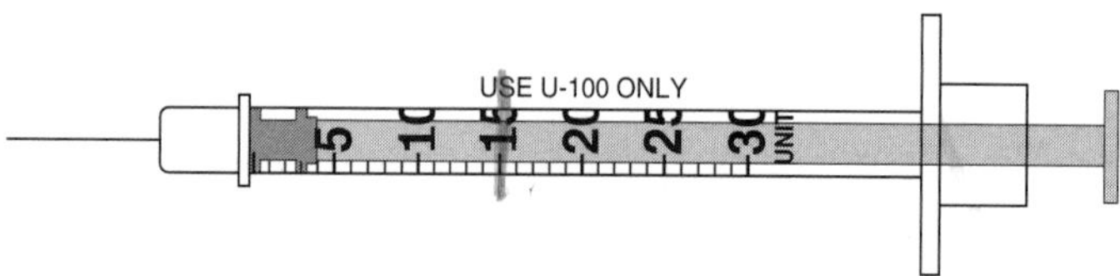

19. 66 units U-100 insulin

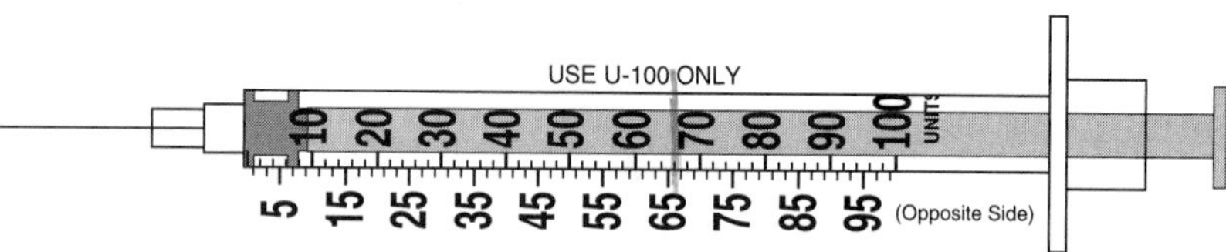

20. 16 units U-100 insulin

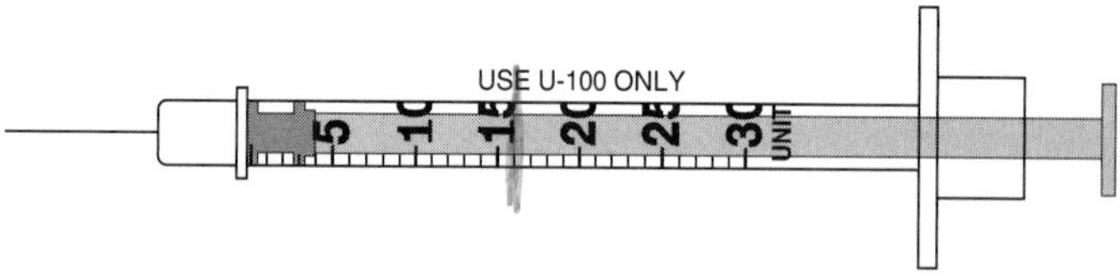

21. 32 units of U-100 insulin

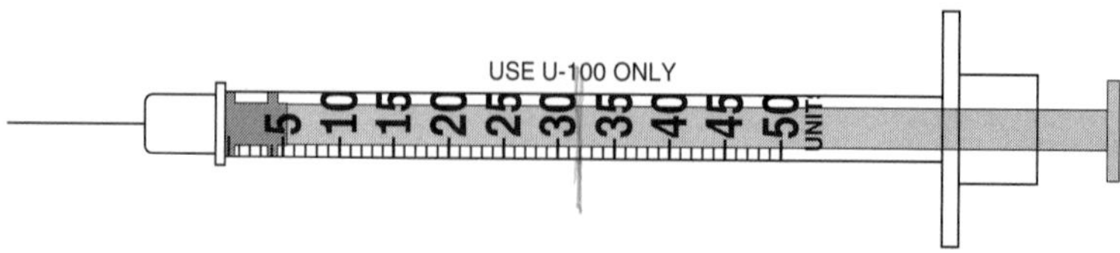

Draw arrows, and label the dosage for each of the combination insulin orders to be measured in the same syringe.

22. *Novolin R Regular U-100 insulin 21 U with Novolin N NPH U-100 insulin 15 U SC stat*

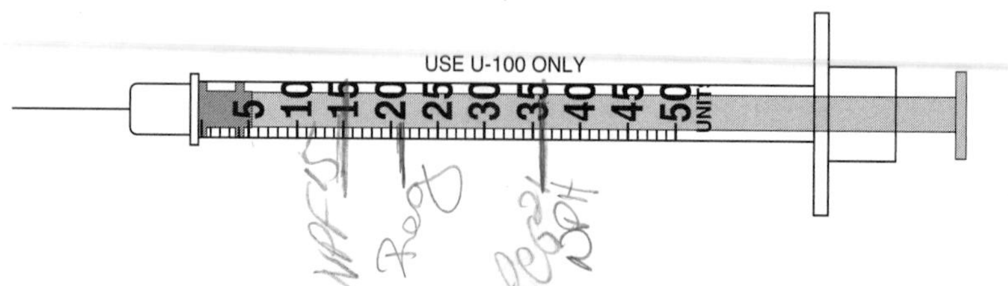

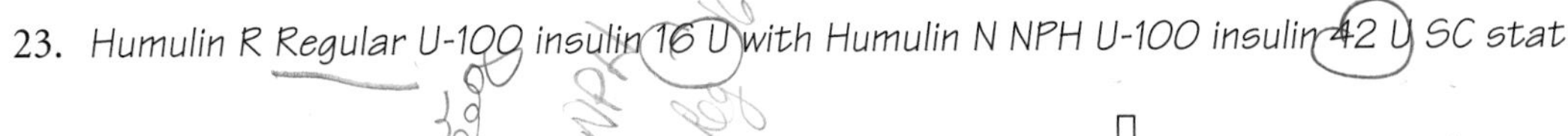

23. *Humulin R Regular U-100 insulin 16 U with Humulin N NPH U-100 insulin 42 U SC stat*

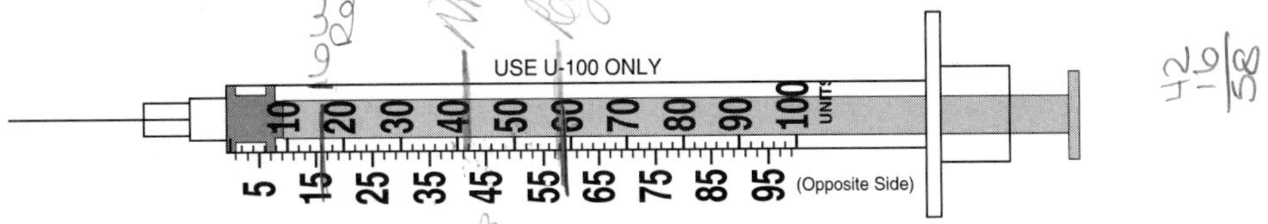

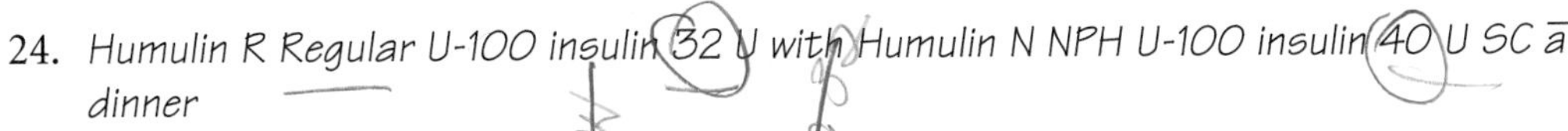

24. *Humulin R Regular U-100 insulin 32 U with Humulin N NPH U-100 insulin 40 U SC ā dinner*

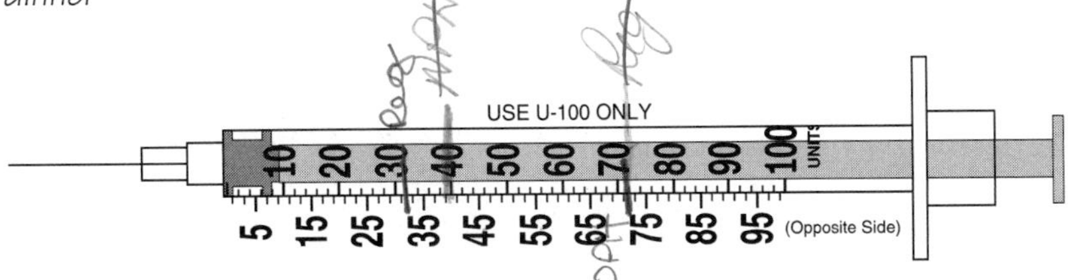

25. *Humulin R Regular U-100 insulin 8 U with Humulin N NPH U-100 insulin 12 U SC stat*

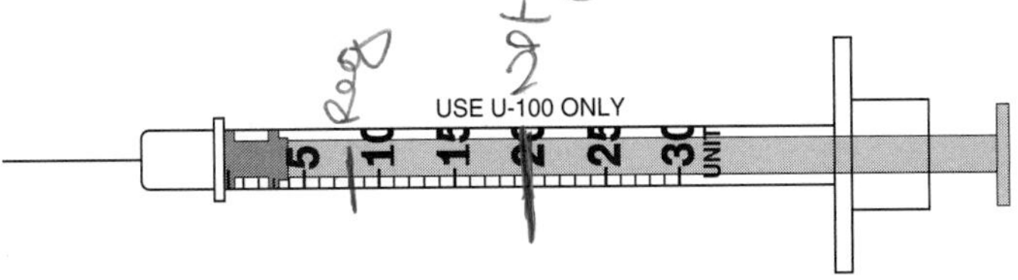

How many mL are supplied in the insulin dosage ordered?

26. *Novolin N NPH U-100 insulin 34 U SC stat* ________ mL
27. *Novolin R Regular U-100 insulin 75 U SC now* ________ mL
28. *Humulin N NPH U-100 insulin 22 U SC ā breakfast* ________ mL
29. *Novolin N NPH U-100 insulin 13 U SC stat* ________ mL
30. *Humulin R Regular U-100 insulin 17 U with Humulin N NPH U-100 insulin 42 U SC stat* ________ mL total

After completing these problems, see pages 434 and 435 to check your answers.

Calculating Parenteral Dosage Expressed as a Ratio or Percent

Occasionally, solutions will be ordered and/or supplied in a dosage strength expressed as a ratio or percent.

rule

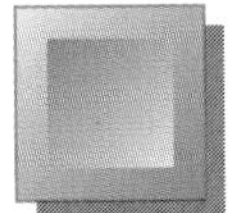

Ratio solutions express the *number of grams* of the drug *per total milliliters of solution.*

Examples:

Epinephrine 1:1000 contains 1 g pure drug per 1000 mL solution, 1 g:1000 mL = 1000 mg:1000 mL = 1 mg:1 mL.

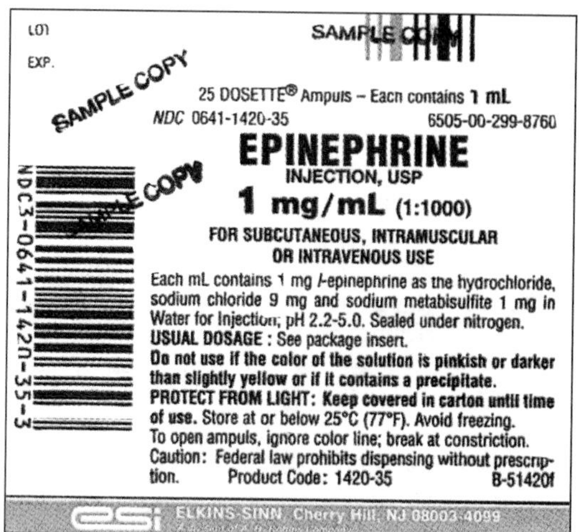

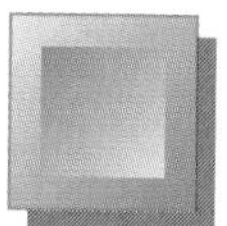

rule

Percentage (%) solutions express the *number of grams* of the drug *per 100 milliliters of solution.*

Examples:

Calcium gluconate 10% contains 10 g pure drug per 100 mL solution, 10 g/100mL = 10,000 mg/100 mL = 100 mg/mL.

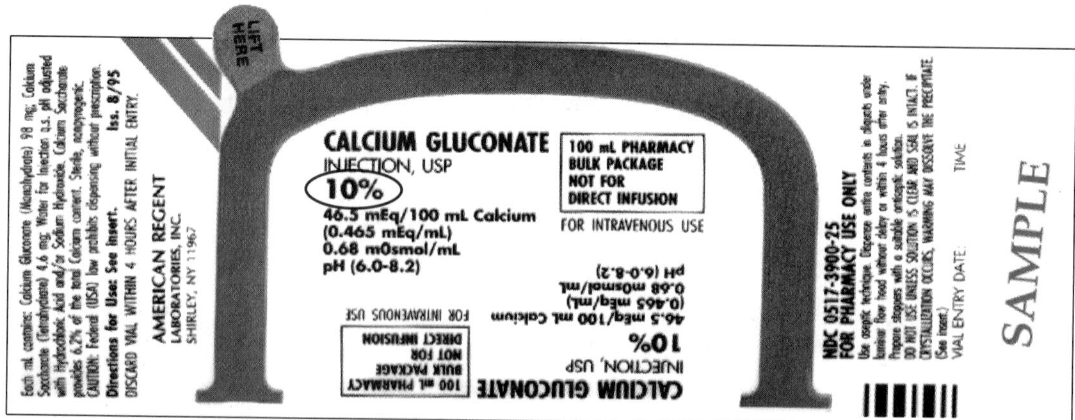

Lidocaine 2% contains 2 g pure drug per 100 mL solution, 2 g/100 mL = 2000 mg/100 mL = 20 mg/mL.

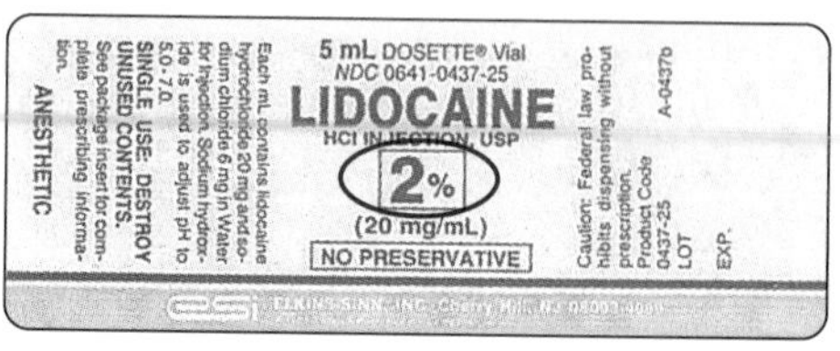

Courtesy of Elkins-Sinn, Inc., a subsidiary of A. H. Robins, Cherry Hill, NJ

remember

Solving dosage problems expressed in ratio and percent is not difficult. Follow the same steps used to calculate all dosages.

STEP 1 **CONVERT** Be sure all units are the same system and same size; that is convert ratio or percent to g or mg per mL.

STEP 2 **THINK** Estimate for the reasonable amount to give.

STEP 3 **CALCULATE** $\frac{D}{H} \times Q = X$

Example 1:

Order: *Epinephrine 0.4 mg SC q.3h p.r.n., asthma*

Supply: *1 mL ampules of Epinephrine 1:1000*

STEP 1 **CONVERT** Epinephrine 1:1000 = 1 g of Epinephrine in 1000 mL = 1000 mg in 1000 mL = 1 mg in 1 mL

The problem now looks like this:

Order: *Epinephrine 0.4 mg*

Supply: Epinephrine 1 mg per 1 mL

STEP 2 **THINK** You have 1 mg per 1 mL and you want to give 0.4 mg; therefore, you want to give 0.4 mL.

STEP 3 **CALCULATE** $\frac{D}{H} \times Q = \frac{0.4\ \cancel{mg}}{\cancel{1}\ \cancel{mg}} \times \cancel{1}\ mL = 0.4\ mL$

Give 0.4 mL of the 1 mL ampule measured in a 0.5 mL tuberculin syringe.

Example 2:

Order: *Calcium gluconate 1 g IV stat*

Supply: *10 mL ampule of 10% calcium gluconate*

STEP 1 **CONVERT** 10% calcium gluconate = 10 g in 100 mL.

Order: *Calcium gluconate 1 g*

Supply: 10 mL ampule of calcium gluconate 10% = 10 g of calcium gluconate in 100 mL

NOTE: "10 mL ampule" simply refers to the volume size of the ampule. The 10% = 10 g per 100 mL.

STEP 2 **THINK** If there are 10 g in 100 mL and you want to give 1 g or one-tenth of 10 g, then you want to give one-tenth of 100 mL or 10 mL.

STEP 3 **CALCULATE** $\frac{D}{H} \times Q = \frac{1\ \cancel{g}}{\underset{1}{\cancel{10}}\ \cancel{g}} \times \overset{10}{\cancel{100}}\ mL = 10\ mL$

Give 10 mL or all of the 10 mL ampule measured in a 10 cc syringe.

quick review

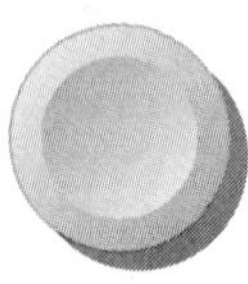

- Ratio solutions = g:mL
- Percent solutions = g/100 mL

review set 30

Calculate the amount you will prepare for one dose.

1. Order: *Magnesium sulfate 4 g IV*

   Supply: 10 mL vial of 20% magnesium sulfate solution

   Give: ______________________ mL

2. Order: *Epinephrine 0.5 mg SC q.3h p.r.n.*

   Supply: 30 mL vial of epinephrine (Adrenalin) 1:2000

   Give: ______________________ mL

3. Order: *Epinephrine 0.3 mg IM*

   Supply: Epinephrine solution 1:1000

   Give: ______________________ mL

4. Order: *Prostigmin 0.25 mg IM*

   Supply: Prostigmin 1:2000 solution

   Give: ______________________ mL

5. Order: *Calcium gluconate gr viiss IV*

   Supply: Calcium gluconate 25% solution

   (Watch this one, it's a little tricky. HINT: Convert gr to g first.)

   Give: ______________________ mL

After completing these problems, see page 436 to check your answers.

critical thinking skills

Many insulin errors occur when the nurse fails to clarify an incomplete order. Let's look at an example of an insulin error when the order did not include the type of insulin to be given.

error 1

Failing to clarify an insulin order when the type of insulin is not specified.

possible scenario

Suppose the physician wrote an insulin order this way:

Humulin insulin 50 U $\bar{a}$ breakfast

Because the physician did not specify the type of insulin, the nurse assumed it was Regular insulin and noted that on the medication administration record. Suppose the patient was given the Regular insulin for three days. On the morning of the third day, the patient developed signs of hypoglycemia (low blood glucose), including shakiness, tremors, confusion, and sweating.

potential outcome

A stat blood glucose would likely reveal a dangerously low glucose level. The patient would be given a glucose infusion to increase the blood sugar. The nurse may not have realized the error until she and the doctor checked the original order and found that the incomplete order had been filled in by the nurse. When the doctor did not specify the type of insulin, the nurse assumed the physician meant Regular, which is short-acting, when in fact intermediate-acting NPH insulin was desired.

prevention

This error could have been avoided by remembering all the essential components of an insulin order: species, type of insulin (such as Regular or NPH), the amount to give in units, and the frequency. When you fill in an incomplete order, you are essentially practicing medicine without a license. This would be a clear malpractice incident. It does not make sense to put you and your patient in such jeopardy. A simple phone call would clarify the situation for everyone involved. Further, the nurse should have double-checked the dosage with another licensed practitioner. Had this occurred the error would have been discovered prior to administration.

critical thinking skills

Many injection medication errors occur by not reading the directions on the label for the correct dilution. Let's look at an example in which the nurse did not select the correct dilution for the amount of medication to be given.

error 2

Choosing the incorrect dilution for injection.

possible scenario

Suppose a physician ordered *Penicillin G 1,000,000 U IM stat* for a patient with a severe staph infection. Look at the label of the medication available on hand.

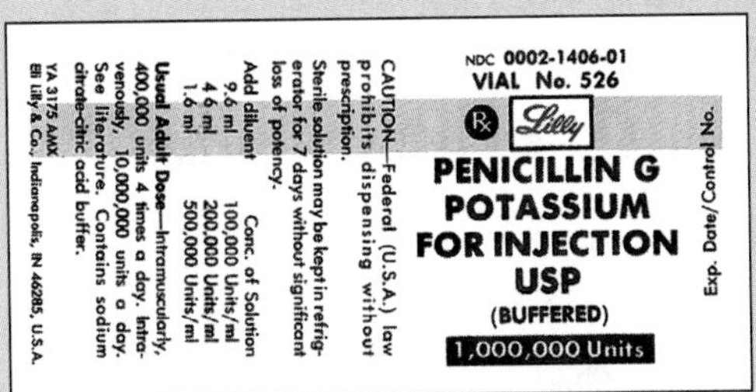

The nurse in a hurry to give the stat medication selected the first concentration given on the label: 100,000 Units/mL concentration. Next the nurse calculated the dosage using the $\frac{D}{H} \times Q = X$ formula.

$$\frac{D}{H} \times Q = \frac{1,000,000 \text{ U}}{100,000 \text{ U}} \times 1 \text{ mL} = 10 \text{ mL}$$

The nurse added 9.6 mL to the vial and drew up 10 mL of medication. It was not until the nurse drew up the 10 mL that the error was recognized. The nurse realized that 10 mL IM should not be administered in one or even in two injection sites. The nurse called the pharmacy for another vial of Penicillin G and prepared the dose again, using 1.6 mL of diluent for a concentration of 500,000 Units/mL. To give 1,000,000 U the nurse easily calculated to give 2 mL, which was a safe volume of medication for IM injection in adults.

potential outcome

Had the nurse given the 10 mL intramuscular injection, the patient would likely have developed an abscess at the site due to the excessive volume of medication being given into the muscle. The patient's hospital stay would likely have been lengthened. Further, the nurse and the hospital may have faced a malpractice suit. The alternative would have been to divide the dose into four injections. Although the patient would have received the correct dosage, to give four injections would have been poor nursing judgment.

prevention

This type of error could have been prevented had the nurse read the label carefully for the correct amount of diluent for the dosage of medication to be prepared. Had the nurse read the label carefully before the medication was prepared, medication and valuable time would have been saved. Additionally, if the nurse had used step 2 of the three-step method, the nurse would have realized sooner (before preparing it) that 10 mL would be an unreasonable volume for an IM injection.

Summary

You are now prepared to solve most of the dosage calculations you will encounter in your health care career. Oral and parenteral drug orders, written in the forms presented thus far, account for the largest percentage of prescriptions. You have learned to think through the process from order to supply to amount administered and to apply the formula $\frac{D}{H} \times Q = X$.

Work the practice problems for Chapter 10. After completing the practice problems, you should feel comfortable and confident working dosage calculations. If not, seek additional instruction. Concentrate on accuracy. Remember, one error in dosage calculation can be a serious mistake for your patient.

practice problems—chapter 10

Calculate the amount you will prepare for one dose. Indicate the syringe you will select to measure the medication.

1. Order: *Demerol 20 mg IM q.3–4h p.r.n., pain*

   Supply: Demerol 50 mg/mL

   Give: ________ mL Select ________ syringe

2. Order: *Morphine sulfate 15 mg IM stat*

   Supply: Morphine sulfate gr $\frac{1}{4}$ per mL

   Give: ________ mL Select ________ syringe

3. Order: *Lanoxin 0.6 mg IV now*

   Supply: Lanoxin 500 mcg/2 mL

   Give: ________ mL Select ________ syringe

4. Order: *Vistaril 15 mg IM stat*

   Supply: Vistaril 25 mg/mL

   Give: ________ mL Select ________ syringe

5. Order: *Penicillin G potassium 500,000 U IM q.4h*

   Supply: Penicillin G potassium 1,000,000 U in 10 mL vial

   Directions: Add 3.6 mL diluent for 250,000 U/mL

   Give: ________ mL Select ________ syringe

6. Order: *Cleocin 300 mg IM q.i.d.*

   Supply: Cleocin 0.6 g/4 mL

   Give: ________ mL Select ________ syringe

7. Order: *Isuprel 3 mg IV drip in 500 mL dextrose and water; run at 5 mcg/minute*

   Supply: Isuprel 1 mg/5 mL

   Add: __________ mL to IV. Select __________ syringe

8. Order: *Ampicillin 500 mg IM q.4h*

   Supply: Polycillin N (ampicillin) 500 mg

   Directions: Reconstitute with 1.8 mL diluent for volume of 2 mL with concentration of 250 mg/mL

   Give: __________ mL Select __________ syringe

9. Order: *Potassium chloride 30 mEq added to each 1000 mL IV fluids*

   Supply: 30 mL multiple dose vial potassium chloride 2 mEq/mL

   Give: __________ mL Select __________ syringe

10. Order: *Atarax 40 mg IM q.4–6h p.r.n., agitation*

    Supply: Atarax 50 mg/mL

    Give: __________ mL Select __________ syringe

11. Order: *Valium 5 mg IM q.4–6h p.r.n., agitation*

    Supply: Valium 10 mg/2 mL

    Give: __________ mL Select __________ syringe

12. Order: *Tigan 100 mg IM q.6h p.r.n., nausea and vomiting*

    Supply: Tigan 200 mg/2 mL

    Give: __________ mL Select __________ syringe

13. Order: *Dilantin 25 mg IV q.8h*

    Supply: Dilantin 100 mg/2 mL ampule

    Give: __________ mL Select __________ syringe

14. Order: *Atropine gr $\frac{1}{100}$ IM on call to O.R.*

    Supply: Atropine 0.4 mg/mL

    Give: __________ mL Select __________ syringe

15. Order: *Valium 3 mg IV stat*

    Supply: Valium 10 mg/2 mL

    Give: __________ mL Select __________ syringe

16. Order: *Heparin 6000 U SC q.12h*

    Supply: Heparin 10,000 U/mL vial

    Give: __________ mL Select __________ syringe

17. Order: *Tobramycin sulfate 75 mg IM q.8h*

    Supply: Nebcin (tobramycin sulfate) 80 mg/2 mL

    Give: __________ mL Select __________ syringe

18. Order: *Morphine sulfate gr $\frac{1}{10}$ IM q.3h p.r.n., pain*

    Supply: Morphine sulfate 10 mg/cc ampule

    Give: __________ mL Select __________ syringe

19. Order: *Atropine gr $\frac{1}{150}$ IM on call to O.R.*

    Supply: Atropine 0.4 mg/mL

    Give: __________ mL Select __________ syringe

20. Order: *Terramycin 120 mg IM q.d.*

    Supply: Terramycin 100 mg/mL

    Give: __________ mL Select __________ syringe

21. Order: *Ancef 500 mg IV q.6h*

    Supply Ancef 1 g

    Directions: Reconstitute with 2.5 mL diluent to yield 3 mL with concentration of 330 mg/mL.

    Give: __________ mL Select __________ syringe

22. Order: *Garamycin 40 mg IM q.8h*

    Supply: Garamycin 80 mg/2 mL

    Give: __________ mL Select __________ syringe

23. Order: *Demerol 60 mg IM q.3h p.r.n., pain*

    Supply: Demerol 75 mg/1.5 mL

    Give: __________ mL Select __________ syringe

24. Order: *Demerol 35 mg IM q.4h p.r.n., pain*

    Supply: Demerol 50 mg/1 mL

    Give: __________ mL Select __________ syringe

25. Order: *Vitamin B_{12} 0.75 mg IM q.d.*

    Supply: Vitamin B_{12} 1000 mcg/mL

    Give: __________ mL Select __________ syringe

26. Order: *Aquamephyton 15 mg IM stat*

    Supply: Aquamephyton 10 mg per mL

    Give: __________ mL Select __________ syringe

27. Order: *Phenergan 35 mg IM q.4h p.r.n., nausea*

    Supply: Phenergan 50 mg/1 mL

    Give: __________ mL Select __________ syringe

28. Order: *Heparin 8000 U SC stat*

    Supply: Heparin 10,000 U/1 mL

    Give: __________ mL Select __________ syringe

29. Order: *Morphine sulfate gr $\frac{1}{10}$ SC q.4h p.r.n., pain*

    Supply: Morphine sulfate 6 mg/1 cc

    Give: __________ mL Select __________ syringe

30. Order: *Cefadyl 750 mg IV PB in 50 mL D_5W q.6h*

    Supply: Cefadyl 2 g

    Directions: Reconstitute with 10 mL diluent for 1 g/5 mL.

    Give: __________ mL Select __________ syringe

31. Order: *Omnipen N 100 mg IM q.8h*

    Supply: Omnipen N 125 mg

    Directions: Reconstitute with 1 mL of sterile water to yield 125 mg/1 mL

    Give: ________ mL Select ________ syringe

32. Order: *Lanoxin 0.4 mg IV stat*

    Supply: Lanoxin 500 mcg/2 cc

    Give: ________ mL Select ________ syringe

33. Order: *Lasix 60 mg IV stat*

    Supply: Lasix 20 mg per 2 mL ampule

    Give: ________ mL Select ________ syringe

34. Order: *Heparin 4000 U SC q.6h*

    Supply: Heparin 5000 U/1 mL

    Give: ________ mL Select ________ syringe

35. Order: *Apresoline 30 mg IV q.6h*

    Supply: Hydralazine (Apresoline) 20 mg per mL

    Give: ________ mL Select ________ syringe

36. Order: *Calcium gluconate 0.5 g IV stat*

    Supply: Calcium gluconate 10%

    Give: ________ mL Select ________ syringe

37. Order: *Potassium penicillin G 400,000 U IM daily for 10 days*

    Supply: 10 mL potassium penicillin G reconstituted to 300,000 U/mL

    Give: ________ mL Select ________ syringe

38. Order: *Calan 2.5 mg IV push stat*

    Supply: Calan 10 mg/4 mL

    Give: ________ mL Select ________ syringe

39. Order: *Heparin 3500 U SC q.12h*

    Supply: Heparin 5000 U/mL

    Give: ________ mL Select ________ syringe

40. Order: *Neostigmine 0.5 mg IM t.i.d.*

    Supply: Neostigmine 1:2000

    Give: ________ mL Select ________ syringe

41. Order: *KCl 60 mEq added to each 1000 mL IV fluid*

    Supply: KCl 2 mEq/1 mL

    Give: ________ mL Select ________ syringe

42. Order: *Novolin R Regular U-100 insulin 16 U SC a.c.*

    Supply: Novolin R Regular U-100 insulin, with standard 100 U and Lo-Dose 30 U U-100 insulin syringes

    Give: ________ U Select ________ syringe

43. Order: *Humulin R Regular U-100 insulin 70 U SC stat*

    Supply: Humulin R Regular U-100 insulin with standard 100 U and Lo-Dose 50 U U-100 insulin syringes

    Give: __________ U   Select __________ syringe

44. Order: *Novolin N NPH U-100 insulin 25 U SC ā breakfast*

    Supply: Novolin N NPH U-100 insulin with standard 100 U and Lo-Dose 50 U U-100 insulin syringes

    Give: __________ U   Select __________ syringe

Calculate one dose of each of the drug orders numbered 45 through 62. Draw an arrow indicating the calibration line on the syringe that corresponds to the dose to be administered. The labels provided on pages 229–232 are the medications you have available. Indicate dosages that need to be divided.

45. *Vistaril 35 mg IM stat*

    Give: __________ mL

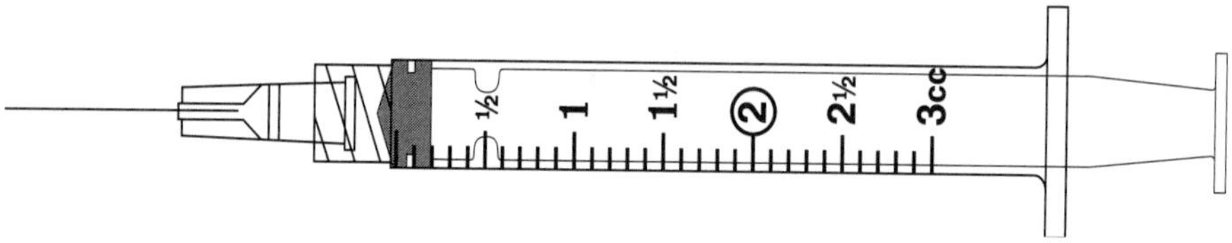

46. *Kefzol 500 mg IV q.8h*

    Give: __________ mL

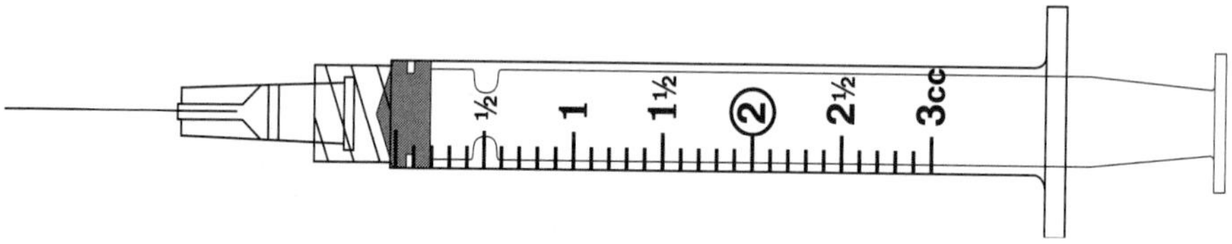

47. *Nebcin 65 mg IM q.8h*

    Give: __________ mL

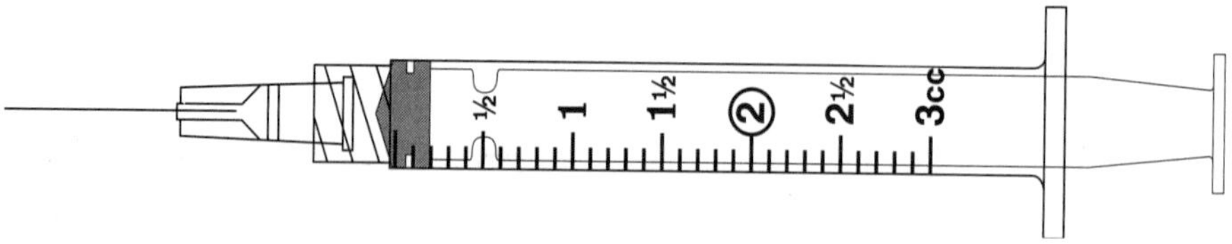

48. *Carbenicillin disodium 2 g IM q.6h*

    Give: __________ mL

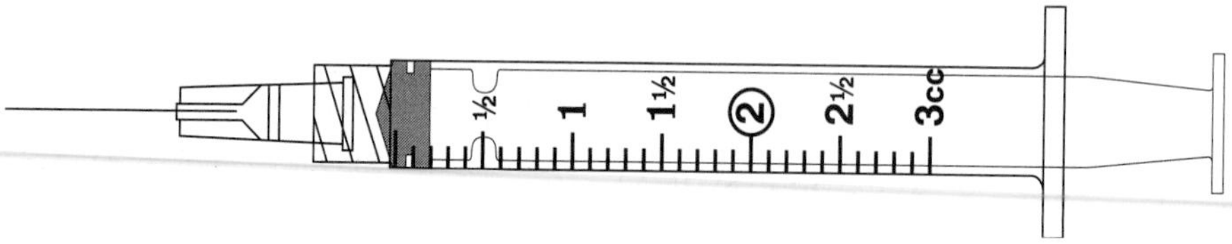

49. *Vitamin B_{12} 0.5 mg IM stat*

Give: __________ mL

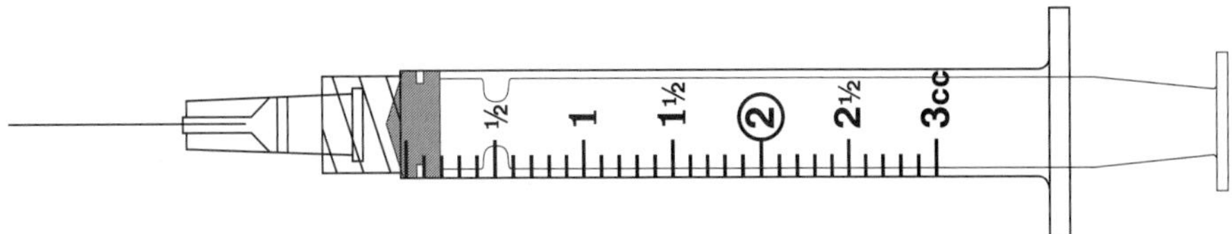

50. *Penicillin G procaine 400,000 U IM q.d.*

Give: __________ mL

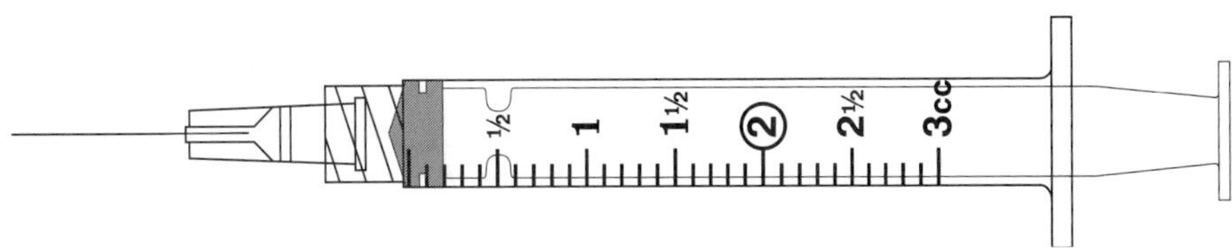

51. *Humulin R Regular U-100 insulin 22 U SC stat*

Give: __________ U

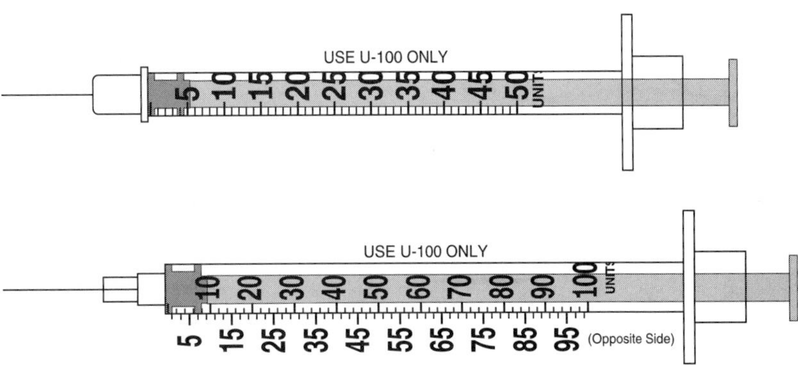

52. *Bentyl 15 mg IM q.i.d.*

Give: __________ mL

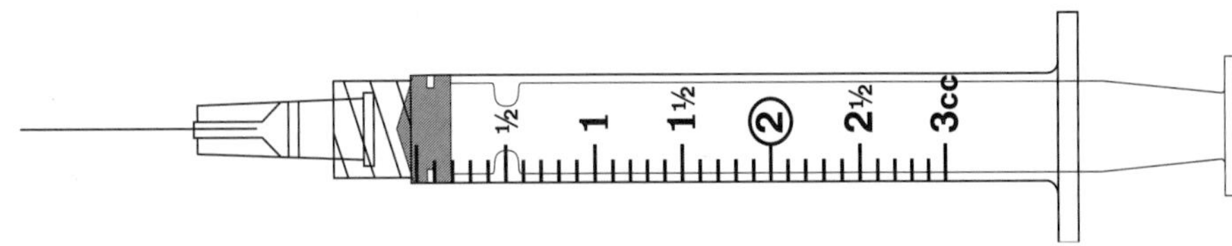

53. *Heparin 8000 U SC q.12h*

Give: __________ mL

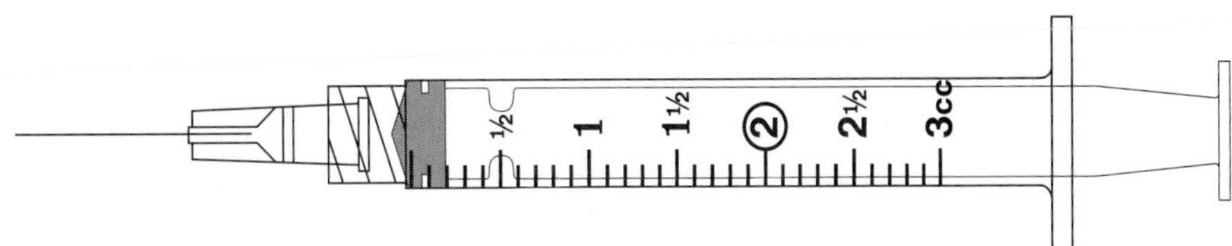

54. *Tazidime 300 mg IM q.12h*

Give: __________ mL

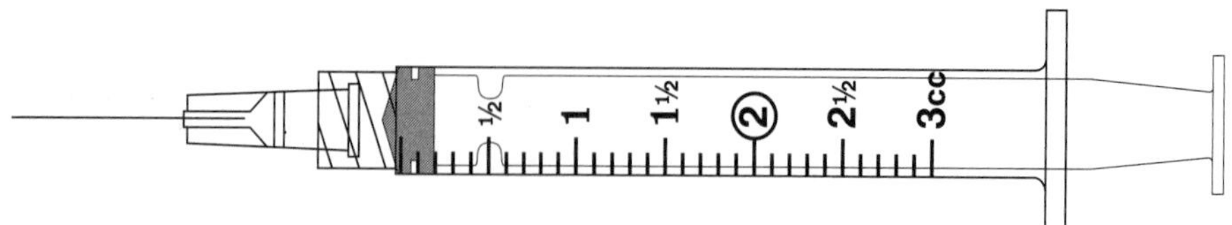

55. *Moxam 0.5 g IM q.8h*

Give: __________ mL

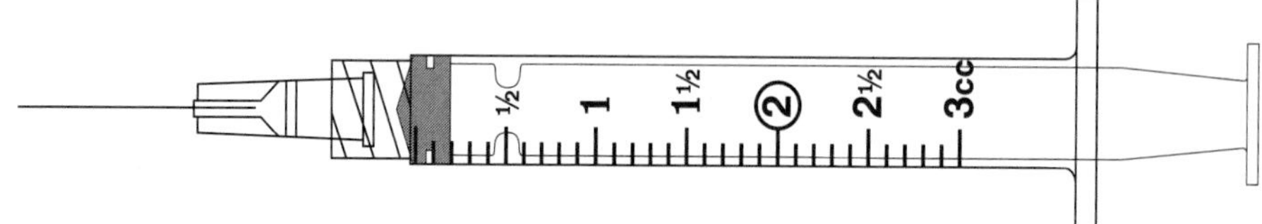

56. *Methylprednisolone 200 mg IM stat*

Give: __________ mL

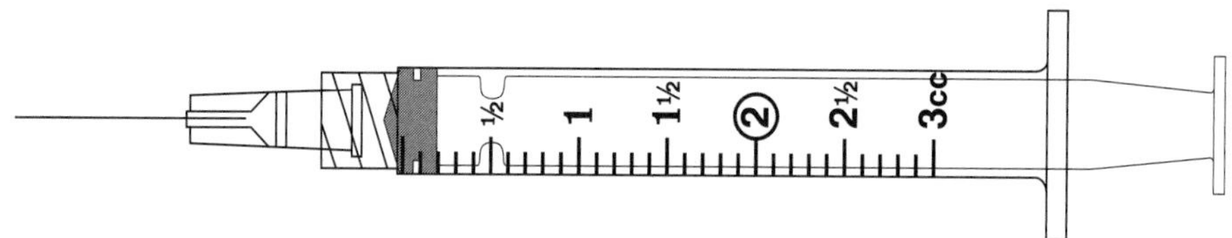

57. *Nafcillin 500 mg IM q.6h*

Give: __________ mL

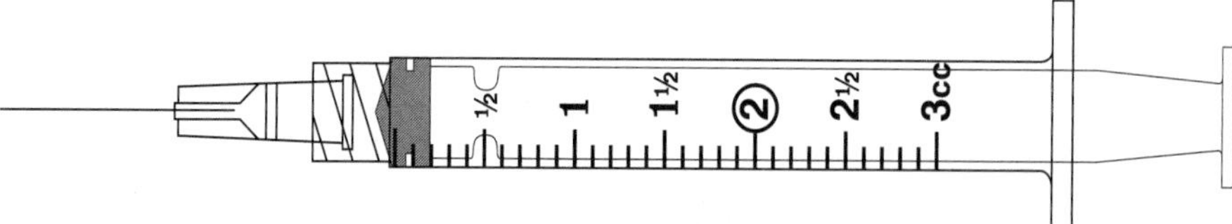

58. *Atropine gr $\frac{1}{300}$ SC stat*

Give: __________ mL

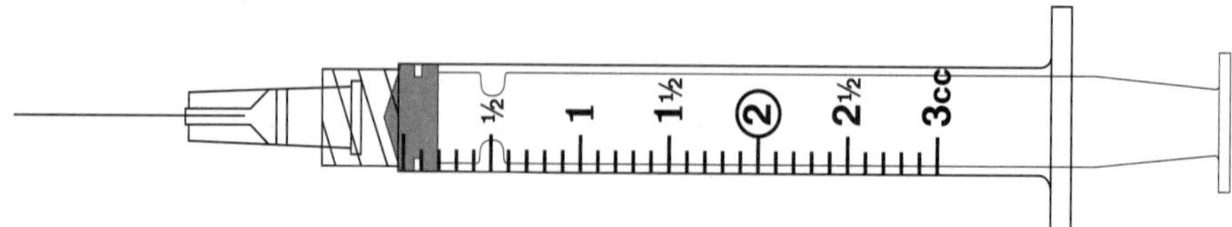

59. *Terramycin 60 mg IM q.12h*

Give: __________ mL

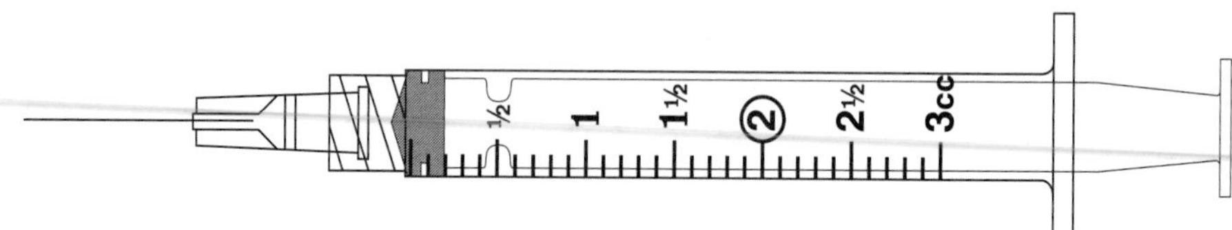

60. *Bricanyl 0.25 mg SC q.30 min × 2 doses*

Give: __________ mL

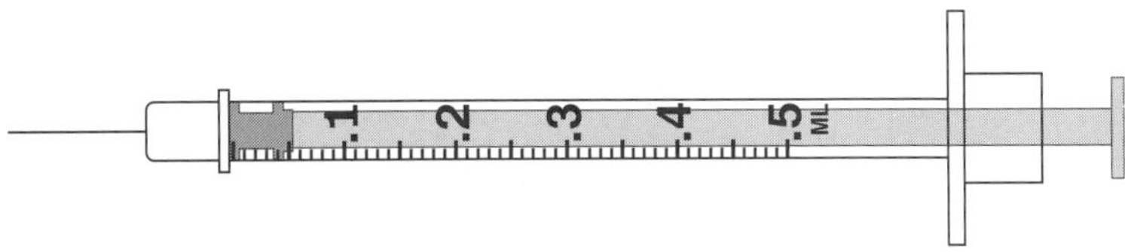

61. *Novolin R Regular U-100 insulin 32 U with Novolin N NPH U-100 insulin 54 U SC ā breakfast*

Give: __________ total U

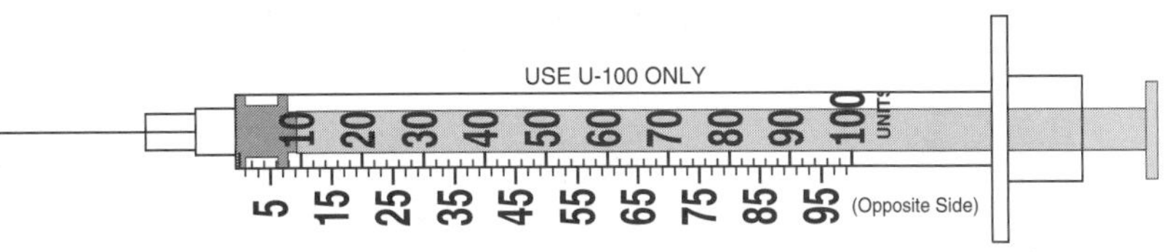

62. *Novolin 70/30 U-100 insulin 46 U SC ā dinner*

Give: __________ U

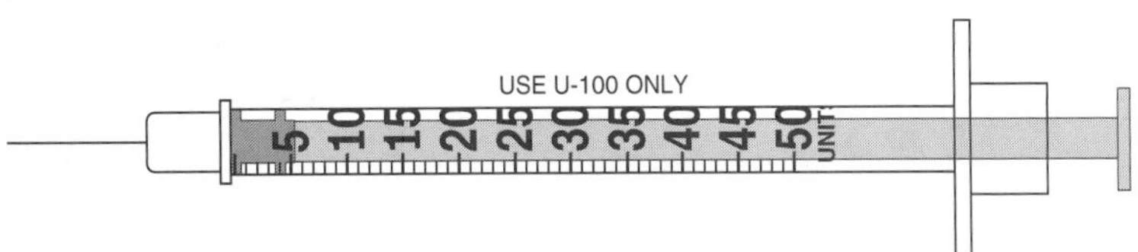

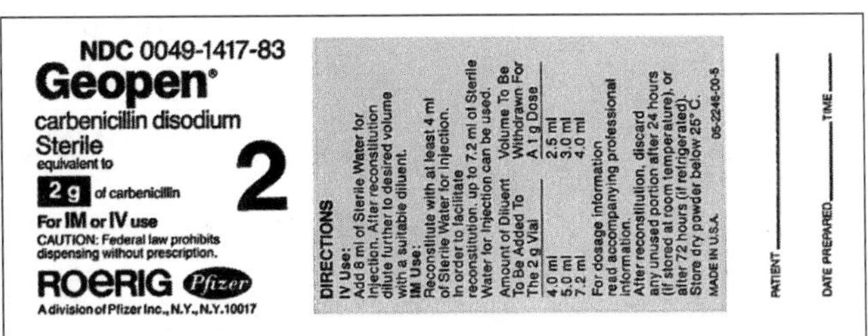

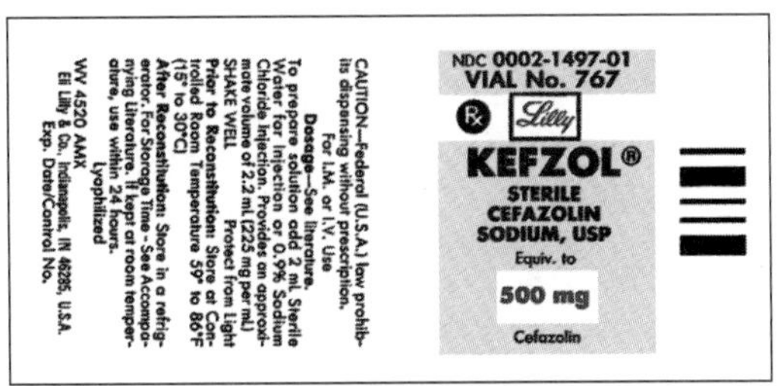

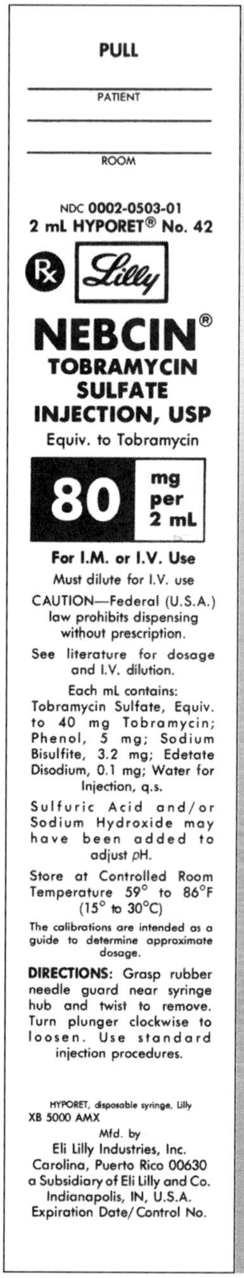

PULL
PATIENT
ROOM
NDC 0002-0503-01
2 mL HYPORET® No. 42
Lilly
NEBCIN®
TOBRAMYCIN
SULFATE
INJECTION, USP
Equiv. to Tobramycin
80 mg per 2 mL
For I.M. or I.V. Use
Must dilute for I.V. use
CAUTION—Federal (U.S.A.) law prohibits dispensing without prescription.
See literature for dosage and I.V. dilution.
Each mL contains:
Tobramycin Sulfate, Equiv. to 40 mg Tobramycin; Phenol, 5 mg; Sodium Bisulfite, 3.2 mg; Edetate Disodium, 0.1 mg; Water for Injection, q.s.
Sulfuric Acid and/or Sodium Hydroxide may have been added to adjust pH.
Store at Controlled Room Temperature 59° to 86°F (15° to 30°C)
The calibrations are intended as a guide to determine approximate dosage.
DIRECTIONS: Grasp rubber needle guard near syringe hub and twist to remove. Turn plunger clockwise to loosen. Use standard injection procedures.
HYPORET, disposable syringe, Lilly
XB 5000 AMX
Mfd. by
Eli Lilly Industries, Inc.
Carolina, Puerto Rico 00630
a Subsidiary of Eli Lilly and Co.
Indianapolis, IN, U.S.A.
Expiration Date/Control No.

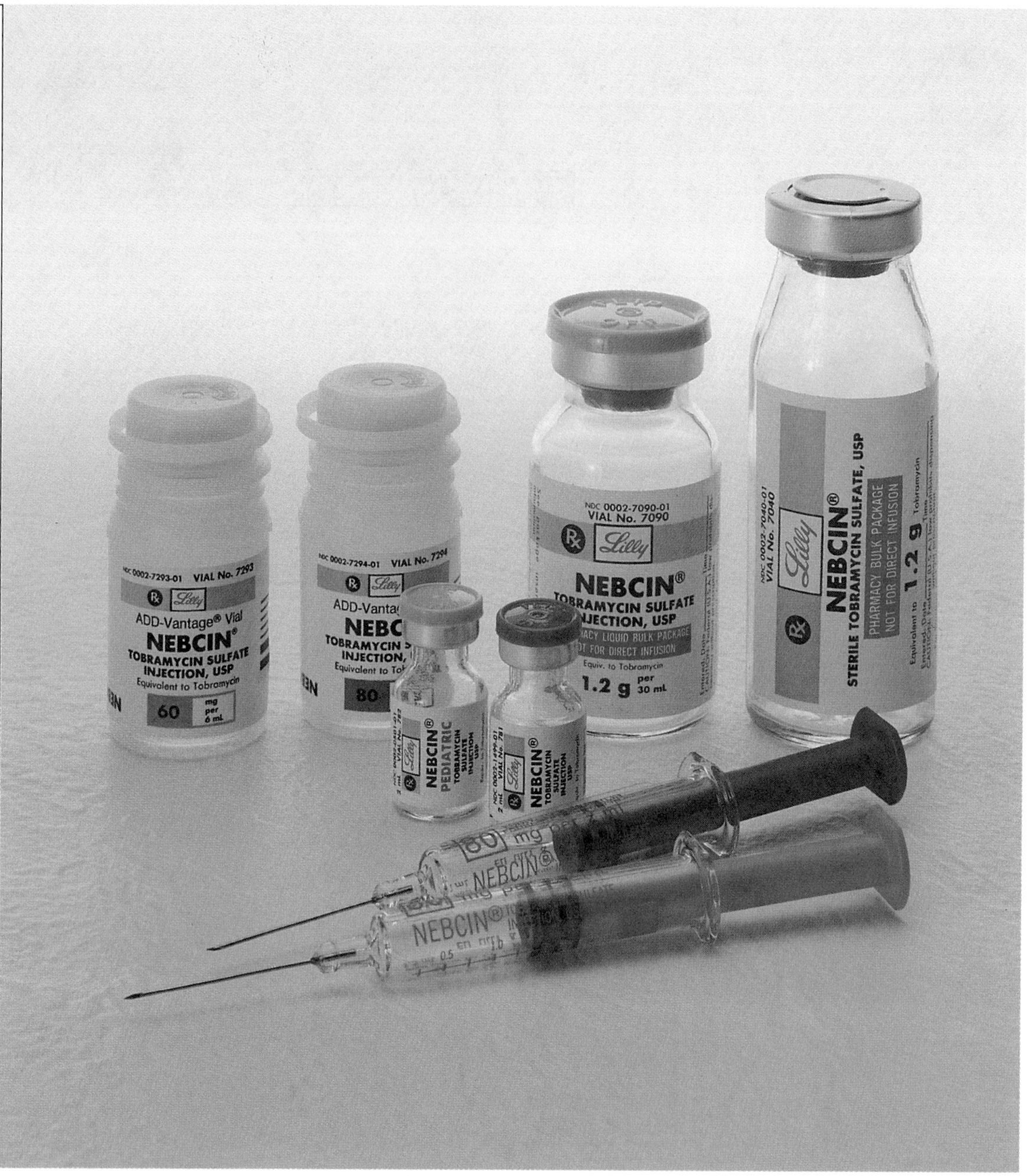

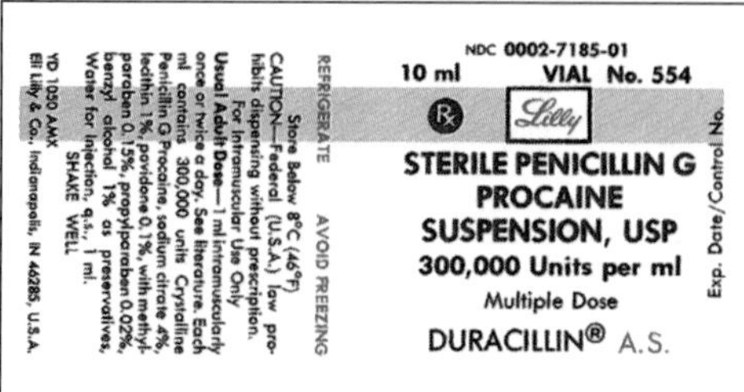

NDC 0002-7293-01 VIAL No. 7293
ADD-Vantage® Vial
NEBCIN®
TOBRAMYCIN SULFATE
INJECTION, USP
60 mg per 6 mL
NDC 0002-7090-01
VIAL No. 7090
NEBCIN®
TOBRAMYCIN SULFATE
INJECTION, USP
1.2 g per 30 mL
NDC 0002-7040-01
VIAL No. 7040
NEBCIN®
STERILE TOBRAMYCIN SULFATE, USP
PHARMACY BULK PACKAGE
NOT FOR DIRECT INFUSION
1.2 g
NEBCIN®
PEDIATRIC

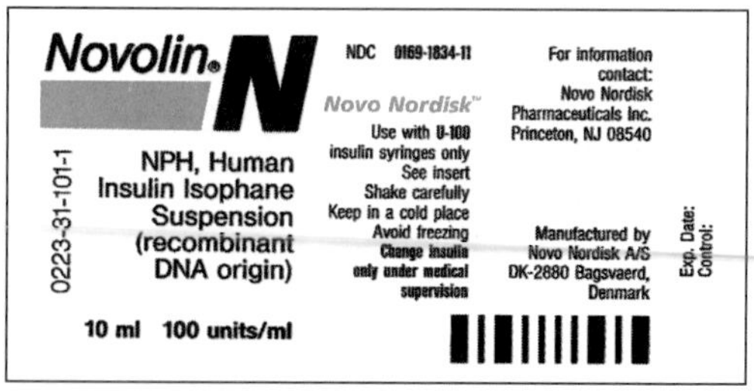

NDC 0002-7185-01
10 ml VIAL No. 554
Lilly
STERILE PENICILLIN G
PROCAINE
SUSPENSION, USP
300,000 Units per ml
Multiple Dose
DURACILLIN® A.S.
Exp. Date/Control No.
REFRIGERATE AVOID FREEZING
Store Below 8°C (46°F)
CAUTION—Federal (U.S.A.) law prohibits dispensing without prescription.
For Intramuscular Use Only
Usual Adult Dose—1 ml intramuscularly once or twice a day. See literature. Each ml contains 300,000 units Crystalline Penicillin G Procaine, sodium citrate 4%, lecithin 1%, povidone 0.1%, with methylparaben 0.15%, propylparaben 0.02%, benzyl alcohol 1% as preservatives, Water for Injection, q.s., 1 ml.
SHAKE WELL
YD 1050 AMX
Eli Lilly & Co., Indianapolis, IN 46285, U.S.A.

Novolin® N
NDC 0169-1834-11
Novo Nordisk™
For information contact:
Novo Nordisk Pharmaceuticals Inc.
Princeton, NJ 08540
0223-31-101-1
NPH, Human
Insulin Isophane
Suspension
(recombinant
DNA origin)
Use with U-100 insulin syringes only
See insert
Shake carefully
Keep in a cold place
Avoid freezing
Change insulin only under medical supervision
Manufactured by
Novo Nordisk A/S
DK-2880 Bagsvaerd, Denmark
Exp. Date:
Control:
10 ml 100 units/ml

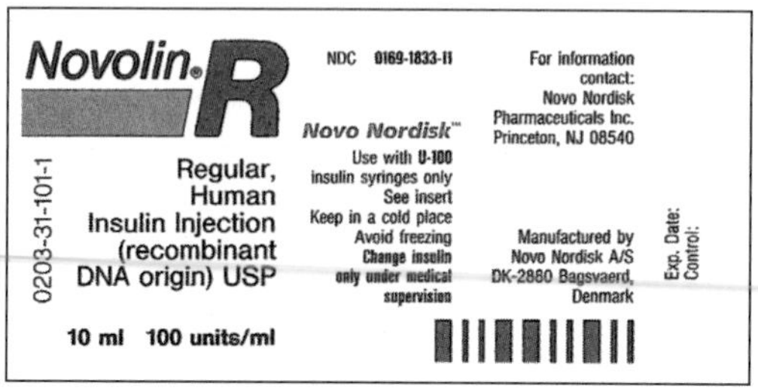

Novolin® R
NDC 0169-1833-11
Novo Nordisk™
For information contact:
Novo Nordisk Pharmaceuticals Inc.
Princeton, NJ 08540
0203-31-101-1
Regular,
Human
Insulin Injection
(recombinant
DNA origin) USP
Use with U-100 insulin syringes only
See insert
Keep in a cold place
Avoid freezing
Change insulin only under medical supervision
Manufactured by
Novo Nordisk A/S
DK-2880 Bagsvaerd, Denmark
Exp. Date:
Control:
10 ml 100 units/ml

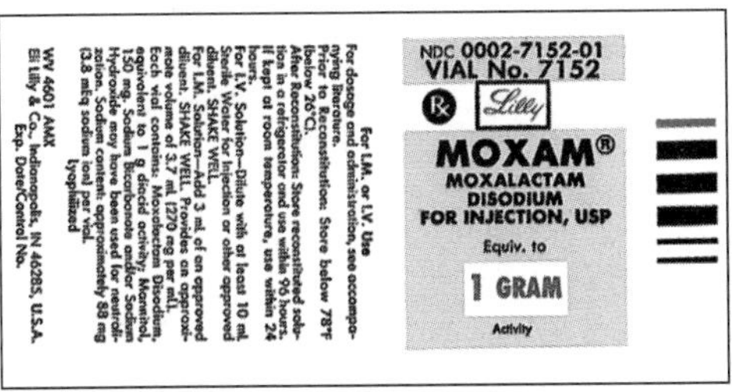

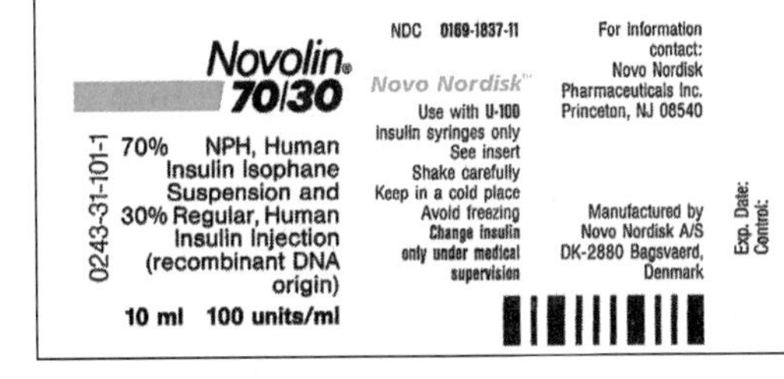

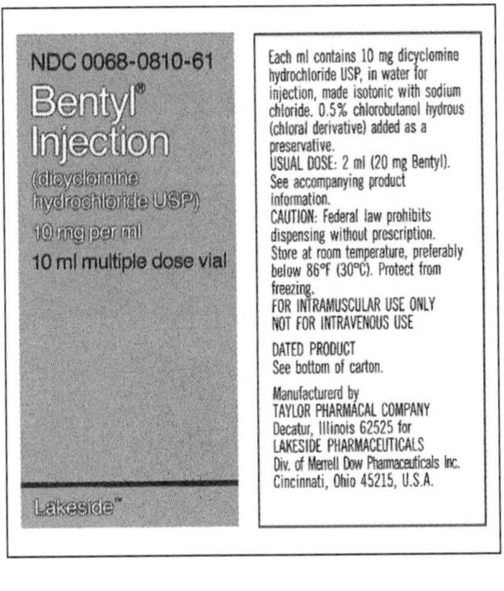

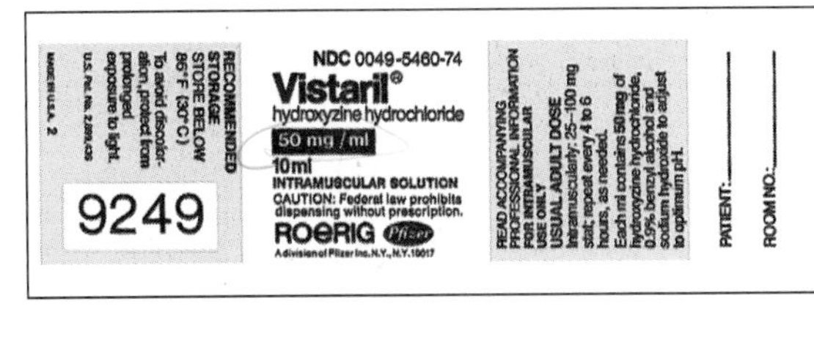

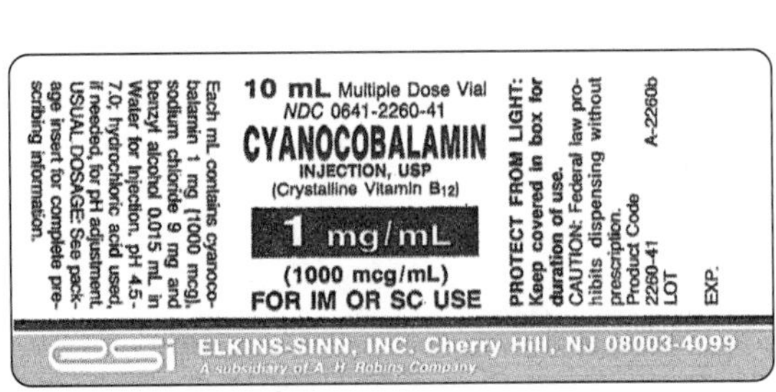

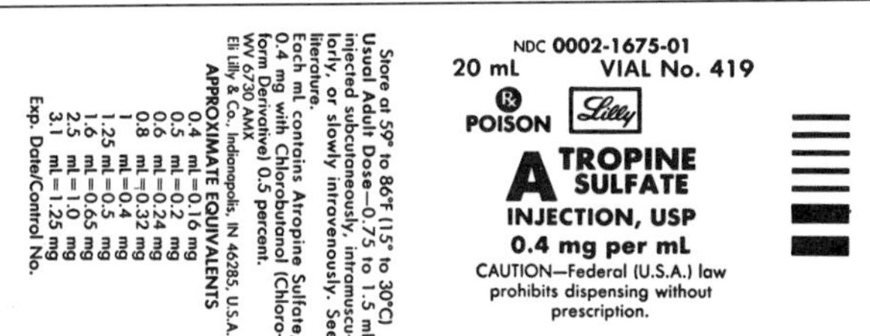

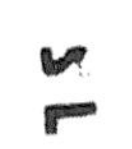

NDC 0009-3389-01 8 mL Act-O-Vial®
Solu-Medrol® 1 gram *
Sterile Powder
methylprednisolone sodium succinate for injection, USP
Single-Dose Vial
For intramuscular or intravenous use

See package insert for complete product information.
Store solution at controlled room temperature 15°-30° C (59°-86° F) and use within 48 hours after mixing.
Each 8 mL (when mixed) contains:
*methylprednisolone sodium succinate equivalent to 1 gram methylprednisolone (125 mg per mL).
Lyophilized in container 814 184 001
The Upjohn Company
Kalamazoo, Michigan 49001, USA

NDC 0002-7217-01
5 ml VIAL No. 520
Lilly
HEPARIN SODIUM INJECTION, USP
10,000 USP Units per ml
Multiple Dose

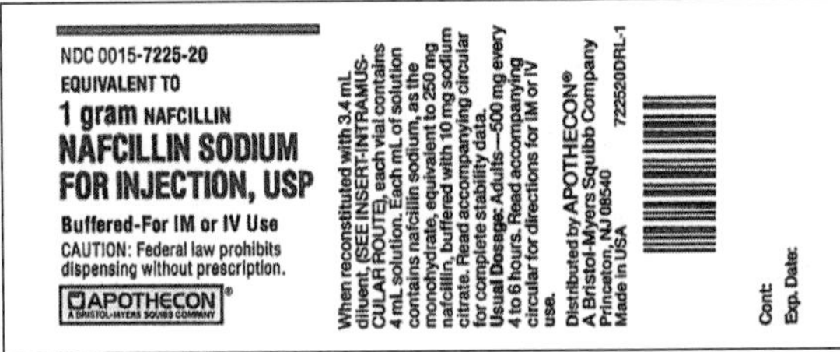

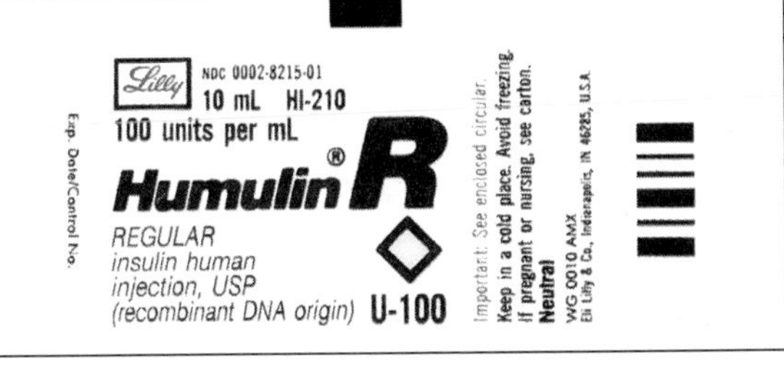

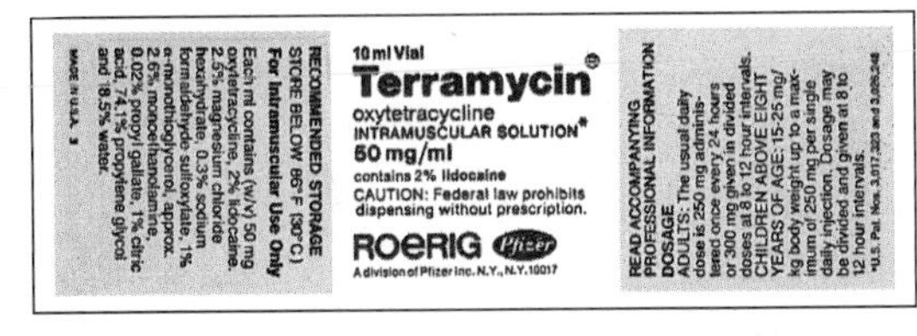

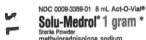

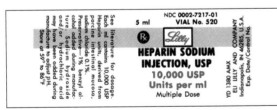

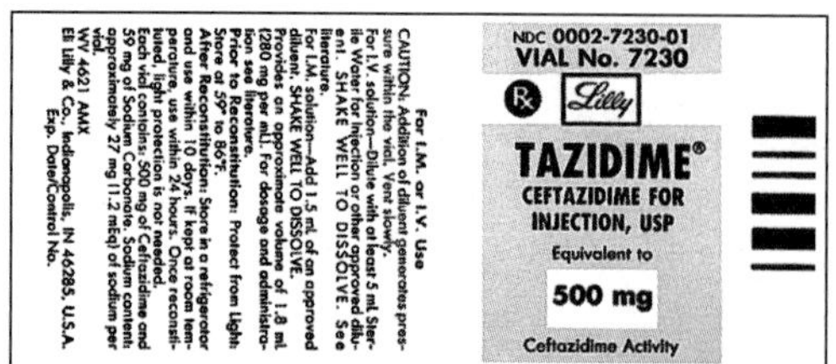

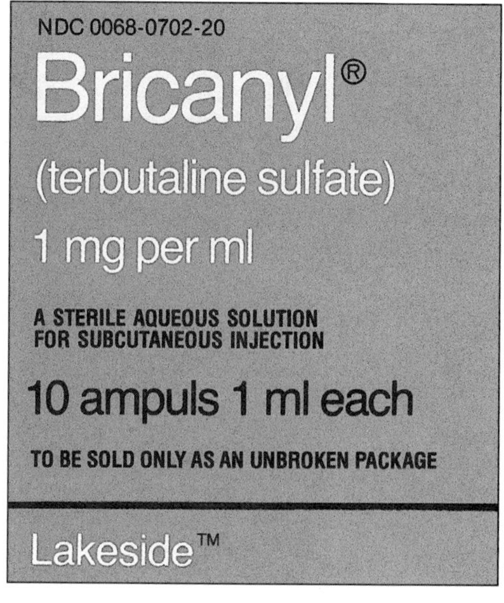

63. Critical Thinking Skill: Describe the strategy you would implement to prevent this medication error.

possible scenario

Suppose the physician ordered Humulin R insulin 20 units mixed with Humulin N insulin 40 units to be administered before breakfast. The nurse selected the vials of Humulin R and Humulin N from the medication drawer and injected 20 units of air in the Humulin N vial and 40 units of air in the Humulin R vial, drew up 40 units of Humulin R and then drew up 20 units of Humulin N.

potential outcome

The patient received the incorrect dose of insulin because the nurse drew up 40 units of Humulin R and 20 units of Humulin N instead of the dosage that was ordered: 20 units of Humulin R and 40 units of Humulin N. Because the patient received too much short-acting insulin (twice the amount ordered), the patient would likely show signs of hypoglycemia such as shakiness, confusion, and diaphoresis.

prevention

____

____

64. Critical Thinking Skill: Describe the strategy you would implement to prevent this medication error.

possible scenario

Suppose the physician ordered 10 units of Novolin R insulin for a patient with a blood glucose of 300. The nurse selected the Novolin R from the patient's medication drawer and selected a tuberculin syringe to administer the dose. The nurse looked at the syringe for the 10-unit mark and was confused as to how much should have been drawn up. The nurse finally decided to draw up 1 mL of insulin into the tuberculin syringe, administered the dose, and then began to question whether the correct dosage was administered. The nurse called the supervisor for advice.

potential outcome

The patient would have received 10 times the correct dosage of insulin. Because this was a short-acting insulin, the patient would likely show signs of severe hypoglycemia, such as loss of consciousness and seizures. The likelihood of a successful outcome is questionable.

prevention

____

____

After completing these problems, see pages 436–439 to check your answers.

CHAPTER

11

Using Ratio-Proportion to Calculate Dosages

objectives

Upon mastery of Chapter 11, you will be able to calculate the dosages of drugs using the ratio-proportion method. To accomplish this, you will also be able to:

- Convert all units of measurement to the same system and same size units.
- Consider the reasonable amount of the drug to be administered.
- Set up and solve the dosage calculation ratio-proportion: ratio for the dosage you have on hand equals the ratio for the desired dosage.

You may prefer to calculate drug dosages by the ratio-proportion method. It is presented here as an alternative to the formula method $\frac{D}{H} \times Q = X$ found in Chapters 9 and 10.

If you preferred to perform conversions by the ratio-proportion method found in Chapter 4, then you will likely want to use ratio-proportion to solve dosage problems. Try both methods: $\frac{D}{H} \times Q = X$ and *ratio-proportion. Choose the one that is easier and more logical to you.*

rule

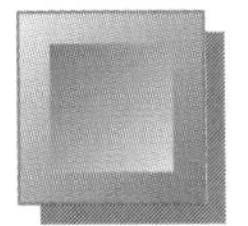

Ratio for the dosage you have on hand equals ratio for the desired dosage.

Recall that a proportion is a relationship comparing two ratios. When setting up the first ratio to calculate a drug dosage, use the supply dosage or drug concentration information available on the drug label. This is the drug you *have on hand.* Set up the second ratio using the drug order or the *desired dosage* and the amount or volume you will give to the patient. (This is the unknown or "X".) Keep the *known* information on the left side of the proportion and the *unknown* on the right. Refer to Chapters 1, 2, and 4 to review information about ratios and proportions, if needed.

remember

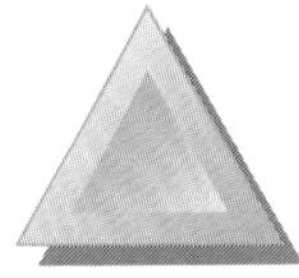

$$\frac{\text{Dosage on hand}}{\text{Amount on hand}} = \frac{\text{Dosage desired}}{\text{X Amount desired}}$$

For example, the physician *orders* 500 milligrams of Amoxil (amoxicillin), and you *have on hand* a drug labeled amoxicillin 250 mg per capsule. The proportion is:

$$\frac{250\text{ mg}}{1\text{ cap}} = \frac{500\text{ mg}}{\text{X cap}} \quad \text{(Cross-multiply and solve for X)}$$

$$250\text{ X} = 500$$

$$\frac{250\text{X}}{250} = \frac{500}{250} \quad \text{(Simplify)}$$

$$\text{X} = 2\text{ capsules}$$

Use the same three steps to calculate dosages learned in Chapters 9 and 10. Substitute the ratio-proportion method for the formula $\frac{D}{H} \times Q = X$ in step 3. Remember that proportions compare like things. Therefore, you must first convert all units to the same system and to the same size. As pointed out in Chapter 4, notice that the ratio must follow the same sequence. The proportion is set up so that like units are across from each other. The numerators of each represent the weight of the dosage, and the denominators represent the amount. It is important to keep like units in order, such as mg as the numerators (on top) and capsules as the denominators (on the bottom). Labeling units helps you to recognize if you have set up the equation in the proper sequence. If you are careful to use the full three-step method and "think through" for the logical dosage, you will also minimize the potential for error.

remember

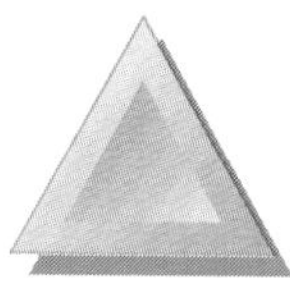

STEP 1	**CONVERT**	All units to the same system, and all units to the same size.
STEP 2	**THINK**	Estimate the reasonable amount.
STEP 3	**CALCULATE**	$\frac{\text{Dosage on hand}}{\text{Amount on hand}} = \frac{\text{Dosage desired}}{\text{X Amount desired}}$

Example 1:

Order: *Thorazine 15 mg IM stat*

Supply: Thorazine (chlorpromazine) 25 mg per mL

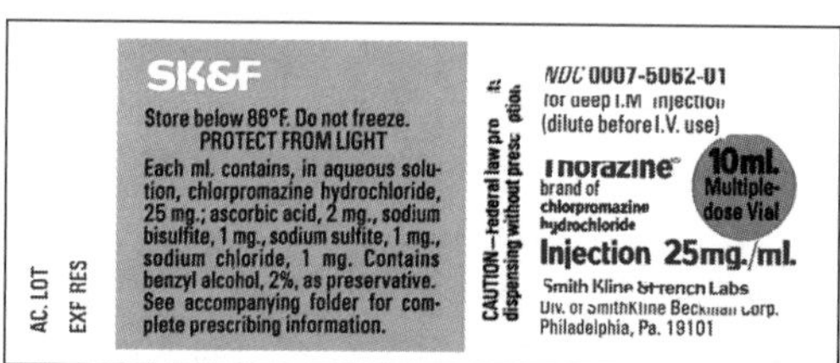

AC. LOT
EXF RES
SK&F
Store below 86°F. Do not freeze.
PROTECT FROM LIGHT
Each ml. contains, in aqueous solution, chlorpromazine hydrochloride, 25 mg.; ascorbic acid, 2 mg., sodium bisulfite, 1 mg., sodium sulfite, 1 mg., sodium chloride, 1 mg. Contains benzyl alcohol, 2%, as preservative. See accompanying folder for complete prescribing information.
NDC 0007-5062-01
(dilute before I.V. use)
brand of chlorpromazine hydrochloride
10ml. Multiple-dose Vial
Injection 25mg./ml.
Philadelphia, Pa. 19101

STEP 1 **CONVERT** No conversion is necessary.

STEP 2 **THINK** You want to give less than 1 mL; in fact, you want to give $\frac{15}{25}$ of a mL or $\frac{3}{5} = 0.6$ mL.

STEP 3 **CALCULATE** $\frac{\text{Dosage on hand}}{\text{Amount on hand}} = \frac{\text{Dosage desired}}{\text{X Amount desired}}$

$$\frac{25 \text{ mg}}{1 \text{ mL}} = \frac{15 \text{ mg}}{\text{X mL}} \quad \text{(Cross-multiply)}$$

$$25X = 15$$

$$\frac{25X}{25} = \frac{15}{25} \quad \text{(Simplify)}$$

$X = \frac{3}{5} = 0.6$ mL given intramuscularly now.

Example 2:

Order: *Ritalin 15 mg p.o. q.d.*

Supply: Ritalin 10 mg tablets

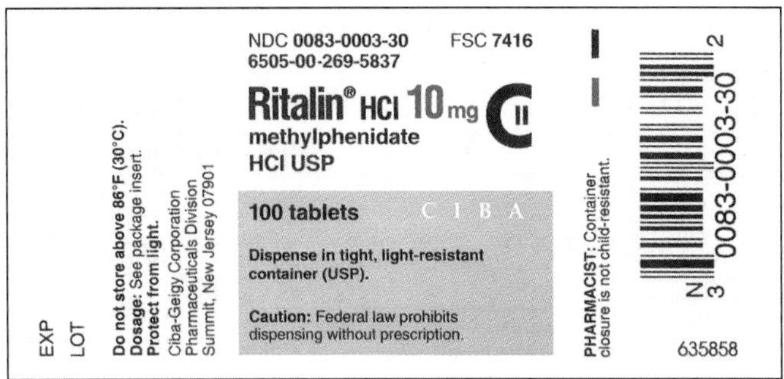

STEP 1 CONVERT No conversion is necessary.

STEP 2 THINK You want to give more than one tablet. In fact, you want to give $1\frac{1}{2}$ times more or $1\frac{1}{2}$ tablets.

STEP 3 CALCULATE

$$\frac{\text{Dosage on hand}}{\text{Amount on hand}} = \frac{\text{Dosage desired}}{\text{X Amount desired}}$$

$$\frac{10 \text{ mg}}{1 \text{ tab}} = \frac{15 \text{ mg}}{\text{X tab}} \text{ (Cross-multiply)}$$

$$10X = 15$$

$$\frac{10X}{10} = \frac{15}{10} \text{ (Simplify)}$$

$X = 1\frac{1}{2}$ tablets given orally once daily.

Example 3:

Order: *Lopid 0.6 g p.o. b.i.d.*

Supply: Lopid 300 mg tablets

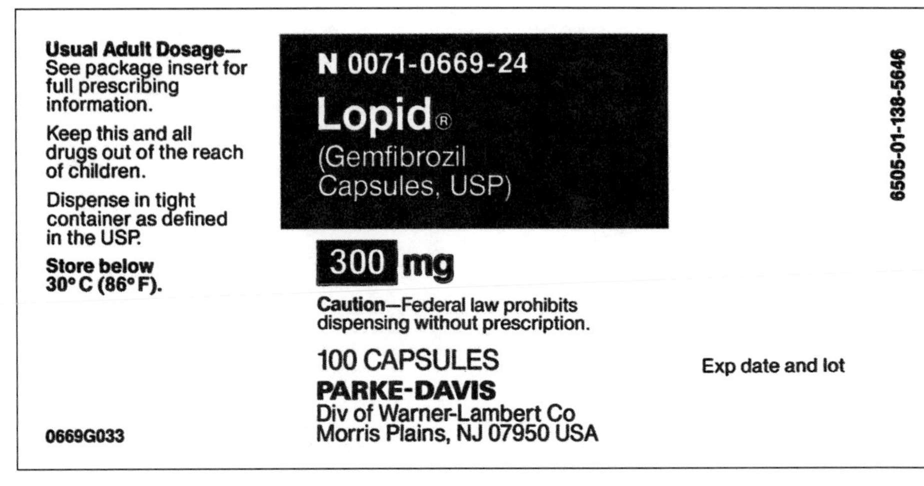

STEP 1 **CONVERT** Equivalent 1 g = 1000 mg

$$\frac{1\text{ g}}{1000\text{ mg}} = \frac{0.6\text{ g}}{X\text{ mg}} \quad \text{(Cross-multiply)}$$

X = 600 mg

0.6 g = 600 mg

STEP 2 **THINK** You want to give 600 mg and each tablet supplies 300 mg. You will need to give 2 tablets.

STEP 3 **CALCULATE**

$$\frac{\text{Dosage on hand}}{\text{Amount on hand}} = \frac{\text{Dosage desired}}{\text{X Amount desired}}$$

$$\frac{300\text{ mg}}{1\text{ tab}} = \frac{600\text{ mg}}{X\text{ tab}} \quad \text{(Cross-multiply)}$$

300X = 600

$$\frac{300X}{300} = \frac{600}{300} \quad \text{(Simplify)}$$

X = 2 tablets, given orally twice daily

Example 4:

Order: *Phenobarbital gr $\frac{1}{8}$ p.o. t.i.d.*

Supply: Phenobarbital 15 mg tablets

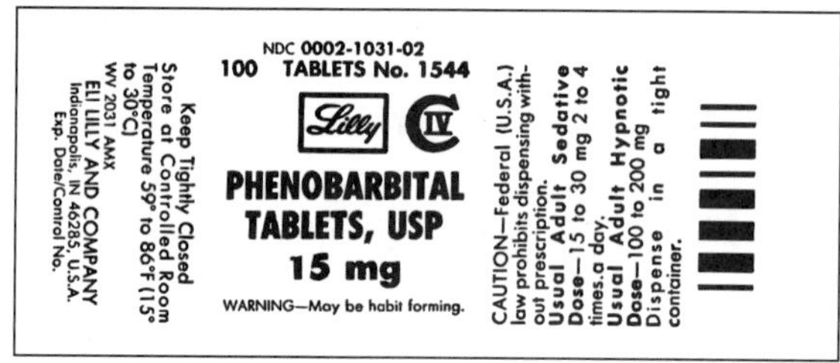

STEP 1 **CONVERT** Equivalent gr i = 60 mg

$$\frac{\text{gr i}}{60\text{ mg}} = \frac{\text{gr }\frac{1}{8}}{X\text{ mg}} \quad \text{(Cross-multiply)}$$

$$X = \frac{1}{8} \times 60 = \frac{60}{8} = 7.5\text{ mg}$$

$$\text{gr }\frac{1}{8} = 7.5\text{ mg}$$

STEP 2 **THINK** You want to give less than one tablet. Actually, you want to give $\frac{1}{2}$ tablet.

STEP 3 **CALCULATE**

$$\frac{\text{Dosage on hand}}{\text{Amount on hand}} = \frac{\text{Dosage desired}}{\text{X Amount desired}}$$

$$\frac{15\text{ mg}}{1\text{ tab}} = \frac{7.5\text{ mg}}{X\text{ tab}} \quad \text{(Cross-multiply)}$$

15X = 7.5

$$\frac{15X}{15} = \frac{7.5}{15} \quad \text{(Simplify)}$$

X = $\frac{1}{2}$ tablet, given orally three times a day

Example 5:

Order: *Lasix 15 mg po in AM*

Supply: Lasix 10 mg/mL oral solution

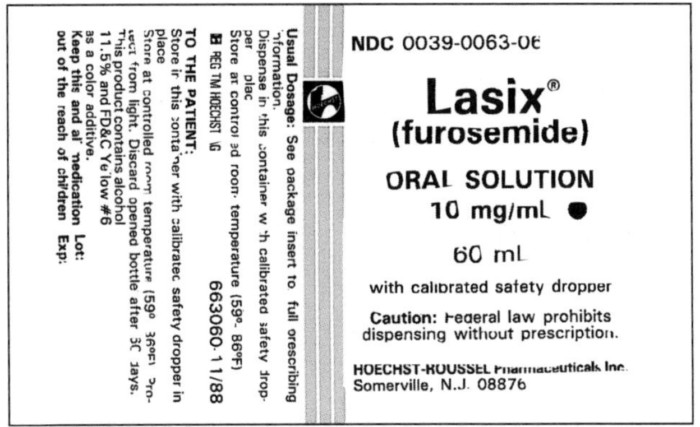

STEP 1 **CONVERT** No conversions are necessary.

STEP 2 **THINK** You want to give more than 1 mL and less than 2 mL.

STEP 3 **CALCULATE**

$$\frac{\text{Dosage on hand}}{\text{Amount on hand}} = \frac{\text{Dosage desired}}{\text{X Amount desired}}$$

$$\frac{10 \text{ mg}}{1 \text{ mL}} = \frac{15 \text{ mg}}{\text{X mL}} \quad \text{(Cross-multiply)}$$

$$10\text{X} = 15$$

$$\frac{10\text{X}}{10} = \frac{15}{10} \quad \text{(Simplify)}$$

$X = \frac{15}{10} = 1\frac{1}{2} = 1.5$ mL, given orally in the morning

quick review

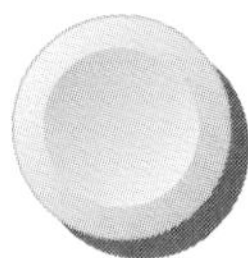

When calculating dosages using the ratio and proportion method:

- Ratio for dosage you have on hand equals ratio for desired dosage.
- $$\frac{\text{Dosage on hand}}{\text{Amount on hand}} = \frac{\text{Dosage desired}}{\text{X Amount desired}}$$
- Drug dosages cannot be accurately calculated until all units of measurement are in the same system and the same size.
- Always **convert** first, then **think** or reason for the logical answer before you finally **calculate**.

review set 31

Use the ratio-proportion method to calculate the amount you will prepare for each dose.

1. Order: *Premarin 1.25 mg p.o. q.d.*

   Supply: Premarin 0.625 mg tablets

   Give: __________ tablet(s)

2. Order: *Tagamet 150 mg p.o. q.i.d. $\bar{c}$ meals & h.s.*

   Supply: Tagamet liquid 300 mg per 5 mL

   Give: __________ mL

3. Order: *Thiamine 80 mg IM stat*

   Supply: Thiamine 100 mg per 1 mL

   Give: __________ mL

4. Order: *Demerol 35 mg IM q.4h p.r.n.*

   Supply: Demerol 50 mg per 1 mL

   Give: __________ mL

5. Order: *Lithium 12 mEq p.o. t.i.d.*

   Supply: Lithium 8 mEq per 5 mL

   Give: __________ mL

6. Order: *Ativan 2.4 mg IM h.s. p.r.n.*

   Supply: Ativan 4 mg per 1 mL

   Give: __________ mL

7. Order: *Prednisone 7.5 mg p.o. q.d.*

   Supply: Prednisone 5 mg (scored) tablets

   Give: __________ tablet(s)

8. Order: *Hydrochlorothiazide 30 mg p.o. b.i.d.*

   Supply: Hydrochlorothiazide 50 mg/5 mL

   Give: __________ mL

9. Order: *Theophylline 160 mg p.o. q.6h*

   Supply: Theophylline 80 mg per 15 mL

   Give: __________ mL

10. Order: *Tofranil 20 mg IM h.s.*

    Supply: Tofranil 25 mg per 2 mL

    Give: __________ mL

11. Order: *Indocin 15 mg p.o. t.i.d.*

    Supply: Indocin Suspension 25 mg/5 mL

    Give: __________ mL

12. Order: *Ativan 2 mg IM 2 h pre-op*

    Supply: Ativan 4 mg per mL

    Give: __________ mL

13. Order: *Luminal gr ss p.o. t.i.d.*

    Supply: Phenobarbital (Luminal) 15 mg tablets

    Give: __________ tablet(s)

14. Order: *Diabinese 125 mg p.o. q.d.*

    Supply: Diabinese 100 mg or 250 mg tablets

    Give: __________ tablet(s)

15. Order: *Thorazine 60 mg IM stat*

    Supply: Thorazine 25 mg per mL

    Give: __________ mL

16. Order: *Synthroid 0.15 mg p.o. q.d.*

    Supply: Synthroid 75 mcg tablets

    Give: __________ tablet(s)

17. Order: *Choledyl Elixir 160 mg p.o. q.6h*

    Supply: 100 mg per 5 mL

    Give: __________ mL

18. Order: *Solu-Medrol 100 mg IV q.6h*

    Supply: Methylprednisolone (Solu-Medrol) 80 mg per mL

    Give: __________ mL

19. Order: *Prolixin Elixir 8 mg p.o. q.8h*

    Supply: Prolixin Elixir 2.5 mg per 5 mL

    Give: __________ mL

20. Order: *Trimox 350 mg p.o. q.8h*

    Supply: Amoxicillin (Trimox) 250 mg per 5 mL

    Give: __________ mL

After completing these problems, see page 440 to check your answers.

For more practice, recalculate the amount you will prepare for each dose in Review Sets 25 through 27 using the ratio-proportion method.

critical thinking skills

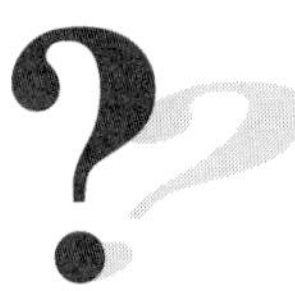

Medication errors are often caused by setting up ratio and proportion problems incorrectly. Let's look at an example to identify the nurse's error.

error

Using the ratio and proportion method of calculation incorrectly.

possible scenario

Suppose the physician ordered *Keflex 80 mg p.o. q.i.d.* for a child with an upper respiratory infection and the Keflex is supplied in an oral suspension with 250 mg per 5 mL. The nurse decided to calculate the dosage using the ratio and proportion method and set up the problem this way:

$$\frac{80\text{ mg}}{5\text{ mL}} = \frac{250\text{ mg}}{X\text{ mL}}$$

$$80X = 1250$$

$$\frac{80X}{80} = \frac{1250}{80}$$

$$X = 15.6\text{ mL}$$

The nurse gave the child 15 mL of Keflex for two doses. The next day as the nurse prepared the medication in the medication room, another nurse observed the nurse pour 15 mL in a medicine cup and asked about the dosage. At that point, the nurse realized the error.

potential outcome

The child would likely have developed complications from overdosage of Keflex, such as renal impairment and liver damage. When the physician was notified of the errors, he would likely have ordered the medication be discontinued, and the child's blood urea nitrogen (BUN) and liver enzymes be monitored. An incident report would be filed and the family notified of the error.

prevention

This type of calculation error occurred because the nurse set up the ratio and proportion problem incorrectly. The dosage on hand and amount on hand were not both set up on the left (or same) side of the proportion. The problem should have been calculated this way:

$$\frac{250\text{ mg}}{5\text{ mL}} = \frac{80\text{ mg}}{X\text{ mL}}$$

$$250X = 400$$

$$\frac{250X}{250} = \frac{400}{250}$$

$$X = 1.6\text{ mL}$$

In addition, had the nurse used step 2 in the calculation process, the nurse would have realized the dose required is less than 5 mL, not more. In calculating ratio and proportion problems remember to keep the weight of medication and the amount of the *known* together on the left side of the proportion, and the weight and the amount of the *unknown* together on the right side. In this scenario the patient would have received almost ten times the amount of medication ordered by the physician each time the nurse committed the error. You know this because there are 250 mg in 5 mL, and the nurse gave 15 mL. You can use ratio and proportion to determine how many mg of Keflex the child received in the scenario.

$$\frac{250 \text{ mg}}{5 \text{ mL}} = \frac{X \text{ mg}}{15 \text{ mL}}$$

5X = 3750

X = 750 mg, not 80 mg as ordered

Obviously the nurse did not think through for the logical amount, and either miscalculated the dosage three times or did not bother to calculate the dosage again, preventing identification of the error.

practice problems—chapter 11

Use the ratio-proportion method to calculate the amount you prepare for each dose.

1. Order: *Lactulose 30 g in 100 mL fluid p.r. t.i.d.*

   Supply: Lactulose 3.33 g per 5 mL

   Give: __________ mL in 100 mL

2. Order: *Penicillin G potassium 500,000 U IM q.i.d.*

   Supply: Penicillin G potassium 5,000,000 U per 20 mL

   Give: __________ mL

3. Order: *Keflex 100 mg p.o. q.i.d.*

   Supply: Keflex oral suspension 250 mg per 5 mL

   Give: __________ mL

4. Order: *Amoxicillin 125 mg p.o. q.i.d.*

   Supply: Amoxicillin 250 mg per 5 mL

   NOTE: You are giving home care instructions.

   Give: __________ t

5. Order: *Benadryl 25 mg IM stat*

   Supply: Diphenhydramine (Benadryl) 10 mg per 1 mL

   Give: __________ mL

6. Order: *Benadryl 40 mg p.o. stat*

   Supply: Diphenhydramine (Benadryl) 12.5 mg per 5 mL

   Give: __________ mL

7. Order: *Penicillin G potassium 350,000 U IM b.i.d.*

   Supply: Penicillin G potassium 500,000 U per 2 mL

   Give: __________ mL

8. Order: *Valium 3.5 mg IM q.6h p.r.n., anxiety*

   Supply: Valium 10 mg per 2 mL

   Give: __________ mL

9. Order: *Tobramycin sulfate 90 mg IM q.8h*

   Supply: Nebcin (tobramycin sulfate) 80 mg per 2 mL

   Give: __________ mL

10. Order: *Heparin 2500 U SC b.i.d.*

    Supply: Heparin 20,000 U per mL

    Give: __________ mL

11. Order: *Compazine 8 mg IM q.6h p.r.n., nausea*

    Supply: Compazine 10 mg per 2 mL

    Give: __________ mL

12. Order: *Gentamycin 60 mg IM q.6h*

    Supply: Garamycin (gentamycin) 80 mg per 2 mL

    Give: __________ mL

13. Order: *Pipracil 500 mg IM b.i.d.*

    Supply: Pipracil 1 g per 2.5 mL

    Give: __________ mL

14. Order: *Nilstat Oral Suspension 250,000 U p.o. q.i.d.*

    Supply: Nilstat Oral Suspension 100,000 U per mL

    Give: __________ mL

15. Order: *Ilosone 80 mg p.o. q.4h*

    Supply: Ilosone 250 mg per 5 mL

    Give: __________ mL

16. Order: *Potassium 10 mEq p.o. stat*

    Supply: Potassium 20 mEq per 15 mL

    Give: __________ mL

17. Order: *Unipen 400 mg IM q.6h*

    Supply: Nafcillin (Unipen) 1 g per 4 mL

    Give: __________ mL

18. Order: *Synthroid 150 mcg p.o. q.d.*

    Supply: Synthroid 0.075 mg tablets

    Give: __________ tablet(s)

19. Order: *Amoxicillin 400 mg p.o. q.8h*

    Supply: Amoxicillin 250 mg per 5 mL

    Give: __________ mL

20. Order: *Dilantin 225 mg IV stat*

    Supply: Dilantin 50 mg per mL

    Give: __________ mL

21. Order: *Elixophyllin 160 mg p.o. q.6h*

    Supply: Elixophyllin 80 mg per 15 mL

    Give: __________ mL

22. Order: *Thorazine 35 mg IM stat*

    Supply: Chlorpromazine (Thorazine) 25 mg per mL

    Give: __________ mL

23. Order: *Add potassium chloride 30 mEq to 1000 mL D_5 W IV*

    Supply: KCl (potassium chloride) 40 mEq per 20 mL

    Add: __________ mL

24. Order: *Phenergan 25 mg via NG tube h.s.*

    Supply: Phenergan 6.25 mg per 5 mL

    Give: __________ mL

25. Order: *Ceclor 300 mg p.o. t.i.d.*

    Supply: Ceclor 125 mg per 5 mL

    Give: __________ mL

26. Critical Thinking Skill: Describe the strategy you would implement to prevent this medication error.

    possible scenario

    The physician ordered *Keflex 50 mg p.o. q.i.d.* for a child with an upper respiratory infection. Keflex is supplied in an oral suspension with 125 mg/5 mL. The nurse calculated the dose this way:

    $$\frac{125 \text{ mg}}{50 \text{ mg}} = \frac{\text{X mL}}{5 \text{ mL}}$$

    $$50\text{X} = 625$$

    $$\frac{50\text{X}}{50} = \frac{625}{50}$$

    $$\text{X} = 12.5 \text{ mL}$$

    potential outcome

    The patient received a large overdose and should have received only 2 mL. The child would likely have developed complications from overdosage of Keflex, such as renal impairment and liver damage. When the physician was notified of the error, he would likely have ordered the medication be discontinued and the patient's blood urea nitrogen (BUN) and liver enzymes be monitored. An incident report would be filed and the family notified of the error.

    prevention

    ____

    ____

After completing these problems, see pages 440 and 441 to check your answers.

CHAPTER

12

Pediatric Dosages

objectives

Upon mastery of Chapter 12, you will be able to calculate drug dosages based on body weight for children and verify safety of pediatric drug orders. To accomplish this you will also be able to:

- Convert pounds to kilograms.
- Consult a reputable drug resource to calculate the recommended safe pediatric dosage per kilogram of body weight.
- Compare the ordered dosage with the recommended safe dosage.
- Determine whether the ordered dosage is safe to administer.
- Apply body weight dosage calculations to patients across the life span.

Only the doctor, dentist, or nurse practitioner (in some states) may prescribe the dosage of medications. However, before administering a drug, the nurse should know if the ordered dosage is safe. This is important for adults and critical for infants and children.

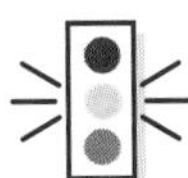

Caution: Those who administer drugs to patients are legally responsible for recognizing incorrect and unsafe dosages and for alerting the physician.

The one who administers an incorrect dosage is just as responsible for the patient's safety as the one who prescribes it. For the protection of the patient and yourself, you must familiarize yourself with the recommended dosage of drugs or consult a reputable drug reference, such as the *package insert* that accompanies the drug or the *Hospital Formulary*.

Standard adult dosage is determined by the drug manufacturer. Dosage is usually recommended based on the requirements of an average-weight adult. Frequently an adult range is given, listing a minimum and maximum safe dosage, allowing the nurse to simply compare what is ordered to what is recommended.

Dosages for infants and children are based on their unique and changing body differences. The prescribing practitioner must consider the weight, height, body surface, age, and condition of the child as contributing factors of safe and effective medication dosages. The two methods currently used for calculating safe pediatric dosages are *body weight* (such as mg/kg), and *body surface area* (BSA measured in m^2). The body weight method is more common in pediatric situations and is emphasized in this chapter. The BSA method is based on both weight and height. It is primarily used in oncology and critical care situations. BSA will be discussed in Chapter 15. Although used most frequently in pediatrics, both the body weight and BSA methods are used for adults, especially in critical care situations. The calculations are the same.

Administering Medications to Children

Numerically, the infant's or child's dosage appears smaller, but *proportionally* pediatric dosages are frequently much larger per kilogram of body weight than the usual adult dosage. Infants, birth to one year, have a greater percentage of body water and diminished absorption of water-soluble drugs, necessitating higher dosages of oral and some parenteral drugs compared to their size. Children, age one to twelve years, metabolize drugs more readily than adults, which necessitates higher dosages as compared to their size. Both infants and children, however, are growing and their organ systems are still maturing. Immature physiological processes related to absorption, distribution, metabolism, and excretion put them continuously at risk for overdose, toxic reactions, and even death. Adolescents, age 13 to 18 years, are often erroneously thought of as adults because of their body weight (greater than 110 pounds or 50 kilograms) and mature physical appearance. But they must still be regarded as physiologically immature with unpredictable growth spurts and hormonal surges. Drug therapy for the pediatric population is further complicated because very little detailed pharmacologic research has been done on children and adolescents. The infant or child, therefore, must be frequently evaluated for desired clinical responses to medications, and serum drug levels are needed to help adjust some drug dosages. It is important to remember that administration of an incorrect dosage to adult patients is dangerous; but with a child, the risk is even greater. Therefore, using a reputable drug reference to verify safe pediatric dosages is a critical health care skill.

Two well-written drug references written especially for pediatrics are *Pediatric Drugs and Nursing Implications* (2nd ed.), by Ruth McGillis Bindler and Linda Berner Howry, 1996, Norwalk, CT: Appleton & Lange, and *Pediatric Medications: A Handbook for Nurses,* by Susan Miller and Joanne Fioravanti, 1997, St. Louis: Mosby-Year Book, Inc. There are also a variety of pocket-size pediatric drug handbooks. Two widely used handbooks are *Johns Hopkins Hospital: The Harriet Lane Handbook* (14th ed.), Michael A. Barone (Ed.), 1996, St. Louis: Mosby-Year Book, Inc., and *Pediatric Dosage Handbook* (4th ed.), by Carol K. Taketomo, et al., 1997, Cleveland: LEXI-COMP.

Converting Pounds to Kilograms

The body weight method is calculated based on the person's weight in kilograms. Recall that the pounds to kilograms conversion was introduced in Chapter 4.

remember

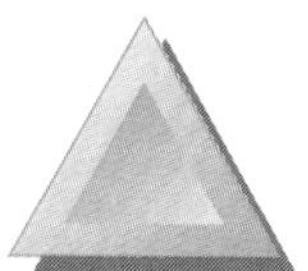

1 kg = 2.2 lb and **1 lb = 16 oz**

Simply stated, weight in pounds is approximately twice the metric weight in kg; or weight in kg is approximately $\frac{1}{2}$ of weight in pounds.

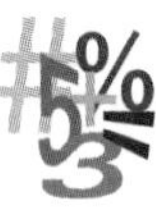

math tip: When converting pounds to kilograms, round kilogram weight to *one* decimal place.

Example 1:

Convert 45 lb to kg

Approximate equivalent: 1 kg = 2.2 lb

Smaller → Larger: (÷)

45 lb = 45 ÷ 2.2 = 20.45 = 20.5 kg

Example 2:

Convert 10 lb 12 oz to kg

Approximate equivalents: 1 kg = 2.2 lb
1 lb = 16 oz

Smaller → Larger: (÷)

$$12 \text{ oz} = 12 \div 16 = \frac{\overset{3}{\cancel{12}}}{\underset{4}{\cancel{16}}} = \frac{3}{4} \text{ lb; so } 10 \text{ lb } 12 \text{ oz} = 10\tfrac{3}{4} \text{ lb}$$

$$10\tfrac{3}{4} \text{ lb} = 10.75 \div 2.2 = 4.88 = 4.9 \text{ kg}$$

Body Weight Method for Calculating Safe Pediatric Dosage

The most common method of prescribing and administering the therapeutic amount of medication that a child needs is to calculate the amount of drug according to the child's body weight in **kilograms**. The nurse then compares the child's *ordered dosage* to the recommended *safe dosage* from a reputable drug resource before administering the medication. The intent is to ensure that the ordered dosage is safe and effective *before* calculating the amount to give and administering the dose to the patient.

rule

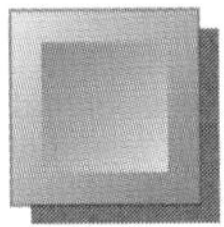

To verify safe pediatric dosing:

1. Convert the child's weight from pounds to kilograms.
2. Calculate the safe dosage in mg/kg or mcg/kg for this weight child as recommended by a reputable drug reference: **multiply mg/kg by child's weight in kg**.
3. Compare the *ordered dose* to the *recommended dose*, and decide if the dosage is safe.
4. If safe, calculate the amount to give and administer the dose; if the dosage seems unsafe, consult with the ordering practitioner before administering the drug.

NOTE: The *dosage per kg* may be mg/kg, mcg/kg, g/kg, mEq/kg, U/kg, mU/kg, etc.

For each pediatric medication order, you must ask yourself, "Is this dosage safe?" Let's work through some examples.

Example 1:

Single-dosage drugs

Single-dosage drugs are intended to be given once or p.r.n. Dosage ordered by the body weight method is based on **mg/kg/dose, calculated by multiplying the recommended mg by the child's kg weight for each dose.**

The physician orders *morphine sulfate 1.8 mg IM stat.* The child weighs 79 lb. Is this dosage safe?

1. **Convert lb to kg.** Approximate equivalent: 1 kg = 2.2 lb.

   Smaller → Larger: (÷)

   Conversion factor: 2.2

   79 lb = 79 ÷ 2.2 = 35.91 = 35.9 kg
2. **Calculate mg/kg as recommended by a reputable drug resource.** A reputable drug resource indicates that the usual IM/SC dosage may be initiated at 0.05 mg/kg/dose.

   Per dose, $\frac{0.05 \text{ mg}}{\cancel{\text{kg}}} \times 35.9 \cancel{\text{kg}} = 1.79 \text{ mg} = 1.8 \text{ mg/dose}$
3. **Decide if the dosage is safe by comparing ordered and recommended dosages.** For this child's weight, 1.8 mg is the recommended dosage and 1.8 mg is the ordered dosage. Yes, the dosage is safe.

4. **Calculate one dose.** Apply the three steps to dosage calculation.
   Order: *Morphine sulfate 1.8 mg IM stat*
   Supply: Morphine sulfate 2 mg/mL

STEP 1 CONVERT No conversion is necessary.

STEP 2 THINK You want to give less than 1 mL. Estimate that you want to give between 0.5 mL and 1 mL.

STEP 3 CALCULATE $\frac{D}{H} \times Q = \frac{\overset{0.9}{\cancel{1.8\text{ mg}}}}{\underset{1}{\cancel{2\text{ mg}}}} \times 1\text{ mL} = 0.9\text{ mL}$

Or, apply the ratio and proportion method.

$\frac{2\text{ mg}}{1\text{ mL}} = \frac{1.8\text{ mg}}{X\text{ mL}}$

$2X = 1.8$

$\frac{2X}{2} = \frac{1.8}{2}$

$X = 0.9\text{ mL}$

Example 2:

Single-dosage range

The recommended dosage of some single-dosage medications indicates a minimum and maximum range.

The practitioner orders *Vistaril 10 mg IM q.4–6h p.r.n., nausea.* The child weighs 44 lb. Is this a safe dosage?

1. **Convert lb to kg.** 44 lb = 44 ÷ 2.2 = 20 kg
2. **Calculate recommended dosage.** A reputable drug resource indicates that the usual IM dosage is 0.5 mg to 1 mg/kg/dose every 4 to 6 hours as needed. Notice that the recommended dosage is represented as a range of "0.5–1 mg/kg/dose" for dosing flexibility. Calculate the minimum and maximum safe dosage range.

   Minimum per dose: $\frac{0.5\text{ mg}}{\cancel{\text{kg}}} \times 20\ \cancel{\text{kg}} = 10\text{ mg/dose}$

   Maximum per dose: $\frac{1\text{ mg}}{\cancel{\text{kg}}} \times 20\ \cancel{\text{kg}} = 20\text{ mg/dose}$

3. **Decide if the ordered dosage is safe.** The recommended dosage range is 10 mg to 20 mg, and the ordered dosage of 10 mg is within this range. Yes, the ordered dosage is safe.
4. **Calculate one dose.** Apply the three steps to dosage calculation.
   Order: *Vistaril 10 mg IM q.4–6 h p.r.n., nausea.*
   Supply: Vistaril 25 mg/mL

STEP 1 CONVERT No conversion is necessary.

STEP 2 THINK Estimate that you want to give less than 0.5 mL.

STEP 3 CALCULATE $\frac{D}{H} \times Q = \frac{\overset{2}{\cancel{10}}\ \text{mg}}{\underset{5}{\cancel{25}}\ \text{mg}} \times 1\ \text{mL} = \frac{2}{5}\ \text{mL} = 0.4\ \text{mL}$

Or, apply the ratio and proportion method.

$$\frac{25\ \text{mg}}{1\ \text{mL}} = \frac{10\ \text{mg}}{X\ \text{mL}}$$

$$25X = 10$$

$$\frac{25X}{25} = \frac{10}{25}$$

$$X = 0.4\ \text{mL}$$

This is a child's dose and a small dose. Measure it in a 0.5 mL tuberculin syringe.

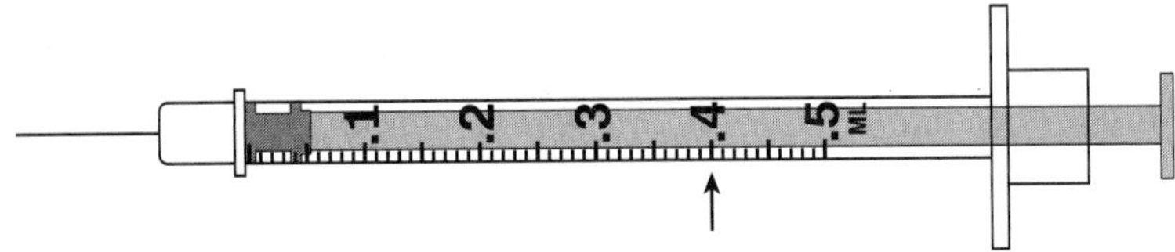

Example 3:

Routine or round-the-clock drugs

Routine or round-the-clock drugs are intended for a continuous effect on the body over 24 hours. They are recommended as a *total daily dosage:* **mg/kg/day to be divided into some number of individual doses.**

The practitioner orders *Ceclor 100 mg p.o. t.i.d.* The child weighs 33 lb. Is this dosage safe?

1. **Convert lb to kg:** 33 lb = 33 ÷ 2.2 = 15 kg
2. **Calculate recommended dosage.** Figure 12-1 shows the recommended dosage on the drug label, "Usual dose: Children, 20 mg per kg a day . . . in three divided doses."

   First, calculate the total daily dosage: $\frac{20\ \text{mg}}{\cancel{\text{kg}}} \times 15\ \cancel{\text{kg}} = 300$ mg/day. Then, divide this total daily dosage into 3 doses: 300 mg ÷ 3 doses = 100 mg/dose.
3. **Decide if the ordered dosage is safe.** Yes, the ordered dosage is safe.

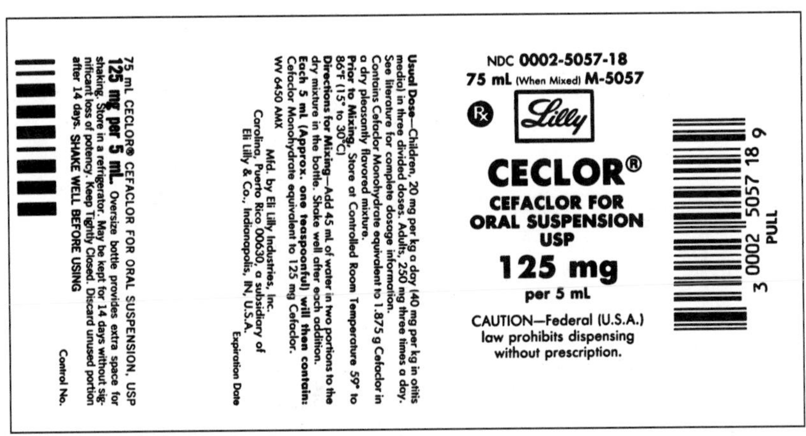

FIGURE 12-1 Ceclor Label

4. **Calculate one dose.** Apply the three steps to dosage calculation.
   Order: *Ceclor 100 mg p.o. t.i.d.*
   Supply: Ceclor 125 mg/5 mL

STEP 1 **CONVERT** No conversion is necessary.

STEP 2 **THINK** You want to give less than 5 mL. Estimate you want to give between 2.5 mL and 5 mL.

STEP 3 **CALCULATE**

$$\frac{D}{H} \times Q = \frac{\overset{4}{\cancel{100}\ \cancel{mg}}}{\underset{5}{\cancel{125}\ \cancel{mg}}} \times 5\text{ mL} = \frac{4}{\cancel{5}} \times \cancel{5}\text{ mL} = 4\text{ mL}$$

Or, apply the ratio and proportion method.

$$\frac{125\text{ mg}}{5\text{ mL}} = \frac{100\text{ mg}}{X\text{ mL}}$$

$$125X = 500$$

$$\frac{125X}{125} = \frac{500}{125}$$

$$X = 4\text{ mL}$$

Example 4:

Total daily dosage range per kg

Many medications are recommended by a minimum and maximum mg/kg range per day to be divided into some number of doses. Amoxicillin is an antibiotic that is used to treat a variety of infections in adults and children. It is a medication that is recommended to be given in divided doses round-the-clock for a total daily dosage.

Suppose the physician orders *Amoxil (amoxicillin) 200 mg p.o. q.8h* for a child who weighs 22 lb. Is this dosage safe?

1. **Convert lb to kg.** 22 lb = 22 ÷ 2.2 = 10 kg
2. **Calculate recommended dosage.** Look at the label for Amoxil (amoxicillin), Figure 12-2. The label describes the recommended dosage as, "usual child dosage: 20–40 mg/kg/day in divided doses every 8 hours . . . ."

   Calculate the minimum and maximum dosage for each single dose. The total daily dosage is recommended to be divided and administered every 8 hours, resulting in 3 doses in 24 hours.

   Minimum total daily dosage: $\frac{20\text{ mg}}{\cancel{kg}} \times 10\ \cancel{kg} = 200$ mg/day

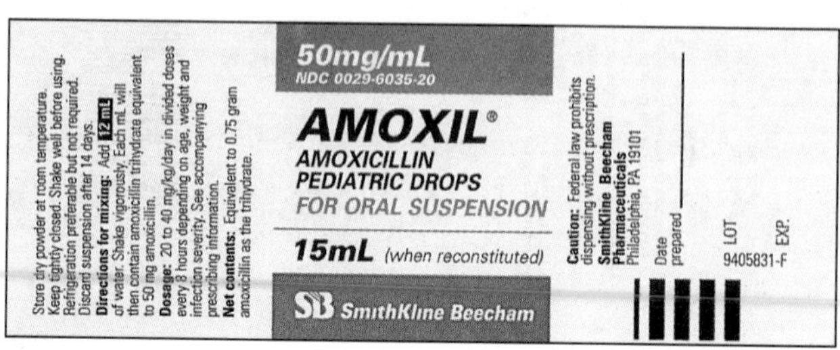

FIGURE 12-2 Amoxil Label

Minimum dosage for each single dose: 200 mg ÷ 3 doses = 66.7 = 67 mg/dose

Maximum total daily dosage: $\frac{40 \text{ mg}}{\cancel{\text{kg}}} \times 10 \cancel{\text{kg}} = 400$ mg/day

Maximum dosage for each single dose: 400 mg ÷ 3 doses = 133.3 = 133 mg/dose

The single dosage range is 67 to 133 mg/dose.

3. **Decide if the ordered dosage is safe.** The ordered dosage is 200 mg, and the allowable, safe dosage is 67 to 133 mg/dose. No, this dosage is too high and is not safe.
4. **Contact the physician to discuss the order.**

Example 5:

Total daily dosage range per kg with maximum daily allowance

Some medications have a range of mg/kg/day recommended, with a maximum allowable total amount per day also specified.

The physician orders *cefazolin 2.1 g IV q.8h* for a child with a serious joint infection. The child weighs 95 lb. The drug reference indicates that the usual IM or IV dosage for infants and children is 50 to 100 mg/kg/day divided every 8 hours; maximum dosage is 6 g/day. This means that regardless of how much the child weighs, the maximum safe allowance of this drug is 6 g per 24 hours.

1. **Convert lb to kg.** 95 lb = 95 ÷ 2.2 = 43.18 = 43.2 kg
2. **Calculate recommended dosage.**

   Minimum mg/kg/day: $\frac{50 \text{ mg}}{\cancel{\text{kg}}} \times 43.2 \cancel{\text{kg}} = 2160$ mg/day

   Minimum mg/dose: 2160 mg ÷ 3 doses = 720 mg/dose or 0.72 g/dose

   Maximum mg/kg/day: $\frac{100 \text{ mg}}{\cancel{\text{kg}}} \times 43.2 \cancel{\text{kg}} = 4320$ mg/day; which is below the maximum allowable per day dosage of 6 g or 6000 mg.

   Maximum mg/dose: 4320 mg ÷ 3 doses = 1440 mg/dose or 1.44 g/dose.
3. **Decide if the dosage is safe.** No, the dosage ordered is too high. It exceeds both the highest mg/kg/dose extreme of the range (1440 mg/dose), and it exceeds the maximum allowable dosage. At 6 g/day, no more than 2 g/dose would be allowed. The ordered dosage of 2.1 g is not safe, because 3 doses/day would deliver 6.3 g of the drug (2.1 g × 3 = 6.3 g). This example points out the importance of carefully reading all dosage recommendations.
4. **Contact the physician to discuss the order.**

Example 6:

Underdosage

Underdosage, as well as overdosage, can be a hazard. If the medication is necessary for the treatment or comfort of the patient, then giving too little can be just as hazardous as giving too much. Dosage that is less than the recommended therapeutic dosage is also considered unsafe, because it may be ineffective.

The nurse notices a baby's fever has not come down below 102.6°F in spite of several doses of ibuprofen that the physician ordered as an antipyretic (fever reducer). The order reads *ibuprofen 40 mg p.o. q.6h p.r.n., temp > 101.6°F*. The 7-month-old baby weighs $17\frac{1}{2}$ lb.

1. **Convert lb to kg.** $17\frac{1}{2}$ lb = 17.5 lb = 17.5 ÷ 2.2 = 7.95 = 8 kg
2. **Calculate safe dosage.** The drug reference states "... Usual dosage ... oral: Children: ... Antipyretic: 6 months–12 years: Temperature < 102.5°F (39°C) 5 mg/kg/dose; temperature > 102.5°F: 10 mg/kg/dose; given every 6–8 hr; Maximum daily dose: 40 mg/kg/day."

   The recommended safe mg/kg dosage to treat this child's fever of 102.6°F is based on 10 mg/kg/dose. For the 8 kg child, per dose, $\frac{10 \text{ mg}}{\cancel{\text{kg}}} \times 8 \cancel{\text{kg}} = 80$ mg/dose.
3. **Decide if the dosage is safe.** The nurse realizes that the dosage as ordered is insufficient to lower the child's fever. Because it is below the recommended therapeutic dosage, it is unsafe.
4. **Contact the physician.** Upon discussion with the physician, the doctor agrees and revises the order to *ibuprofen 80 mg p.o. q.6h p.r.n., Temp > 102.5°F*. Underdosage with an antipyretic may result in serious complications of hyperthermia. Likewise, consider how underdosage with an antibiotic may lead to a superinfection and underdosage of a pain reliever may be inadequate to effectively treat the patient's pain, delaying recovery. Remember, the information in the drug reference provides important details related to specific use of medications and appropriate dosages for certain age groups to provide safe, therapeutic dosing. Both the physician and nurse must work together to ensure accurate and safe dosages that are within the recommended parameters as stated by the manufacturer on the label, in a drug insert, or in a reputable drug reference.

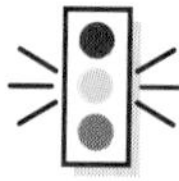

Caution: Once an adolescent attains a weight of 50 kg (110 lb) or greater, the standard adult dosage is frequently prescribed instead of a calculated dosage by weight. Care must be taken when verifying a child's dosage that the order *does not exceed* the maximum adult dosage recommended by the manufacturer.

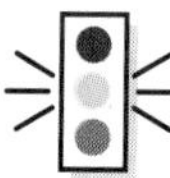

Caution: Many over-the-counter preparations, such as fever reducers and cold preparations, have printed dosing instructions that show the recommended child dose *per pound*, Figure 12-3. Manufacturers understand that most parents measure their child's weight in pounds and are most familiar with household measurement. The recommended dosage is measured in teaspoons. Recall that pounds and teaspoons are primarily used for measurement in the home setting. In the clinical setting, you should measure body weight in kg and calculate dosage by the body weight method using recommended dosage in metric measurement, such as mg/kg, not mg/lb.

Combination Drugs

Some medications contain two drugs combined into one solution or suspension. To calculate the safe dosage of these medications, the nurse should consult a pediatric drug reference. Often the nurse will need to calculate the *safe* dosage for each of the medications combined in the solution or suspension. Combination drugs are usually ordered by the amount to give or dose volume.

Example 1:

The physician orders *Pediazole 6 mL p.o. q.6h* for a child weighing 44 lb. The pediatric drug reference states that Pediazole is a combination drug containing 200 mg of erythromycin ethylsuccinate with 600 mg of sulfisoxazole acetyl in every 5 mL oral suspension. The usual dosage for Pediazole is 50 mg erythromycin and 150 mg

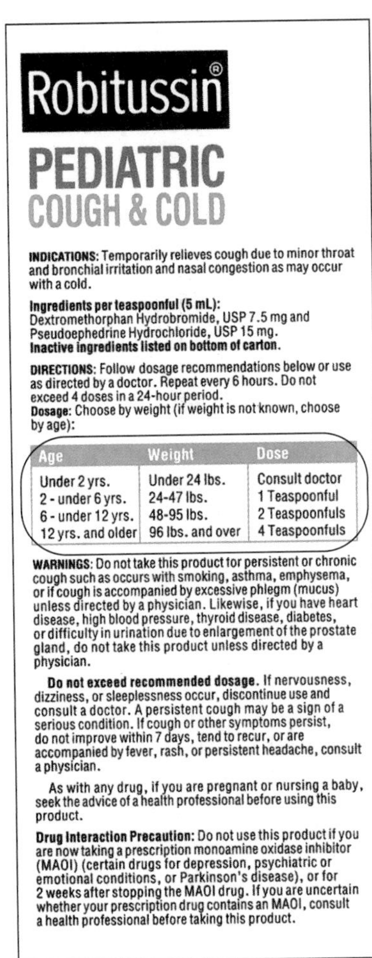

FIGURE 12-3 Label with Dosage-Per-Lb Instructions

sulfisoxazole/kg/day in equally divided doses administered every 6 hours. Is the dose volume ordered safe?

Because this is a combination drug, notice that the order is for the dose volume (6 mL). To verify that the dose is safe, you must calculate the recommended dosage and the recommended quantity to give to supply that dosage for each drug component.

1. **Convert lb to kg.** 44 lb = 44 ÷ 2.2 = 20 kg
2. **Calculate the safe dosage for each drug component.**

   erythromycin per day: $\frac{50 \text{ mg}}{\cancel{\text{kg}}} \times 20 \cancel{\text{kg}} = 1000$ mg/day; divided into 4 doses/day

   1000 mg ÷ 4 doses = 250 mg/dose

   sulfisoxazole per day: $\frac{150 \text{ mg}}{\cancel{\text{kg}}} \times 20 \cancel{\text{kg}} = 3000$ mg/day; divided into 4 doses/day

   3000 mg ÷ 4 doses = 750 mg/dose
3. **Calculate the volume of medication recommended for one dose for each drug component.**

   erythromycin: 250 mg is the recommended dosage; the supply has 200 mg/5 mL.

   $$\frac{D}{H} \times Q = \frac{\overset{5}{\cancel{250 \text{ mg}}}}{\underset{4}{\cancel{200 \text{ mg}}}} \times 5 \text{ mL} = \frac{25}{4} \text{ mL} = 6.25 = 6 \text{ mL recommended}$$

   Or, use ratio and proportion.

$$\frac{200\text{ mg}}{5\text{ mL}} = \frac{250\text{ mg}}{X\text{ mL}}$$

$200X = 1250$

$$\frac{200X}{200} = \frac{1250}{200}$$

X = 6.25 = 6 mL recommended

sulfisoxazole: 750 mg is the recommended dosage; 600 mg/5 mL is the supply.

$$\frac{D}{H} \times Q = \frac{\overset{5}{\cancel{750\text{ mg}}}}{\underset{4}{\cancel{600\text{ mg}}}} \times 5\text{ mL} = \frac{25}{4}\text{ mL} = 6.25 = 6\text{ mL recommended}$$

Or, use ratio and proportion.

$$\frac{600\text{ mg}}{5\text{ mL}} = \frac{750\text{ mg}}{X\text{ mL}}$$

$600X = 3750$

$$\frac{600X}{600} = \frac{3750}{600}$$

X = 6.25 = 6 mL recommended

4. **Decide if the dose volume ordered is safe.** The ordered dose is 6 mL, and the appropriate dose based on the recommended dosage for each component is 6 mL. The dose is safe. **Realize that because this is a combination product; 6 mL contains *both* medications delivered in this suspension.**

Example 2:

The physician orders *Septra suspension (co-trimoxazole) 7.5 cc ($1\frac{1}{2}$t) p.o. q.12h* for a child who weighs 22 kg. The drug reference states that Septra is a combination drug containing trimethoprim (TMP) 40 mg and sulfamethoxazole 200 mg in 5 mL oral suspension. It further states that the usual dose of Septra is based on the TMP component, which is 6 to 12 mg/kg/day p.o. in divided doses q.12h for a mild to moderate infection. Is this dose volume safe?

1. **Convert lb to kg.** 22 ~~kg~~ lbs = 22 ÷ 2.2 = 10 kg
2. **Calculate the safe dose for the TMP range.**

   TMP minimum daily dosage: $\frac{6\text{ mg}}{\cancel{\text{kg}}} \times 10\ \cancel{\text{kg}} = 60$ mg/day; divided into 2 doses/day

   60mg ÷ 2 doses = 30 mg/dose

   TMP maximum daily dose: $\frac{12\text{ mg}}{\cancel{\text{kg}}} \times 10\ \cancel{\text{kg}} = 120$ mg/day; divided into 2 doses:

   120 mg ÷ 2 doses = 60 mg/dose
3. **Calculate the volume of medication for the dosage range.**

   Minimum dose volume: $\frac{D}{H} \times Q = \frac{\overset{3}{\cancel{30\text{ mg}}}}{\underset{4}{\cancel{40\text{ mg}}}} \times 5\text{ mL} = \frac{15}{4}\text{ mL} = 3.75\text{ mL}$

   Or, use ratio and proportion.

   $$\frac{40\text{ mg}}{5\text{ mL}} = \frac{30\text{ mg}}{X\text{ mL}}$$

   $40X = 150$

   $$\frac{40X}{40} = \frac{150}{40}$$

   X = 3.75 mL, minimum per dose

Maximum dose volume: $\frac{D}{H} \times Q = \frac{\overset{3}{\cancel{60 \text{ mg}}}}{\underset{2}{\cancel{40 \text{ mg}}}} \times 5 \text{ mL} = \frac{15}{2} \text{ mL} = 7.5 \text{ mL}$

Or, use ratio and proportion.

$$\frac{40 \text{ mg}}{5 \text{ mL}} = \frac{60 \text{ mg}}{X \text{ mL}}$$

$$40X = 300$$

$$\frac{40X}{40} = \frac{300}{40}$$

X = 7.5 mL, maximum per dose

4. **Decide if the dose volume is safe.** Because the physician ordered 7.5 mL, it falls within the safe range and is a safe dose.
   What dosage of TMP did the physician actually order per dose for this child? Using the formula, $\frac{D}{H} \times Q = X$, write in the quantities you already know.

$\frac{D \text{ mg}}{40 \text{ mg}} \times 5 \text{ mL} = 7.5 \text{ mL}$ Solve for the unknown "D", desired dosage.

$\frac{5D}{40} = \frac{7.5}{1}$ Notice you now have a ratio and proportion.

$5D = 300$

$\frac{5D}{5} = \frac{300}{5}$

$D = 60 \text{ mg}$ This is the dosage of TMP you would give in one 7.5 mL dose.

Or, you could have started with a ratio and proportion: ratio for dosage on hand equals ratio for desired dosage.

$\frac{40 \text{ mg}}{5 \text{ mL}} = \frac{D \text{ mg}}{7.5 \text{ mL}}$ The unknown "D" is the desired dosage.

$5D = 300$

$\frac{5D}{5} = \frac{300}{5}$

$D = 60 \text{ mg}$

Example 3:

The pediatric oral surgeon orders *Tylenol and codeine (acetaminophen and codeine phosphate) suspension 10 mL p.o. q.4–6h p.r.n., pain* for a child weighing 42 lb, who had 2 teeth repaired. The drug reference states that Tylenol and Codeine is a combination drug containing 120 mg of acetaminophen and 12 mg of codeine phosphate per 5 mL. Safe dosage is based on the codeine component, which is 0.5–1 mg/kg/dose every 4 to 6 hours as needed. Is this dose volume safe?

1. **Convert lb to kg.** 42 lb = 42 ÷ 2.2 = 19.09 = 19.1 kg
2. **Calculate the safe dosage range for the codeine.**

   codeine minimum per dose: $\frac{0.5 \text{ mg}}{\cancel{\text{kg}}} \times 19.1 \cancel{\text{kg}} = 9.55 = 9.6 \text{ mg/dose}$

   codeine maximum per dose: $\frac{1 \text{ mg}}{\cancel{\text{kg}}} \times 19.1 \cancel{\text{kg}} = 19.1 \text{ mg/dose}$

3. **Calculate the volume of medication for the minimum and maximum dose.**

Minimum dose volume: $\frac{D}{H} \times Q = \frac{9.6 \text{ mg}}{12 \text{ mg}} \times 5 \text{ mL} = 4 \text{ mL minimum}$

Or, use ratio and proportion

$\frac{12 \text{ mg}}{5 \text{ mL}} = \frac{9.6 \text{ mg}}{X \text{ mL}}$

$12X = 48$

$\frac{12X}{12} = \frac{48}{12}$

$X = 4 \text{ mL minimum}$

Maximum dose volume: $\frac{D}{H} \times Q = \frac{19.1 \text{ mg}}{12 \text{ mg}} \times 5 \text{ mL} = 7.96 \text{ or } 8 \text{ mL maximum}$

Or, use ratio and proportion.

$\frac{12 \text{ mg}}{5 \text{ mL}} = \frac{19.1 \text{ mg}}{X \text{ mL}}$

$12X = 95.5$

$\frac{12X}{12} = \frac{95}{12}$

$X = 7.96 \text{ or } 8 \text{ mL maximum}$

4. **Decide if the dose volume is safe.** The ordered dose of 10 mL exceeds the maximum safe dose range; the dose is not safe. Contact the physician to discuss the order.

Be sure to take the time to doublecheck pediatric dosage. The health care provider who administers the medication has the last opportunity to ensure safe drug therapy.

quick review

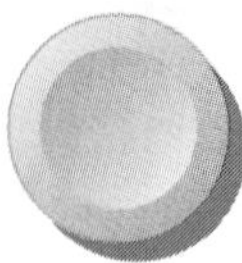

To use the body weight method to verify the safety of pediatric dosages:

- Convert child's weight from pounds and ounces to kilograms: 1 kg = 2.2 lb; 1 lb = 16 oz.
- Calculate the recommended safe dosage in mg/kg.
- Compare the ordered dosage with the recommended dosage to decide if the dosage is safe.
- If the dosage is safe, calculate the amount to give for one dose; if not, notify the physician.
- Combination drugs are ordered by dose volume. Check a reputable drug reference to be sure the dose ordered contains the safe amount of each drug as recommended.

review set 32

Calculate the following pediatric dosages.

1. Order: *Pathocil 125 mg p.o. q.6h* for a 55 lb child. The recommended dosage of Pathocil (dicloxacillin sodium) for children weighing less than 40 kg is 12.5 to 50 mg/kg/day p.o. in equally divided doses q.6h for moderate to severe infections. Calculate the minimum and maximum dosage range per single dose for this child. ________ to ________ mg. Is this dosage safe? ________

2. The dicloxacillin sodium is available as an oral suspension of 62.5 mg per 5 mL. If the dosage ordered in question #1 is safe, calculate one dose. ________ mL

3. Order: *Chloromycetin 55 mg IV q.12h* for an 8-day-old infant who weighs 2200 g. The recommended dosage for Chloromycetin (chloramphenicol) is 50 mg/kg/day IV divided q.12h. Is this dosage safe? ________

4. The chloramphenicol is available as a solution for injection of 1 g/20 mL. If the dosage ordered in question #3 is safe, calculate one dose. ________ mL

5. Order: *Suprax 120 mg p.o. q.d.* for a 33 lb child. The recommended dosage of Suprax (cefixime) for children under 50 kg is 8 mg/kg/day p.o. as a single dose. Is this dosage safe? ________

6. Suprax is available as a suspension of 100 mg/5 mL. If the dosage ordered in question #5 is safe, calculate one dose. ________ mL. How many full doses will a 50 mL bottle of Suprax provide? ________ full doses

7. Order: *Panadol 480 mg p.o. q.4–6h p.r.n. for temperature ≥ 101.6°F.* The child's weight is 32 kg. The recommended dosage of Panadol (acetaminophen) is 10 to 15 mg/kg/dose p.o. q.4–6 h p.r.n., for fever. Calculate the minimum and maximum recommended dosage range for this child. ________ to ________ mg. This dosage is based on the ________ recommended safe dosage. Panadol is available as a suspension of 160 mg/5 mL. Calculate one dose. ________ mL

8. Order: *Nebcin (tobramycin) 10 mg IM q.8h.* The neonate weighs 4000 g. The recommended dosage of tobramycin is 2.5 mg/kg/dose IM q.8h. Is this dosage safe? ________

9. Nebcin (tobramycin) is available in a solution of 40 mg/mL. If the dosage in question #8 is safe, calculate one dose. ________ mL. Indicate the volume on the syringe using an arrow.

.1 .2 .3 .4 .5 ML

10. Order: *Keflex 125 mg p.o. q.6h* for a 44 lb child. If the recommended dosage is 25 mg/kg/day in four divided doses, is this dosage safe? ________ Keflex is available in an oral suspension of 250 mg per 5 mL. If the dosage is safe, give ________ mL/dose.

Use the following order and accompanying label to answer questions 11 through 15.

Order: *Polymox suspension 75 mg p.o. q.8h × 10 days* for a 15 lb child. The following label represents the medication available.

Cont:
Exp. Date of Powder:

To the Pharmacist: Prepare suspension at time of dispensing. Add 9 mL water to the bottle and shake well. This provides 15 mL of suspension. When prepared as directed, each mL contains amoxicillin trihydrate equivalent to 50 mg amoxicillin. Dropper delivers 25 mg (1/2 full), or 50 mg (full). **Usual Dosage:** Children—20 to 40 mg/kg/day in divided doses every 8 hours, depending on severity of infection. • KEEP BOTTLE TIGHTLY CLOSED. SHAKE WELL BEFORE USING. • Discard unused portion after 14 days storage at either room temperature or refrigeration. • NDC 0015-7277-16 **READ ACCOMPANYING CIRCULAR**

APOTHECON®
A Bristol-Myers Squibb Company
Princeton, NJ 08540 Made in USA
727716DRL-1

NDC 0015-**7277-16** **15 mL BOTTLE**

EQUIVALENT TO
50 mg per mL
when reconstituted according to directions.

POLYMOX®
Amoxicillin For Oral Suspension, USP Pediatric Drops

CAUTION: Federal law prohibits dispensing without prescription.

11. What is the recommended dosage range as stated on the label? ________ to ________ mg/kg/day

12. How many doses are recommended per day? ________ doses

13. Is this order safe? ________ Explain. ________________________________

14. If safe, how much should you give the child to administer one dose? ________ mL

15. Can you administer the full 10 day order from this bottle? yes Explain.
4.5 mL/Day x 10 days = 45 mL

Use the following order and accompanying label to answer questions 16 through 18.

Order: *Kantrex 34 mg IM t.i.d.* for a 7 lb 8 oz infant.

Available: Kantrex Pediatric Injection 75 mg per 2 mL

Intramuscular Route: The recommended maximum dosage for children is 15 mg/kg/day in two equally divided doses.

16. What is the recommended maximum single dosage? __________ mg
17. Is the order safe? __________
18. If safe, how much should you administer per dose? __________ mL

Use the following order to answer questions 19 through 22. *Claforan 300 mg IV q.6h* for a child who weighs 8 kg. The reference guide states the safe dose of Claforan is 50 to 80 mg/kg/day/ q.6–8h.

19. What is the minimum safe daily dosage for this child? __________ mg/day
20. What is the maximum safe daily dosage for this child? __________ mg/day
21. What is the safe dosage range per dose that this child can receive if the drug is ordered q.6h? __________ to __________ mg per dose
22. Is the dosage ordered safe for this child? __________
23. The physician orders Septra IV for a child weighing 15 kg. The pediatric reference states that Septra IV solution is a combination medication containing 16 mg/mL of trimethoprim (TMP) and 80 mg/mL of sulfamethoxazole (SMZ). The safe dosage of Septra is based on the TMP component and is recommended at a dosage range of 6 to 12 mg/kg of TMP per day. What dosage range of the TMP component of Septra should this child receive daily? __________ to __________ mg/day
24. If the physician ordered *Septra 6 mL IV q.12h* for the child in question #23, is the dose volume safe? __________

Use the following order to answer questions 25 through 27.

Order for a 66 lb child: *Depakene (valproic acid) 450 mg p.o. at 8 AM; Depakene 900 mg p.o. at 8 PM.* (NOTE: The child is taking a safe, individualized dosage verified with blood levels.)

Supply: 480 mL bottle of Depakene syrup 250 mg/5 mL

25. How many mg/kg/day does this child receive? __________ mg/kg/day
26. Calculate the amount to be given for each of the two daily doses. __________ mL for the AM dose; __________ mL for the PM dose.
27. How many full days will this bottle last? __________ days

After completing these problems, see pages 441 and 442 to check your answers.

critical thinking skills

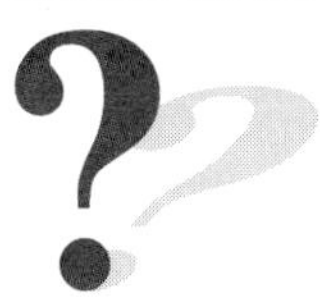

Medication errors in pediatrics often occur when the nurse fails to properly identify the child before administering the dose.

error

Failing to identify the child before administering a medication.

possible scenario

Suppose the physician ordered *ampicillin 500 mg IV q.6h* for a child with pneumonia. The nurse calculated the dosage to be safe, checked to be sure the child had no allergies, and prepared the medication. The child had been assigned to a semi-private room. The nurse entered the room and noted only one child in the room and administered the IV ampicillin to that child, without checking the identification of the child. Within an hour of the administered ampicillin the child began to break out in hives and had signs of respiratory distress. The nurse asked the child's mother, "Does Johnny have any known allergies?" The mother replied, "This is James, not Johnny, and yes, James is allergic to penicillin. His roommate, Johnny, is in the playroom." At this point the nurse realized the ampicillin was given to the wrong child, who was allergic to penicillin.

potential outcome

James' physician would have been notified and he would likely have ordered epinephrine SC stat (given for anaphylactic reactions), followed by close monitoring of the child. Anaphylactic reactions can range from mild to severe. Ampicillin is a derivative of penicillin and would not have been prescribed for a child such as James.

prevention

This error could have easily been avoided had the nurse remembered the cardinal rule of identifying the child before administering any and all medications. Children are very mobile, and you cannot assume the identity of a child simply because he is in a particular room. The correct method of identifying the child is to check the wrist or ankle band and compare it to the medication administration record with the child's name, room number, physician, and account number. Finally, remember that the first of the *five rights* of medication administration is the *right patient*.

practice problems—chapter 12

Convert the following weights to kilograms. Round to one decimal place.

1. 12 lb = ________ kg
2. 8 lb 4 oz = ________ kg
3. 1,570 g = ________ kg
4. 2,300 g = ________ kg
5. 34 lb = ________ kg
6. 6 lb 10 oz = ________ kg
7. 52 lb = ________ kg
8. 64 lb = ________ kg
9. 71 lb = ________ kg
10. 890 g = ________ kg

Calculate the following dosages.

11. Order: *Gentamicin sulfate 18 mg IVPB q.8h* for a 9 kg child

    Supply: Gentamicin sulfate 20 mg/2 mL

    Recommended dose: Gentamicin sulfate 2 mg/kg/dose IV q.8h

    If safe, give ________ mL/dose.

12. The doctor orders *theophylline 105 mg p.o. q.6h* for a 66 lb child. The drug insert recommends 3 mg/kg per dosage given four times per day. Theophylline is supplied in a dosage strength of 105 mg per 5 mL. Is the order safe and reasonable according to the recommended dosage? __________ What would you do next? __________

13. Order: *Prednisone 13 mg p.o. q.12 h × 4 days.* The recommended dosage range is 1 mg to 2 mg/kg/day p.o. in divided doses q.12h for 3 to 5 days. Calculate the safe oral dosage range per administration of Prednisone for a 13 kg child with acute asthma. Minimum dosage: __________ mg/dose; maximum dosage: __________ mg/dose. What is the total milligrams of prednisone this child should receive if drug therapy lasts 4 days? __________ mg

Use the following information to answer questions 14 through 18.

Order: *Cefzil (cefprozil) 75 mg p.o. b.i.d. for otitis media*

Package insert recommended dosage: Cefzil 30 mg/kg/dose given q.12h

Supply: Cefprozil 125 mg/5 mL

Child's weight: 11 lb

14. What is the child's weight in kg? __________ kg
15. What should the child's dosage of cefprozil be per day? __________ mg/day
16. What should each q.12h dosage be? __________ mg
17. Is the order safe according to the recommended dosage? __________
18. What should the nurse do? __________
19. Order: *Ampicillin 125 mg p.o. q.6h* for a child who weighs 22 pounds with a respiratory infection. Refer to the package insert in Figure 12-4. Is this dosage safe? __________
20. Order: *Zinacef 500 mg IM q.8h* for a 44 lb child. Recommended dosage from the package insert: 75 to 150 mg/kg/day divided into three equal doses. Is this order safe? __________
21. The physician orders a drug according to the recommended dosage: *Tylenol 10 mg/kg/dose q.3–4h p.r.n., fever > 99°F* for a child weighing 12 kg. How many milligrams of Tylenol per dose should the child receive? __________ mg
22. Tylenol elixir is provided in a solution with 80 mg/2.5 cc. How much would you prepare for one dose for the child in question #21? __________ mL

Wyeth® A.H.F.S. Category 8:12.16

Omnipen® Drops

(ampicillin)

for oral suspension

Pediatric

Description

Omnipen (ampicillin) is a semisynthetic penicillin derived from the basic penicillin nucleus, 6-amino-penicillanic acid.

Omnipen Pediatric Drops for oral administration is a powder which when reconstituted as directed yields a suspension of 100 mg ampicillin per mL. The inactive ingredients present are artificial and natural flavors, colloidal silicon dioxide, D&C Yellow 10, methylparaben, propylparaben, simethicone, sodium benzoate, sodium citrate, sucrose, and water.

Dosage and Administration

Infection	Total Daily Dose* (Give in equal doses q. 6h.)
Respiratory Tract	50 mg/kg/24 hours
Gastrointestinal Tract	100 mg/kg/24 hours
Genitourinary Tract	100 mg/kg/24 hours

FIGURE 12-4 Portion of an Omnipen Drops Package Insert

23. The physician orders *digoxin elixir 0.048 mg p.o. q.d.* for a one-month-old infant weighing 4 kg. The pediatric reference guide states the safe dosage of digoxin is 10 to 12 mcg/kg/day for a child under 2 years. Is the dosage ordered safe? ________

24. The physician orders *Versed 1 mg IM stat* preoperatively for a child weighing 14 kg. The recommended dosage of Versed is 0.05 to 0.1 mg/kg per dose preoperatively. Is the dosage ordered safe? ________

25. If the safe dosage range of Fentanyl IV preoperatively is 1 to 2 mcg/kg/dose, how many milligrams of Fentanyl could a child weighing 40 kg receive per dose? Minimum: ________ mg; Maximum: ________ mg

26. If the Fentanyl is available as 0.05 mg/mL, how much would the nurse draw up to give the maximum dose calculated in question #25? ________ mL

27. The safe dosage of Tobramycin is 7.5 mg/kg/day IV given q.8h. Calculate the safe daily dosage for a child weighing 25 kg. ________ mg

28. How many milligrams of Tobramycin should the child in question #27 receive per dose? ________ mg

29. The recommended dosage range of Solu-Medrol is 1 to 2 mg/kg/day. Calculate the safe dosage range per day of Solu-Medrol for a child weighing 22 kg. ________ to ________ mg

30. Order: *Codeine 20 mg p.o. q.4h p.r.n., pain* for a child who weighs 40 kg. The recommended dosage is 0.5 mg/kg/dose not to exceed 6 doses per day. Is this ordered dosage safe? ________

31. The available supply of codeine liquid is 15 mg/mL. If the dosage ordered is safe, calculate one dose for the child in question #30. ________ mL

Questions 32–34 refer to a 25 kg child with an order for IV Septra.

32. The pediatric reference guide states that Septra IV solution is a combination medication containing 16 mg/mL of trimethroprim (TMP) and 80 mg/mL of sulfamethoxazole (SMZ). A dose of Septra is based on the TMP component and is recommended at a dosage range of 6 to 10 mg/kg/day of TMP given q.12h. What dosage range of the TMP component should the child receive daily? ________ to ________ mg

33. What dosage range of TMP should the child receive for each dose? ________ mg – ________ mg

34. If the physician ordered *Septra 7.5 mL IV q.12h* for the child, is the dose volume safe? ________

35. Order: *Albuterol 1.2 mg p.o. t.i.d.* for an 18 kg child with severe asthma. Recommended dosage from the manufacturer: 0.2 mg/kg/day orally in three equally divided doses. Is the ordered dosage safe? ________

Questions 36 through 39 refer to the following order and Figure 12-5 on page 262. Order: *Augmentin 350 mg p.o. q.8h* for a 30 kg child with an upper respiratory tract infection.

36. What is the ordered daily dosage? ________ mg/kg/day

37. Augmentin is a combination antibiotic containing amoxicillin and clavulanic acid. The usual dosage is based upon the amoxicillin at a dosage range of 20 to 40 mg/kg/day in three equally divided doses. Is the ordered dosage safe? ________

38. Calculate one dose of Augmentin for the child. ________ mL

39. Calculate the total volume of Augmentin required for the child, if the therapy lasts 10 days. ________ mL

40. *Carbamazepine 150 mg p.o. q.i.d.* is ordered for a child who has a history of seizures. The dosage is safe for the child's weight. Calculate one dose of this drug with each of these available preparations: *scored, 100 mg chewable tablets:* ________ tablet(s); or, *oral suspension 100 mg/5 mL:* ________ mL

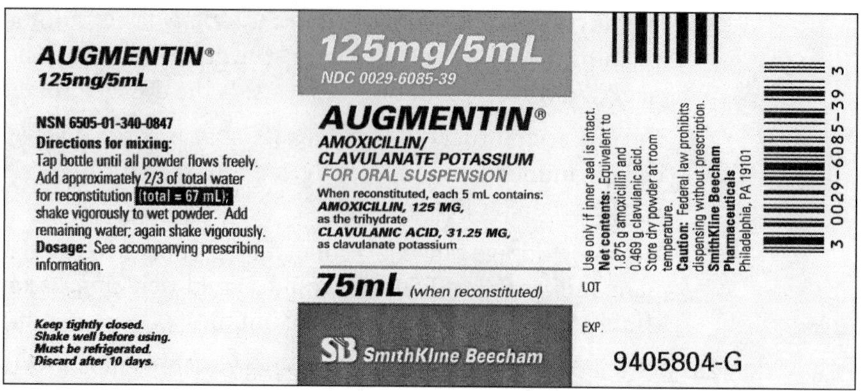

FIGURE 12-5 Augmentin Label

Calculate one dose of each of the following pediatric medication orders.

41. Order: *Klonopin 0.32 mg p.o. t.i.d.*

    Supply: Klonopin 1 mg/mL

    Give: ______ mL

42. Order: *Diuril 80 mg p.o. b.i.d.*

    Supply: Diuril 100 mg/5 mL

    Give: ______ mL

43. Order: *Ceclor 60 mg p.o. q.8h*

    Supply: Ceclor 187 mg/5 mL

    Give: ______ mL

44. Order: *Digoxin 0.175 mg p.o. b.i.d.*

    Supply: Digoxin 50 mcg/mL

    Give: ______ mL

45. Order: *Reglan 3.6 mg p.o. q.i.d. a.c. & h.s.*

    Supply: Reglan 10 mg/mL

    Give ______ mL

46. The physician orders *Ritalin 25 mg p.o. b.i.d.* Ritalin 5 mg, 10 mg, and 20 mg tablets are available. What would you give this school-age child and why? ______________________

    ____

47. Order: *Lasix 13 mg p.o. q.6h.* Calculate one dose of each available preparation: *40 mg/5 mL*, give ______ mL; and *10 mg/mL*, give ______ mL.

Questions #48 and #49 refer to the following medication order.

The physician orders *Biaxin (clarithromycin) 230 mg p.o. q.12h* for a 23 kg child with AIDS. The recommended dosage of Biaxin is 15 to 30 mg/kg/day orally in two equally divided doses.

48. What minimum and maximum dosages per administration would be appropriate for this child? Minimum dosage: ______ mg; maximum dosage: ______ mg. Is the ordered dosage safe? ______

49. If safe calculate one minimum dose and one maximum dose if Biaxin is supplied as a suspension that is 250 mg/5 mL. Minimum dose: ______ mL; maximum dose: ______ mL.

50. Critical Thinking Skill: Describe the strategy you would implement to prevent this medication error.

possible scenario

Suppose the family practice resident ordered *tobramycin 110 mg IV q.8h* for a child with cystic fibrosis who weighs 10 kg. The pediatric reference guide states that the safe dosage of tobramycin for a child with severe infections is 7.5 mg/kg/day in three equally divided doses. The nurse received five admissions the evening of this order and thought, "I'm too busy to calculate the safe dosage this time." The pharmacist prepared and labeled the medication in a syringe and the nurse administered the first dose of the medication. An hour later the resident arrived on the pediatric unit and inquired if the nurse had given the first dose. When the nurse replied "yes," the resident became pale and stated, "I just realized that I ordered an adult dose of tobramycin. I had hoped you hadn't given the medication yet."

potential outcome

The resident's next step would likely have been to discontinue the Tobramycin and order a stat tobramycin level. The level would most likely be elevated and the child would have required close monitoring for renal damage and hearing loss.

prevention

____

____

After completing these problems, see pages 442 and 443 to check your answers.

Section 3 Self-Evaluation

Chapter 9—Oral Dosage Calculations and Chapter 11—Using Ratio and Proportion to Calculate Dosages

Calculate the following dosages using either the formula method ($\frac{D}{H} \times Q = X$) or the ratio-proportion method.

1. A patient's medication is available as "gr viss tablets." If he is told to take 195 mg, how many tablet(s) should he take? __________ tablet(s)

2. A patient who is being treated for chronic pain is given gr $\frac{3}{4}$ of morphine sulphate every 3 hours. How many milligrams will he receive in 24 hours? __________ mg

3. Your patient uses nitroglycerin for chest pain. If 0.2 mg tablets are available and gr $\frac{1}{300}$ is ordered, how many tablet(s) should she take? __________ tablet(s)

4. The patient has an order for *Lactulose 15 g NG b.i.d. q.d.* Lactulose is available as 10 g/15 mL. Give __________ mL

5. Order: *Lanoxin elixir 0.15 mg p.o. q.d.*

   Supply: Lanoxin elixir 50 mcg/ml

   Give: __________ mL

6. Tylenol and codeine suspension is a combination liquid. It contains 120 mg acetaminophen and 12 mg codeine per 5 mL of suspension. If the doctor orders 9.5 mL per dose, the child will receive __________ mg acetaminophen and __________ mg codeine per dose.

7. Cedax (ceftibuten) is concentrated as 90 mg/5 mL and is supplied in a 60 mL bottle. If the doctor orders *Cedax 40 mg p.o. q.d.*, how many full days will the supply of Cedax in the 60 mL bottle last? __________ days

8. Order: *Inderal 30 mg p.o. b.i.d.*

   Supply: Inderal 60 mg tablets

   Give: __________ tablet(s)

9. Order: *Orinase 250 mg p.o. b.i.d.*

   Supply: Orinase 0.5 g tablets

   Give: __________ tablet(s)

10. Order: *Levothroid 0.3 mg p.o. q.d.*

    Supply: Levothroid 150 mcg tablets

    Give: __________ tablet(s)

11. Order: *Sudafed 60 mg p.o. q.d.*

    Supply: Sudafed 30 mg tablets

    Give: __________ tablet(s)

12. Order: *Pen Vee K 600,000 U p.o. q.8h*

    Supply: Pen Vee K 250 mg (400,000 U) per 5 mL

    Give: __________ mL

13. Order: *Rimactane 0.6 g p.o. q.d.*

    Supply: Rimactane 300 mg capsules

    Give: __________ capsule(s)

14. Order: *Codeine gr ss p.o. q.4h p.r.n., pain*

    Supply: Codeine 30 mg tablets

    Give: __________ tablet(s)

15. Order: *Plendil gr $\frac{1}{6}$ p.o. q.d.*

    Supply: Plendil 10 mg tablets

    Give: __________ tablet(s)

16. Order: *Ceclor 175 mg p.o. q.8h*

    Supply: Ceclor 250 mg per 5 mL

    Give: __________ mL

17. Order: *Synthroid 150 mcg p.o. q.d.*

    Supply: Synthroid 0.05 mg tablets

    Give: __________ tablet(s)

18. Order: *Erythromycin oral suspension 600 mg p.o. q.6h*

    Supply: E-Mycin E (erythromycin) Liquid 400 mg/5 mL

    Give: __________ mL

    State the discharge instructions you should give: include dosage in household measure, route, and frequency.

    ____

19. Order: *Amoxicillin 0.5 g p.o. q.8h*

    Supply: Amoxicillin 250 mg tabs

    Give: __________ tablet(s)

20. Order: *Provera (medroxyprogesterone) p.o. q.d. × 10 days, as follows:*

    Day #1, 2, 3—10 mg

    Day #4, 5, 6—7.5 mg

    Day #7, 8—5 mg

    Day #9, 10—2.5 mg

    Supply: Provera 5 mg scored tablets

    How many total tablets will the patient need dispensed to take this complete course of Provera? __________ tablets

Chapter 10 Parenteral Dosage Calculations

21. Order: *Morphine sulfate 12 mg IM q.4h p.r.n., pain*

    Supply: Morphine sulfate gr $\frac{1}{4}$ per mL

    Give: __________ mL

22. Order: *Atropine 0.4 mg IM on call to O.R.*

    Supply: Atropine gr $\frac{1}{150}$ per mL

    Give: __________ mL

23. Order: *Demerol 65 mg IM on call to O.R.*

    Supply: Demerol 75 mg per 1.5 mL

    Give: __________ mL

24. Order: *Vistaril 35 mg IM q.3–4h p.r.n., nausea*

    Supply: Vistaril 50 mg/cc

    Give: __________ mL

25. Order: *Vistaril 25 mg IM stat*

    Supply: Hydroxyzine (Vistaril) 100 mg per 2 cc

    Give: __________ mL

26. Order: *Thorazine 15 mg IM q.4h p.r.n., agitation*

    Supply: Thorazine 25 mg/mL

    Give: __________ mL

27. Order: *Cleocin 0.3 g IM q.i.d.*

    Supply: Cleocin 300 mg per 2 mL

    Give: __________ mL

28. Order: *Vitamin B_{12} 0.5 mg IM today*

    Supply: Vitamin B_{12} 1000 mcg/mL

    Give: __________ mL

29. Order: *Garamycin 50 mg IM q.8h*

    Supply: Garamycin 40 mg/mL

    Give: __________ mL

Calculate one dose of each the drugs ordered in questions 30 through 34. Draw an arrow indicating the calibration line on the syringe that corresponds to the dose to be administered.

30. Order: *Humulin R Regular U-100 insulin 19 U SC stat*

    Give: __________ U

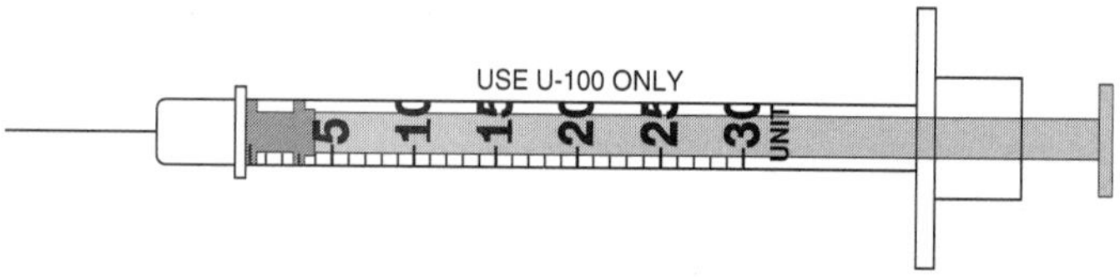

USE U-100 ONLY
5 10 15 20 25 30 UNIT

31. Order: *Novulin R Regular U-100 insulin 22 U and Novulin N NPH U-100 insulin 31 U SC ā dinner*

    Give: __________ total U

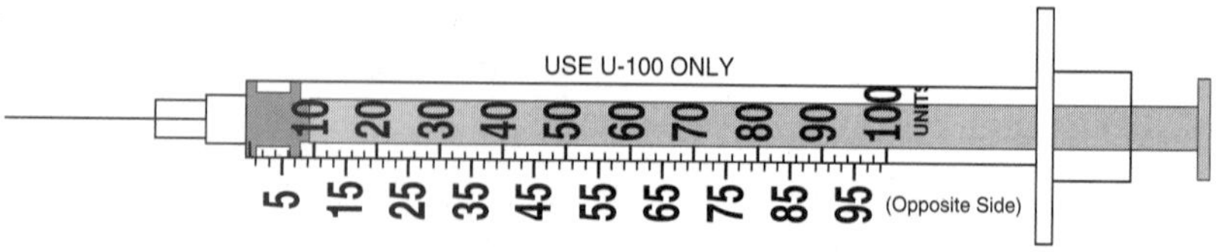

USE U-100 ONLY
10 20 30 40 50 60 70 80 90 100 UNITS
5 15 25 35 45 55 65 75 85 95 (Opposite Side)

32. Order: *Humulin 50/50 U-100 insulin 36 U SC stat.*

    The patient is actually receiving __________ units of NPH and __________ units of regular insulin for a total of __________ units.

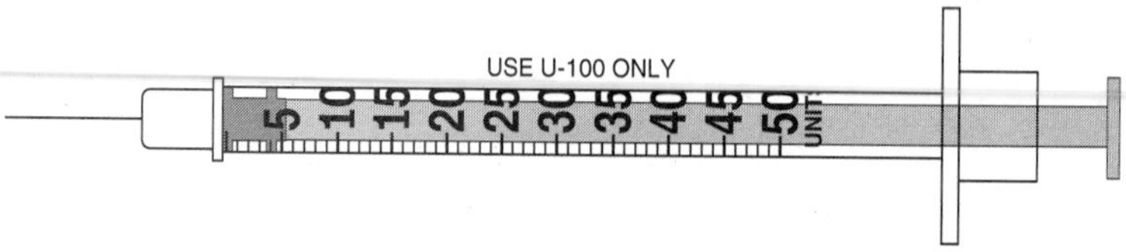

USE U-100 ONLY
5 10 15 20 25 30 35 40 45 50 UNIT

33. Order: *Cefizox 1 g IM q.6h*

    Supply: 2 g Cefizox powder

    Reconstitution directions: "Add 4 mL of sterile water to provide 500 mg per mL."

    Give: __________ mL

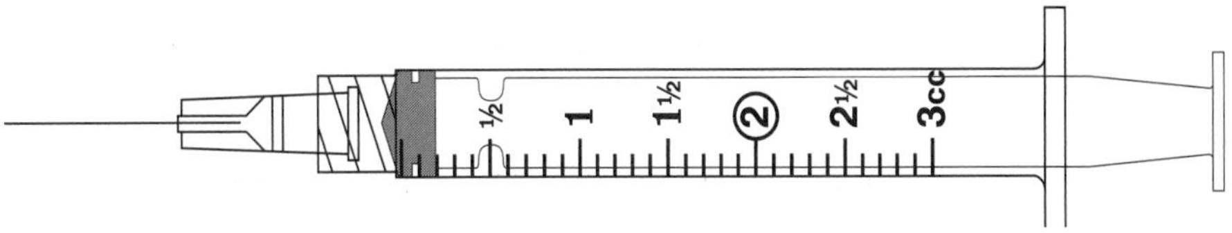

34. Order: *Carbenicillin 1.2 g IM q.6h*

    Supply: 5 g carbenicillin powder

    Reconstitution directions: "Add 9.5 mL normal saline to provide 1 g in 2.5 mL."

    Give: __________ mL

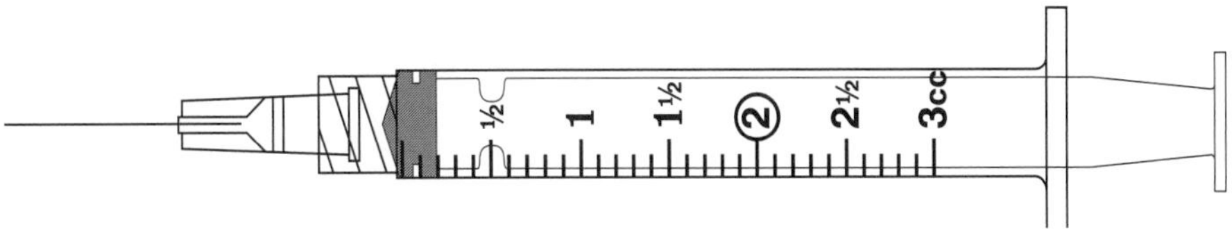

Chapter 12—Pediatric Dosages

Verify that each ordered dosage is safe. If safe, calculate the weight-based dosages as requested.

35. Order: *Calcijex (calcitriol) 0.24 mcg IV q.d. on Monday, Wednesday, and Friday* for a child on hemodialysis who weighs 8 kg. The recommended dosage is 0.01 to 0.05 mcg/kg/day, 3 times per week. Calculate the safe minimum and maximum daily dosage range. __________ to __________ mcg/day

36. Calcijex (calcitriol) is available as a 1 mcg/mL ampule. If the order is safe, calculate one dose from question #35. __________ mL

37. Using the ordered dosage from question #35, calculate the number of full doses that could be obtained from a 2 mL vial of Calcijex that contained 1 mcg/mL. __________ doses

38. Order: *Human Antihemophilic Factor 858 U IV at 0800* for a child who weighs 63 lb. The recommended dosage is 30 U/kg/dose IV. This drug is supplied for injection as 1000 units/50 mL. If the order is safe, calculate one dose. __________ mL

39. Order: *Ceftriaxone 850 mg IV q.12h* for a child weighing 17 kg. The recommended dosage is 100 mg/kg/day in two divided doses for a severe infection. Ceftriaxone is supplied as 1 g/5 mL for injection. If the dosage is safe, you would give __________ mL/dose and __________ mL/day.

40. Order: *Potassium phosphate 2.7 mmol IV stat.* The recommended dosage is 0.25 mmol/kg/dose IV. The patient weighs 23 lb 12 oz. Potassium phosphate is supplied as 3 mmol/15 mL for injection. If the dosage is safe, you would give __________ mL/dose.

41. Order: *Nuromax 64 mcg IV (given in surgery)* to a child who weighs 14 lb. The recommended dosage of Nuromax is 10 mcg/kg/dose IV for anesthesia induction. Nuromax is available for injection as 1 mg/5 mL. If the dosage is safe, you would give __________ mL/dose.

42. Order: *Opium tincture 0.18 mL p.o. q.4h p.r.n., diarrhea* for a 24 kg child. The recommended dosage is 0.0075 mL/kg/dose for a maximum of 6 doses/24 hours for diarrhea. If the dosage is safe, you would give __________ mL/day if the child takes the maximum number of doses.

43. Order: *Urokinase 195,800 U IV stat, infused over 10 minutes* for a child weighing 98 lb. The recommended dosage is to initiate therapy with 4400 units/kg IV over 10 minutes. Urokinase is supplied as 250,000 units/5 mL. If the dosage is safe, you would give __________ mL/dose.

44. Order: *Ranitidine HCl 4 mg p.o. q.6h* for a child weighing 5.7 kg. The recommended dosage is 2 to 4 mg/kg/day given orally in four divided doses. Ranitidine is supplied as 150 mg/10 mL. The safe minimum daily dosage is __________ mg; the safe maximum daily dosage is __________ mg. If the ordered dosage is safe, you would give __________ mL to provide a single-ordered dose.

45. Order: *Nystatin 2 mL p.o. q.i.d., 1 mL to inside of each cheek for thrush.* This term infant weighs 15 lb 8 oz. The recommended dosage of Nystatin for a term infant is 1 mL to the inside of each cheek in the mouth q.i.d. Nystatin suspension is supplied as 100,000 U/mL. If the dosage is safe and if the infant receives Nystatin for 5 days, calculate the total number of units given. __________ U

    Calculate the total volume received over 5 days. __________ mL

46. Order: *Sandostatin 900 mcg SC q.12h* for a 9 kg patient with severe diarrhea. The recommended dosage is 1 to 10 mcg/kg/day in two equally divided doses; the maximum dosage is 1500 mcg/day. Discuss the safety of this dosage. ____________________

    ____

47. Order: *Prilosec 3.8 mg p.o. q.i.d.* for a 42 lb child. The recommended minimum dosage is 0.7 mg/kg/dose orally four times per day. Discuss the safety of this dosage.

    ____

48. Order: *Ticarcillin/clavulanate 2.4 g IV q.6h* for a 32 kg child with a serious infection. The recommended dosage is based on the ticarcillin component as 300 mg/kg/day divided q.6h with a maximum dosage of 24 g/day. Discuss the safety of this order.

    ____

    ____

49. Order: *Morphine sulfate 0.9 mg IV stat* for a child in the recovery room who weighs 13 lb 3 oz. The recommended dosage is 0.1 to 0.2 mg/kg/dose q.2–4h p.r.n. for pain. The minimum safe dosage is ________ mg; the maximum safe dosage is ________ mg.

50. Morphine sulfate is supplied as 2 mg/mL. If the dosage ordered in question #49 is safe, calculate one dose. __________ mL. Select the better syringe for a child, and draw an arrow to indicate the correct amount to give: __________ mL.

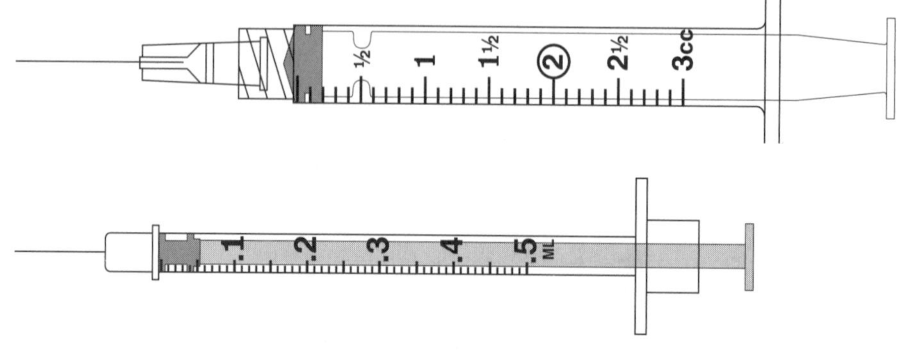

After completing these problems, see pages 443–446 to check your answers.

Perfect Score = 100%   My score = __________

Minimum mastery score = 86% (43 correct)

SECTION

4

Advanced Calculations

CHAPTER

13

Reconstitution of Noninjectable Solutions

objectives

Upon mastery of Chapter 13, you will be prepared to reconstitute noninjectable solutions. To accomplish this you will also be able to:

- Define and apply the terms *solvent, solute,* and *solution.*
- Calculate the amount of solute and solvent needed to prepare a desired strength and quantity of an irrigating solution or enteral feeding.

As more health care is provided in the home setting, nurses and other health care workers must prepare topical irrigants, soaks, and nutritional formulas and feedings. They must also instruct family members in the preparation of these solutions. In most hospitals and long-term care settings, a pharmacy and nutrition service will provide ordered solutions for irrigants, soaks, nutrition, and so on. However, on occasion it is the nurse's responsibility to prepare or add to these solutions, too.

Recall that in Chapter 10 you learned how to reconstitute powder-form drugs into injectable solutions. The manufacturer provided specific instructions on the label or in a drug reference like the *Hospital Formulary.* That previous information should serve as a primer for your understanding of the solutions you will calculate in this chapter.

Solution Strength

As you look at Figure 13-1, let's review the terms of reconstitution and their definitions.

- *Solute*—a substance to be dissolved or diluted. It can be in solid or liquid form.
- *Solvent*—a substance (liquid) that dissolves another substance to prepare a solution. *Diluent* is a synonymous term.
- *Solution*—the resulting mixture of a solute plus a solvent.

To prepare a therapeutic *solution,* you will *add a solvent* or diluent (usually normal saline or water) *to a solute* (concentrated stock solution or solid substance) to obtain the required strength of a stated volume of a solution. This means that the stock solution or solid substance, called a *solute,* is diluted with a *solvent* to obtain a reconstituted *solution* of a weaker strength. However, the amount of the drug that was in the pure solute or concentrated stock solution still equals the amount of pure drug in the diluted solution. Only the solvent has been added to the solute, expanding the total volume.

Figure 13-1 shows that the amount of pure drug (solute) remains the same in the concentrated form as well as in the resulting solution. However, in solution, notice the solute particles are dispersed or suspended throughout the resulting weaker solution.

The *strength of a solution* or *concentration* was briefly discussed in Chapter 10. Solution strength indicates the ratio of solute to solvent. Consider how each of these substances—solute and solvent—contributes a certain number of parts to the total solution. Look again at the label for 500 mg of Kefzol powder (Figure 13-2). The label directions indicate that 2 mL of sterile water (*solvent*) should be added to the powder (*solute*) to make 2.2 mL of reconstituted *solution.* The resulting solution strength would be 225 mg of solute (Kefzol) per 1 mL of solution.

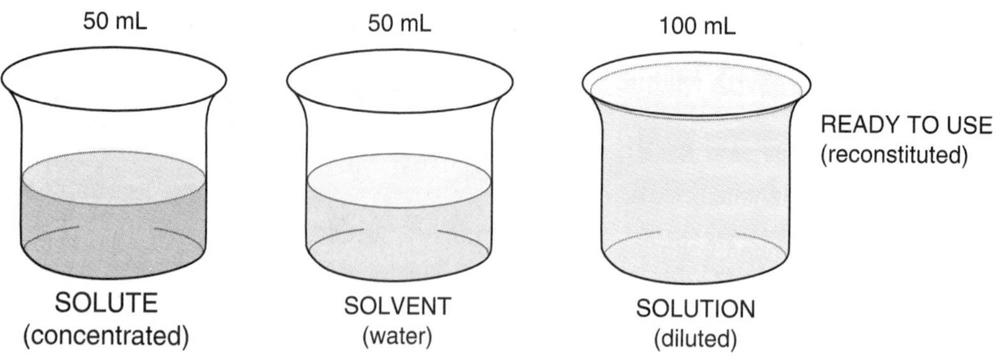

FIGURE 13-1 50 milliliters of concentrated solute diluted with 50 milliliters of solvent make 100 milliliters of diluted solution.

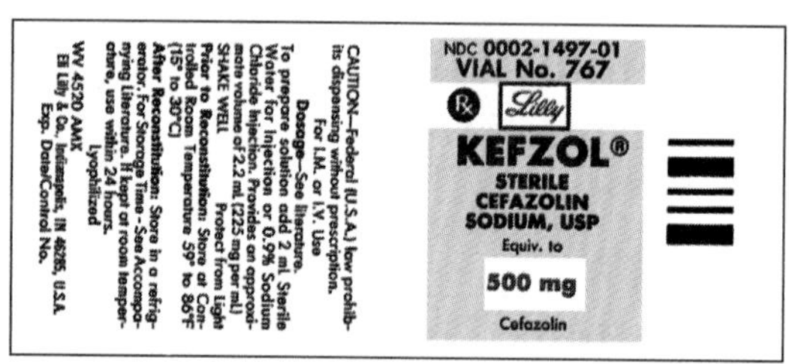

DOSAGE AND ADMINISTRATION

Kefzol may be administered intramuscularly or intravenously after reconstitution. Total daily dosages are the same for either route of administration.

Intramuscular Administration—Reconstitute as directed by Table 3 with 0.9% Sodium Chloride Injection, Sterile Water for Injection, or Bacteriostatic Water for Injection. Shake well until dissolved. Kefzol should be injected into a large muscle mass. Pain on injection is infrequent with Kefzol.

TABLE 3. DILUTION TABLE

Vial Size	Diluent to Be Added	Approximate Available Volume	Approximate Average Concentration
250 mg	2 mL	2 mL	125 mg/mL
→ 500 mg	2 mL	2.2 mL	225 mg/mL
1 g*	2.5 mL	3 mL	330 mg/mL

*The 1-g vial should be reconstituted only with Sterile Water for Injection or Bacteriostatic Water for Injection.

Intravenous Administration—Kefzol may be administered by intravenous injection or by continuous or intermittent infusion.

Intermittent intravenous infusion: Kefzol can be administered along with primary intravenous fluid management programs in a volume control set or in a separate, secondary IV bottle. Reconstituted 500 mg or 1 g of Kefzol may be diluted in 50 to 100 mL of 1 of the following intravenous solutions: 0.9% Sodium Chloride Injection, 5% or 10% Dextrose Injection, 5% Dextrose in Lactated Ringer's Injection, 5% Dextrose and 0.9% Sodium Chloride Injection (also may be used with 5% Dextrose and 0.45% or 0.2% Sodium Chloride Injection), Lactated Ringer's Injection, 5% or 10% Invert Sugar in Sterile Water for Injection, Ringer's Injection, Normosol®-M in D5-W, Ionosol® B with Dextrose 5%, or Plasma-Lyte® with 5% Dextrose.

ADD-Vantage Vials of Kefzol are to be reconstituted *only* with 0.9% Sodium Chloride Injection or 5% Dextrose Injection in the 50-mL or 100-mL Flexible Diluent Containers.

Intravenous injection (Administer solution directly into vein or through tubing): Dilute the reconstituted 500 mg or 1 g of Kefzol in a minimum of 10 mL of Sterile Water for Injection. Inject solution slowly over 3 to 5 minutes. Do not inject in less than 3 minutes. (NOTE: ADD-VANTAGE VIALS ARE NOT TO BE USED IN THIS MANNER.)

Dosage—The usual adult dosages are given in Table 4.

TABLE 4. USUAL ADULT DOSAGE

Type of Infection	Dose	Frequency
Pneumococcal pneumonia	500 mg	q12h
Mild infections caused by susceptible gram-positive cocci	250 to 500 mg	q8h
Acute uncomplicated urinary tract infections	1 g	q12h
Moderate to severe infections	500 mg to 1 g	q6 to 8h
Severe, life-threatening infections (eg, endocarditis, and septicemia)*	1 g to 1.5 g	q6h

*In rare instances, doses up to 12 g of cefazolin per day have been used.

FIGURE 13-2 Kefzol Label with Portion of the Package Insert

An important concept for understanding solution strength is that the amount of solvent used to decrease the total concentration is determined by the desired final strength of the solution. The *less* solvent added, the more concentrated the final solution strength; the *more* solvent added, the less concentrated the final solution strength. Think of orange juice concentrate as a way to illustrate this concept. The directions call for 3 cans of water to be added to 1 can of orange juice concentrate. The result is what we associate as "reconstituted juice," a ready-to-drink beverage. If you like a stronger orange taste, you might only add 2 cans of water, making it a *more* concentrated juice, but you get *less total volume* to drink. If you have several people wanting to drink orange juice, you might choose to add 4 cans of water to the final total volume. You get *more* volume, but the orange juice is *less* concentrated; therefore, it is more dilute, because you have increased the water (solvent) content. Note that in either case, the amount of orange juice concentrate in the final solution is the same.

Medical notation to express the strength of a solution uses either a ratio, percent, or fraction. The fraction is the preferred form because it is easily applied in calculation and helps explain the ratio of solute to total solution. Recall that a ratio or percent can also be expressed as a fraction.

rule

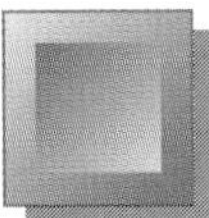

When a fraction expresses the strength of a solution made from a liquid concentrate:

- The *numerator* of the fraction is the number of parts of *solute.*
- The *denominator* of the fraction is the total number of parts of total *solution.*
- The *difference* between the denominator (final solution) and the numerator (parts of solute) is the number of parts of *solvent.*

Let's describe some solutions made from liquid concentrates.

Example 1:

$\frac{1}{4}$ *strength reconstituted orange juice* made from canned frozen concentrate

$$\frac{1}{4} \text{ strength} = \frac{\text{1 part (can) of frozen orange juice concentrate}}{\text{4 parts (cans) of total reconstituted orange juice}}$$

- 1 part (can) frozen orange juice concentrate (*solute*, numerator)
- 4 parts of total reconstituted orange juice (*solution*, denominator)
- $4 - 1 = 3$ parts (cans) of water (*solvent*)

Three cans of water added to one can frozen orange juice concentrate makes four cans of a final reconstituted orange juice solution. The resulting $\frac{1}{4}$ strength reconstituted orange juice is comparable to the strength of fresh juice.

Example 2:

$\frac{1}{3}$ *strength nutritional formula*

- 1 part concentrate formula as the solute
- 3 parts of total solution
- $3 - 1 = 2$ parts solvent (water)

Example 3:

1:20 boric acid solution (This is the same as $\frac{1}{20}$ *boric acid solution.*)

- 1 part stock boric acid solute
- 20 parts total solution
- $20 - 1 = 19$ parts solvent (water)

Example 4:

25% acetic acid solution (This is the same as $\frac{25}{100}$ *acetic acid solution.*)

- 25 parts stock acetic acid as the solute
- 100 parts total solution
- 100 – 25 = 75 parts solvent (water)

When the solute is a solid or dry form (tablet, powder, salt), the fraction or ratio that represents the solution strength consists of some number of *grams of solute* per the total number of *milliliters of solution*. See Chapter 10 to review this information. Recall from the parenteral solutions chapter (Chapter 10) that *solutions expressed as a percent mean X g per 100 mL solution.*

Example 1:

1:20 sodium chloride solution means there is 1 g of salt to 20 mL of solution.

Example 2:

5% sodium chloride solution means there are 5 g of salt to 100 mL of solution.

Calculating Solutions

To prepare a prescribed solution of a certain strength from a solute, you can apply a similar formula to the one you learned for calculating dosages, $\frac{D}{H} \times Q = X$.

rule

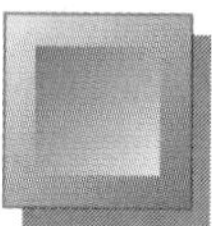

To prepare solutions,

1. D (Desired solution strength) × Q (Quantity of desired solution) = X (Amount of solute)

   or you can apply ratio-proportion to find the amount of solute:

   $$\text{Ratio for desired solution strength} = \frac{\text{Amount of solute}}{\text{Quantity of desired solution}}$$

2. Quantity of desired solution – Amount of liquid solute = Amount of solvent

In this application, "D" is the strength of desired solution, which is written as a fraction. "Q" is the amount of solution you desire to prepare, usually expressed as mL or ounces. The unknown "X" you are solving for is the quantity or amount of solute you will need to add to the solvent to prepare the desired solution. Let's look at how this rule and formula are applied in health care.

Topical Solutions/Irrigants

Topical or irrigating solutions may be mixed from powders, salts, or liquid concentrates. Asepsis in mixing, storage, and use is essential. Liquids can quickly harbor microorganisms. Our focus here is to review the essentials of reconstitution, but nurses need to be alert at all times to the chain of infection.

Most often nurses will further dilute ready-to-use solutions, which are called *full-strength* or stock solutions, to create a less concentrated liquid. Consider the desired solution strength as well as the final volume needed for the task.

Example 1:

Hydrogen peroxide, which is usually available full strength as a 3% solution, can be very drying to the skin and should not be directly applied undiluted. For use as a topical antiseptic, the therapeutic protocol is to reconstitute hydrogen peroxide to $\frac{1}{2}$ strength with normal saline used as the solvent. You decide to make 4 ounces that can be kept in a sterile container at the patient's bedside for traction pin care.

STEP 1 CONVERT No conversion is necessary.

STEP 2 THINK The fraction represents the desired solution strength: $\frac{1}{2}$ strength means 1 part solute (hydrogen peroxide) to 2 total parts solution. The amount of solvent is 2 – 1 = 1 part saline. Because you need 4 oz of solution, you estimate that you will need $\frac{1}{2}$ of it as solute and $\frac{1}{2}$ of it as solvent, or 2 oz hydrogen peroxide and 2 oz saline to make a total of 4 oz of $\frac{1}{2}$ strength hydrogen peroxide.

STEP 3 CALCULATE $D \times Q = X$

$\frac{1}{2}$ (Strength of desired solution) × **4 oz** (Quantity desired) =

X (Amount of solute)

$\frac{1}{2} \times 4 \text{ oz} = 2 \text{ oz solute}$

You could also use ratio-proportion, if you prefer.

Remember that $\frac{1}{2}$ strength $= \frac{\text{1 part solute}}{\text{2 parts total solution}}$. Here, the desired solution strength is $\frac{1}{2}$. The quantity of solution desired is 4 oz. You want to know how much solute (X oz) you will need.

$$\frac{1}{2} = \frac{X \text{ oz}}{4 \text{ oz}} \quad \begin{matrix}\text{(solute)} \\ \text{(solution)}\end{matrix}$$

$$2X = 4$$

$$\frac{2X}{2} = \frac{4}{2}$$

$$X = 2 \text{ oz}$$

X (2 oz) is the quantity of solute (full-strength hydrogen peroxide) you will need to prepare the desired solution (4 oz of $\frac{1}{2}$ strength hydrogen peroxide). The amount of solvent is: 4 oz – 2 oz = 2 oz. If you add 2 ounces of full-strength hydrogen peroxide (solute) to 2 ounces of normal saline (solvent) you will prepare 4 ounces of a $\frac{1}{2}$ strength hydrogen peroxide topical antiseptic.

Example 2:

Suppose a physician orders a patient's wound irrigated with $\frac{2}{3}$ strength hydrogen peroxide and normal saline solution q.4h while awake. The nurse needs 60 mL per irrigation and will do 3 irrigations during her 12 hour shift. She will need to prepare 60 mL × 3 irrigations = 180 mL total solution. How much stock hydrogen peroxide and normal saline are needed?

STEP 1 CONVERT No conversion is necessary.

STEP 2 THINK You want to make $\frac{2}{3}$ strength, which means 2 parts solute (concentrated hydrogen peroxide) to 3 total parts solution.

The amount of solvent is 3 – 2 =1 part saline. Because you need 180 mL of solution, you estimate that you will need $\frac{2}{3}$ of it as solute ($\frac{2}{3} \times 180 = 120$ mL) and $\frac{1}{3}$ of it as solvent ($\frac{1}{3} \times 180 = 60$ mL).

STEP 3 CALCULATE $D \times Q = \frac{2}{3} \times 180 \text{ mL} = 120$ mL of solute

Or, use ratio-proportion, if you prefer.

$$\frac{2}{3} = \frac{X \text{ mL}}{180 \text{ mL}} \quad \begin{matrix}\text{(Solute)}\\ \text{(Solution)}\end{matrix}$$

$$3X = 360$$

$$\frac{3X}{3} = \frac{360}{3}$$

$$X = 120 \text{ mL of solute}$$

"X" (120 mL) is the quantity of solute (hydrogen peroxide) you will need to prepare the desired solution (180 mL of $\frac{2}{3}$ strength). Because you desire to make a total of 180 mL of solution for wound irrigation, the amount of solvent you need is 180 – 120 = 60 mL of normal saline. Therefore, to make 180 mL of $\frac{2}{3}$-strength hydrogen peroxide, mix 120 mL full-strength hydrogen peroxide and 60 mL normal saline.

Example 3:

The physician orders a patient to irrigate his mouth every 2 hours after oral surgery. He needs to do this for 12 hours (6 irrigations), and the physician asks the nurse to mix up *1 quart of physiologic (0.9%) saline* using table salt so the patient can take it home and have it ready to use.

STEP 1 CONVERT 1 qt = 1000 mL

STEP 2 THINK The fraction for 0.9% saline is $\frac{0.9}{100}$. Salt is solid and pure form, so the strength of the desired solution is 0.9 g salt per 100 mL.

STEP 3 CALCULATE $D \times Q = \frac{0.9 \text{ g}}{100 \text{ mL}} \times 1000 \text{ mL} =$

$$\frac{0.9 \text{ g}}{\cancelto{1}{100 \text{ mL}}} \times \cancelto{10}{1000 \text{ mL}} = 9 \text{ g of solid solute}$$

Or, use ratio-proportion, if you prefer.

$$\frac{0.9 \text{ g}}{100 \text{ mL}} = \frac{X \text{ g}}{1000 \text{ mL}}$$

$$100X = 900$$

$$\frac{100X}{100} = \frac{900}{100}$$

$$X = 9 \text{ g of solid solute}$$

Because 1 mL of water weighs 1 g, grams and milliliters are used interchangeably when making saline or salt water. So 9 g = 9 mL or approximately 2 t (because 1 t = 5 mL). To make 1 qt of physiologic saline, add 2 t of salt to 1 qt or 1000 mL of water.

quick review

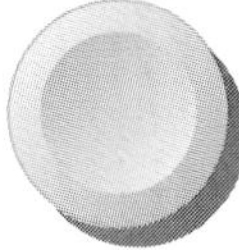

- *Solute*—a concentrated or solid substance to be dissolved or diluted.
- *Solvent*—a liquid substance that dissolves another substance to prepare a solution.
- *Solution*—the resulting mixture of a solute plus a solvent.
- Solution strengths can be expressed as a fraction, ratio, or percent. Examples $\frac{1}{2}$, 1:2, 50%.
- When a fraction expresses the strength of a solution made from a liquid concentrate:
  - The *numerator* of the fraction is the number of parts of *solute.*
  - The *denominator* of the fraction is the total number of parts of *solution.*
  - The *difference between the denominator and the numerator* is the number of parts of *solvent.*
- To prepare solutions,
  1. D (Desired solution strength) × Q (Quantity of desired solution) = X (Amount of solute)

     or, Ratio for desired solution strength = $\frac{\text{Amount of solute}}{\text{Quantity of desired solution}}$
  2. Quantity of desired solution – Amount of solute = Amount of solvent.

review set 33

Explain how you would prepare each of the following solutions from liquid stock hydrogen peroxide, with saline as the solvent.

1. 480 mL of $\frac{1}{3}$ strength for wound irrigation. ______
2. 4 ounces of $\frac{1}{4}$ strength for skin cleansing. ______
3. 240 mL of $\frac{3}{4}$ strength for skeletal pin care. ______
4. 16 ounces of $\frac{1}{2}$ strength for wound care. ______

Calculate the following solutions.

5. 500 mL 3% sodium chloride (saline) solution. ______ g or ______ mL or ______ t table salt; ______ mL water
6. 300 mL 20% acetic acid solution. ______ mL stock acetic acid; ______ mL water
7. 500 mL 50% betadine solution using normal saline. ______ mL stock betadine; ______ mL normal saline
8. 1 pt $\frac{1}{4}$ strength acetic acid solution. ______ oz stock acetic acid; ______ oz water

After completing these problems, see page 446 to check your answers.

Oral and Enteral Feedings

The principles of reconstitution are frequently applied to nutritional liquids for children and adults with special needs. Premature infants require increased calories for growth yet cannot take large volumes. Children who suffer from intestinal malabsorption require incremental changes as their bodies adjust to more concentrated formulas. Adults, especially the elderly, also experience nutritional problems that can be remedied with liquid nutrition. Prepared solutions that are taken orally or through feeding tubes are usually available and ready to use from manufacturers. Nutritional solutions may also be mixed from powders or liquid concentrates. Figure 13-3 shows examples of the three forms of one nutritional formula. Directions on the label detail how much water needs to be added to the powdered form or liquid concentrate. Nutritionists further provide expertise in creating complex solutions for special patient needs.

As mentioned previously, nurses must be alert at all times to the chain of infection. Asepsis in mixing, storage, and use of nutritional liquids is essential. Because they contain sugars, there is an increased risk for contamination during preparation and spoilage during storage and use.

Diluting Ready-to-Use Nutritional Liquids

Ready-to-use nutritional liquids are those solutions that are normally administered directly from the container without any further dilution. Most ready-to-use formulas contain 20 calories per ounce and are used for children and adults. The manufacturer balances the solute (nutrition) and solvent (water) to create a balanced, full strength solution. However, some children and adults require less than full-strength formula for a short period to normalize intestinal absorption. Nutritional formulas are diluted with sterile water or tap water for oral use. Consult the facility policy regarding the use of tap water to reconstitute nutritional formulas. Let's look at a few typical examples.

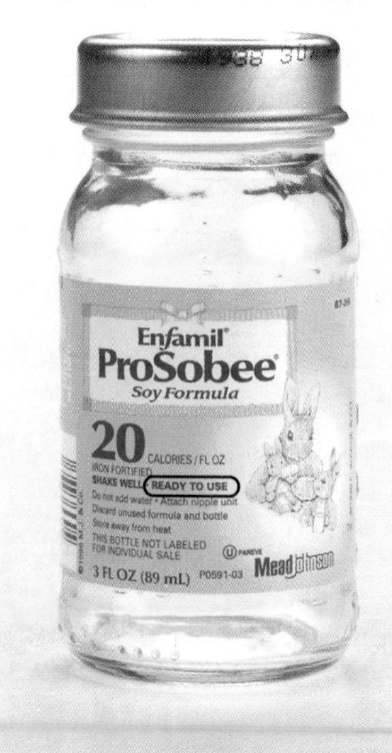

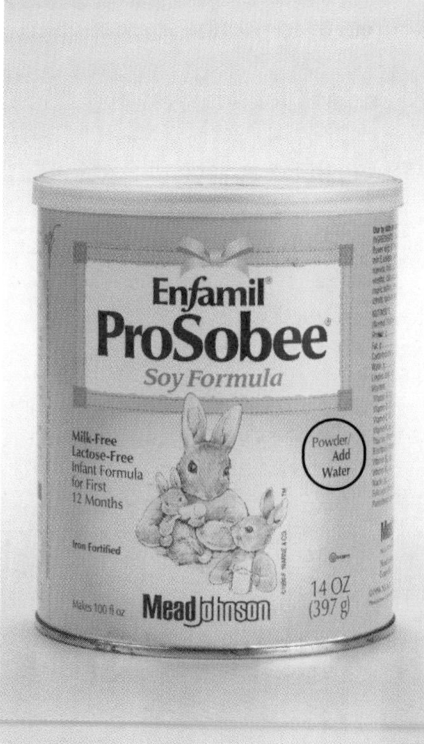

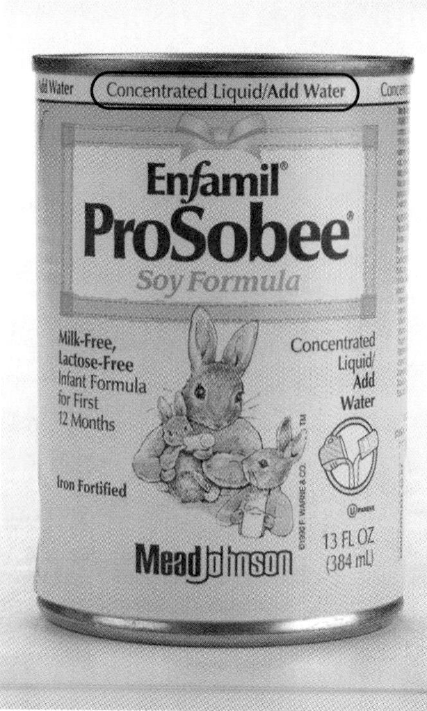

FIGURE 13-3 Nutritional Formulas

Example 1:

A physician orders *Ensure $\frac{1}{4}$ strength 120 mL q.2h via NG tube × 3 feedings* for a patient who is recovering from gastric surgery. Available are 4 and 8 ounce cans of Ensure, ready-to-use formula.

STEP 1 CONVERT Approximate equivalent: 1 oz = 30 mL; Larger → Smaller: (x); 4 oz = 4 × 30 = 120 mL and 8 oz = 8 × 30 = 240 mL.

STEP 2 THINK You need 120 mL total reconstituted formula for each of 3 feedings. This is a total of 120 × 3 = 360 mL. But you must dilute the full-strength formula to $\frac{1}{4}$ strength. You know that $\frac{1}{4}$ strength means 1 part formula to 4 parts solution. The solvent needed is 4 – 1 = 3 parts water. You will need $\frac{1}{4}$ of the solution as solute ($\frac{1}{4} \times 360$ mL = 90 mL) and $\frac{3}{4}$ of the solution as solvent ($\frac{3}{4} \times 360$ mL = 240 mL). Therefore, if you mix 90 mL of full-strength formula with 240 mL of water, you will have 360 mL of $\frac{1}{4}$ strength formula.

STEP 3 CALCULATE $D \times Q = \frac{1}{4} \times 360 \text{ mL} = 90 \text{ mL}$ full-strength Ensure

Or, use ratio-proportion.

$$\frac{1}{4} = \frac{X \text{ mL}}{360 \text{ mL}}$$

$$4X = 360$$

$$\frac{4X}{4} = \frac{360}{4}$$

X = 90 mL of full-strength Ensure

You need 90 mL of the formula (solute). Use 90 mL from the 4 oz can because it contains 120 mL. (You will have 30 mL left over.) The amount of solvent needed is 360 – 90 = 270 mL water. Add 270 mL water to 90 mL, full-strength Ensure to make a total of 360 mL of $\frac{1}{4}$ strength Ensure. You now have enough for 3 full feedings. Administer 120 mL to the patient for each feeding.

Example 2:

The physician orders *800 mL of $\frac{3}{4}$ strength Sustacal through a gastrostomy tube over 8 hours* to supplement a patient while he sleeps. Sustacal ready-to-use formula comes in 10 ounce cans.

STEP 1 CONVERT 1 oz = 3 mL; 10 oz = 10 × 30 = 300 mL

STEP 2 THINK The ordered solution strength is $\frac{3}{4}$. This means 3 parts solute to 4 total parts in solution. You know that $\frac{3}{4}$ of the 800 mL will be solute or full-strength Sustacal ($\frac{3}{4} \times 800$ mL = 600 mL) and $\frac{1}{4}$ of the solution will be solvent or water ($\frac{1}{4} \times 800$ mL = 200 mL). This proportion of solute to solvent will reconstitute the Sustacal to the required $\frac{3}{4}$ strength and total volume of 800 mL.

STEP 3 CALCULATE $D \times Q = \frac{3}{4} \times 800 \text{ mL} = 600 \text{ mL}$ of full-strength Sustacal

Or, use ratio-proportion.

$$\frac{3}{4} = \frac{X \text{ mL}}{800 \text{ mL}}$$

$$4X = 2400$$

$$\frac{4X}{4} = \frac{2400}{4}$$

$X = 600$ mL of full-strength Sustacal

You need 600 mL of the formula (solute). Because the 10 oz can contains 300 mL, you will need 2 cans (600 mL) to prepare the $\frac{3}{4}$ strength Sustacal as ordered. The amount of solvent needed is 800 mL – 600 mL = 200 mL water. Add 200 mL water to 600 mL (or 2 cans) of full-strength Ensure to make a total of 800 mL of $\frac{3}{4}$ strength Sustacal for the full feeding.

quick review

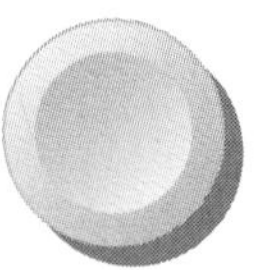

- To prepare solutions,
  1. D (Desired solution strength) × Q (Quantity of desired solution) = X (Amount of solute)

     or, Ratio for desired solution strength = $\frac{\text{Amount of solute}}{\text{Quantity of desired solution}}$
  2. Quantity of desired solution – Amount of solute = Amount of liquid solvent

review set 34

Explain how you would prepare each of the following from ready-to-use nutritional formulas for the specified time period. Note which supply would require the least discard of unused formula.

1. $\frac{1}{3}$ *strength Ensure 900 mL via NG tube over 9 h.* Supply: Ensure 4, 8, 12 ounce cans.
2. $\frac{1}{4}$ *strength Isomil 4 oz. p.o. q.4h for 24 h.* Supply: Isomil 3, 6, 12 ounce cans.
3. $\frac{2}{3}$ *strength Sustacal 300 mL p.o. q.i.d.* Supply: Sustacal 5 and 10 ounce cans.
4. $\frac{1}{2}$ *strength Ensure 26 oz. via gastrostomy tube over 5 h.* Supply: 4, 8, 12 ounce cans.
5. $\frac{1}{2}$ *strength Sustacal 250 mL p.o. q.i.d.* Supply: Sustacal 5 and 10 ounce cans.
6. $\frac{3}{4}$ *strength Isomil 8 oz. p.o. q.4h for 24 h.* Supply: Isomil 3, 6, 12 ounce cans.
7. $\frac{2}{3}$ *strength Ensure 6 oz. via gastrostomy tube over 2 h.* Supply: Ensure 4, 8, 12 ounce cans.

8. $\frac{1}{4}$ *strength Ensure 16 oz. via NG tube over 6 h.* Supply: Ensure 4, 8, 12 ounce cans.

4 oz Ensure 12 oz water use (1) 4 oz can

After completing these problems, see page 447 to check your answers.

critical thinking skills

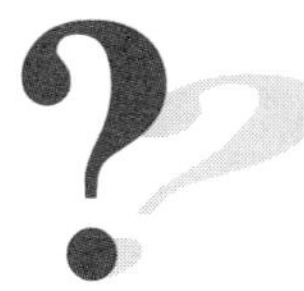

Errors in formula dilution occur when the nurse fails to correctly calculate the amount of solute and solvent needed for the required solution strength.

error

Incorrect calculation of solute and solvent.

possible scenario

Suppose the physician ordered $\frac{1}{3}$ *strength Isomil 90 mL p.o. q.3h for four feedings* for an infant recovering from gastroenteritis. The concentration will be increased after these feedings. The nurse knows she will give all four feedings during her 12 hour shift, so she makes up 360 mL of formula. She takes a 3 ounce bottle of ready-to-use Isomil and adds three, 3 ounce bottles of water for oral use. She thinks, "One-third means 1 bottle of formula and 3 bottles of water. The amount I need even works out!"

potential outcome

What the nurse has actually mixed is a $\frac{1}{4}$ strength solution. Because the infant is getting a more dilute solution than intended, the amount of water to solute is increased and the incremental tolerance of more concentrated formula could be jeopardized. Thinking the child is tolerating $\frac{1}{3}$ strength, the physician might increase it to $\frac{2}{3}$ strength, and the infant may have problems digesting this more concentrated formula. His progress could be slowed or even set back.

prevention

The nurse should have thought through the meaning of the terms of a solution. If so, she would have recognized that $\frac{1}{3}$ strength meant 1 part solute (formula) to 3 total parts of solution with 2 parts water; not 1 part formula to 3 parts water. She should have applied the calculation formula or ratio and proportion to determine the amount of solute (full strength Isomil) needed and the amount of solvent (water). If she did not know how to prepare the formula, she should have conferred with another nurse or called the pharmacy or dietary services for assistance. Never guess. Think and calculate with accuracy.

practice problems—chapter 13

H_2O_2

Explain how you would prepare each of the following hydrogen peroxide (solute) and normal saline (solvent) irrigation solutions.

1. 240 mL of $\frac{1}{2}$ strength solution 120 mL Solute & 120 mL NS
2. 16 ounces of $\frac{1}{8}$ strength solution 2 oz H_2O_2 & 14 oz NS
3. 320 mL of $\frac{3}{8}$ strength solution 120 mL H_2O_2 200 mL NS
4. 80 mL of $\frac{5}{8}$ strength solution 50 mL H_2O_2 & 30 mL NS

5. 18 ounces of $\frac{2}{3}$ strength solution ______________________

6. 8 ounces of $\frac{7}{8}$ strength solution ______________________

7. 2 ounces of $\frac{1}{4}$ strength solution ½ oz solute 1½ oz solvent.

Explain how you would prepare each of the following from ready-to-use nutritional formulas for the specified time period. Note how many cans or bottles of supply are needed and how much unused formula would remain from the used supply.

8. Order: $\frac{1}{4}$ *strength Enfamil 12 mL via NG tube q.h. for 10 hours*

   Supply: Enfamil 3 ounce bottles.

   ____

9. Order: $\frac{3}{4}$ *strength Sustacal 360 mL over 4 hours via gastrostomy*

   Supply: Sustacal 10 ounce cans

   270 mL solute 90 mL solvent discard 30 mL

10. Order: $\frac{2}{3}$ *strength solution Ensure. Give 90 mL q.h. for 5 hours via NG tube.*

    Supply: Ensure 8 ounce cans

    ____

11. Order: $\frac{5}{8}$ *strength solution Isomil 36 mL via NG tube hourly for 8 feedings.*

    Supply: Isomil 3 ounce bottles

    ____

12. Order: $\frac{3}{8}$ *strength solution Enfamil.* Three patients need 32 ounces of the $\frac{3}{8}$ strength Enfamil for one feeding each

    Supply: Enfamil 6 ounce bottles

    ____

13. Order: $\frac{1}{8}$ *solution Ensure. Give 160 mL stat via NG tube.*

    Supply: Ensure 4 ounce cans

    ____

14. Order: $\frac{1}{2}$ *strength solution Ensure 55 mL hourly for 10 hours via gastrostomy tube.*

    Supply: Ensure 12 ounce cans

    ____

The nurse is making up $\frac{1}{4}$ strength Enfamil formula for several infants in the nursery.

15. If she has 8 ounce cans of ready-to-use Enfamil, how many cans of formula will she need to make 48 ounces of reconstituted $\frac{1}{4}$ strength Enfamil? __________

16. How many ounces of water will she add to the Enfamil in #15 to correctly reconstitute the $\frac{1}{4}$ strength Enfamil? __________

Prepare the following saline solutions from table salt:

17. 2 L 0.9% saline. ______

18. 1 quart 0.45% saline. ______

19. 500 mL 2% saline. ______

Prepare the following solution from concentrated liquid stock.

20. 500 mL 1:20 boric acid solution. ______

After completing these problems, see pages 447 and 448 to check your answers.

most Common

U-100 / 1mL

U-500 – not common

CHAPTER

14

Intravenous Solutions, Equipment, and Calculations

objectives

Upon mastery of Chapter 14, you will be able to calculate intravenous (IV) solution flow rate for electronic or manual infusion systems. To accomplish this you will also be able to:

- Identify common IV solutions and equipment.
- Calculate the amount of specific components in common IV fluids.
- Define the following terms: IV, peripheral line, central line, primary IV, secondary IV, saline/heparin locks, IV PB, and IV push.
- Calculate milliliters per hour: mL/h.
- Recognize the calibration or drop factor in gtt/mL as stated on the IV tubing package.
- Apply the formula method to calculate IV flow rate in gtt/min.:

$$\frac{\text{V (volume)}}{\text{T (time in min)}} \times \text{C (drop factor calibration)} = \text{R (rate of flow)}$$

- Apply the short cut method to calculate IV flow rate in gtt/min.:

$$\frac{\text{mL / h}}{\text{drop factor constant}} = \text{gtt / min}$$

- Recalculate the flow rate when the IV is off schedule.
- Calculate small volume piggyback IVs (IV PB).
- Calculate IV infusion time.
- Calculate IV infusion volume.

Intravenous means the administration of fluids or medication through a vein. Intravenous (IV) fluids are ordered for a variety of reasons. They may be ordered for replacement of lost fluids, to maintain fluid and electrolyte balance, or to administer IV medications. *Replacement fluids* are often ordered due to losses that may occur from hemorrhage, vomiting, or diarrhea. *Maintenance fluids* sustain normal fluid and electrolyte balance. They may be used for the patient who is not yet depleted but is beginning to show symptoms of depletion. They may also be ordered for the patient who has the potential to become depleted, such as the patient who is allowed nothing by mouth (NPO) for surgery.

Intravenous fluids and drugs may be administered by two methods: *continuous* and *intermittent* infusion. Continuous IV infusions replace or maintain fluid and electrolytes and serve as a vehicle for drug administration. Intermittent, such as IV piggyback and IV push, infusions are used for IV administration of drugs and supplemental fluids. Saline or heparin locks are used to maintain venous access without continuous fluid infusion.

Intravenous therapy is an important and challenging nursing role. This chapter will cover the essential information and calculations presented step by step for your thorough understanding and mastery. Let's begin by analyzing IV solutions.

IV Solutions

IV solutions are ordered by the physician; however, they are administered and monitored by the nurse. It is the responsibility of the nurse to ensure that the correct IV fluid is administered to the correct patient. IV fluids can be prepared in plastic solution bags or glass bottles with the volume of the IV fluid container varying from 50 mL to 1000 mL. The IV solution bag or bottle will be labeled with the exact components and amount of the IV solution. Health care practitioners often use abbreviations when communicating about the IV solution. It is important for the nurse to know the common IV solution components and the solution concentration strengths represented by such abbreviations.

Solution Components

Glucose (dextrose), water, saline (sodium chloride or NaCl), and selected electrolytes and salts are found in IV fluids. Dextrose and sodium chloride are the two most common solute components. Learn these common IV component abbreviations.

remember

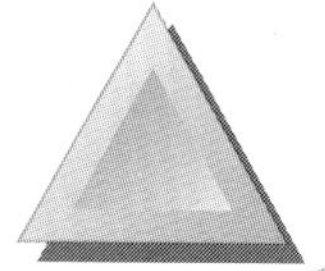

COMMON IV COMPONENT ABBREVIATIONS

Abbreviation	Solution Component
D	Dextrose
W	Water
S	Saline
NS	Normal Saline
RL	Ringer's Lactate
LR	Lactated Ringer's

Solution Strength

The abbreviation letters indicate the solution components, and the numbers indicate the solution strength or concentration of the components.

Example 1:

Suppose an order includes *D_5W*. This abbreviation means "Dextrose 5% in Water" and is supplied as 5% Dextrose Injection, Figure 14-1. This means the solution strength of the solute (dextrose) is 5%. The solvent is water. Recall from Chapter 10 that parenteral solutions expressed in a percent indicate X g per 100 mL. Read the IV bag label and notice that "each 100 mL contains 5 g dextrose . . . ." For every 100 mL of solution, there are 5 g of dextrose.

Example 2:

Suppose a nurse writes *D_5LR* in the nurse's notes. This abbreviation means "Dextrose 5% in Lactated Ringer's" and is supplied as 5% Dextrose and Lactated Ringer's Injection, Figure 14-2.

Example 3:

An order states, *D_5NS 1000 mL IV q.8h*. This order means "administer 1000 mL 5% dextrose in normal saline intravenously every 8 hours" and is supplied as 5% Dextrose

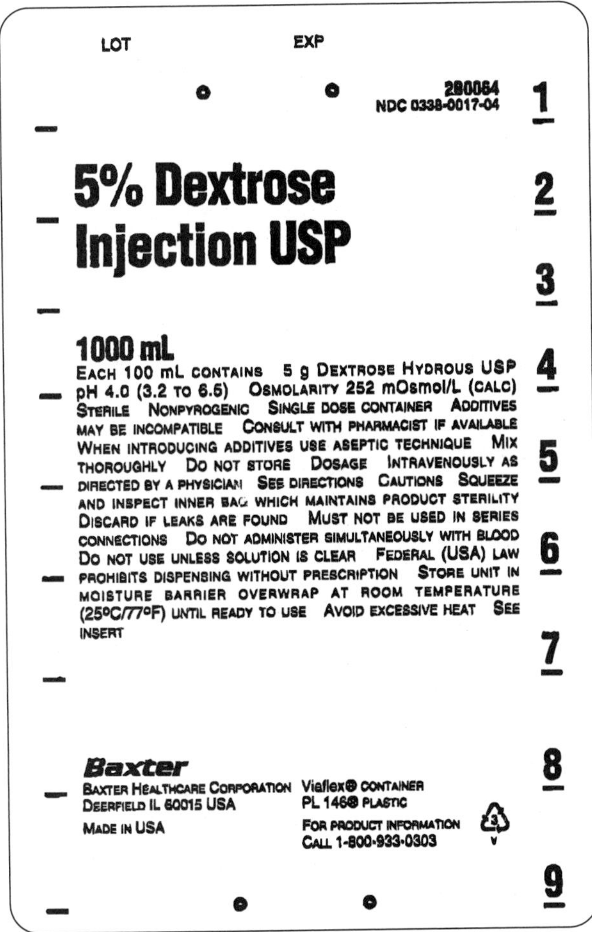

FIGURE 14-1 IV Bag Label (Courtesy of Baxter International Inc., I.V. Systems Division)

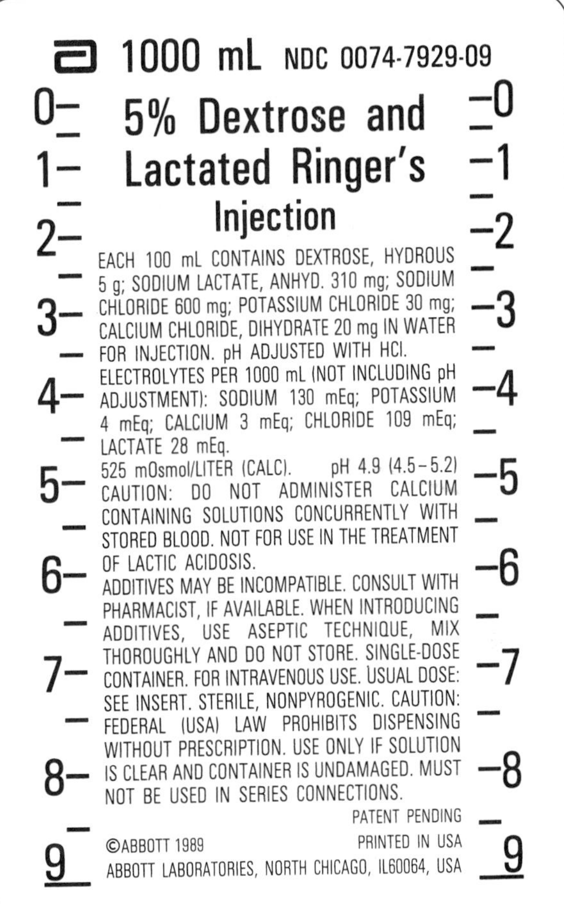

FIGURE 14-2 IV Bag Label (Courtesy of Abbott Laboratories)

and 0.9% Sodium Chloride, Figure 14-3. *Normal saline is the common term for 0.9% sodium chloride.* Another name is *physiologic saline.* The concentration of sodium chloride in normal saline is 0.9 g per 100 mL of solution.

Another common saline IV concentration is 0.45% Sodium Chloride (NaCl), Figure 14-4. Notice that 0.45% NaCl is $\frac{1}{2}$ the strength of 0.9% NaCl, which is normal saline. Thus, it is typically written as "$\frac{1}{2}$ NS" for $\frac{1}{2}$ normal saline. Other saline solution strengths include 0.33% NaCl (also abbreviated as $\frac{1}{3}$ NS) and 0.225% NaCl (also abbreviated as $\frac{1}{4}$ NS).

The goal of intravenous therapy, achieved through fluid infusion, is to maintain or regain fluid and electrolyte balance. When dextrose or saline (*solute*) is diluted in water for injection (*solvent*), a *solution* results that can be administered to maintain or approximate the normal blood plasma. Blood or serum concentration is called *tonicity* or *osmolarity* and is measured in milliOsmols per liter or mOsm/L. IV fluids are concentrated and classified as *isotonic* (the same tonicity or osmolarity as blood and other body serums), *hypotonic* (lower tonicity or osmolarity as blood and other body serums), or *hypertonic* (higher tonicity or osmolarity as blood and other body serums). Normal saline (0.9% NaCl or physiologic saline) is an isotonic solution. The osmolarity of a manufactured solution is detailed on the printed label. Look for the mOsm/L in the fine print under the solution name in Figures 14-1 through 14-4.

Figure 14-5 compares the three solution concentrations to normal serum osmolarity. Parenteral therapy is determined by unique patient needs but these basic factors must be considered when ordering IV solutions.

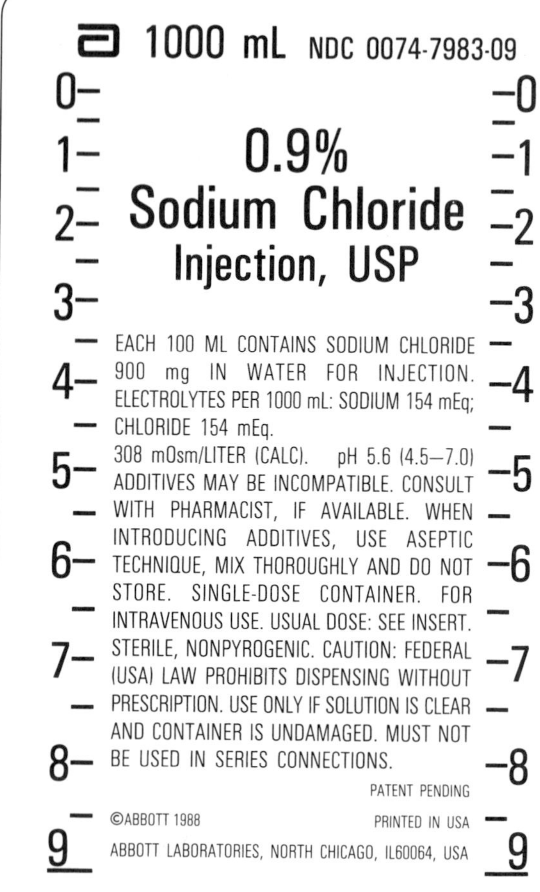

FIGURE 14-3 IV Solution Label (Courtesy of Abbott Laboratories)

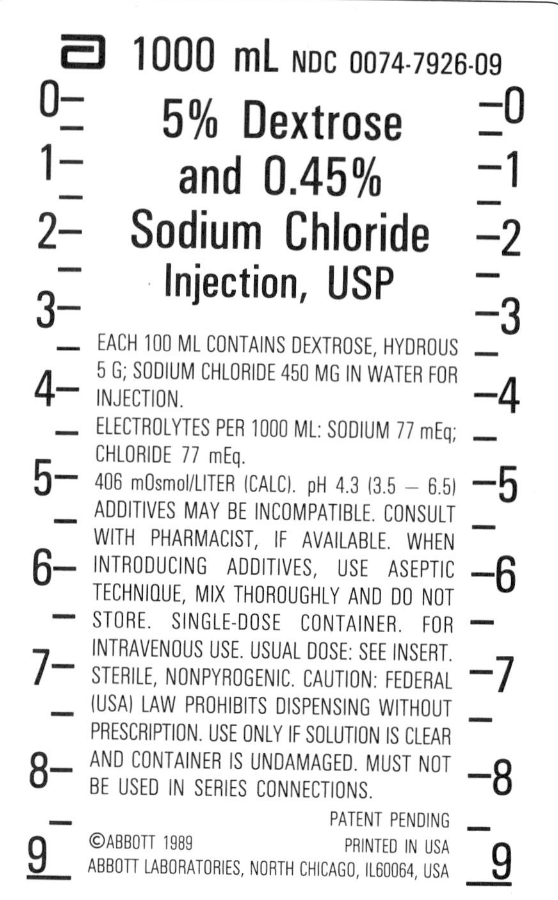

FIGURE 14-4 IV Solution Label (Courtesy of Abbott Laboratories)

NORMAL SERUM OSMOLARITY
(NORMAL AVERAGE TONICITY—ALL AGES)
280–320 mOsm/L

Hypotonic (< 200 mOsm/L)	**Isotonic** (200–400 mOsm/L)	**Hypertonic** (> 400 mOsm/L)
Solvent exceeds solute—used to dilute excess serum electrolytes, as in hyperglycemia	*Solvent and solute are balanced*—used to expand volume and maintain normal tonicity	*Solute exceeds solvent*—used to correct electrolyte imbalances, as in loss from excess vomiting and diarrhea
Example of IV solution: *0.45% Saline* (154 mOsm/L)	Examples of IV solution: *0.9% Saline* (308 mOsm/L) *Lactated Ringer's* (273 mOsm/L) 5% Dextrose in Water (252 mOsm/L)	Example of IV solution *5% Dextrose and 0.9% NaCl* (560 mOsm/L) *5% Dextrose and Lactated Ringer's* (525 mOsm/L)

FIGURE 14-5 Comparison of IV Solution Concentrations by Osmolarity

Solution Additives

Electrolytes also may be added to the basic IV fluid. Potassium chloride (KCl) is a common IV additive and is measured in *milliequivalents* (mEq). The order is usually written to indicate the amount of milliequivalents *per liter* (1000 mL) to be added to the IV fluid.

Example 1:

The physician orders *D_5NS c̄ 20 mEq KCl/L*. This means to add 20 milliequivalents potassium chloride per liter of 5% dextrose and 0.9% sodium chloride.

quick review

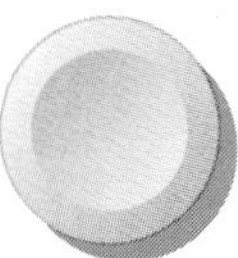

- Pay close attention to IV abbreviations: *letters* indicate the solution components and *numbers* indicate the concentration or solution strength.
- Dextrose and sodium chloride (NaCl) are common IV solutes.
- Solution strength expressed as a percent (%) indicates X g per 100 mL.
- Normal saline is 0.9% sodium chloride: 0.9 g NaCl/100 mL solution.
- IV solution tonicity or osmolarity is measured in mOsm/L.
- Normal saline is a common isotonic solution.

review set 35

For each of the following IV solutions labeled A through H:

a. Specify the *letter* of the illustration corresponding to the fluid abbreviation.

b. List the *solute(s)* of each solution, and identify the *strength (g/mL)* of each solute.

c. Identify the *osmolarity (mOsm/L)* of each solution.

d. Identify the *tonicity (isotonic, hypotonic, or hypertonic)* of each solution.

	a. Letter of Matching Illustration	b. Components and Strength	c. Osmolarity (mOsm/L)	d. Tonicity
1. NS	______	______	______	______
2. D_5W	______	______	______	______
3. D_5NS	______	______	______	______
4. $D_5 \frac{1}{2}NS$	______	______	______	______
5. $D_5 \frac{1}{4}NS$	______	______	______	______
6. D_5LR	______	______	______	______
7. $D_5 \frac{1}{2}NS$ c̄ 20 mEq KCl/L	______	______	______	______
8. $\frac{1}{2}NS$	______	______	______	______

After completing these problems, see page 448 to check your answers.

500 mL NDC 0074-7924-03

5% Dextrose and 0.225% Sodium Chloride Injection, USP

EACH 100 ML CONTAINS DEXTROSE, HYDROUS 5 G; SODIUM CHLORIDE 225 MG IN WATER FOR INJECTION. ELECTROLYTES PER 1000 ML: SODIUM 38.5 mEq; CHLORIDE 38.5 mEq. 329 mOsmol/LITER (CALC). pH 4.3 (3.5 – 6.5) ADDITIVES MAY BE INCOMPATIBLE. CONSULT WITH PHARMACIST, IF AVAILABLE. WHEN INTRODUCING ADDITIVES, USE ASEPTIC TECHNIQUE, MIX THOROUGHLY AND DO NOT STORE. SINGLE-DOSE CONTAINER. FOR INTRAVENOUS USE. USUAL DOSE: SEE INSERT. STERILE, NONPYROGENIC. CAUTION: FEDERAL (USA) LAW PROHIBITS DISPENSING WITHOUT PRESCRIPTION. USE ONLY IF SOLUTION IS CLEAR AND CONTAINER IS UNDAMAGED. MUST NOT BE USED IN SERIES CONNECTIONS.

PATENT PENDING

©ABBOTT 1989 PRINTED IN USA

ABBOTT LABORATORIES, NORTH CHICAGO, IL60064, USA

A

20 mEq POTASSIUM

1000 mL NDC 0074-7902-09

20 mEq POTASSIUM CHLORIDE

in 5% Dextrose and 0.45% Sodium Chloride Inj., USP

EACH 100 mL CONTAINS POTASSIUM CHLORIDE 149 mg; SODIUM CHLORIDE 450 mg; DEXTROSE, HYDROUS 5 g IN WATER FOR INJECTION. MAY CONTAIN HCl FOR pH ADJUSTMENT. ELECTROLYTES PER 1000 mL (NOT INCLUDING IONS FOR pH ADJUSTMENT): POTASSIUM 20 mEq; SODIUM 77 mEq; CHLORIDE 97 mEq.
447 mOsmol/LITER (CALC). pH 4.2 (3.5 – 6.5)

ADDITIVES MAY BE INCOMPATIBLE. CONSULT WITH PHARMACIST, IF AVAILABLE. WHEN INTRODUCING ADDITIVES, USE ASEPTIC TECHNIQUE, MIX THOROUGHLY AND DO NOT STORE.

SINGLE-DOSE CONTAINER. FOR INTRAVENOUS USE. USUAL DOSE: SEE INSERT. STERILE, NONPYROGENIC. CAUTION: FEDERAL (USA) LAW PROHIBITS DISPENSING WITHOUT PRESCRIPTION. USE ONLY IF SOLUTION IS CLEAR AND CONTAINER IS UNDAMAGED. MUST NOT BE USED IN SERIES CONNECTIONS.

U.S. PAT. NO. 4,368,765

©ABBOTT 1994 PRINTED IN USA

ABBOTT LABORATORIES, NORTH CHICAGO, IL 60064, USA

B

1000 mL NDC 0074-7983-09

0.9% Sodium Chloride Injection, USP

EACH 100 ML CONTAINS SODIUM CHLORIDE 900 mg IN WATER FOR INJECTION. ELECTROLYTES PER 1000 mL: SODIUM 154 mEq; CHLORIDE 154 mEq.
308 mOsm/LITER (CALC). pH 5.6 (4.5–7.0) ADDITIVES MAY BE INCOMPATIBLE. CONSULT WITH PHARMACIST, IF AVAILABLE. WHEN INTRODUCING ADDITIVES, USE ASEPTIC TECHNIQUE, MIX THOROUGHLY AND DO NOT STORE. SINGLE-DOSE CONTAINER. FOR INTRAVENOUS USE. USUAL DOSE: SEE INSERT. STERILE, NONPYROGENIC. CAUTION: FEDERAL (USA) LAW PROHIBITS DISPENSING WITHOUT PRESCRIPTION. USE ONLY IF SOLUTION IS CLEAR AND CONTAINER IS UNDAMAGED. MUST NOT BE USED IN SERIES CONNECTIONS.

PATENT PENDING

©ABBOTT 1988 PRINTED IN USA

ABBOTT LABORATORIES, NORTH CHICAGO, IL60064, USA

C

1000 mL NDC 0074-7926-09

5% Dextrose and 0.45% Sodium Chloride Injection, USP

EACH 100 ML CONTAINS DEXTROSE, HYDROUS 5 G; SODIUM CHLORIDE 450 MG IN WATER FOR INJECTION.
ELECTROLYTES PER 1000 ML: SODIUM 77 mEq; CHLORIDE 77 mEq.
406 mOsmol/LITER (CALC). pH 4.3 (3.5 – 6.5) ADDITIVES MAY BE INCOMPATIBLE. CONSULT WITH PHARMACIST, IF AVAILABLE. WHEN INTRODUCING ADDITIVES, USE ASEPTIC TECHNIQUE, MIX THOROUGHLY AND DO NOT STORE. SINGLE-DOSE CONTAINER. FOR INTRAVENOUS USE. USUAL DOSE: SEE INSERT. STERILE, NONPYROGENIC. CAUTION: FEDERAL (USA) LAW PROHIBITS DISPENSING WITHOUT PRESCRIPTION. USE ONLY IF SOLUTION IS CLEAR AND CONTAINER IS UNDAMAGED. MUST NOT BE USED IN SERIES CONNECTIONS.

PATENT PENDING

©ABBOTT 1989 PRINTED IN USA

ABBOTT LABORATORIES, NORTH CHICAGO, IL60064, USA

D

LOT EXP

2B0063
NDC 0338-0017-03

5% Dextrose Injection USP

500 mL

EACH 100 mL CONTAINS 5 g DEXTROSE HYDROUS USP pH 4.0 (3.2 TO 6.5) OSMOLARITY 252 mOsmol/L (CALC) STERILE NONPYROGENIC SINGLE DOSE CONTAINER ADDITIVES MAY BE INCOMPATIBLE CONSULT WITH PHARMACIST IF AVAILABLE WHEN INTRODUCING ADDITIVES USE ASEPTIC TECHNIQUE MIX THOROUGHLY DO NOT STORE DOSAGE INTRAVENOUSLY AS DIRECTED BY A PHYSICIAN SEE DIRECTIONS CAUTIONS SQUEEZE AND INSPECT INNER BAG WHICH MAINTAINS PRODUCT STERILITY DISCARD IF LEAKS ARE FOUND MUST NOT BE USED IN SERIES CONNECTIONS DO NOT ADMINISTER SIMULTANEOUSLY WITH BLOOD DO NOT USE UNLESS SOLUTION IS CLEAR FEDERAL (USA) LAW PROHIBITS DISPENSING WITHOUT PRESCRIPTION STORE UNIT IN MOISTURE BARRIER OVERWRAP AT ROOM TEMPERATURE (25°C/77°F) UNTIL READY TO USE AVOID EXCESSIVE HEAT SEE INSERT

Baxter
BAXTER HEALTHCARE CORPORATION
DEERFIELD IL 60015 USA
MADE IN USA

VIAFLEX® CONTAINER
PL 146® PLASTIC
FOR PRODUCT INFORMATION
CALL 1-800-933-0303

E

EXP

2B1313
NDC 0338-0043-03

0.45% Sodium Chloride Injection USP

500 mL

EACH 100 mL CONTAINS 450 mg SODIUM CHLORIDE USP pH 5.0 (4.5 TO 7.0) mEq/L SODIUM 77 CHLORIDE 77 HYPOTONIC OSMOLARITY 154 mOsmol/L (CALC) STERILE NONPYROGENIC SINGLE DOSE CONTAINER ADDITIVES MAY BE INCOMPATIBLE CONSULT WITH PHARMACIST IF AVAILABLE WHEN INTRODUCING ADDITIVES USE ASEPTIC TECHNIQUE MIX THOROUGHLY DO NOT STORE DOSAGE INTRAVENOUSLY AS DIRECTED BY A PHYSICIAN SEE DIRECTIONS CAUTIONS SQUEEZE AND INSPECT INNER BAG WHICH MAINTAINS PRODUCT STERILITY DISCARD IF LEAKS ARE FOUND MUST NOT BE USED IN SERIES CONNECTIONS DO NOT USE UNLESS SOLUTION IS CLEAR FEDERAL (USA) LAW PROHIBITS DISPENSING WITHOUT PRESCRIPTION STORE UNIT IN MOISTURE BARRIER OVERWRAP AT ROOM TEMPERATURE (25°C/77°F) UNTIL READY TO USE AVOID EXCESSIVE HEAT SEE INSERT

F

1000 mL NDC 0074-7941-09

5% Dextrose and 0.9% Sodium Chloride Injection, USP

EACH 100 ML CONTAINS DEXTROSE, HYDROUS 5 G; SODIUM CHLORIDE 900 MG IN WATER FOR INJECTION.
ELECTROLYTES PER 1000 ML: SODIUM 154 mEq; CHLORIDE 154 mEq.
560 mOsmol/LITER (CALC). pH 4.3 (3.5 – 6.5) ADDITIVES MAY BE INCOMPATIBLE. CONSULT WITH PHARMACIST, IF AVAILABLE. WHEN INTRODUCING ADDITIVES, USE ASEPTIC TECHNIQUE, MIX THOROUGHLY AND DO NOT STORE. SINGLE-DOSE CONTAINER. FOR INTRAVENOUS USE. USUAL DOSE: SEE INSERT. STERILE, NONPYROGENIC. CAUTION: FEDERAL (USA) LAW PROHIBITS DISPENSING WITHOUT PRESCRIPTION. USE ONLY IF SOLUTION IS CLEAR AND CONTAINER IS UNDAMAGED. MUST NOT BE USED IN SERIES CONNECTIONS.
PATENT PENDING
©ABBOTT 1989 PRINTED IN USA
ABBOTT LABORATORIES, NORTH CHICAGO, IL60064, USA

G

500 mL NDC 0074-7929-03

5% Dextrose and Lactated Ringer's Injection

EACH 100 mL CONTAINS DEXTROSE, HYDROUS 5 G; SODIUM LACTATE, ANHYD. 310 mg; SODIUM CHLORIDE 600 mg; POTASSIUM CHLORIDE 30 mg; CALCIUM CHLORIDE, DIHYDRATE 20 mg IN WATER FOR INJECTION. pH ADJUSTED WITH HCl. ELECTROLYTES PER 1000 mL (NOT INCLUDING pH ADJUSTMENT): SODIUM 130 mEq; POTASSIUM 4 mEq; CALCIUM 3 mEq; CHLORIDE 109 mEq; LACTATE 28 mEq. 525 mOsmol/LITER (CALC). pH 4.9 (4.5 – 5.2). CAUTION: DO NOT ADMINISTER CALCIUM CONTAINING SOLUTIONS CONCURRENTLY WITH STORED BLOOD. NOT FOR USE IN THE TREATMENT OF LACTIC ACIDOSIS. ADDITIVES MAY BE INCOMPATIBLE. CONSULT WITH PHARMACIST, IF AVAILABLE. WHEN INTRODUCING ADDITIVES, USE ASEPTIC TECHNIQUE, MIX THOROUGHLY AND DO NOT STORE. SINGLE-DOSE CONTAINER. FOR INTRAVENOUS USE. USUAL DOSE: SEE INSERT. STERILE, NONPYROGENIC. CAUTION: FEDERAL (USA) LAW PROHIBITS DISPENSING WITHOUT PRESCRIPTION. USE ONLY IF SOLUTION IS CLEAR AND CONTAINER IS UNDAMAGED. MUST NOT BE USED IN SERIES CONNECTIONS. PATENT PENDING
©ABBOTT 1989 PRINTED IN USA
ABBOTT LABORATORIES, NORTH CHICAGO, IL60064, USA

H

(A, B, C, D, G, and H Courtesy of Abbott Laboratories. E and F Courtesy of Baxter International Inc., I.V. Systems Division)

Calculating Dosage Expressed as a Percent in IV Fluids

You know that solution strength expressed as a percent (%) indicates X g per 100 mL, so you can calculate the total amount of solute per IV order.

Example 1:

Order: *D_5W 1000 mL*

Calculate the amount of dextrose in 1000 mL D_5W.

This can be calculated using ratio-proportion.

Recall that % indicates g per 100 mL; therefore, 5% dextrose is 5 g dextrose per 100 mL.

$$\frac{5 \text{ g}}{100 \text{ mL}} \times \frac{X \text{ g}}{1000 \text{ mL}}$$

$$100X = 5000$$

$$\frac{100X}{100} = \frac{5000}{100}$$

$$X = 50 \text{ g}$$

1000 mL of D_5W contains 50 g of dextrose.

Example 2:

Order: *NS 1000 mL*

Calculate the amount of sodium chloride (NaCl) in 1000 mL NS.

0.9% = 0.9 g NaCl per 100 mL

$$\frac{0.9 \text{ g}}{100 \text{ mL}} \times \frac{X \text{ g}}{1000 \text{ mL}}$$

$$100X = 900$$

$$\frac{100X}{100} = \frac{900}{100}$$

$$X = 9 \text{ g NaCl}$$

1000 mL of NS contains 9 g of sodium chloride.

Example 3:

Order: *$D_5 \frac{1}{4}$NS 500 mL*

Calculate the amount of dextrose and sodium chloride in 500 mL.

D_5 = Dextrose 5% = 5 g dextrose per 100 mL

$$\frac{5 \text{ g}}{100 \text{ mL}} \times \frac{X \text{ g}}{500 \text{ mL}}$$

$$100X = 2500$$

$$\frac{100X}{100} = \frac{2500}{100}$$

$$X = 25 \text{ g dextrose}$$

$\frac{1}{4}$NS = 0.225% NaCl = 0.225 g NaCl per 100 mL.

$$\frac{0.225\ g}{100\ mL} \times \frac{X\ g}{500\ mL}$$

$$100X = 112.5$$

$$\frac{100X}{100} = \frac{112.5}{100}$$

$$X = 1.125\ g\ NaCl$$

500 mL $D_5\frac{1}{4}$NS contains 25 g dextrose and 1.125 g sodium chloride.

It is important that you know what you are giving your patient when the physician orders IV fluids, such as D_5W. Think, "I am hanging D_5W. Do I know what that fluid contains?" Now you can answer, "Yes."

quick review

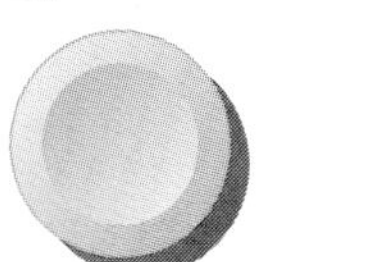

- Solution concentration expressed as a percent is g of solute per 100 mL solution.

review set 36

Calculate the amount of dextrose and/or sodium chloride in each of the following IV solutions.

1. 1000 mL of D_5NS
   dextrose ________ g
   sodium chloride ________ g
2. 500 mL of $D_5\frac{1}{2}$NS
   dextrose ________ g
   sodium chloride ________ g
3. 250 mL of $D_{10}W$
   dextrose ________ g
4. 750 mL of NS
   sodium chloride ________ g
5. 500 mL of D_5 0.33% NaCl
   dextrose ________ g
   sodium chloride ________ g
6. 3 L of D_5 NS
   dextrose ________ g
   sodium chloride ________ g
7. 0.5 L of $D_{10}\frac{1}{4}$NS
   dextrose ________ g
   sodium chloride ________ g
8. 300 mL of D_{12} 0.9% NaCl
   dextrose ________ g
   sodium chloride ________ g
9. 2 L of D_5 0.225% NaCl
   dextrose ________ g
   sodium chloride ________ g
10. 0.75 L of 0.45% NaCl
    sodium chloride ________ g

After completing these problems, see page 448 to check your answers.

IV Sites

IV fluids may be ordered via a *peripheral line,* such as a vein in the arm, leg, or sometimes a scalp vein for infants, if other sites are inaccessible. Blood flowing through these veins can usually dilute the components in IV fluids. Glucose or dextrose usually is concentrated between 5 and 10% for short-term IV therapy. Peripheral veins can maximally accommodate a glucose concentration up to 12%. The rate of infusion in peripheral veins should not exceed 200 mL in one hour.

IV fluids that are transparent flow smoothly into relatively small peripheral veins. When blood transfusion or replacement is needed, a larger vein is preferred to facilitate ease of blood flow. Whole blood or its components, especially packed cells, can be viscous and must be infused within a short period of time.

IV fluids may also be ordered via a *central line,* in which a special catheter is inserted to access a large vein in the chest. The subclavian vein, for example, may be used for a central line. Central lines may be accessed either directly through the chest wall or indirectly via a neck vein or peripheral vein in the arm. Larger veins can accommodate higher concentrations of glucose (up to 35%) and other nutrients, and faster rates of IV fluids (> 200 mL in one hour). They are often utilized if the patient is expected to need IV therapy for an extended period of time.

Monitoring IVs

The nurse is responsible for monitoring the patient regularly during an IV infusion.

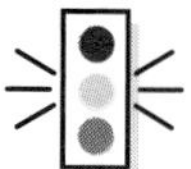

Caution: Generally the IV site and infusion should be checked *at least every 30 minutes to one hour* (according to hospital policy) for volume of remaining fluids, correct infusion rate, and signs of complications.

The major complications associated with IV therapy are phlebitis and infiltration. *Phlebitis* occurs when the vein becomes irritated, red, or painful. (Think: *warm and cordlike vein.*) *Infiltration* is when the IV catheter becomes dislodged from the vein and IV fluid escapes into the subcutaneous tissue. (Think: *cool and puffy skin.*) Should phlebitis or infiltration occur, the IV is discontinued and another IV site chosen to restart the IV. The patient should be instructed to notify the nurse if any pain or swelling is noticed.

Primary and Secondary IVs

Primary IV tubing packaging is shown in Figure 14-6. This IV set is used to set up a typical or *primary IV*. Primary IV tubing includes a drip chamber, injection port, and roller clamp, and is long enough to be attached to the hub of the IV catheter positioned in the patient's vein. The drip chamber is squeezed until it is half full of IV fluid. The nurse can either regulate the rate manually using the roller clamp (Figure 14-7a) or place the tubing in an electronic infusion pump, Figures 14-12, 14-13, 14-14, and 14-15.

Secondary IV tubing is used when giving medications and is "piggybacked" into the primary line (Figure 14-8). This type of tubing (Figure 14-9) generally is shorter and also contains a drip chamber and roller clamp. This gives access to the primary IV catheter without having to start another IV. You will notice that in this type of setup, the *secondary IV* set or *piggyback* is hung higher than the primary IV to allow the secondary set of medication to infuse first. When administering primary IV fluids, choose primary IV tubing; when hanging piggybacks, select secondary IV tubing. IV piggybacks are discussed further at the end of this chapter.

IV bags are often labeled with an infusion label (Figure 14-7b) that gives the nurse a visual check to monitor if the IV infusion is infusing on time as prescribed. These labels are attached to the IV bag and indicate the start and stop times of the infusion as well as how the IV should be progressing, such as at 25 gtt/min.

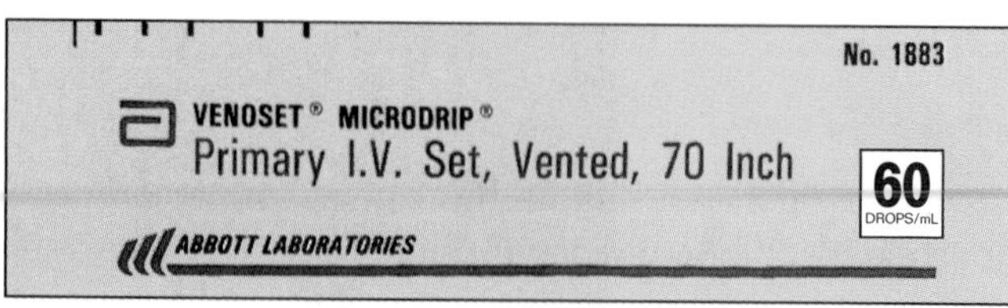

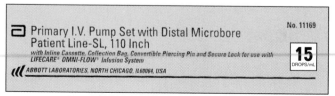

FIGURE 14-6 Intravenous Infusion Tubing: Microdrop = 60 Drops/mL; Macrodrop = 15 Drops/mL

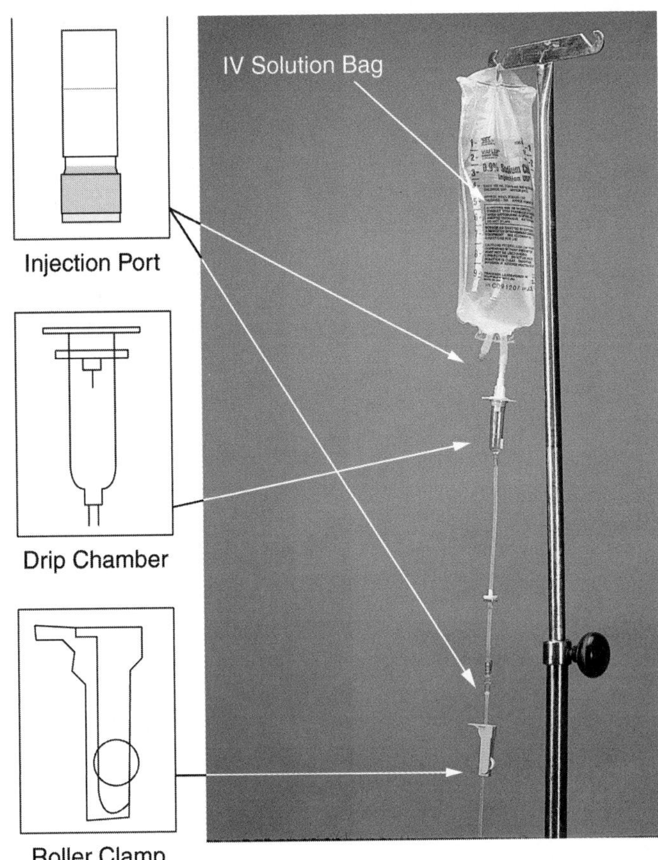

FIGURE 14-7(a) Standard Straight Gravity Flow IV System

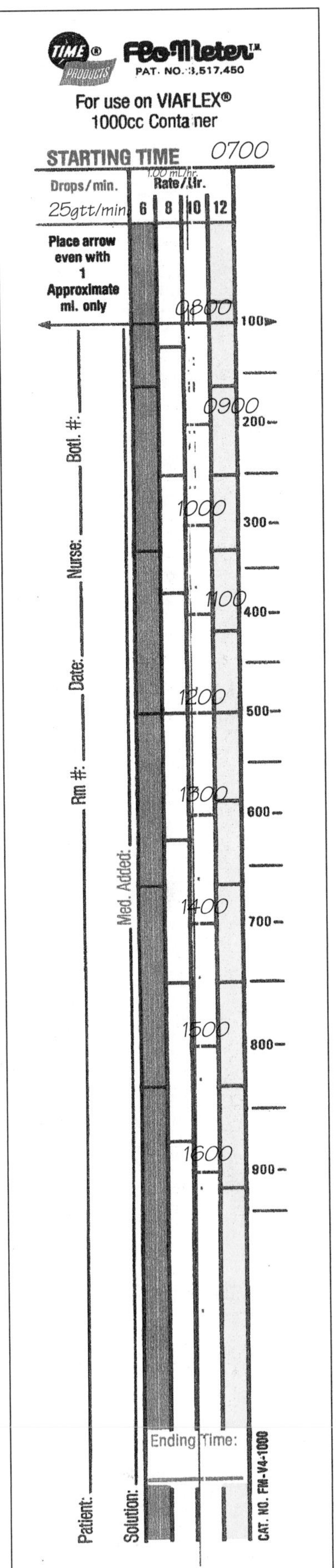

FIGURE 14-7(b) Infusion Label

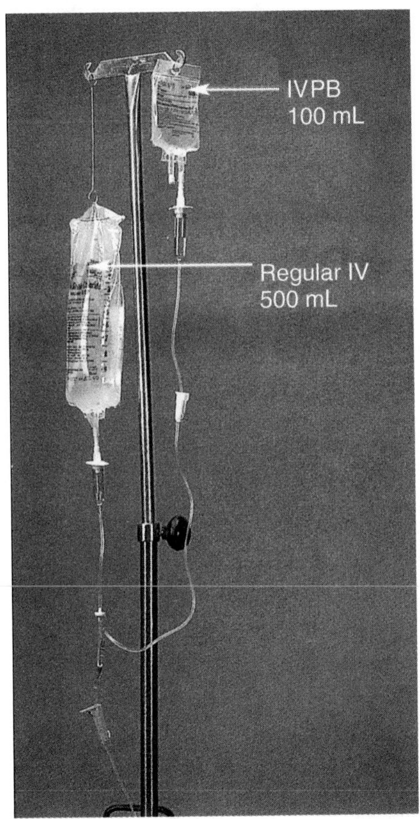

FIGURE 14-8 IV with Piggyback (IV PB)

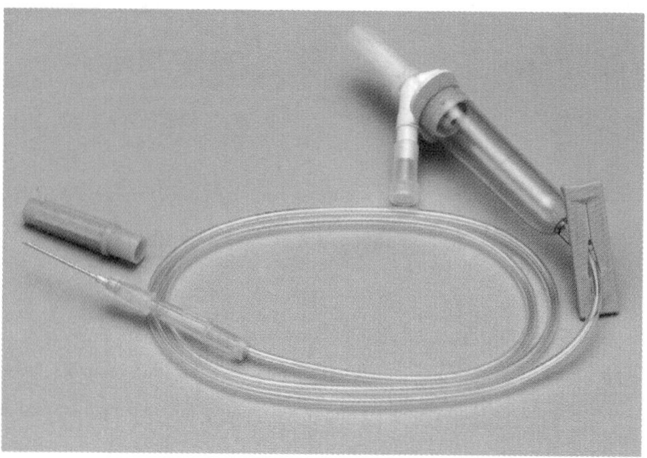
FIGURE 14-9 Secondary IV Set

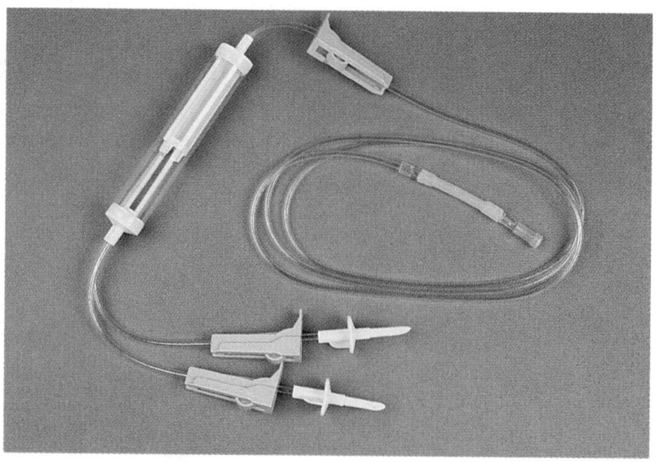
FIGURE 14-10 Y-Type Blood Administration Set

Blood Administration Tubing

When blood is administered, a Y-type blood administration set (Figure 14-10) is commonly used. The "Y" refers to the two spikes that are attached above the drip chamber. One spike is attached to the blood container, and the other spike is attached to normal saline. Normal saline is used to dilute packed cells and to flush the IV tubing at the beginning and at the end of the transfusion. Blood is usually infused manually by gravity, and the roller clamp on the line is used to adjust the rate. Blood infusion is calculated the same as any other IV fluid.

IV Flow Rate

The *flow rate* of an intravenous (IV) infusion is ordered by the physician. It is the nurse's responsibility to regulate, monitor, and maintain this flow rate. Regulation of intravenous therapy is a critical skill in nursing. Because the fluids administered are infusing directly into the patient's circulatory system, careful monitoring is essential to be sure the patient does not receive too much or too little IV fluid and medication. It is important for the nurse to accurately set and maintain the flow rate to administer the prescribed volume of the IV solution within the specified time period. The IV fluids administered and IV flow rates are recorded on the IV administration record (IVAR), Figure 14-11.

IV solutions are usually ordered for a certain volume to run for a stated period of time, such as *125 mL/h or 1000 mL/8 h.* The nurse will use electronic or manual regulating equipment to monitor the flow rate. The calculations you must perform to set the flow rate will depend on the equipment used to administer the IV solutions.

Electronically Regulated IVs

Frequently IV solutions are regulated electronically by an infusion device, such as a controller or pump. The use of an electronic infusion device will be determined by the need to strictly regulate the IV. Manufacturers supply special volumetric tubing that must be used with their infusion devices. This special tubing ensures accurate, consistent IV infusions. Each device can be set for a specific flow rate and will alarm if this rate is interrupted. Electronic units today are powered by direct (wall) current as well as an internal rechargeable battery. The battery takes over when the unit is unplugged, to allow for portability and patient ambulation.

Controllers (Figure 14-12) depend on gravity to maintain the desired flow rate by a compression/decompression mechanism that pinches the IV tubing, rather than forcing IV fluid into the system. They are often referred to as electronic flow clamps, because they monitor the

Page: of

DATE: 11/10/xx through

Correct	I.V. Order	Rate	Time	Initial	Site / Infusion Port	Pump / Other	Tubing Change
✓	$D_5\ ^1\!/_2\ NS$	100ml/hr	0900	GP	LH / PIV	☑	✓
					/	☐	
					/	☐	
					/	☐	
					/	☐	

CIRCULATORY ACCESS SITE

Time	Gauge	Length	Type	Site	# Attempts	Dressing Change	Site Condition	IV Lock	Initial	Time Catheter D/C	Intact	Site Condition	Reason Code	Initial
0800	22	1½"	I	LH	1	✓	0	☐	GP					
								☐						
								☐						
								☐						

Type:
I - Insyte
B - Butterfly
C - Cathlon
CVC - CVC
T - Tunnelled
IP - Implanted Port
PICC - PICC
A - Arterial Line
SG - Swan Ganz
DL - Dual Lumen Peripheral
UAC - UAC
UVC - UVC

Site:
L - Left
R - Right
H - Hand
FA - Forearm
UA - Upper Arm
SC - Subclavian
C - Chest
A - Antecubital
F - Femoral
J - Jugular
FT - Foot
S - Scalp
U - Umbilical
RA - Radial

Dressing Change:
T - Transparent
A - Air Occlusive
B - Bandaid
PR - Pressure Dressing

Reason Code:
1 - Infiltrate
2 - Physician Order
3 - Patient Removed
4 - Clotted
5 - Phlebitis
6 - Site Rotation
7 - Leaking
8 - Positional
9 - Not Patent
10 - Family Refused

Other:
D - Dial-a-flow

Infusion Port:
PIV - Peripheral IV
CVC - CVC
SG - Swan Ganz
D - Distal
M - Middle
P - Proximal
R - Red
BL - Blue
V - Venous
S - Sideport
AN - Access Needle
A - Arterial

Site Condition:
0
1+
2+
3+
4+
5+

Tubing Change:
P - Primary
S - Secondary
E - Extension
T - 3 Way Stopcock
H - Hemodynamic

ALLERGIES:

Initial / Signature - Circulatory Access Site(s) checked hourly.

GP / G. Pickar, R.N. /
/ /
/ /

Reconciled by:

Smith, James 43y M
Dr. Jones Medical Service
Admitted 01-01-xx Rm 237-1
Adm. # 6634297

IV ADMINISTRATION RECORD

602-0203 (2-94)dlg)MPC#32258)

FIGURE 14-11 Intravenous Administration Record

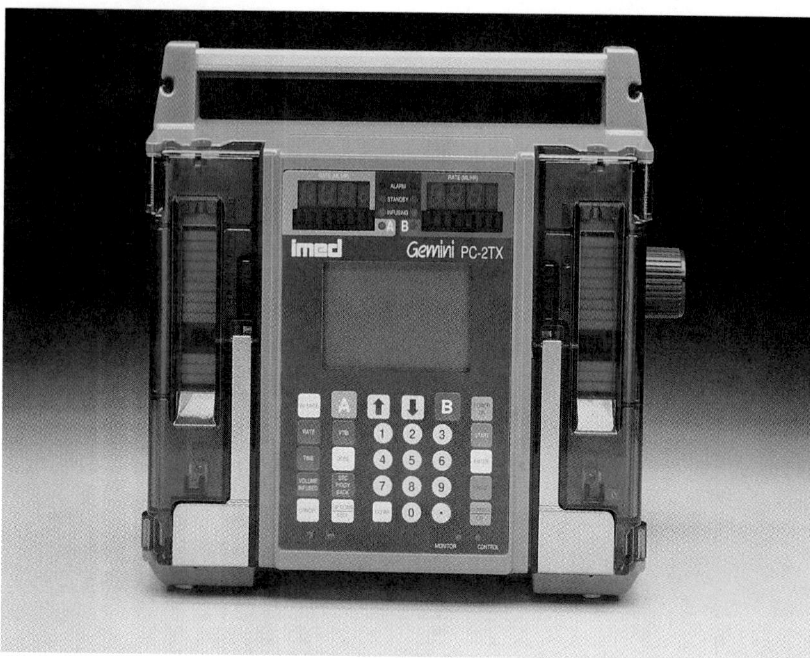

FIGURE 14-12 Volumetric Infusion Controller

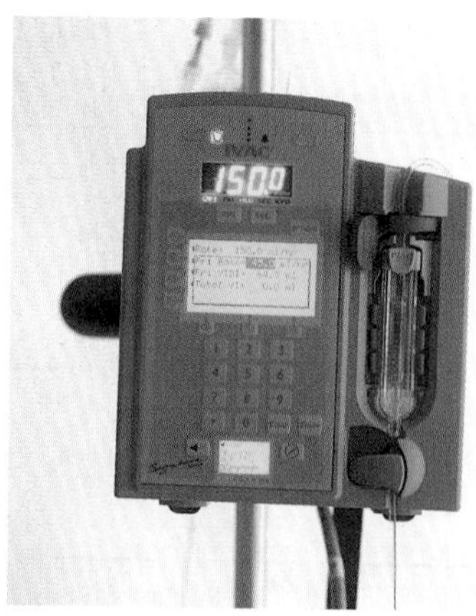

FIGURE 14-13 Infusion Pump (Photo courtesy of Alaris Medical System)

selected rate of infusion by either drop counting (drops per minute) or volumetric delivery (milliliters per hour).

Positive-pressure infusion pumps (Figure 14-13) do not rely on gravity but maintain the flow by adding pressure to the system to continue the flow at the preselected rate. Since pumps operate under pressure, they may continue to infuse, without alarming, in the presence of infiltration or phlebitis. They are designed to infuse IV volumes set at whole *mL per hour.* Therefore, if a mL calculation results in a decimal fraction, round it to a whole mL.

A *syringe pump* (Figure 14-14) is a type of electronic infusion pump. It is used to infuse fluids or medications directly from a syringe. It is most often used in pediatrics when a small volume of medication is being delivered, and in critical care when the drug cannot be mixed with other

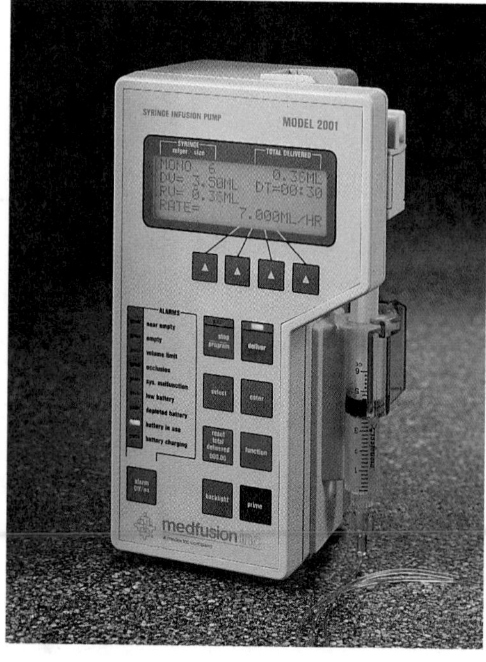

FIGURE 14-14 Syringe Pump (Photo courtesy of Medex, Inc.)

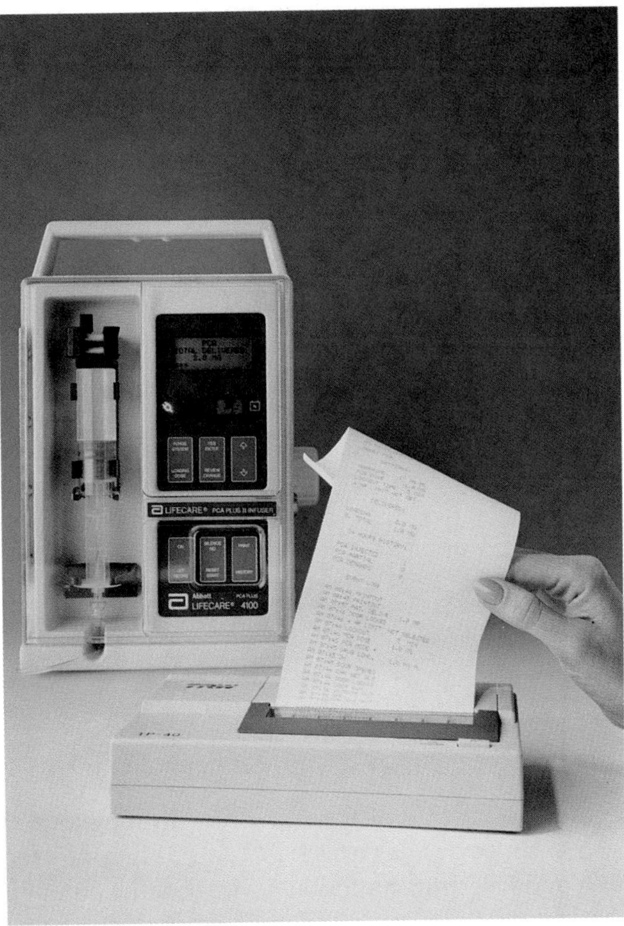

FIGURE 14-15 Abbotts Lifecare PCA (Patient-Controlled Analgesia) Plus II Infusion System (Photo courtesy of Abbott Laboratories)

solutions or medications. Another advantage of the syringe pump is that a prescribed volume can be delivered over a prescribed time. This allows the fluid or medication to be given over less than one hour and is generally used when the desired time is 30 minutes or less. Syringe pumps also infuse IV volumes set at *mL per hour.*

A *patient-controlled analgesia (PCA) pump* (Figure 14-15) is used to allow the patient to self-administer IV medication to control postoperative and other types of severe pain. The physician orders the pain medication, which is contained in a prefilled syringe locked securely in the IV pump. The patient presses the control button and receives the pain medication immediately rather than waiting for someone to bring it. The dose, frequency, and a safety "lock out" time are ordered and programmed into the pump, which delivers an individual therapeutic dose. The pump stores information about how much drug is requested by and delivered to the patient. The nurse can display and print this information to document and evaluate pain management effectiveness.

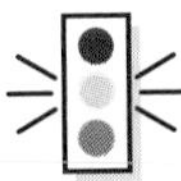

Caution: All electronic infusion devices must be monitored frequently (every 30 minutes to 1 hour) to ensure proper and safe functioning. Check the policy in your facility.

Calculating Flow Rates for Electronic Regulators in mL/h

When an electronic infusion regulator is used, the IV volume is ordered by the physician and programmed into the device by the nurse. These devices are regulated in mL/h. Usually the physician orders the IV volume to be delivered in mL/h. If not, the nurse must calculate it.

rule

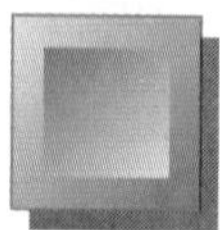

To regulate an IV volume by electronic infusion pump or controller calibrated in mL/h,

$$\frac{\text{Total mL ordered}}{\text{Total h ordered}} = \text{mL/h (rounded to a whole number)}$$

Example 1:

Order reads: *D_5W 250 mL IV over the next 2 h by infusion pump.*

STEP 1 Think. The pump is set by the rate of mL per hour. So, if 250 mL is to be infused in two hours, how much will be infused in one hour? Yes, 125 mL will be infused in one hour. You would set the pump at 125 mL per hour.

STEP 2 Use the formula:

$$\frac{\text{Total mL ordered}}{\text{Total h ordered}} = \text{mL / h}$$

$$\frac{250 \text{ mL}}{2 \text{ h}} = \frac{125 \text{ mL}}{1 \text{ h}}$$

Therefore, set the pump at 125 mL per hour (125 mL/h).

In most cases it is easy to calculate mL/h by dividing total mL by total h. However, an IV with medication added or a piggyback IV (IV PB) may be ordered to be administered in *less than one hour* by an electronic infusion device, but the pump or controller must still be set in mL/h. When the order is for an infusion of less than one hour (or less than 60 minutes), use ratio-proportion to find mL/h.

Example 2:

Order reads: *Ampicillin 500 mg IV in 50 mL $D_5 \frac{1}{2}$ NS in 30 min by controller*

STEP 1 Think. The controller is set by the rate of mL per hour. If 50 mL is to be infused in 30 minutes, then set the controller at the rate of 100 mL per 60 min or 100 mL/h. (The total IV ampicillin will be infused within 30 minutes.)

STEP 2 Use ratio-proportion to check your thinking.

Remember: 1 h = 60 min

$$\frac{50 \text{ mL}}{30 \text{ min}} \times \frac{X \text{ mL}}{60 \text{ min}}$$

$$30X = 3000$$

$$\frac{30X}{30} = \frac{3000}{30}$$

$$X = 100 \text{ mL/60 min or } 100 \text{ mL/h}$$

quick review

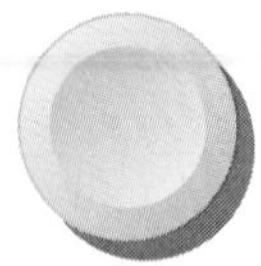

- $\frac{\text{Total mL ordered}}{\text{Total h ordered}} = \text{mL/h}$

review set 37

Calculate the flow rate you will program the electronic infusion regulator for the IVs ordered.

1. *1 L D_5W IV to infuse in 10 h by infusion pump*

   Flow rate: 100 mL/h

2. *1800 mL Normal Saline IV to infuse in 15 h by controller*

   Flow rate: 120 mL/h

3. *2000 mL D_5W IV in 24 h by controller*

   Flow rate: 83 mL/h

4. *100 mL NS IV PB in 30 min by infusion pump*

   Flow rate: 200 mL/h

5. *30 mL antibiotic in D_5W IV in 15 min by infusion pump*

   Flow rate: 120 mL/h

6. *2.5 L NS IV in 20 h by controller*

   Flow rate: 125 mL/h

7. *500 mL D_5LR IV in 4 h by controller*

   Flow rate: 125 mL/h

8. *600 mL 0.45% NaCl IV in 3 h by infusion pump*

   Flow rate: 200 mL/h

9. *150 mL antibiotic in D_5W IV in 2 h by infusion pump*

   Flow rate: 75 mL/h

10. *3 L NS IV in 24 h by controller*

    Flow rate: 125 mL/h

11. *1.5 L LR Injection IV in 24 h by infusion pump*

    Flow rate: 63 mL/h

12. *240 mL $D_{10}W$ IV in 10 h by controller*

    Flow rate: 24 mL/h

13. *750 mL D_5W IV in 5 h by infusion pump*

    Flow rate: 150 mL/h

14. *1.5 L D_5NS IV in 12 h by controller*

    Flow rate: 125 mL/h

15. *380 mL D_5 0.45% NaCl in 9 h by infusion pump*

    Flow rate: 42 mL/h

After completing these problems, see page 449 to check your answers.

Manually Regulated IVs

When an electronic infusion device is not used, the nurse manually regulates the IV rate. To do this the nurse must calculate the ordered IV rate based on a certain *number of drops per minute (gtt/min)*. This actually represents the ordered milliliters per hour as you will shortly see in the calculation.

The number of drops dripping per minute into the IV drip chamber (Figures 14-7a and 14-16) are counted and regulated by opening or closing the roller clamp. You actually place your watch at the level of the drip chamber and count the drops as they fall during a one-minute period (referred to as the *watch count*). This manual, gravity flow rate depends upon the IV tubing calibration called the *drop factor*.

rule

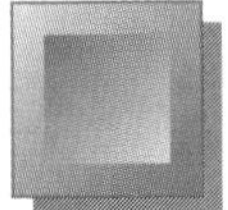

Drop factor = gtt/mL

The drop factor is the number of drops per milliliter (gtt/mL) a particular IV tubing set will deliver. It is stated on the IV tubing package (Figure 14-6) and varies according to the

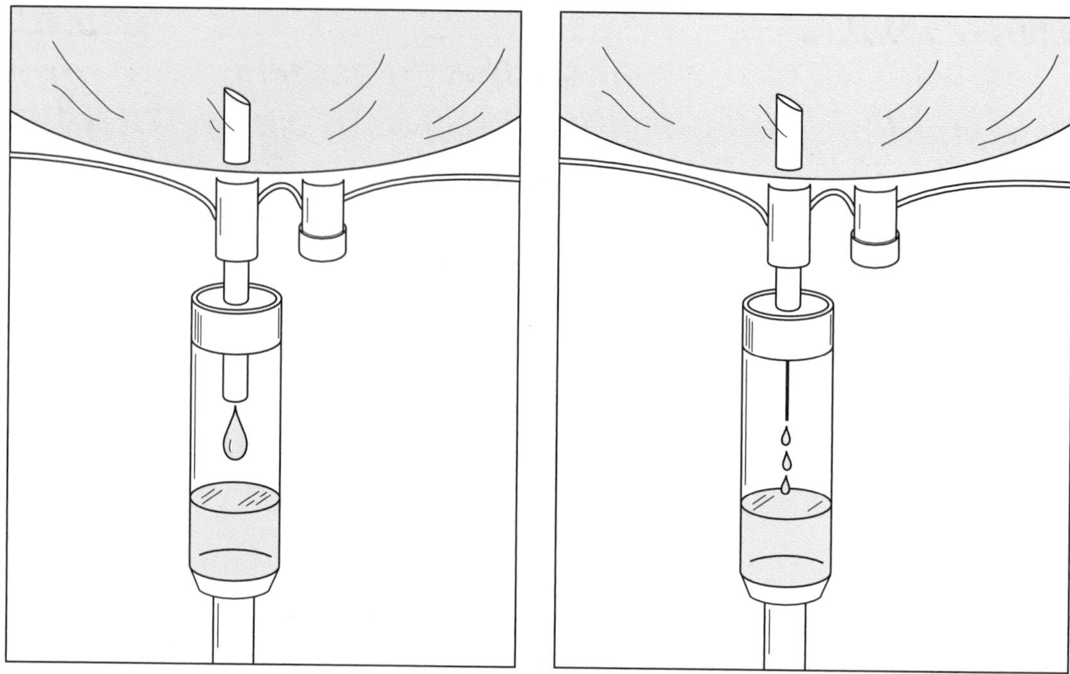

FIGURE 14-16 Intravenous Drip Chambers: Comparison of (A) Macro and (B) Microdrops

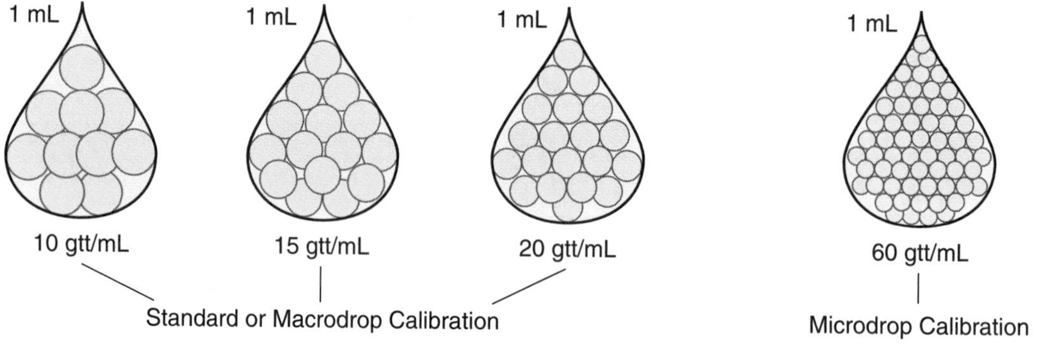

FIGURE 14-17 Comparison of Calibrated Drop Factors

manufacturer of the IV equipment. Standard or *macrodrop* IV tubing sets have a drop factor of 10, 15, or 20 gtt/mL. All microdrip (or minidrip) IV tubing has a drop factor of 60 gtt/mL. Hospitals typically stock one macrodrop tubing for routine adult IV administration and the microdrip tubing for situations requiring more exact measurement.

Figure 14-16 compares macro- and microdrops. Figure 14-17 demonstrates the size and number of drops in 1 mL for each drop factor. Notice that the smaller the number of drops per milliliter, the larger the actual drop size.

quick review

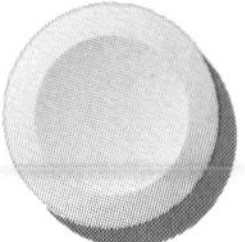

- Drop factor = gtt/mL
- The drop factor is stated on the IV tubing package.
- Macrodrop factors: 10, 15, or 20 gtt/mL
- Microdrop factor: 60 gtt/mL

review set 38

Identify the drop factor calibration of the primary IV tubing pictured.

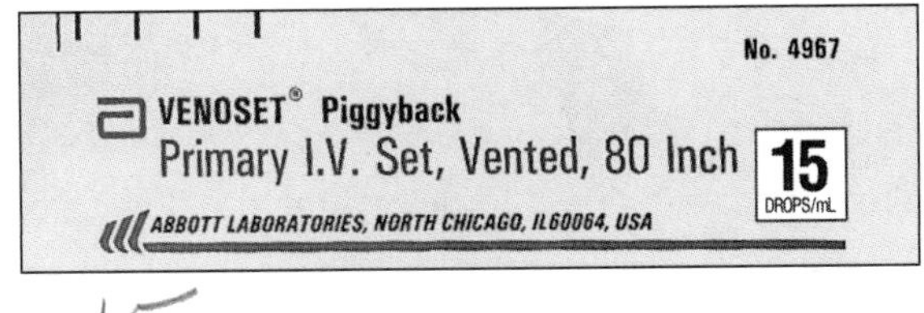

1. 15 gtt/mL

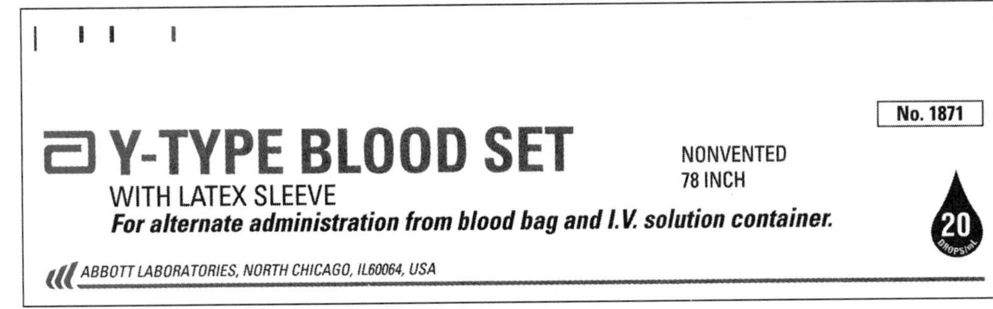

2. 20 gtt/mL

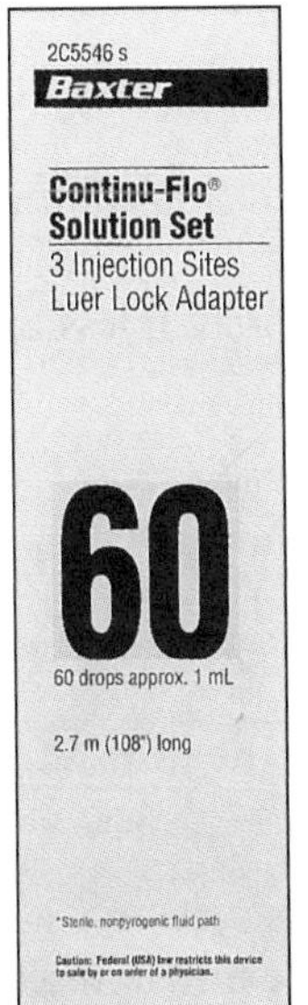

3. 60 gtt/mL

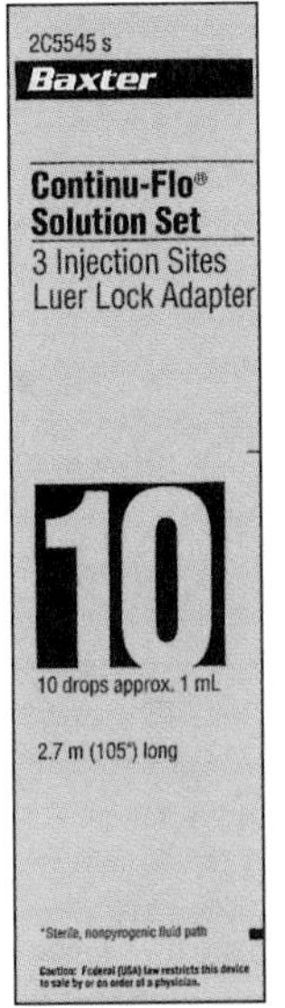

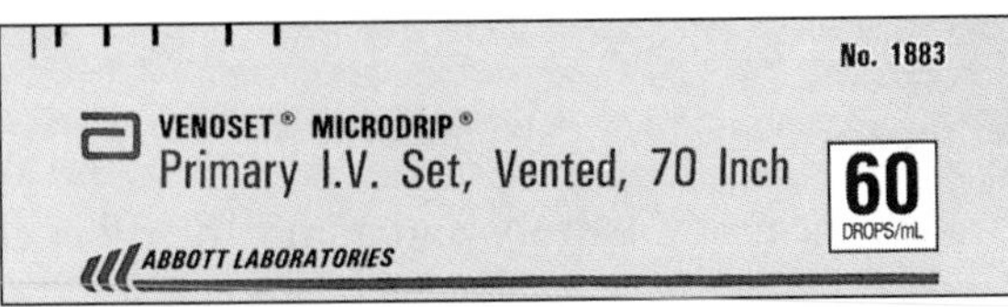

4. 60 gtt/mL

5. 10 gtt/mL

After completing these problems, see page 449 to check your answers.

Calculating Flow Rates for Manually Regulated IVs in gtt/min

In this section you will learn two methods to calculate IV flow rate for manually regulated IVs: the formula method and the shortcut method.

Formula Method

The formula method can be used to determine the flow rate in drops per minute (*gtt/min*).

rule

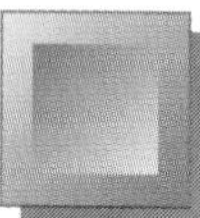

The formula method to calculate IV flow rate for manually regulated IVs ordered in mL/h or for a prescribed number of minutes is:

$$\frac{V}{T} \times C = R$$

$$\frac{\text{Volume (mL)}}{\text{Time (min)}} \times \text{Calibration or drop factor (gtt/mL)} = \text{Rate (gtt/min)}$$

In this formula:

V = *volume* per hour ordered by the physician to be infused in mL.

C = *calibration* of tubing (drop factor) in gtt/mL.

T = *time* ordered by the physician or pharmacy converted to minutes.

R = *rate* of flow in gtt/min. Think: The unknown is the "watch count."

IV fluid and medication orders are written as a specific volume to be infused in a certain time period. Most IV fluid orders are written as "X mL/h," and the time is obviously 60 minutes. However, some IV medications are to be administered in less than one hour, for example over 30 minutes.

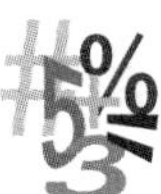

math tip: Carry calculations to one decimal place. Round gtt/min to nearest whole number, because you can only watch count whole drops.

Let's look at some examples of how to calculate the flow rate or "watch count" in gtt/min.

Example 1:

The physician orders *D_5W IV @ 125 mL/h.* The infusion set is calibrated for a drop factor of 10 gtt/mL. Calculate the IV flow rate in gtt/min.

$$\frac{V}{T} \times C = \frac{125 \text{ mL}}{60 \text{ min}} \times 10 \text{ gtt/mL} = \frac{125 \cancel{\text{mL}}}{\underset{6}{\cancel{60}} \text{ min}} \times \frac{\overset{1}{\cancel{10}} \text{ gtt}}{1 \cancel{\text{mL}}} = \frac{125 \text{ gtt}}{6 \text{ min}} = 20.8 = 21 \text{ gtt/min}$$

Notice that the mL cancel out, leaving *gtt/min.*

Use your watch to count the drops and adjust the roller clamp to deliver 21 gtt/min.

Example 2:

Order reads: *Lactated Ringer's IV @ 150 mL/h.* The drop factor is 15 gtt/mL.

$$\frac{V}{T} \times C = \frac{150 \cancel{\text{mL}}}{\underset{4}{\cancel{60}} \text{ min}} \times \overset{1}{\cancel{15}} \text{ gtt/}\cancel{\text{mL}} = \frac{150}{4} = 37.5 = 38 \text{ gtt/min}$$

Example 3:

Order reads: *Ampicillin 500 mg IV in 100 mL of NS, infuse over 45 min.*

The drop factor is 20 gtt/mL.

$$\frac{V}{T} \times C = \frac{100\ \cancel{mL}}{45\ min} \times 20\ gtt/\cancel{mL} = \frac{2000}{45} = 44.4 = 44\ gtt/min$$

Example 4:

Order reads: *D_5W NS IV @ 50 mL/h.* The drop factor is 60 gtt/mL.

$$\frac{V}{T} \times C = \frac{50\ \cancel{mL}}{\cancel{60}\ min} \times \cancel{60}\ gtt/\cancel{mL} = 50\ gtt/min$$

Notice that the order, 50 mL/h, is *the same as the flow rate* of 50 gtt/min when the drop factor is 60 gtt/mL.

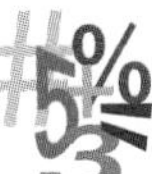

math tip: When the IV drop factor is 60 gtt/mL (microdrip sets), then the flow rate in gtt/min is the same as the volume ordered in mL/h.

Sometimes the physician will order a total IV volume to be infused over a total number of hours. In such cases, first calculate the mL/h, then calculate gtt/min.

rule

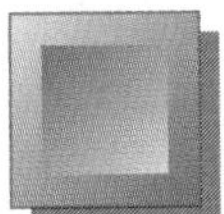

The formula method to calculate IV flow rate for manually regulated IVs ordered in total volume and total hours is:

STEP 1 $\frac{\text{Total mL}}{\text{Total hours}} = \text{mL/h}$

STEP 2 $\frac{V}{T} \times C = R$

Example:

Order: *NS IV 3000 mL/24 h.* Drop factor is 15 gtt/min.

STEP 1 $\frac{\text{Total mL}}{\text{Total h}} = \frac{3000\ mL}{24\ h} = 125\ mL/h$

STEP 2 $\frac{V}{T} \times C = \frac{125\ mL}{60\ min} \times 15\ gtt/mL = \frac{125\ \cancel{mL}}{\underset{4}{\cancel{60}}\ min} \times \frac{\overset{1}{\cancel{15}}\ gtt}{1\ \cancel{mL}} = \frac{125}{4} = 31.2 = 31\ gtt/min$

quick review

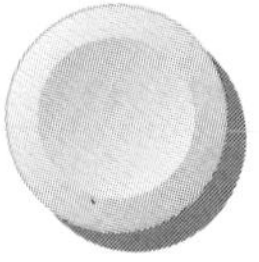

- The formula method to calculate the flow rate, or watch count, in gtt/min for manually regulated IV rates ordered in mL/h or minutes is

  $\frac{\text{Volume (mL)}}{\text{Time (min)}} \times \text{Calibration or drop factor (gtt/mL)} = \text{Rate (gtt/min)}$

- When total volume and total hours are ordered, first calculate mL/h.
- When the drop factor calibration is 60 (microdrop sets), then the flow rate in gtt/min is the same as the ordered volume in mL/h.
- Round gtt/min to a whole number.

review set 39

1. State the rule for the formula method to calculate IV flow rate in gtt/min when mL/h are known.

____

Calculate the flow rate or watch count in gtt/min.

2. Order: *3000 mL D_5W IV @ 125 mL/h*
   Drop factor: 10 gtt/mL
   ________ gtt/min

3. Order: *250 mL LR IV @ 50 mL/h*
   Drop factor: 60 gtt/mL
   ________ gtt/min

4. Order: *100 mL NS bolus IV to infuse in 60 min*
   Drop factor: 20 gtt/mL
   ________ gtt/min

5. Order: *$D_5 \frac{1}{2}$ NS IV with 20 mEq KCl per liter to run at 25 mL/h*
   Drop factor: 60 gtt/mL
   ________ gtt/min

6. Order: *Two 500 mL units of whole blood IV to be infused in 4 h*
   Infusion rate is calibrated to 20 drops per milliliter.
   ________ gtt/min

7. Hyperalimentation solution is ordered for 1240 mL to infuse in 12 h using an infusion set with tubing calibrated to 15 gtt/mL
   ________ gtt/min

8. Order: *D_5NS IV @ 150 mL/h*
   Drop factor: 20 gtt/mL
   ________ gtt/min

9. Order: *150 mL NS bolus IV to infuse in 45 min*
   Drop factor: 15 gtt/mL
   ________ gtt/min

10. Order: *80 mL D_5W antibiotic solution IV to infuse in 60 min*
    Drop factor: 60 gtt/mL
    ________ gtt/min

11. Order: *480 mL packed red blood cells IV to infuse in 4 h*
    Drop factor: 10 gtt/mL
    ________ gtt/min

12. Order: *D_5W IV @ 120 mL/h*
    Drop factor: 15 gtt/mL
    ________ gtt/min

13. Order: *D_5 0.33% NaCl IV @ 50 mL/h*
    Drop factor: 20 gtt/mL
    ________ gtt/min

14. Order: *2500 mL LR IV @ 165 mL/h*
    Drop factor: 20 gtt/mL
    ________ gtt/min

15. Order: *3500 mL D_5LR IV to run at 160 mL/h*
    Drop factor: 15 gtt/mL
    ________ gtt/min

After completing these problems, see page 449 to check your answers.

Short-Cut Method

By converting the volume and time in the formula method to mL/h (or mL/60 min), you can use a short cut to calculate flow rate. This short cut is derived from the drop factor (C), which cancels out each time and reduces the 60 minutes (T). You are left with the *drop factor constant*. Look at this example.

Example 1:

Administer *Normal Saline 1000 mL IV at 125 mL/h* with a microdrop infusion set calibrated for *60 gtt/mL*. Use the formula $\frac{V}{T} \times C = R$.

$$\frac{125 \cancel{\text{mL}}}{\underset{1}{\cancel{60}} \text{ min}} \times \overset{1}{\cancel{60}} \text{ gtt}/\cancel{\text{mL}} = \frac{125}{①} = 125 \text{ gtt/min}$$

The drop factor constant for an infusion set with 60 gtt/mL is 1. Therefore, to administer 125 mL/h, set the flow rate at 125 gtt/min.

Example 2:

Administer 125 mL/h IV with *20 gtt/mL* infusion set.

$$\frac{125 \text{ mL}}{\underset{3}{\cancel{60}} \text{ min}} \times \overset{1}{\cancel{20}} \text{ gtt/mL} = \frac{125}{③} = 41.6 = 42 \text{ gtt/min}$$

Drop factor constant = 3

Each drop factor constant is obtained by dividing 60 by the drop factor calibration from the infusion set.

remember

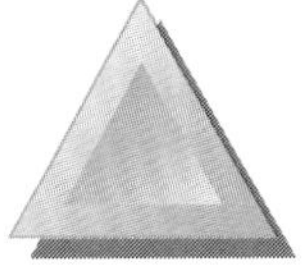

Manufacturer	Drop Factor	Drop Factor Constant
Baxter-Travenol	10 gtt/mL	$\frac{60}{10} = 6$
Abbott	15 gtt/mL	$\frac{60}{15} = 4$
Armour	20 gtt/mL	$\frac{60}{20} = 3$
Any micro or minidrop	60 gtt/mL	$\frac{60}{60} = 1$

Most hospitals consistently use infusion equipment manufactured by one company. You will become very familiar with the one used where you work; therefore, the shortcut method is very practical, quick, and simple to use.

rule

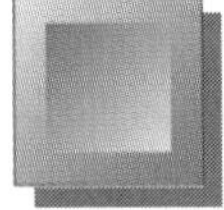

The short cut method to calculate IV flow rate is:

$$\frac{\text{mL/h}}{\text{Drop factor constant}} = \text{gtt/min}$$

Let's re-examine the previous four examples using the short-cut method.

Example 1:

The IV order reads: *D_5W IV @ 125 mL/h.* The infusion set is calibrated for a drop factor of 10 gtt/mL. Drop factor constant: 6

$$\frac{\text{mL / h}}{\text{Drop factor constant}} = \text{gtt/min}$$

$$\frac{125 \text{ mL/h}}{6} = 20.8 = 21 \text{ gtt/min}$$

Example 2:

Order reads *LR IV @ 150 mL/h.* The drop factor is 15 gtt/mL. Drop factor constant: 4

$$\frac{\text{mL / h}}{\text{Drop factor constant}} = \text{gtt/min}$$

$$\frac{150 \text{ mL/h}}{4} = 37.5 = 38 \text{ gtt/min}$$

Example 3:

Order reads: *200 mL $D_5 \frac{1}{2}$ NS IV in 2 h*

Drop factor: 20 gtt/mL

Drop factor constant: 3

STEP 1 $\frac{\text{Total mL}}{\text{Total h}} = \text{mL/h}$

$$\frac{200}{2} = 100 \text{ mL/h}$$

STEP 2 $\frac{\text{mL / h}}{\text{Drop factor constant}} = \text{gtt/min}$

$$\frac{100 \text{ mL/h}}{3} = 33.3 = 33 \text{ gtt/min}$$

Example 4:

Order reads: *D_5W NS IV @ 50 mL/h.* The drop factor is 60 gtt/mL. Drop factor constant: 1

$$\frac{\text{mL / h}}{\text{Drop factor constant}} = \text{gtt/min}$$

$$\frac{50 \text{ mL/h}}{1} = 50 \text{ gtt/min}$$

Remember, when the drop factor is 60 (microdrip), set the flow rate at the same gtt/min as the mL/h.

quick review

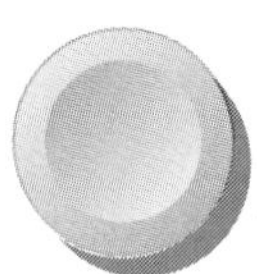

- The drop factor constant is 60 ÷ drop factor.

Drop Factor	Drop Factor Constant
10	6
15	4
20	3
60	1 ⟶ Set the flow rate at the same gtt/min as the mL/h.

- $\frac{\text{mL/h}}{\text{Drop factor constant}} = \text{gtt/min}$

review set 40

1. The drop factor constant is derived by dividing ____60____ by the drop factor calibration.

Determine the drop factor constant for each of the following infusion sets.

2. 60 gtt/mL ________
3. 20 gtt/mL ________
4. 15 gtt/mL ________
5. 10 gtt/mL ________
6. State the rule for the short-cut method to calculate the IV flow rate in gtt/min.

____

Calculate the IV flow rate in gtt/min using the short-cut method.

7. Order: *1000 mL D_5W IV to infuse @ 200 mL/h*

   Drop factor: 15 gtt/mL

   ________ gtt/min

8. Order: *750 mL D_5W to infuse @ 125 mL/h*

   Drop factor: 20 gtt/mL

   ________ gtt/min

9. Order: *500 mL D_5W 0.45% Saline IV to infuse @ 165 mL/h*

   Drop factor: 10 gtt/mL

   ________ gtt/min

10. Order: *2 L NS IV to infuse at 60 cc/h with microdrop infusion set of 60 gtt/mL*

    ________ gtt/min

11. Order: *400 cc D_5W IV to infuse @ 50 cc/h*

    Drop factor: 10 gtt/mL

    Flow rate: ________ gtt/min

12. Order: *3 L NS IV to infuse @ 125 mL/h*

    Drop factor: 15 gtt/mL

    Flow rate: ________ gtt/min

13. Order: *500 mL D_5LR to infuse for 6 h*

    Drop factor: 20 gtt/mL

    Flow rate: ________ gtt/min

14. Order: *0.5 L 0.45% NaCl IV infuse in 20 h*

    Drop factor: 60 gtt/mL

    Flow rate: ________ gtt/min

15. Order: *650 mL D_5 0.33% NaCl IV infuse in 10 h*

    Drop factor: 10 gtt/mL

    Flow rate: ________ gtt/min

After completing these problems, see pages 449 and 450 to check your answers.

Calculating mL/h to program electronic infusion devices and gtt/min to watch count manually regulated IVs are the majority of the IV calculations you need to know. Further, you have learned to calculate the supply dosage of certain IV solutes. These important topics warrant additional reinforcement and review.

quick review

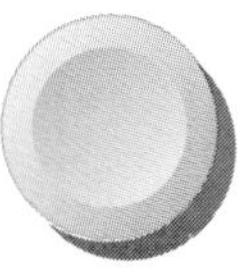

- Solution strength expressed as a percent (%) indicates X g of solute per 100 mL of solution.
- When regulating IV flow rate for an electronic infusion device, calculate mL/h.
- When calculating IV flow rate to regulate an IV manually, calculate mL/h, find the drop factor, and calculate gtt/min by using the:

  Formula Method

  $\frac{V}{T} \times C = R$

  or Short-Cut Method

  $\frac{\text{mL/h}}{\text{Drop factor constant}} = \text{gtt/min}$

- Carefully monitor patients receiving intravenous fluids at least hourly.
- Check remaining IV fluids.
- Check IV flow rate.
- Observe IV site for complications.

review set 41

Calculate the IV flow rate.

1. Order: *3000 mL 0.45% NaCl IV for 24 h*

   Drop factor: 15 gtt/mL

   Flow rate: ________ gtt/min

2. Order: *200 mL D_5W IV to run @ 100 mL/h*

   Drop factor: Microdrop, 60 gtt/mL

   Flow rate: ________ gtt/min

3. Order: *800 cc $D_5\frac{1}{3}$ NS IV for 8 h*

   Drop factor: 20 gtt/mL

   Flow rate: ________ gtt/min

4. Order: *1000 cc NS IV @ 50 cc/h*

   Drop factor: 60 gtt/mL

   Flow rate: ________ gtt/min

5. Order: *1500 mL D_5W IV for 12 h*

   Drop factor: 15 gtt/mL

   Flow rate: ________ gtt/min

6. Order: *Aminophylline 0.5 g IV in 250 mL D_5W to run for 2 h by infusion pump*

   Drop factor: 60 gtt/mL

   Flow rate: ________ gtt/min

7. Order: *2500 mL D_5 0.45% NaCl IV @ 105 mL/h*

   Drop factor: 20 gtt/mL

   Flow rate: ________ gtt/min

8. Order: *500 mL D_5 0.45% NaCl IV @ 100 mL/h*

   Drop factor: 10 gtt/mL

   Flow rate: ________ gtt/min

9. Order: *1200 mL NS IV @ 150 mL/h*

   Drop factor: 10 gtt/mL

   Flow rate: ________ gtt/min

10. Order: *1000 cc D_5 0.45% NaCl to infuse over 8 h*

    Drop factor: On electronic infusion pump

    Flow rate: ________ mL/h

11. Order: *2000 cc D_5NS to infuse over 24 h*

    Drop factor: On electronic infusion controller

    Flow rate: ________ mL/h

12. Order: *500 cc LR to infuse over 4 h*

    Drop factor: On electronic infusion controller

    Flow rate: ________ mL/h

13. Order: *100 mL IV antibiotic to infuse in 30 min via electronic infusion pump*

    Flow rate: ________ mL/h

14. Order: *50 mL IV antibiotic to infuse in 20 min via electronic infusion pump*

    Flow rate: ________ mL/h

15. Order: *150 mL IV antibiotic to infuse in 45 min via electronic infusion pump*

    Flow rate: ________ mL/h

What is the total dosage of the solute(s) the patient will receive for each of the following orders?

16. *3000 mL $\frac{1}{2}$ NS IV* NaCl: ________ g
17. *200 mL D_{10} NS IV* D: ________ g NaCl: ________ g
18. *2500 mL NS IV* NaCl: ________ g
19. *650 mL D_5 0.33% NaCl IV* D: ________ g NaCl: ________ g
20. *1000 mL $D_5\frac{1}{4}$ NS IV* D: ________ g NaCl: ________ g

After completing these problems, see page 450 to check your answers.

Adjusting IV Flow Rate

IV fluids, especially those with medicines added (called additives), are viewed as medications with specific dosages (rates of infusion, in this case). It is the responsibility of the nurse to maintain this rate of flow through careful calculations and close observation at regular intervals.

Various circumstances, such as gravity, condition, and movement of the patient can alter the set flow rate of an IV causing the IV to run ahead of or behind schedule.

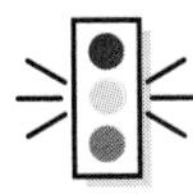

Caution: It is not at the discretion of the nurse to arbitrarily speed up or slow down the flow rate to catch up the IV. This practice can result in serious conditions of over or underhydration and electrolyte imbalance.

If during your regular monitoring of the IV, you find that the rate is not progressing as schedule or is significantly ahead of or behind schedule, the physician may need to be notified as warranted by the patient's condition, hospital policy, or good nursing judgment. However, as allowed by hospital policy, the flow rate per minute may be adjusted by *up to 25 percent more or less* than the original rate depending on the condition of the patient. In such cases, assess the patient and if stable recalculate the flow rate to administer the total milliliters remaining over the number of hours remaining of the original order.

rule

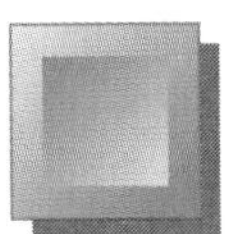

The variation between ordered and adjusted IV flow rate may not exceed 25%, as permitted by agency policy.

$$\frac{\text{Adjusted gtt/min} - \text{Ordered gtt/min}}{\text{Ordered gtt/min}} = \%\text{ of variation}$$

The *% of variation* will be positive (+) if administration is slow and needs to have rate increased and negative (–) if administration is too fast and rate needs to be decreased.

Example 1:

The order reads: *1000 mL D_5W IV @ 125 mL/h for 8 h.* The drop factor is 10 gtt/mL, and the IV is correctly set at 21 gtt/min. You would expect that after 4 hours, one-half of the total or 500 mL of the solution would be infused (125 mL/h × 4 h = 500 mL). However, checking the IV bag the fourth hour after starting the IV, you find 600 milliliters remaining. The rate of flow is *behind schedule.* You would compute a new flow rate for 600 milliliters to complete the IV fluid order in the remaining 4 hours.

STEP 1

$$\frac{\text{Remaining volume}}{\text{Remaining hours}} = \text{Recalculated mL/h}$$

$$\frac{600\text{ mL}}{4\text{ h}} = 150\text{ mL/h}$$

STEP 2

$$\frac{V}{T} \times C = \frac{150\text{ mL}}{\overset{6}{\cancel{60}}\text{ min}} \times \overset{1}{\cancel{10}}\text{ gtt/mL} = \frac{150}{6} = 25\text{ gtt/min (Adjusted flow rate)}$$

You could also use the short-cut method.

$$\frac{\text{mL / h}}{\text{Drop factor constant}} = \text{gtt / min}$$

$$\frac{150\text{ mL}}{6\text{ h}} = 25\text{ gtt/min}$$

STEP 3 $\frac{\text{Adjusted gtt/min} - \text{Ordered gtt/min}}{\text{Ordered gtt/min}} = \%$ of variation

$\frac{25-21}{21} = \frac{4}{21} = 0.19 = 19\%$; within the acceptable 25% of variation depending on policy and patient's condition

Compare 25 gtt/min (in the last example) with the start flow rate of 21 gtt/min. You can see that adjusting the total remaining volume over the total remaining hours changes the flow rate per minute very little. Most patients can tolerate this small amount of increase per minute over several hours. However, trying to catch up the lost 100 milliliters in one hour can be very dangerous. To infuse an extra 100 milliliters in one hour, with a drop factor of 10, you would need to speed up the IV to a much faster rate.

$$\frac{V}{T} \times C = \frac{100 \not{mL}}{\not{60}_{6} \text{ min}} \times \not{10}^{1} \text{ gtt}/\not{mL} = \frac{100}{6} = 16.6 = 17 \text{ gtt/min}$$

To catch up the IV over the next hour, the flow rate would need to be 17 drops per minute faster than the original 21 drops per minute rate. The infusion would need to be set at 17 + 21 = 38 gtt/min for one hour and then slowed to the original rate. Such an increase would be $\frac{38-21}{21} = \frac{17}{21} = 81\%$ greater than the ordered rate. For a child or a seriously ill patient, this can present a serious problem. **Do not do it! If permitted by hospital policy, the flow rate must be recalculated when the IV is off schedule.**

Example 2:

The order reads: *500 mL LR to run over 10 h @ 50 mL/h.* The drop factor is 60 gtt/mL and the IV is correctly infusing at 50 gtt/min. After $2\frac{1}{2}$ hours, you find 300 mL remaining. Almost half of the total volume has already infused in about one-quarter the time. This IV infusion is *ahead of schedule.* You would compute a new flow rate for 300 mL to complete the IV fluid order in the remaining $7\frac{1}{2}$ hours. The patient would require close assessment for fluid overload.

STEP 1 $\frac{\text{Remaining volume}}{\text{Remaining hours}} = \text{Recalculated mL/h}$

$\frac{300 \text{ mL}}{7.5 \text{ h}} = 40 \text{ mL/h}$

STEP 2 $\frac{V}{T} \times C = \frac{40 \not{mL}}{\not{60} \text{ min}} \times \not{60} \text{ gtt}/\not{mL} = 40$ gtt/min (Adjusted flow rate)

Or, you know when drop factor is 60, then mL/h = gtt/min.

STEP 3 $\frac{\text{Adjusted gtt/min} - \text{Ordered gtt/min}}{\text{Ordered gtt/min}} = \%$ of variation

$\frac{40-50}{50} = \frac{-10}{50} = -0.2 = -20\%$ within the acceptable 25% of variation

Remember, the negative percent of variation (–20%) indicates the adjusted flow rate will be decreased.

A good rule of thumb is that the recalculated flow rate should not vary from the original rate by more than 25 percent. If the recalculated rate does vary from the original by more than 25 percent, contact your supervisor or the doctor for further instructions. The original order may need to be revised. Regular monitoring helps to prevent or minimize this problem.

Patients who require close monitoring for IV fluids will most likely have the IV regulated by an electronic infusion device. Because of the nature of their condition, "catching up" these IVs, if off schedule, is not recommended. If an IV regulated by an infusion pump or controller is off schedule or inaccurate, consider that the infusion pump may need recalibration. Consult with your supervisor, as needed.

quick review

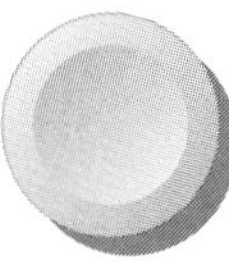

- For manually regulated IVs, recalculate flow rate when off schedule, if permitted by the hospital policy.
- Recalculated flow rate must not be increased or decreased by more than 25% from the original rate, if allowed by hospital policy. Do not arbitrarily speed up or slow down to catch up.
- $\frac{\text{Adjusted gtt/min} - \text{Ordered gtt/min}}{\text{Ordered gtt/min}}$ = % of variation

review set 42

Compute the flow rate in drops per minute. Hospital policy permits recalculating IVs when off schedule with a maximum variation in rate of 25%. Compute the % of variation.

1. Order: *1500 mL Lactated Ringer's IV for 12 hours @ 125 mL/h*

   Drop factor: 20 gtt/mL

   Flow rate: 42 gtt/min

   After 6 hours, there are 850 mL remaining; describe your action at this time.

   Reset to 47 gtt 12% increase

2. Order: *1000 mL Lactated Ringer's IV for 6 hours @ 167 mL/h*

   Drop factor: 15 gtt/mL

   Flow rate: 42 gtt/min

   After 4 hours, there are 360 mL remaining; describe your action now.

   Reset to 45 gtt 7% increase

3. Order: *1000 mL D_5W IV for 8 hours @ 125 mL/h*

   Drop factor: 20 gtt/mL

   Flow rate: 42 gtt/min

   After 4 hours, there are 800 mL remaining; describe your action now.

   Reset 67 gtt/min, 60% to High - Contact Physician

4. Order: *2000 mL NS IV for 12 hours @ 167 mL/h*

   Drop factor: 10 gtt/mL

   Flow rate: 28 gtt/min

   After 8 hours, there are 750 mL remaining; describe your action now.

   Reset to 31 gtt, 10% increase

5. Order: *1000 mL NS IV for 8 h @ 125 mL/h*

   Drop factor: 10 gtt/min

   Flow rate: 21 gtt/min

   After 4 hours, there are 750 mL remaining; describe your action now.

   Reset to 31 gtt, 48% - To High Call Physician

6. Order: *2000 mL NS IV for 16 h @ 125 mL/h*

   Drop factor: 15 gtt/mL

   Flow rate: 31 gtt/min

   After 6 hours, 650 mL of fluid have infused; describe your action now.

   reset to 34, 9% increase

7. Order: *900 mL NS IV for 6 h @ 150 mL/h*

   Drop factor: 20 gtt/mL

   Flow rate: 50 gtt/min

   After 3 hours, there are 700 mL remaining; describe your action now.

   reset to 78 gtt, 55% increase Call physician

8. Order: *500 mL D5NS IV for 5 h @ 100 mL/h*

   Drop factor: 20 gtt/mL

   Flow rate: 33 gtt/min

   After 2 hours, there are 250 mL remaining; describe your action now.

   reset to 28, -15% decrease

9. Order: *1 L NS IV for 20 h @ 50 mL/h*

   Drop factor: 15 gtt/mL

   Flow rate: 13 gtt/min

   After 10 hours, there are 600 mL remaining; describe your action now.

   reset to 15, 15% increase

10. Order: *1000 mL D_5W IV for 10 h @ 100 mL/h*

    Drop factor: 60 gtt/mL

    Flow rate: 100 gtt/min

    After 5 hours, there are 500 mL remaining; describe your action now.

    No change necessary

After completing these problems, see pages 450 and 451 to check your answers.

Intermittent IV Infusions

Sometimes the patient needs to receive supplemental fluid therapy and/or IV medications but does not need continuous replacement or maintenance IV fluids. Several intermittent IV infusion systems are available to administer IV drugs. These include IV piggyback, IV locks for IV push drugs, the Add-Vantage system, elastomeric balloon infusion devices, and volume control sets (such as Buretrol). Volume control sets will be discussed in the next chapter.

IV Piggybacks

A medication may be ordered to be dissolved in a small amount of intravenous fluid (usually 50 to 100 mL) and run "piggyback" the regular intravenous fluids (Figure 14-8, page 295). Recall that the piggyback IV (or secondary IV) requires a secondary IV set (Figure 14-9, page 296).

The IV piggyback (IV PB) medication may come premixed by the manufacturer or pharmacy or may be the nurse's responsibility to properly prepare. Whichever the case, it is always the responsibility of the nurse to accurately administer the medication. The infusion time is usually less than 60 minutes.

Sometimes the physician's order for the IV PB medication will not include an infusion time or rate. It is understood, when this is the case, that the nurse will follow the manufacturer's guidelines for infusion rates, keeping in mind the amount of fluid accompanying the medication and any standing orders that limit fluid amounts or rates. Appropriate infusion times are readily available in many drug books. Reference books are readily available on most nursing units, or you can consult with the hospital pharmacist.

Example 1:

Order: *Kefzol 0.5 g in 100 mL D_5W IV PB to run over 30 min*

Drop factor: 20 gtt/mL

What is the flow rate in gtt/min?

$$\frac{V}{T} \times C = \frac{100 \text{ mL}}{\overset{}{\cancel{30}}_{3} \text{ min}} \times \overset{2}{\cancel{20}} \text{ gtt/}\cancel{\text{mL}} = \frac{200}{3} = 66.67 = 67 \text{ gtt/min}$$

Example 2:

If an infusion pump or controller is used to administer the same order as in Example 1, remember that you would need to program the device in *mL/h.*

STEP 1 THINK If 100 mL will be administered in 30 minutes or one-half hour, then 200 mL will be administered in 60 minutes or one hour.

STEP 2 CALCULATE Use ratio-proportion to calculate mL/h.

$$\frac{100 \text{ mL}}{30 \text{ min}} = \frac{X \text{ mL}}{60 \text{ min}} \quad (1 \text{ h} = 60 \text{ min})$$

$$30X = 6000$$

$$\frac{30X}{30} = \frac{6000}{30}$$

$$X = 200 \text{ mL/h}$$

Set the electronic IV PB regulator to 200 mL/h

Saline and Heparin IV Locks for IV Push Drugs

IV locks can be attached to the hub of the IV catheter that is positioned in the vein. The lock may be referred to as a *saline lock,* meaning saline is used to flush or maintain the IV catheter patency, or a *heparin lock* if heparin is used to maintain the IV catheter patency. Medications can be given *IV push,* meaning that a syringe is attached to the lock and medication is pushed in. An *IV bolus,* usually a quantity of IV fluid, can be run in over a specified period of time through an IV setup that is attached to the lock. Using either a saline or heparin lock allows for intermittent medication and fluid infusion. Heparin and saline locks are also used for outpatient and home care medication therapy. Refer to the policy at your hospital or health care agency regarding the frequency, volume, and concentration of saline or heparin to be used to maintain the IV lock.

Caution: Heparin lock flush solution usually is concentrated 10 units/mL or 100 units/mL. Much higher concentrations of heparin are given IV or SC, so carefully check the concentration.

Dosage calculation for IV push injections are the same as calculations for intramuscular (IM) injections. The IV push route of administration is often preferred when immediate onset of action is desired for persons with small or wasted muscle mass, poor circulation, or for drugs that have limited absorption from body tissues. Drug literature recommends an acceptable rate (per minute) of IV push drug administration.

Example:

Order: *Ativan 3 mg IV Push 20 min preoperatively*

Supply: Ativan 4 mg/mL with drug literature guidelines of "IV infusion not to exceed 2 mg/min"

How much Ativan should you prepare?

STEP 1 **CONVERT** No conversion is necessary.

STEP 2 **THINK** You want to give less than 1 mL.

STEP 3 **CALCULATE** $\frac{D}{H} \times Q = \frac{3 \cancel{mg}}{4 \cancel{mg}} \times 1 \text{ mL} = 0.75 \text{ mL}$

What is a safe infusion time?

Use $\frac{D}{H} \times Q$ to calculate the time required to administer the drug as ordered. In this problem "Q" represents the quantity (or amount) of time of the supply rate: 1 min.

$$\frac{D}{H} \times Q = \frac{3 \cancel{mg}}{2 \cancel{mg}} \times 1 \text{ min} = \frac{3}{2} \text{ min} = 1\frac{1}{2} \text{ min}$$

Or use ratio-proportion to calculate the time required to administer the drug as ordered.

$$\frac{2 \text{ mg}}{1 \text{ min}} \times \frac{3 \text{ mg}}{X \text{ min}}$$

$$2X = 3$$

$$\frac{2X}{2} = \frac{3}{2}$$

$$X = 1\frac{1}{2} \text{ min}$$

Administer 0.75 mL over $1\frac{1}{2}$ min.

Elastomeric Balloon Devices

An elastomeric device is made of soft, rubberized, disposable material that inflates to a predetermined volume to hold and dispense a single dose of IV medication. Baxter's Intermate (Figure 14-18) is a medication balloon reservoir that is protected inside a rigid, transparent container. The medication is prepared and dispensed in the Intermate, ready to use. It can be set for a fixed infusion rate and does not need an IV pole or electric current to operate. It holds 50 to 100 mL and is for one-time use only. Elastomeric devices are being used mainly in outpatient and home care settings for single-dose infusion therapies.

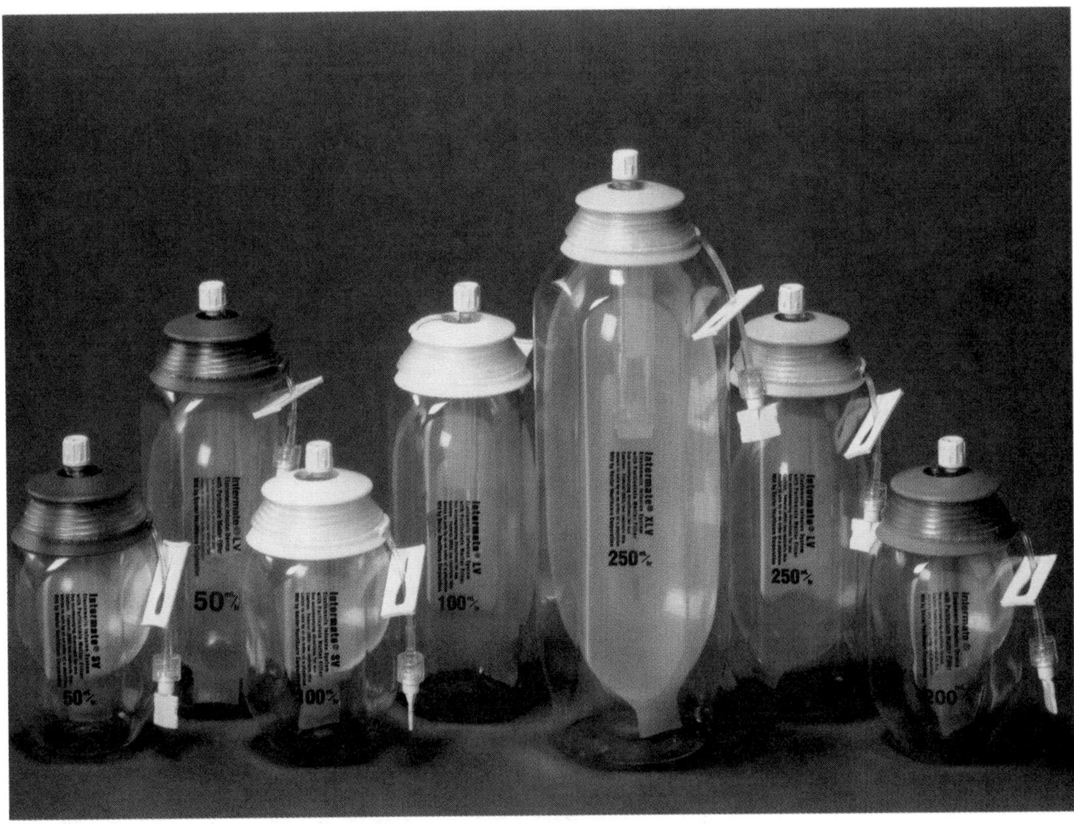

FIGURE 14-18 Elastometric Balloon Devices (Photo courtesy of Baxter International Inc., I.V. Systems Division)

ADD-Vantage System

Another type of IV medication setup commonly used in hospitals is the ADD-Vantage system by Abbott Laboratories (Figure 14-19). In this system a specially designed IV bag with a medication vial port is used. The medication vial comes with the ordered dosage and medication prepared in a powder form. The medication vial is attached to the special IV bag, and together they become the IV piggyback container. The powder is dissolved by the IV fluid and used within a specified time. This system maintains asepsis and eliminates the extra time and equipment (syringe and diluent vials) associated with reconstitution of powder medications. Several drug manufacturers currently market many common IV antibiotics using the ADD-Vantage system.

quick review

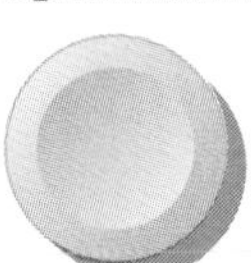

- Intermittent IV infusions typically require less than 60 minutes of infusion time.
- Calculate IV PB flow rate in gtt/min: $\frac{V}{T} \times C = R$.
- Use a proportion to calculate IV PB flow rate in mL/h for electronic infusion device.
- Use the three-step dosage calculation method to calculate the amount to give for IV push medications: convert, think, calculate ($\frac{D}{H} \times Q = X$).
- Use $\frac{D}{H} \times Q$ or ratio-proportion to calculate safe IV push time in minutes as recommended by a reputable drug reference.

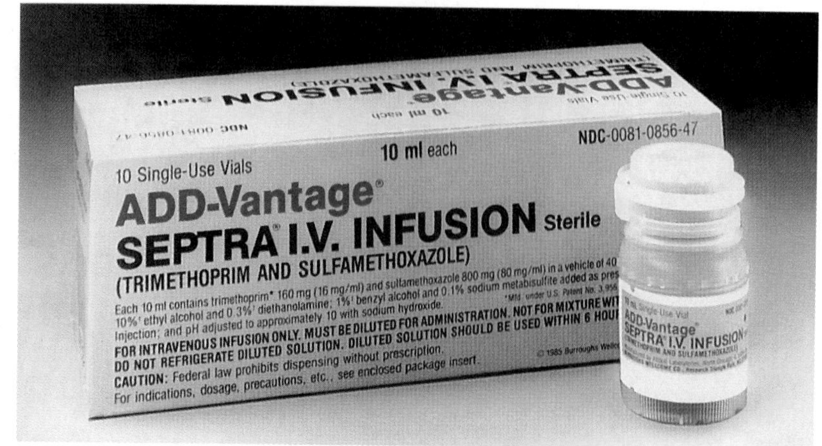

FIGURE 14-19 ADD-Vantage System: Medications can be added to another solution being infused. (Reproduced with permission of Burroughs Wellcome Co.)

SEPTRA® I.V. INFUSION ADD-Vantage® Vials
(trimethoprim and sulfamethoxazole)

To Assemble ADD-Vantage® Vial and Flexible Diluent Container:
(Use Aseptic Technique)

1. Remove the protective covers from the top of the vial and the vial port on the diluent container as follows:
   a. To remove the breakaway vial cap, swing the pull ring over the top of the vial and pull down far enough to start the opening (see Figure 1), then pull straight up to remove the cap (see Figure 2). **NOTE:** Once the breakaway cap has been removed, do not access vial with syringe.

Fig. 1

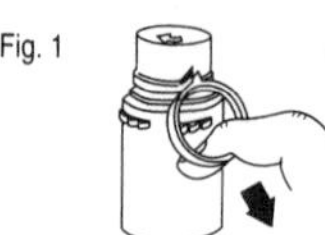

Fig. 2

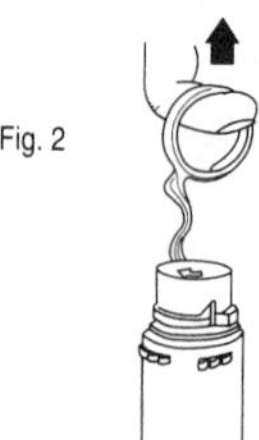

   b. To remove the vial port cover, grasp the tab on the pull ring, pull up to break the three tie strings, then pull back to remove the cover (see Figure 3).
2. Screw the vial into the vial port until it will go no further. THE VIAL MUST BE SCREWED IN TIGHTLY TO ASSURE A SEAL. This occurs approximately ½ turn (180°) after the first audible click (see Figure 4). The clicking sound does not assure a seal; the vial must be turned as far as it will go. **NOTE:** Once vial is seated, do not attempt to remove (see Figure 4).
3. Recheck the vial to assure that it is tight by trying to turn it further in the direction of assembly.
4. Label appropriately.

Fig. 3

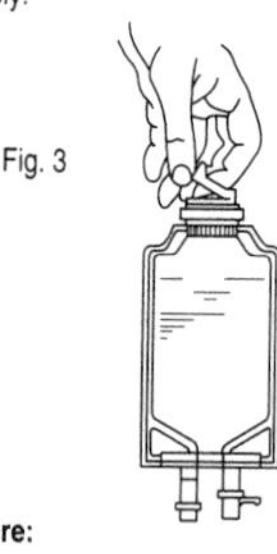

Fig. 4

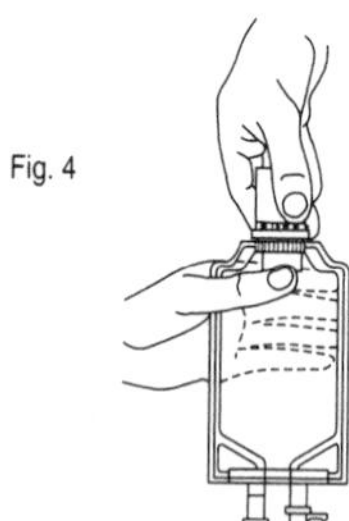

To Prepare Admixture:

1. Squeeze the bottom of the diluent container gently to inflate the portion of the container surrounding the end of the drug vial.
2. With the other hand, push the drug vial down into the container telescoping the walls of the container. Grasp the inner cap of the vial through the walls of the container (see Figure 5).
3. Pull the inner cap from the drug vial (see Figure 6). Verify that the rubber stopper has been pulled out, allowing the drug and diluent to mix.
4. Mix container contents thoroughly and use within the specified time.

Fig. 5

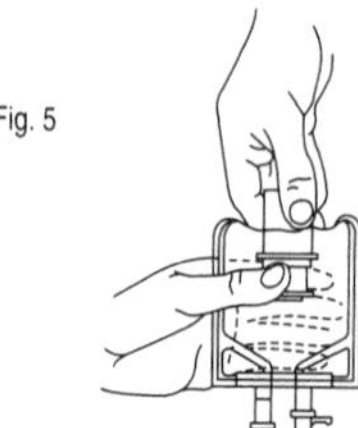

Fig. 6

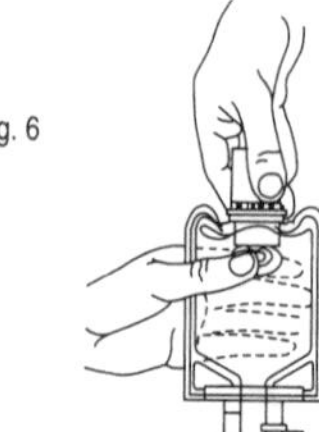

Preparation for Administration:
(Use Aseptic Technique)

1. Confirm the activation and admixture of vial contents.
2. Check for leaks by squeezing container firmly. If leaks are found, discard unit as sterility may be impaired.
3. Close flow control clamp of administration set.
4. Remove cover from outlet port at bottom of container.

review set 43

Calculate the IV PB flow rate.

1. Order: *Ancef 1 g in 100 cc D_5W IV PB to be infused over 45 min*

   Drop factor: 60 gtt/mL

   Flow rate: __________ gtt/min

2. Order: *Ancef 1 g in 100 cc D_5W IV PB to be administered by electronic infusion controller to infuse in 45 min*

   Flow rate: __________ mL/h

3. Order: *Geopen (carbenicillin disodium) 2 g IV PB diluted in 50 mL D_5W to infuse in 15 min*

   Drop factor: 15 gtt/mL

   Flow rate: __________ gtt/min

4. Order: *Geopen (carbenicillin disodium) 2 g IV PB diluted in 50 mL D_5W to infuse in 15 min by an electronic infusion pump*

   Flow rate: __________ mL/h

5. Order: *50 mL IV PB antibiotic solution to infuse in 30 min*

   Drop factor: 60 gtt/mL

   Flow rate: __________ gtt/min

6. Order: *Zosyn 3 g in 100 mL D_5W IV PB to be infused over 40 min*

   Drop factor: 10 gtt/mL

   Flow rate: __________ gtt/min

7. Order: *Unasyn 1.5 g in 50 mL D_5W IV PB to be infused over 15 min*

   Drop factor: 15 gtt/mL

   Flow rate: __________ gtt/min

8. Order: *Merram 1 g in 100 mL D_5W IV PB to be infused over 30 min*

   Use infusion pump.

   Flow rate: __________ mL/h

9. Order: *Keflin 750 mg in 50 mL NS IV PB to be infused over 20 min*

   Use infusion pump.

   Flow rate: __________ mL/h

10. Order: *Oxacillin Sodium 900 mg in 125 mL D_5W IV PB to be infused over 45 min*

    Use infusion pump.

    Flow rate: __________ mL/h

11. Order: *Unasyn 0.5 g in 100 mL D_5W IV PB to be infused over 15 min*

    Drop factor: 20 gtt/mL

    Flow rate: __________ gtt/min

12. Order: *Keflin 500 mg in 50 mL NS IV PB to be infused over 20 min*

    Drop factor: 10 gtt/mL

    Flow rate: __________ gtt/min

13. Order: *Merram 1 g in 100 mL D_5W IV PB to be infused over 50 min*

    Use infusion pump.

    Flow rate: __________ mL/h

14. Order: *Oxacillin Sodium 900 mg in 125 mL D_5W IV PB to be infused over 45 min*

    Drop factor: 20 gtt/mL

    Flow rate: __________ gtt/min

15. Order: *Zosyn 1.3 g in 100 mL D_5W IV PB to be infused over 30 min*

    Drop factor: 60 gtt/mL

    Flow rate: __________ gtt/min

16. Order: *Lasix 120 mg IV push stat*

    Supply: Lasix 10 mg/mL with drug insert, which states, "IV infusion not to exceed 40 mg/min."

    Give: __________ mL

    Infusion time: __________ min

17. Order: *Dilantin 150 mg IV push stat*

    Supply: Dilantin 250 mg/5 mL with drug insert, which states, "IV infusion not to exceed 50 mg/min."

    Give: __________ mL

    Infusion time: __________ min

18. Order: *Morphine sulfate gr $\frac{1}{10}$ IV push q.3h, prn*

    Supply: Morphine sulfate 10 mg/mL with drug reference recommendation, which states, "IV infusion not to exceed 2.5 mg/min."

    Give: __________ mL

    Infusion time: __________ min and __________ seconds

19. The purpose of intermittent IV infusions is ______________________.

20. Elastomeric balloon devices are used primarily in inpatient settings. (True) or (False)

After completing these problems, see pages 451 and 452 to check your answers.

Calculating IV Infusion Time

Intravenous solutions are usually ordered to be administered at a prescribed number of milliliters per hour, such as *1000 mL Lactated Ringer's IV to run at 125 mL per hour.* You may need to calculate the total infusion time in order to anticipate when to add a new bag or bottle, or when to discontinue the IV.

rule

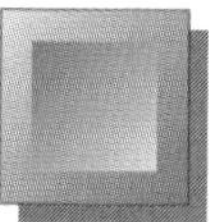

To calculate IV infusion time:

$$\frac{\text{TOTAL volume}}{\text{mL/h}} = \text{TOTAL hours}$$

Or use ratio-proportion: ratio for prescribed flow rate in mL/h = Ratio for total mL to X total hours

$$\frac{\text{mL}}{\text{h}} = \frac{\text{Total mL}}{\text{X Total h}}$$

Example 1:

1000 mL LR IV to run at 125 mL/h. How long will this IV last?

$$\frac{1000 \text{ mL}}{125 \text{ mL/h}} = 8 \text{ h}$$

Or, use ratio-proportion.

$$\frac{125 \text{ mL}}{1 \text{ h}} = \frac{1000 \text{ mL}}{\text{X h}}$$

$$125\text{X} = 1000$$

$$\frac{125\text{X}}{125} = \frac{1000}{125}$$

$$\text{X} = 8 \text{ h}$$

Example 2:

1000 mL D_5W IV to infuse at 60 mL/h to begin at 0600. At what time will this IV be complete?

$$\frac{1000 \text{ mL}}{60 \text{ mL/h}} = 16.67 \text{ h} = 16\tfrac{2}{3} \text{ h} = 16 \text{ h and } 40 \text{ min}$$

Or, use ratio-proportion:

$$\frac{60 \text{ mL}}{1 \text{ h}} = \frac{1000 \text{ mL}}{\text{X h}}$$

$$60\text{x} = 1000$$

$$\frac{60\text{X}}{60} = \frac{1000}{60}$$

$$\text{X} = 16.67 \text{ h}$$

The IV will be complete at 0600 + 1640 = 2240 or 10:40 PM.

You can also determine the infusion time if you know the volume, flow rate in gtt/min, and drop factor. Calculate the infusion time by using the $\frac{V}{T} \times C = R$ formula; T time in minutes is unknown.

rule

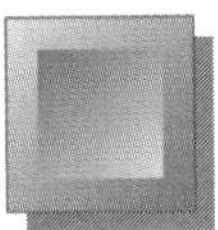

Use the formula method to calculate time (T):

$$\frac{V}{T} \times C = R$$

Example:

80 mL D_5W IV at 20 microdrops/min

The drop factor is 60 gtt/mL. Calculate the infusion time.

STEP 1 $\frac{V}{T} \times C = \frac{80 \text{ mL}}{\text{T min}} \times 60 \text{ gtt/mL} = 20 \text{ gtt/min}$

$$\frac{80 \text{ mL}}{\text{T min}} \times 60 \text{ gtt/mL} = \frac{20 \text{ gtt}}{\text{min}}$$

Now you can apply ratio-proportion.

$$\frac{4800}{T} \times \frac{20}{1}$$

$$20T = 4800$$

$$\frac{20T}{20} = \frac{4800}{20}$$

$$T = 240 \text{ minutes}$$

STEP 2 Convert: minutes to hours

$$240 \text{ min} = \frac{240}{60} = 4$$

Calculating IV Fluid Volumes

If you have an IV that is regulated at a particular flow rate (gtt/min) and you know the drop factor (gtt/mL) and the amount of time, you can determine the volume to be infused.

Apply the flow rate formula; V (volume) is unknown.

rule

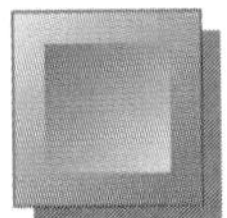

To calculate IV volume (V):

$$\frac{V}{T} \times C = R$$

Example:

When you start your shift at 7 AM, there is an IV bag of *D_5W infusing at the rate of 25 gtt/min*. The infusion set is calibrated for a drop factor of *15 gtt/mL*. How much can you anticipate the patient will receive during your 8-hour shift?

$$8\text{ h} = 8 \times 60\text{ min} = 480\text{ min}$$

$$\frac{V}{T} \times C = R$$

$$\frac{V\text{ mL}}{480\text{ min}} \times 15\text{ gtt/mL} = 25\text{ gtt/min}$$

$$\frac{V\text{ mL}}{480\text{ min}} \times 15\text{ gtt/mL} = \frac{25\text{ gtt}}{1\text{ min}}$$

$$\frac{15V}{480} \times \frac{25}{1}$$

$$15V = 12{,}000$$

$$\frac{15V}{15} = \frac{12{,}000}{15}$$

$$V = 800\text{ mL to be infused in 8 h}$$

If the IV is regulated in mL/h, you can also calculate the total volume that will infuse over a specific time.

rule

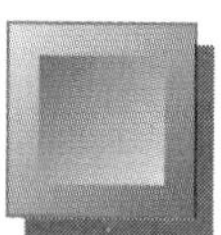

To calculate IV volume:

Total hours × mL/h = Total volume

Or use ratio-proportion:
Ratio for ordered mL/h = Ratio for X total volume to total hours

$$\frac{\text{mL}}{\text{h}} = \frac{\text{X Total mL}}{\text{Total h}}$$

Example:

Your patient's IV is running on an infusion pump set at the rate of 100 mL/h. How much will be infused during the next 8 hours?

$$8\text{ h} \times 100\text{ mL/h} = 800\text{ mL}$$

Or, use ratio-proportion:

$$\frac{100\text{ mL}}{1\text{ h}} = \frac{X\text{ mL}}{8\text{ h}}$$

$$X = 800\text{mL}$$

quick review

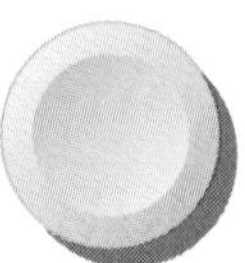

- The formula to calculate IV infusion time, when mL is known: $\frac{\text{Total volume}}{\text{mL/h}} = \text{Total hours}$
  or use ratio-proportion: $\frac{\text{mL}}{\text{h}} = \frac{\text{Total mL}}{\text{X total h}}$
- The formula to calculate IV infusion time, when flow rate in gtt/min, drop factor, and volume are known: $\frac{V}{T} \times C = R$; "T" is the unknown.
- The formula to calculate total infusion volume, when mL/h are known:

  Total hours × mL/h = Total volume

  Or, use ratio-proportion: $\frac{\text{mL}}{\text{h}} = \frac{\text{X total mL}}{\text{Total h}}$

- The formula to calculate IV volume, when flow rate (gtt/min), drop factor, and time are known: $\frac{V}{T} \times C = R$; "V" is the unknown.

review set 44

Calculate the infusion time and rate for the following IV orders:

1. Order: *500 mL D_5W at 30 gtt/min*

   Drop factor: 20 gtt/mL

   Time: __________

2. Order: *1000 mL Lactated Ringer's at 25 gtt/min*

   Drop factor: 10 gtt/mL

   Time: __________

3. Order: *800 mL D_5 Lactated Ringer's at 25 gtt/min*

   Drop factor: 15 gtt/mL

   Time: __________

4. Order: *120 mL Normal Saline to run at 20 mL/h*

   Drop factor: 60 microdrops/mL

   Time: __________

   Flow rate: __________ gtt/min

5. Order: *80 mL D_5W to run at 20 mL/h*

   Drop factor: 60 microdrops/mL

   Time: __________

   Flow rate: __________ gtt/min

Calculate the completion time for the following IVs.

6. At 1600 hours the nurse started an IV of 1200 mL D_5W at 27 gtt/min. The infusion set used is calibrated for a drop factor of 15 gtt/mL. Time: __________

7. At 1530 hours the nurse starts 2000 mL of D_5W to run at 125 mL/h. The infusion set used is calibrated for a drop factor of 10 gtt/mL. The IV rate should be set at __________ gtt/min, and the IV should be completed at __________.

Calculate the total volume (mL) to be infused per 24 hours.

8. A 1000 mL bag of D_5 Lactated Ringer's is infusing on an electronic infusion pump @ 125 mL/h. __________ mL

9. An IV is flowing at 12 gtt/min and the infusion set has a drop factor of 15 gtt/mL. __________ mL

10. IV: D_5W

    Flow rate: 21 gtt/min

    Drop factor: 10 gtt/mL

    __________ mL

Calculate IV volume for the following IVs.

11. *0.9% sodium chloride IV infusing at 65 mL/h for 4 h*

    Volume: __________ mL

12. *D_5W IV infusing at 150 mL/h for 2 h*

    Volume: __________ mL

13. *D_5LR IV at 75 mL/h for 8 h*

Volume: __________ mL

14. *D_5 0.225 NaCl IV at 40 gtt/min for 8 h*

Drop factor: 60 gtt/mL

Volume: __________ mL

15. *0.45% NaCl IV at 45 gtt/min for 4 h*

Drop factor: 20 gtt/mL

Volume: __________ mL

After completing these problems, see pages 452 and 453 to check your answers.

critical thinking skills

It is important to know the equipment you are using. Let's look at an example in which the nurse was unfamiliar with the IV piggyback setup.

error

Failing to follow manufacturer's directions when using a new IV piggyback system.

possible scenario

Suppose the physician ordered Rocephin 1 g IV q.12h for an elderly patient with streptococcus pneumonia. The medication was sent to the unit by pharmacy utilizing the ADD-Vantage system. Rocephin 1 gram was supplied in a powder form and attached to a 50 mL IV bag of D_5W. The directions for preparing the medication were attached to the label. The nurse, who was unfamiliar with the new ADD-Vantage system, hung the IV medication, calculated the drip rate, and infused the 50 mL of fluid. The nurse cared for the patient for three days. During walking rounds on the third day, the on-coming nurse noticed that the Rocephin powder remained in the vial and never was diluted in the IV bag. The nurse realized that the vial stopper inside of the IV bag was not open. Therefore, the medication powder was not mixed in the IV fluid during this shift for the past three days.

potential outcome

The omission by the nurse resulted in the patient missing three doses of the ordered IV antibiotic. The delay in the medication administration could have serious consequence for the patient, such as worsening of the pneumonia, septicemia, and even death, especially in the elderly. The patient received only one-half of the daily dose ordered by the physician for three days. The physician would be notified of the error and likely order additional diagnostic studies, such as chest X ray, blood cultures, and an additional one-time dose of Rocephin.

prevention

This error could easily have been avoided had the nurse read the directions for preparing the medication or consulted with another nurse familiar with the system.

practice problems—chapter 14

Compute the flow rate in drops per minute or milliliters per hour as requested. Hospital policy permits recalculating IVs when off schedule with a maximum variation in rate of 25 percent.

1. Order: *Ampicillin 500 mg dissolved in 200 mL D_5W IV to run for 2 h*

   Drop factor: 10 gtt/mL

   Flow rate: __________ gtt/min

2. Order: *1000 mL D_5W IV per 24 h KVO (keep vein open)*

   Drop factor: 60 gtt/mL

   Flow rate: __________ gtt/min

3. Order: *1500 mL D_5LR IV to run for 12 h*

   Drop factor: 20 gtt/mL

   Flow rate: __________ gtt/min

4. Order: *200 mL D_5RL IV to run KVO for 24 h*

   Drop factor: 60 gtt/mL

   Flow rate: __________ gtt/min

5. Order: *1 L $D_{10}W$ IV to run from 1000 to 1800*

   Drop factor: On electronic infusion pump

   Flow rate: __________ mL/h

6. See # 5. At 1100 there are 800 mL remaining. Describe your nursing action now.

   ____

7. Order: *1000 mL NS followed by 2000 mL D_5W IV to run for 24 h*

   Drop factor: 15 gtt/mL

   Flow rate: __________ gtt/min

8. Order: *2.5 L NS IV to infuse at 125 mL/h*

   Drop factor: 20 gtt/mL

   Flow rate: __________ gtt/min

9. Order: *1000 mL D_5W IV for 6 h*

   Drop factor: 15 gtt/mL

   After 2 hours, 800 mL remain. Describe your nursing action now.

   ____

The IV tubing package below is the IV system available in your hospital for manually regulated, straight gravity flow IV administration with macrodrop. The patient has an order for *500 mL D_5W IV q.4h* The order was written at 1515 and you start the IV at 1530. Questions 10 through 20 refer to this situation.

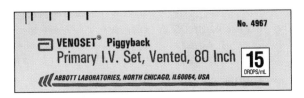

10. How much IV fluid will the patient receive in 24 hours? __________ mL
11. Who is the manufacturer of the IV infusion set tubing? __________
12. What is the drop factor calibration for the IV infusion set tubing? __________
13. What is the drop factor constant for the IV infusion set tubing? __________
14. Using the short cut (drop factor constant) method, calculate the flow rate of the IV as ordered. Show your work.

    Short cut method calculation: ______________________________

    Flow rate: __________ gtt/min
15. Using the formula method, calculate the flow rate of the IV as ordered. Show your work.

    Formula method calculation: ______________________________

    Flow rate: __________ gtt/min
16. At what time should you anticipate the first IV bag of 500 mL D_5W will be completely infused? __________.
17. How much IV fluid should be infused by 1730? __________ mL
18. At 1730 you notice that the IV has 210 mL remaining. After assessing your patient and confirming that his condition is stable, what should you do?

    ____
19. After consulting the physician you decide to use an electronic controller to better regulate the flow rate. The physician orders that the controller be set to infuse 500 mL every 4 hours. You should set the controller for __________ mL/h.
20. The next day the physician adds the order *Amoxicillin 250 mg in 50 mL D_5W IV PB to infuse in 30 min. q.i.d.* The patient is still on the IV controller. To infuse the IV PB, set the controller for __________ mL/h.
21. List the components and concentration strengths of the IV fluid $D_{2.5}\frac{1}{2}$NS.

    ____
22. Calculate the amount of dextrose and sodium chloride in D_5NS 500 mL.

    dextrose __________ g

    NaCl __________ g
23. Define a central line.

    ____
24. Define a primary line.

    ____
25. Describe the purpose of a saline or heparin lock.

    ____
26. A safe IV push infusion rate of protamine sulfate is 5 mg/min. What is a safe infusion time to administer 50 mg? __________ min
27. Describe the purpose of the PCA pump.

    ____
28. Identify two advantages of the syringe pump.

    ____

29. List two complications of IV sites.

____

30. How often should the IV site be monitored?

____

31. Describe the purpose of the Y-set IV system.

____

For each IV order in #32 through 47, use the four different possible drop factors to calculate the respective flow rate in gtt/min.

Order: *1 L hyperalimentation solution IV to infuse in 12 h*

32. Drop factor 10 gtt/mL Flow rate: _______ gtt/min
33. Drop factor 15 gtt/mL Flow rate: _______ gtt/min
34. Drop factor 20 gtt/mL Flow rate: _______ gtt/min
35. Drop factor 60 gtt/mL Flow rate: _______ gtt/min

Order: *2 L D_5NS IV to infuse in 20 h*

36. Drop factor 10 gtt/mL Flow rate: _______ gtt/min
37. Drop factor 15 gtt/mL Flow rate: _______ gtt/min
38. Drop factor 20 gtt/mL Flow rate: _______ gtt/min
39. Drop factor 60 gtt/mL Flow rate: _______ gtt/min

Order: *Give 1000 mL of 0.45% NaCl IV @ 200 mL/h*

40. Drop factor 10 gtt/mL Flow rate: _______ gtt/min
41. Drop factor 15 gtt/mL Flow rate: _______ gtt/min
42. Drop factor 20 gtt/mL Flow rate: _______ gtt/min
43. Drop factor 60 gtt/mL Flow rate: _______ gtt/min

Order: *Give 540 mL D_5 0.33% NaCl IV @ 45 mL/h*

44. Drop factor 10 gtt/mL Flow rate: _______ gtt/min
45. Drop factor 15 gtt/mL Flow rate: _______ gtt/min
46. Drop factor 20 gtt/mL Flow rate: _______ gtt/min
47. Drop factor 60 gtt/mL Flow rate: _______ gtt/min
48. You make rounds before your lunch break and find that a patient has 150 mL of IV fluid remaining. The flow rate is 25 gtt/min. The drop factor is 10 gtt/mL. What volume will be infused during the hour that you are at lunch? _______ mL What should you alert your relief nurse to watch for while you are off the unit? _______

    ____

49. Your shift is 0700–1500. You make rounds at 0730 and find an IV of D_5 0.45% NaCl is regulated on an electronic infusion pump at the ordered rate of 75 mL/h with 400 mL remaining. The order specifies a continuous infusion. At what time should you anticipate hanging the next IV bag? _______
50. Critical Thinking Skill: Describe the strategy you would implement to prevent this medication error.

possible scenario

Suppose the physician ordered *D_5LR IV at 125 mL/h* for an elderly patient just returning from the OR following abdominal surgery. The nurse gathered the IV solution and IV tubing, which had a drop factor of 20 gtt/mL. The nurse did not check the package for the drop factor and assumed it was 60 gtt/mL. The manual rate was calculated this way:

$$\frac{125\ \cancel{mL}}{\cancel{60}\ min} \times \cancel{60}\ gtt/\cancel{mL} = 125\ gtt/\ min$$

The nurse infused the D_5LR at 125 gtt/min for 8 hours. While giving report to the oncoming nurse, the patient called for the nurse complaining of shortness of breath. On further assessment the nurse heard crackles in the patient's lungs and noticed the patient's third 1000 mL bag of D_5LR this shift was nearly empty again. At this point the nurse realized the IV rate was in error. The nurse was accustomed to using the 60 gtt/mL IV set and therefore calculated the drip rate using the 60 gtt/mL (microdrip) drop factor. However, the tubing used delivered 20 gtt/mL (macrodrip) drop factor. The nurse never looked at the drop factor on the IV set package and assumed it was a 60 gtt/mL set.

potential outcome

The patient developed signs of fluid overload and possibly could have developed congestive heart failure due to the excessive IV rate. The physician would have been notified and likely ordered Lasix (a diuretic) to help eliminate the excess fluid. The patient probably would have been transferred to the ICU for closer monitoring.

prevention:

____

____

Upon completion of these problems, see pages 453 and 454 to check your answers.

CHAPTER 15

Advanced Pediatric Calculations

objectives

Upon mastery of Chapter 15, you will be able to perform advanced calculations for children and apply these advanced concepts across the life span. To accomplish this you will also be able to:

- Determine the body surface area (BSA) of children and adults using a calculation formula or a nomogram scale.
- Compute the safe amount of drug to be administered when ordered according to the BSA.
- Calculate pediatric intermittent IV medications administered with IV infusion control sets.
- Calculate the amount to mix proportionate IV additive medications into pediatric volume IV solutions.
- Calculate the minimal and maximal dilution in which an IV medication can be safely prepared and delivered to a child, such as via a syringe pump.
- Calculate pediatric IV maintenance fluids.

This chapter will focus on additional and more advanced calculations used frequently by pediatric nurses. It will help you understand the unique drug and fluid management required by the growing child. Further, these concepts, which are most commonly related to children, are also applied to adults in special situations. Let's start by looking at the body surface area (BSA) method of calculating a dosage or checking for accuracy and safety of a particular drug order.

Body Surface Area (BSA) Method

The Body Surface Area (BSA) is an important measurement in calculating dosages for infants and children. BSA is also used for selected adult populations, such as those undergoing open-heart surgery or radiation therapy, severe burn victims, and those with renal disease. Regardless of age, antineoplastic agents (chemotherapy drugs) and an increasing number of other highly potent drug classifications are being prescribed based on BSA.

BSA is a mathematical estimate using the patient's *height* and *weight*. BSA is expressed in square meters (**m^2**). Most practitioners use a chart called a nomogram that *estimates* the BSA by plotting the height and weight and simply connecting the dots with a straight line. Figure 15-1 shows the most well-known BSA chart, the West Nomogram. It is used for both children and adults for heights up to 240 cm (95 inches) and weights up to 80 kg (180 lb).

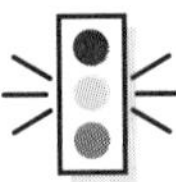

Caution: Notice that the increments of measurement and the spaces on the BSA nomogram are not consistent. Be sure you correctly read the numbers and the calibration values between them.

For a child of normal height and weight, the BSA can be determined on the West Nomogram using the weight alone. Notice the enclosed column to the center left.

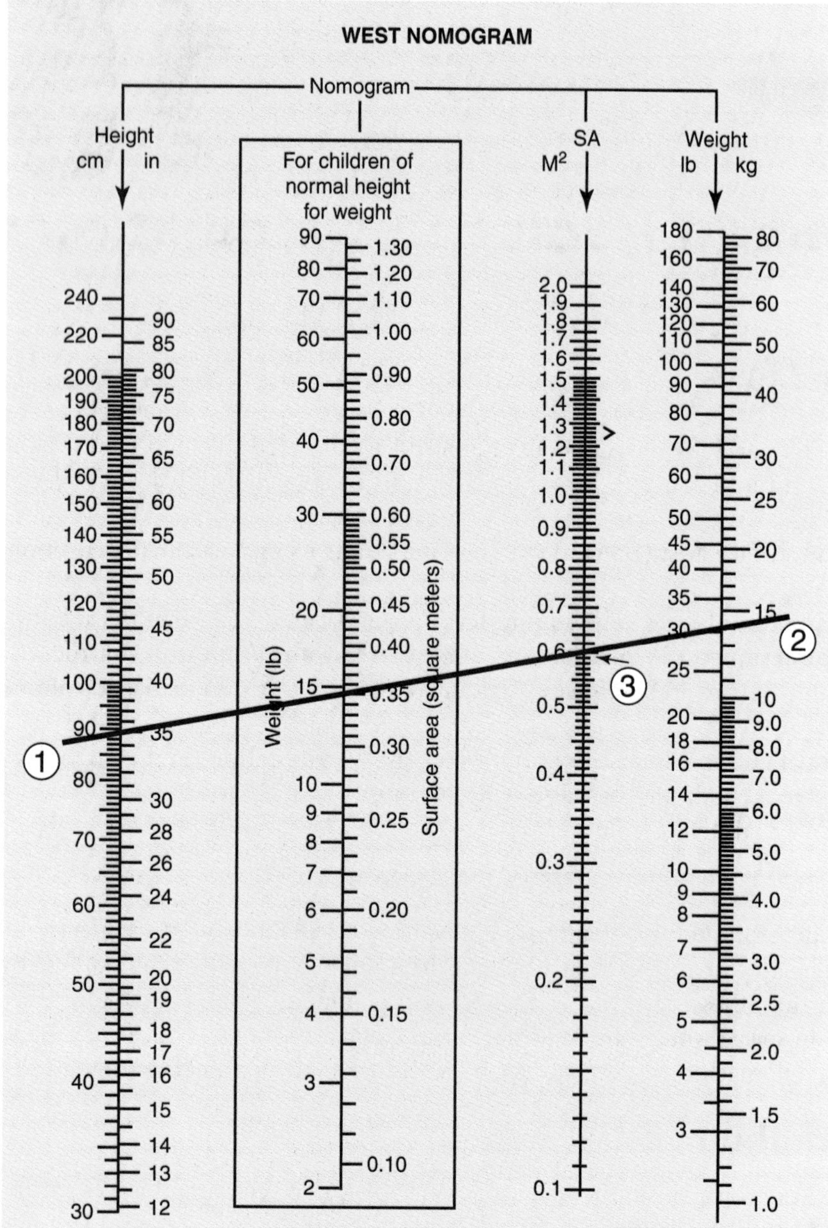

FIGURE 15-1 Body surface area (BSA) is determined by drawing a straight line from the patient's height (1) in the far left column to his or her weight (2) in the far right column. Intersection of the line with body surface area (BSA) column (3) is the estimated BSA (m^2). For infants and children of normal height and weight BSA may be estimated from weight alone by referring to the enclosed area. (From *Nelson Textbook of Pediatrics* (15th ed.) by R. E. Behrman, R. M. Kleigman, & A. M. Arvin, 1996, Philadelphia: Saunders. Reprinted with permission.)

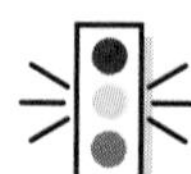

Caution: To use the normal column on the West Nomogram, you must be familiar with normal height and weight standards for children. If you are unsure, use both height and weight to estimate BSA. Do not guess.

Figure 15-2 shows another nomogram specific for children up to 120 cm and 40 kg, whose height and weight may or may not be considered average. Figure 15-3 shows a nomogram specific for adults up to 150 kg (330 lb) and 200 cm (79 inches), measurements that should include most adults.

BSA can also be calculated using two easy formulas and the square root function on a calculator. One formula is based on metric measurement of height in centimeters and weight in kilograms. The other uses household measurement of height in inches and the weight in pounds. Of course, the formulas are more accurate than the nomograms, which are based on estimates of height and weight.

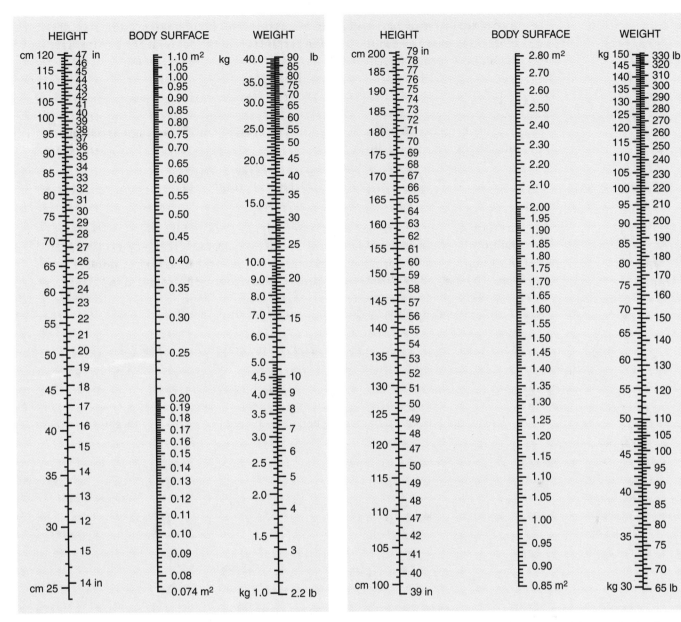

FIGURE 15-2 Nomogram for Determining Body Surface of Children from Height and Weight. (From *Oncology Pocket Guide to Chemotherapy*, by L. Balter and R. Berkery, 1994, St. Louis, MO: Mosby Year-Book. Reprinted with permission.)

FIGURE 15-3 Nomogram for Determining Body Surface or Adults from Height and Weight (From *Oncology Pocket Guide to Chemotherapy*, by L. Balter and R. Berkery, 1994, St. Louis, MO: Mosby Year-Book. Reprinted with permission.)

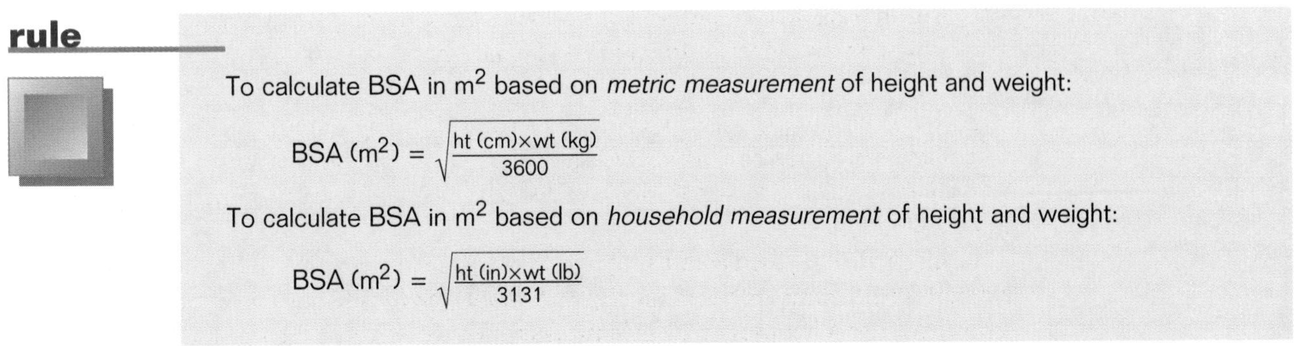

rule

To calculate BSA in m² based on *metric measurement* of height and weight:

$$\text{BSA } (m^2) = \sqrt{\frac{\text{ht (cm)} \times \text{wt (kg)}}{3600}}$$

To calculate BSA in m² based on *household measurement* of height and weight:

$$\text{BSA } (m^2) = \sqrt{\frac{\text{ht (in)} \times \text{wt (lb)}}{3131}}$$

Let's apply both formulas, and see how the BSA measurements compare.

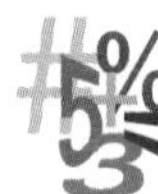

math tip: Notice that in addition to metric versus household measurement, the other difference between the two BSA formulas is in the denominators of the fraction within the square root sign.

Example 1:

Use the metric formula to calculate the BSA of an infant whose length is 50 cm (20 in) and weight is 6.8 kg (15 lb).

$$\text{BSA} = \sqrt{\frac{50 \text{ cm} \times 6.8 \text{ kg}}{3600}} = \sqrt{\frac{340}{3600}} = \sqrt{0.094} = 0.31 \text{ m}^2$$

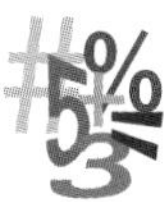

math tip: To perform BSA calculations on most calculators, follow this sequence: multiply height in *cm* by weight in *kg*, divide by 3600, press =, then press √ to arrive at m^2. Round m^2 to hundredths (2 decimal places). For the preceding example, BSA = enter 50 × 6.8 ÷ 3600 = 0.094, and press √ to arrive at 0.307, rounded to 0.31 m^2.

Or use the BSA formula based on household measurement.

$$\text{BSA} = \sqrt{\frac{20 \text{ in} \times 15 \text{ lb}}{3131}} = \sqrt{\frac{300}{3131}} = \sqrt{0.096} = 0.31 \text{ m}^2$$

Example 2:

Calculate the BSA of a child whose height is 105 cm (42 inches) and weight is 31.8 kg (70 lb).

Metric:

$$\text{BSA} = \sqrt{\frac{105 \text{ cm} \times 31.8 \text{ kg}}{3600}} = \sqrt{\frac{3339}{3600}} = \sqrt{0.928} = 0.96 \text{ m}^2$$

Household:

$$\text{BSA} = \sqrt{\frac{42 \text{ in} \times 70 \text{ lb}}{3131}} = \sqrt{\frac{2940}{3131}} = \sqrt{0.939} = 0.97 \text{ m}^2$$

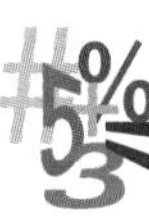

math tip: There is a slight variation in m^2 calculated by the metric and household BSA methods because of the rounding used to convert centimeters and inches; 1 in = 2.54 cm, which is rounded to 2.5 cm.

Example 3:

Calculate the BSA of an adult whose height is 173 cm (69 inches) and weight is 88.6 kg (195 lb).

Metric:

$$\text{BSA} = \sqrt{\frac{173 \text{ cm} \times 88.6 \text{ kg}}{3600}} = \sqrt{\frac{15327.8}{3600}} = \sqrt{4.258} = 2.06 \text{ m}^2$$

Household:

$$\text{BSA} = \sqrt{\frac{68 \text{ in} \times 195 \text{ lb}}{3131}} = \sqrt{\frac{13260}{3131}} = \sqrt{4.235} = 2.06 \text{ m}^2$$

These examples show that either metric or household measurements of height and weight result in essentially the same calculated BSA value.

quick review

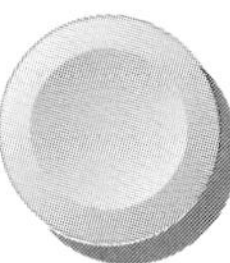

- BSA is used to calculate select dosages across the life span, most often for children.
- BSA is calculated by height and weight and expressed in m^2.
- Nomograms can be used to estimate BSA, by correlating height and weight measurements to m^2.
- The *normal height and weight* column on the West Nomogram for estimating BSA should only be used when the child's height and weight are within normal limits.
- The formula methods to calculate more exact BSA are:

$$BSA\ (m^2) = \sqrt{\frac{ht\ (cm) \times wt\ (kg)}{3600}}\ \text{(metric)}$$

$$BSA\ (m^2) = \sqrt{\frac{ht\ (in) \times wt\ (lb)}{3131}}\ \text{(household)}$$

review set 45

Use the formula method to determine the BSA. Round to two decimal places.

1. A child measures 36 inches tall and weighs 40 lb. __________ m^2
2. An adult measures 190 cm tall and weighs 105 kg. __________ m^2
3. A child measures 94 cm tall and weighs 18 kg. __________ m^2
4. A teenager measures 153 cm tall and weighs 46 kg. __________ m^2
5. An adult measures 175 cm tall and weighs 85 kg. __________ m^2
6. A child measures 41 inches tall and weighs 76 lb. __________ m^2
7. An adult measures 62 inches tall and weighs 140 lb. __________ m^2
8. A child measures 28 inches tall and weighs 18 lb. __________ m^2
9. A teenager measures 160 cm tall and weighs 64 kg. __________ m^2
10. A child measures 65 cm tall and weighs 15 kg. __________ m^2
11. A child measures 55 inches tall and weighs 70 lb. __________ m^2
12. A child measures 92 cm tall and weighs 24 kg. __________ m^2

Find the BSA on the West Nomogram (Figure 15-1, p. 330) for a child of normal height and weight.

13. 4 lb __________ m^2 14. 42 lb __________ m^2 15. 17 lb __________ m^2

Find the BSA on the West Nomogram (Figure 15-1, p. 330) for children with the following height and weight.

16. 41 inches and 32 lb __________ m^2
17. 21 inches and 8 lb __________ m^2
18. 140 cm and 30 kg __________ m^2
19. 80 cm and 11 kg __________ m^2
20. 106 cm and 25 kg __________ m^2

After completing these problems, see page 454 to check your answers.

BSA Dosage Calculations

Once the BSA is obtained, the drug dosage can be verified by consulting a reputable drug resource for the recommended dosage. Package inserts, the *Hospital Formulary*, or other dosage handbooks contain pediatric and adult dosages. Remember to carefully read the reference to verify if the drug dosage is calculated in m^2 *per dose* or m^2 *per day.*

rule

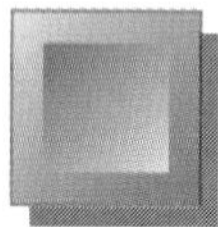

To verify safe pediatric dosing based on BSA:

1. Determine BSA in m^2.
2. Calculate the safe dosage based on BSA: **multiply recommended dosage in mg/m^2 by BSA measured in m^2: $mg/m^2 \times m^2 = X$ mg**
3. Compare the ordered dosage to the recommended dosage, and decide if the dosage is safe.
4. If the dosage is safe, calculate the amount to give and administer the dose. If the dosage seems unsafe, consult with the ordering practitioner before administering the drug.

Example 1:

A child is 126 cm tall and weighs 23 kg. The drug order reads: *Oncovin (vincristine) 1.8 mg IV at 10 AM.* Is this dosage safe for this child? The recommended dosage as noted on the package instructions is 2 mg/m^2, Figure 15-4. Supply: Oncovin 2 mg/2 mL

1. **Determine BSA.** The child's BSA is 0.9 m^2 (using the West Nomogram, Figure 15-1).
2. **Calculate recommended dosage.** $mg/m^2 \times m^2 = \frac{2 \text{ mg}}{\cancel{m^2}} \times 0.9 \cancel{m^2} = 1.8$ mg
3. **Decide if the dosage is safe.** The dosage is safe. How much should you give?

10:00

ONCOVIN®

VINCRISTINE SULFATE INJECTION, USP

SOLUTION

Oncovin must be administered via an intact, free-flowing intravenous needle or catheter. Care should be taken that there is no leakage or swelling occurring during administration (*see* Caution statement *under* Description).

The solution may be injected either directly into a vein or into the tubing of a running intravenous infusion (*see* Drug Interactions below). Injection of Oncovin should be accomplished within 1 minute.

The drug is administered intravenously *at weekly intervals*.

The usual dose of Oncovin for children is 2 mg/m^2. For children weighing 10 kg or less, the starting dose should be 0.05 mg/kg, administered once a week.

DOSAGE AND ADMINISTRATION

This preparation is for intravenous use only (see Warnings).

Neurotoxicity appears to be dose related. Extreme care must be used in calculating and administering the dose of Oncovin since overdosage may have a very serious or fatal outcome.

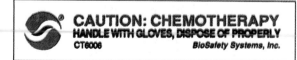

FIGURE 15-4 Portion of Oncovin Package Insert

4. **Calculate one dose**

STEP 1	**CONVERT**	No conversion is necessary.
STEP 2	**THINK**	You want to give more than 1 mL and less than 2 mL.
STEP 3	**CALCULATE**	$\frac{D}{H} \times Q = \frac{1.8 \text{ mg}}{2 \text{ mg}} \times 2 \text{ mL} = 1.8 \text{ mL}$

Or, use ratio-proportion.

$$\frac{2 \text{ mg}}{2 \text{ mL}} \times \frac{1.8 \text{ mg}}{X \text{ mL}}$$

$2X = 3.6$

$\frac{2X}{2} = \frac{3.6}{2}$

$X = 1.8 \text{ mL}$

Example 2:

The child is 35 inches tall and weighs 30 lb. The drug order reads, *Periactin syrup 5 mg po b.i.d.* Is this dosage safe? The drug reference recommended 8 mg/m^2/day divided into 3 equal doses. Periactin syrup is supplied as 2 mg/5 mL.

1. **Determine BSA.** The child's BSA is 0.6 m^2 (using the West Nomogram, Figure 15-1).
2. **Calculate recommended dosage.** $\text{mg/m}^2 \times \text{m}^2 = \frac{8 \text{ mg}}{\text{m}^2} \times 0.6 \text{ m}^2$

   $= 4.8$ mg (per day; divided into 3 doses)

   $\frac{4.8 \text{ mg}}{3 \text{ doses}} = 1.6$ mg per dose.
3. **Decide if dosage is safe.** The dosage is too high and is not safe.
4. **Confer with the prescribing practitioner.** Perhaps the practitioner meant 5 mL, which would have been a more reasonable dose, but you must not assume anything.

quick review

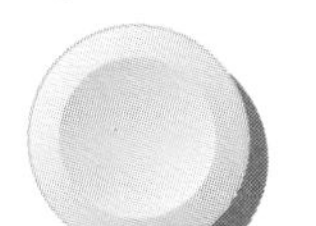

Safe dosage is based on BSA: mg/m^2 × m^2, compared to recommended dosage.

review set 46

1. What is the dosage of one dose of Interferon Alpha-2b required for a child with a BSA of 0.82 m^2 if the recommended dosage is 2 million units/m^2? __________ units
2. What is the total daily dosage range of Mitomycin required for a child with a BSA of 0.59 m^2 if the recommended dosage range is 10 to 20 mg/m^2/day? __________ to __________ mg/day
3. What is the dosage of Calcium EDTA required for an adult with a BSA of 1.47 m^2 if the recommended dosage is 500 mg/m^2? __________ mg
4. What is the total daily dosage of Thioplex required for an adult with a BSA of 2.64 m^2 if the recommended dosage is 6 mg/m^2/day? __________ mg. After 4 full days of therapy, this patient will have received a total of __________ mg of Thioplex.

5. What is the dosage of acyclovir required for a child with a BSA of 1 m^2, if the recommended dosage is 250 mg/m^2? __________ mg

6. Child is 30 inches tall and weighs 25 pounds.

   Order: *Zovirax (acyclovir) 250 mg/m^2 IV q.8h*

   Supply: Acyclovir 50 mg/mL

   Give: __________ mL

7. Child is 45 inches tall and weighs 55 pounds.

   Order: *Methotrexate 3.3 mg/m^2 IV q.d.*

   Supply: Methotrexate 5 mg/2 mL

   Give: __________ mL

8. Order: *Give Benoject (diphenhydramine hydrochloride) 22 mg IV q.8h.* Child has BSA of 0.44 m^2. Recommended safe dosage of Benoject is 150 mg/m^2/day in divided dosages every 6 to 8 hours. Is this a safe dosage? __________

9. Order: *Give quinidine 198 mg p.o. q.d. for 5 days.* Child has BSA of 0.22 m^2. Recommended safe dosage of quinidine is 900 mg/m^2/day given in 5 daily doses. Verify safe dosage, and calculate total milligrams received over 5 days of therapy. __________ mg.

10. Order: *Deferoxamine mesylate IV per protocol.* Child has BSA of 1.02 m^2.

    Protocol: 600 mg/m^2 initially followed by 300 mg/m^2 at 4 hour intervals for 2 doses; then give 300 mg/m^2 q.12h for 2 days. Calculate the total dosage received. __________ mg

11. Order: *Fludara (fludarabine phosphate) 10 mg/m^2 bolus over 15 minutes followed by a continuous IV infusion of 30.5 mg/m^2/day.* Child has BSA of 0.81 m^2. The bolus dosage is __________ mg, and the continuous 24-hour IV infusion will contain __________ mg of Fludara.

12. Order: *Accutane (isotretinoin) 83.75 mg IV q.12h for a child with a BSA of 0.67m^2.* The recommended safe dosage range is 100 to 250 mg/m^2/day in 2 divided doses. Is this dosage safe? __________

13. Order: *Cerubidine (daunorubicin hydrochloride) 9.6 mg IV on day 1 and day 8 of cycle.*

    Protocol: 25 to 45 mg/m^2 on days 1 and 8 of cycle. Child has BSA of 0.32 m^2. Is this dosage safe? __________

Answer items #14 and 15 based on the following information.

The recommended dosage of Oncaspar is 2500 units/m^2/dose IV daily for adults and children.

Supply: Oncaspar 750 units/mL with directions to give in total of 100 mL D_5W over 2 hours. You will administer the drug via infusion pump.

14. Order: *Give Oncaspar (pegaspargase) 2050 units IV today @ 1600.* Child is 100 cm tall and weighs 24 kg. The child's BSA is __________ m^2. Is the ordered dosage of Oncaspar safe? __________ If yes, the amount added to IV fluid is __________ mL, and the IV pump would be set for __________ mL/h.

15. An adult patient is 162 cm tall and weighs 128 pounds. The patient's BSA is __________ m^2. The safe dosage of Oncaspar for this adult is __________ mg. The amount to be added to the IV fluid for this infusion is __________ mL.

After completing these problems, see page 455 to check your answers.

Pediatric Volume Control Sets

Volume control sets, Figure 15-5, are most frequently used to administer hourly fluids and intermittent IV medications to children. They are usually referred to by their trade names, Buretrol, Volutrol, or Soluset. The fluid chamber will hold 100 to 150 milliliters of fluid to be infused in a specified time period as ordered, usually 60 minutes or less. The medication is added to the IV fluid in the chamber for a prescribed dilution volume.

The volume of fluid in the chamber is filled by the nurse every 1 to 2 hours or as needed. Only small, ordered quantities of fluid are added, and the clamp above the chamber is fully closed. The IV bag only acts as a reservoir to hold future fluid infusions. This differs from adult IV infusions that run directly from the IV bag through the drip chamber and IV tubing into the patient's vein. The patient is protected from receiving more volume than intended. This is especially important for children, because they can tolerate only a narrow range of fluid volume.

Volume control sets like Buretrol may also be used to administer intermittent IV medications to adults with fluid restrictions, such as for heart or kidney disease. An electronic controller or pump may also be used to regulate the flow rate. When used, the electronic device will alarm when the Buretrol chamber empties.

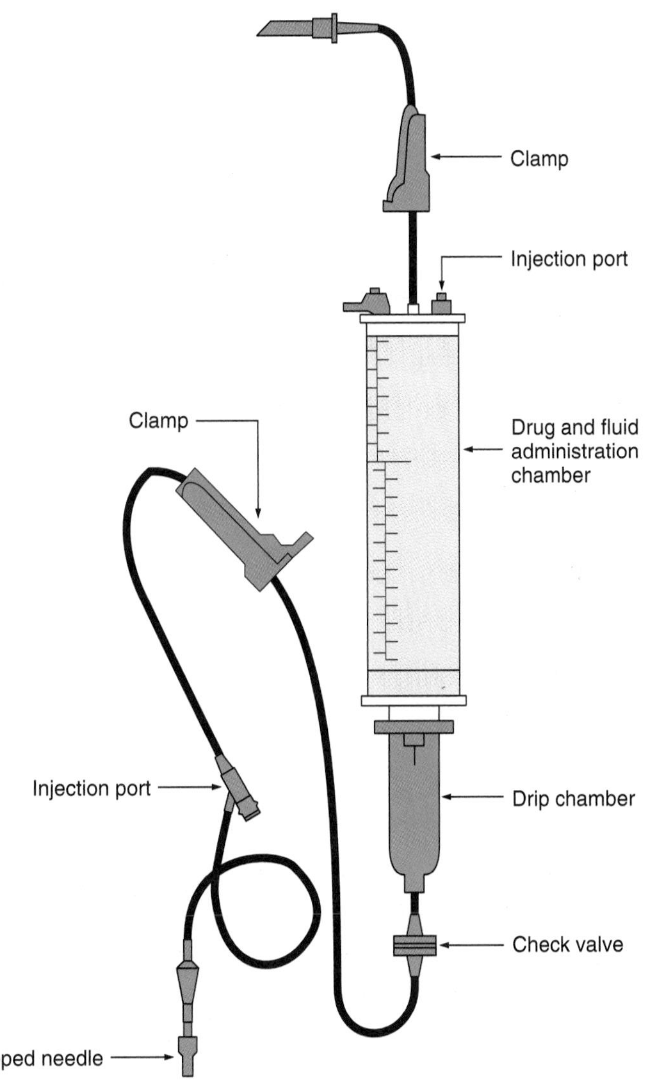

FIGURE 15-5 Volume Control Set (Buretrol, Volutrol, or Soluset)

Intermittent IV Medication Infusion via Volume Control Set Chamber

Children receiving IV medications frequently have a saline or heparin lock in place of a continuous IV infusion. The nurse will inject the medication into the volume control set chamber, add an appropriate volume of IV fluid to dilute the drug, and attach the IV tubing to the child's IV lock to infuse over a specified period of time. After the chamber has emptied and the medication has infused, a flush of IV fluid is given to be sure all the medication has cleared the tubing. Realize that when the chamber empties, some medication still remains in the drip chamber, IV tubing, and the IV lock above the child's vein. There is no standard amount of fluid used to flush peripheral or central IV lines. Because tubing varies by manufacturer, the flush can vary from 15 mL to as much as 50 mL, according to the overall length of the tubing and extra extensions added. Verify your hospital policy on the correct volume to flush peripheral and central IV lines in children. For the purpose of sample calculations, this text uses a 15 mL volume to flush a peripheral IV line, unless specified otherwise.

To calculate the IV flow rate for the volume control set, you must consider the total fluid volume of the medication, the IV fluid used for dilution, and the volume of IV flush fluid. Volume control sets are microdrip sets with a drop factor of 60 gtt/mL.

Example:

Order: *Kefzol 250 mg q.8h in 50 mL $D_5 \frac{1}{4}$ NS to infuse in 60 min followed by a 15 mL flush.* Child has a saline lock.

Supply: Kefzol is reconstituted to 125 mg/mL.

STEP 1 Calculate the total volume of the intermittent IV medication and the IV flush.

50 mL + 15 mL = 65 mL

STEP 2 Calculate the flow rate of the IV medication and IV flush. Remember: the drop factor is 60 gtt/mL. Think: mL/h = gtt/min when drop factor is 60 gtt/mL.

$$\frac{V}{T} \times C = \frac{65 \text{ \cancel{mL}}}{60 \text{ min}} \times 60 \text{ gtt/\cancel{mL}} = 65 \text{ gtt/min}$$

STEP 3 Calculate the volume of the medication to be administered.

$$\frac{D}{H} \times Q = \frac{\overset{2}{\cancel{250} \text{ \cancel{mg}}}}{\underset{1}{\cancel{125} \text{ \cancel{mg}}}} \times 1 \text{ mL} = 2 \text{ mL}$$

STEP 4 Calculate the volume of IV fluid needed to add to the volume control set (Buretrol) chamber for a dilution volume of 50 mL. 50 mL – 2 mL = 48 mL. Run a total of 48 mL 0.9% NaCl into the Buretrol chamber, and add 2 mL of Kefzol. This provides the prescribed volume of 50 mL in the chamber.

STEP 5 Set the flow rate of the 50 mL of intermittent IV medication for 65 gtt/min. Follow with the 15 mL flush also set at 65 gtt/min. When complete, detach IV tubing, and follow saline lock policy.

The patient may also have an intermittent medication ordered as part of a continuous infusion at a prescribed IV volume per hour. In such cases the patient is to receive the same fluid volume each hour, regardless of the addition of intermittent medications. This means that the total prescribed fluid volume must include the intermittent IV medication volume.

EXAMPLE:

Order: *D_5NS IV at 30 mL/h for continuous infusion and Ancef 125 mg IV q.6h*

Supply: Ancef 125 mg/mL with instructions to "add to Buretrol and infuse over 30 minutes"

An infusion controller is in use with the Buretrol.

STEP 1 Calculate the dilution volume required to administer the Ancef at the prescribed continuous flow rate of 30 mL/h.

THINK If 30 mL infuses in 1 h, then $\frac{1}{2}$ of 30, or 15 mL, will infuse in $\frac{1}{2}$ h or 30 min.

CALCULATE Use ratio-proportion to verify your estimate.

$$\frac{30 \text{ mL}}{60 \text{ min}} \times \frac{X \text{ mL}}{30 \text{ min}}$$

$$60X = 900$$

$$\frac{60X}{60} = \frac{900}{60}$$

$$X = 15 \text{ mL}$$

Therefore, the IV fluid dilution volume required to administer 125 mg of Ancef in 30 minutes is 15 mL to maintain the prescribed, continuous infusion rate of 30 mL/h.

STEP 2 Determine the volume of Ancef and IV fluid to add to the Buretrol. 125 mg/mL Ancef available and 125 mg ordered. Add 14 mL D_5NS and 1 mL Ancef for a total volume of 15 mL.

STEP 3 Set the controller to 30 mL/h to deliver 15 mL of intermittent IV Ancef solution in 30 minutes. Resume the regular IV, which will also flush out the tubing. The continuous flow rate will remain at 30 mL/h.

quick review

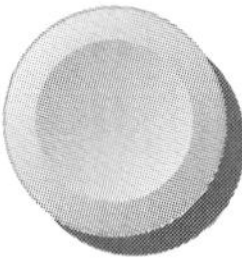

- Volume control sets have a drop factor of 60 gtt/mL.
- The total volume of the medication, IV dilution fluid, and the IV flush fluid must be considered to calculate flow rates when using sets like Buretrol.
- Use ratio-proportion to calculate flow rates for intermittent medications when a continuous IV rate in mL/h is prescribed.

review set 47

Calculate the IV flow rate to administer the following IV medications by using a volume control set, and determine the amount of IV fluid and medication to be added to the chamber. The ordered time includes the flush volume.

1. Order: *Antibiotic X 60 mg IV q.8h in 50 mL $D_5 \frac{1}{3}$NS over 45 min. Flush with 15 mL.*

   Supply: Antibiotic X 60 mg/2 mL

   Flow rate: __________ gtt/min

   Add __________ mL medication and __________ mL IV fluid.

2. Order: *Medication Y 75 mg IV q.6h in 60 mL $D_5\frac{1}{4}$NS over 60 min. Flush with 15 mL.*

   Supply: Medication Y 75 mg/3 mL

   Flow rate: __________ gtt/min

   Add __________ mL medication and __________ mL IV fluid.

3. Order: *Antibiotic Z 15 mg IV b.i.d. in 25 mL 0.9% NaCl over 20 min. Flush with 15 mL.*

   Supply: Antibiotic Z 15 mg 3 mL

   Flow rate: __________ gtt/min

   Add __________ mL medication and __________ mL IV fluid.

4. Order: *Ancef (cefazolin) 0.6 g IV q.12h in 50 mL D_5NS over 60 min on an infusion pump. Flush with 30 mL.*

   Supply: Ancef 1 g/10 mL

   Flow rate: __________ mL/h.

   Add __________ mL medication and __________ mL IV fluid.

5. Order: *Cleocin (clindamycin) 150 mg IV q.8h in 32 mL D_5NS over 60 min on an infusion pump. Flush with 28 mL.*

   Supply: Cleocin 150 mg/mL

   Flow rate: __________ mL/h.

   Add __________ mL medication and __________ mL IV fluid.

   Total IV volume after 3 doses are given is __________ mL.

Calculate the amount of medication and IV fluid to be added to the volume control chamber.

6. Order: *0.9% NaCl at 50 mL/h for continuous infusion with Ancef 250 mg IV q.8h to be infused over 30 min by Buretrol.*

   Supply: Ancef 125 mg/mL

   Add __________ mL medication and __________ mL IV fluid.

7. Order: *D_5W at 30 mL/h for continuous infusion with Medication X 60 mg q.6h to be infused over 20 min by Buretrol.*

   Supply: Medication X 60 mg/2 mL

   Add __________ mL medication and __________ mL IV fluid.

8. Order: *D_5 0.225% NaCl IV at 85 mL/h with Erythromycin 600 mg IV q.6h to be infused over 40 min by Buretrol.*

   Supply: Erythromycin 50 mg/mL.

   Add __________ mL medication and __________ mL IV fluid.

9. Order: *D_5 0.33% NaCl IV at 66 mL/h with Fortaz 720 mg IV q.8h to be infused over 40 min by Buretrol.*

   Supply: Fortaz 1 g/10 mL.

   Add __________ mL medication and __________ mL IV fluid.

10. Order: *D_5 0.45% NaCl IV at 48 mL/h with Vibramycin 75 mg IV q.12h to be infused over 2 h by Buretrol.*

    Supply: Vibramycin 100 mg/10 mL.

    Add __________ mL medication and __________ mL IV fluid.

After completing these problems, see pages 455 and 456 to check your answers.

Preparing Pediatric IVs

The physician may order a medication such as potassium chloride (KCl) to be added to an IV fluid for continuous infusion. The volume of the IV solution bag selected for children is usually smaller than that for adults, since the total volume required per 24 hours is less. Therefore, the amount of medication to be added must be adjusted proportionately to the total volume of the IV bag. Use ratio-proportion to determine the appropriate amount of medication to add to the prescribed dilution.

Example 1:

Order: *$D_5 \frac{1}{2}$ NS IV c̄ 20 mEq KCl/L to infuse at 30 mL/h*

1. Should you choose a 1 liter (1000 mL) or 500 mL bag of IV fluid?

   30 mL/h × 24 h = 720 mL

   At the rate of 30 mL/h, the child would receive only 720 mL in 24 hours, so you should choose a 500 mL bag of $D_5 \frac{1}{2}$ NS rather than a one liter or 1000 mL bag.
2. How many mEq of KCl should you add to the 500 mL bag?

STEP 1 CONVERT 1 L = 1000 mL

STEP 2 THINK 500 mL is $\frac{1}{2}$ of 1000 mL so you would need $\frac{1}{2}$ of the 20 mEq of KCl or 10 mEq.

STEP 3 CALCULATE

$$\frac{20 \text{ mEq}}{1000 \text{ mL}} \times \frac{X \text{ mEq}}{500 \text{ mL}}$$

$$1000X = 10,000$$

$$\frac{1000X}{1000} = \frac{10,000}{1000}$$

$$X = 10 \text{ mEq}$$

3. Potassium chloride is available in 2 mEq per mL. How much KCl should you add to the 500 mL IV bag?

STEP 1 CONVERT No conversions are needed.

STEP 2 THINK You want to give more than 1 mL. In fact, you want to give 5 times 1 mL or 5 mL.

STEP 3 CALCULATE

$$\frac{D}{H} \times Q = \frac{\overset{5}{\cancel{10} \text{ mEq}}}{\underset{1}{\cancel{2} \text{ mEq}}} \times 1 \text{ mL} = 5 \text{ mL}$$

Example 2:

Child is 9 years old and weighs 64 pounds.

Order: *$D_5 \frac{1}{3}$NS c̄ aminophylline 1 g/L at 30 mL/h*

Supply: aminophylline 500 mg/20 mL and a 500 mL bag of $D_5 \frac{1}{3}$NS

1. How many mg aminophylline should be added to the 500 mL bag?

STEP 1 CONVERT 1 g = 1000 mg; 1 L = 1000 mL

STEP 2 THINK You will use a bag that is $\frac{1}{2}$ of 1 L (500 mL), so you will add $\frac{1}{2}$ of 1000 mg or 500 mg.

STEP 3 CALCULATE

$$\frac{1000 \text{ mg}}{1000 \text{ mL}} \times \frac{X \text{ mg}}{500 \text{ mL}}$$

$$1000X = 500,000$$

$$\frac{1000X}{1000} = \frac{500,000}{1000}$$

$$X = 500 \text{ mg}$$

2. How many mL aminophylline should be added to the 500 mL bag?

STEP 1 CONVERT No conversions are needed.

STEP 2 THINK The answer is obvious. There are 500 mg/20 mL; you need 500 mg, so you will add 20 mL.

STEP 3 CALCULATE No calculations are necessary.

3. How many mg of aminophylline will the child receive per hour?

Total IV volume: 500 mL + 20 mL = 520 mL

$$\frac{500 \text{ mg}}{520 \text{ mL}} \times \frac{X \text{ mg/h}}{30 \text{ mL/h}}$$

$$520X = 15,000$$

$$\frac{520X}{520} = \frac{15,000}{520}$$

$$X = 28.8 \text{ or } 29 \text{ mg/h}$$

4. The recommended maintenance dosage of aminophylline for children 1 to 9 years is 1 mg/kg/h. Based on the recommended maintenance dosage, is 29 mg/h a safe dosage?

   1. **Convert lb to kg.** 1 kg = 2.2 lb; 64 lb = $\frac{64}{2.2}$ = 29.09 = 29.1 kg
   2. **Calculate recommended dosage.** 1 mg/~~kg~~/h × 29.1 ~~kg~~ = 29.1 or 29 mg/h
   3. **Decide if the dosage is safe.** Yes, 29 mg/h is recommended, and the rate of 30 mL/h will deliver 29 mg/h.

quick review

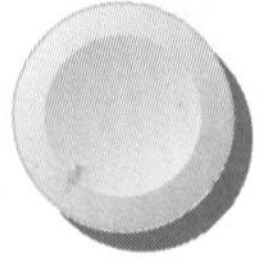

To determine the drug dosage required to prepare a prescribed dilution:

- use ratio-proportion

review set 48

Order: *$D_5W\frac{1}{2}$ NS IV c̄ 20 mEq KCl per L to infuse at 15 mL/h*

Supply: 250 mL $D_5W\frac{1}{2}$ NS and KCl 2 mEq/mL

1. How many mEq KCl should be added to the 250 mL bag? __________ mEq

2. How many mL KCl should

3. How many mEq of KCl wi

Order: *D_5NS IV c̄ aminophyllin*

Supply: Aminophylline 500 m

Child is 8 years old and wei

4. How many mg amin

5. How many mL ami

6. How many mg of

7. The recommend
1 mg/kg/h. Base
aminophylline

8. Is the dosage

Calculate the ordered ... centration. Supply: KCl 2 mEq/...

9. Order: *Add 10 mEq KCl/L of IV fluid.*

   Supply: 480 mL IV solution __________ mEq; __________

10. Order: *Add 20 mEq KCl/L of IV fluid.*

    Supply: 260 mL IV solution __________ mEq; __________ mL

11. Order: *Add 30 mEq KCl/L of IV fluid.*

    Supply: 600 mL IV solution __________ mEq; __________ mL

12. Order: *Add 15 mEq KCl/L of IV fluid.*

    Supply: 850 mL IV solution __________ mEq; __________ mL

After completing these problems, see page 456 to check your answers.

Minimal Dilutions for IV Medications

Intravenous medications in infants and young children (including adults on limited fluids) are often ordered to be given in the smallest volume or *maximal safe concentration* to prevent fluid overload. Consult a pediatric reference, *Hospital Formulary*, or drug insert to assist you in problem-solving. These types of medications are usually given via an electronic pump.

Many pediatric IV medications allow a dilution *range* or a minimum and maximum allowable concentration. A solution of *lower* concentration may be given if the patient can tolerate the added volume (called *minimal safe concentration, maximal dilution, or largest volume*). A solution of *higher* concentration (called *maximal safe concentration, minimal dilution, or smallest volume*) must not exceed the recommended dilution instructions. Recall that the greater the volume of diluent or solvent, the less concentrated is the resulting solution. Likewise, less volume of diluent or solvent results in a more concentrated solution.

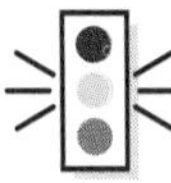

Caution: An excessively high concentration of an IV drug can cause vein irritation and potentially life-threatening toxic effects. Dilution calculations are critical skills.

to follow the drug reference recommendations for a minimal IV drug
imal and maximal range is given for an IV drug dilution.

ommended drug dilution equals ratio for desired drug dilution.

ample 1:

The physician orders 40 mg of Vancocin IV for an infant who weighs 4000 g. What is the minimal amount of IV fluid in which the vancomycin can be safely diluted? The package insert is provided for your reference, Figure 15-6. It states that a "concentration of no more than 10 mg/mL is recommended." This is the *maximal safe concentration.*

$$\frac{10 \text{ mg}}{1 \text{ mL}} \times \frac{40 \text{ mg}}{\text{X mL}}$$

$$10\text{X} = 40$$

$$\frac{10\text{X}}{10} = \frac{40}{10}$$

$$\text{X} = 4 \text{ mL}$$

8:12 PA 8289 AMP

VIALS

VANCOCIN® HCl

STERILE VANCOMYCIN HYDROCHLORIDE, USP

INTRAVENOUS

DOSAGE AND ADMINISTRATION

A concentration of no more than 10 mg/mL is recommended. An infusion of 10 mg/min or less is associated with fewer infusion-related events (*see* Adverse Reactions).

Patients With Normal Renal Function

Adults—The usual daily intravenous dose is 2 g divided either as 500 mg every 6 hours or 1 g every 12 hours. Each dose should be administered over a period of at least 60 minutes. Other patient factors, such as age or obesity, may call for modification of the usual daily intravenous dose.

Children—The total daily intravenous dosage of Vancocin HCl, calculated on the basis of 40 mg/kg of body weight, can be divided and incorporated into the child's 24-hour fluid requirement. Each dose should be administered over a period of at least 60 minutes.

Infants and Neonates—In neonates and young infants, the total daily intravenous dosage may be lower. In both neonates and infants, an initial dose of 15 mg/kg is suggested, followed by 10 mg/kg every 12 hours for neonates in the 1st week of life and every 8 hours thereafter up to the age of 1 month. Close monitoring of serum concentrations of vancomycin may be warranted in these patients.

FIGURE 15-6 Portion of Vancocin Package Insert

Example 2:

The physician orders cefotaxime sodium (Claforan) 1.2 g IV q.8h for a child who weighs 36 kg. The recommended safe administration of Claforan for intermittent IV administration is a final concentration of 20 to 60 mg/mL to infuse over 15 to 30 minutes. What is the minimal amount of IV fluid to safely dilute this dosage? (Remember this represents the maximal safe concentration.)

STEP 1 CONVERT 1.2 g = 1200 mg

STEP 2 THINK 1200 is more than 10 times 60, in fact it is 20 times 60. So you need at least 20 mL to dilute the drug.

STEP 3 CALCULATE

$$\frac{60\text{ mg}}{1\text{ mL}} \times \frac{1200\text{ mg}}{X\text{ mL}}$$

$$60X = 1200$$

$$\frac{60X}{60} = \frac{1200}{60}$$

X = 20 mL (minimal dilution for maximal safe concentration)

What is the maximal amount of IV fluid recommended to safely dilute this drug to the minimal safe concentration?

STEP 1 CONVERT 1.2 g = 1200 mg

STEP 2 THINK 1200 is more than 50 times 20, in fact it is 60 times 20. So you can use up to 60 mL to dilute the drug.

STEP 3 CALCULATE

$$\frac{20\text{ mg}}{1\text{ mL}} \times \frac{1200\text{ mg}}{X\text{ mL}}$$

$$20X = 1200$$

$$\frac{20X}{20} = \frac{1200}{20}$$

X = 60 mL (maximal dilution for minimal safe concentration)

Calculation of Daily Volume for Maintenance Fluids

Another common pediatric IV calculation is to calculate 24-hour maintenance IV fluids for children.

rule

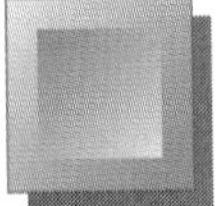

Use this formula to calculate the daily rate of pediatric maintenance IV fluids.

100 mL/kg/day for first 10 kg of body weight

50 mL/kg/day for next 10 kg of body weight

20 mL/kg/day for each kg above 20 kg of body weight

This formula uses the child's weight in kilograms to estimate the 24-hour total fluid need, including oral intake. It does not include replacement for losses, such as diarrhea, vomiting, or fever. This only accounts for fluid needed to maintain normal cellular metabolism and fluid turnover.

Pediatric IV solutions that run over 24 hours usually include a combination of glucose, saline, and potassium chloride and are *hypertonic* solutions, Figure 14-1, page 287. Dextrose (glucose) for energy, is usually concentrated between 5% and 12% for peripheral infusions. Sodium chloride is usually concentrated between 0.225% and 0.9% ($\frac{1}{4}$ NS up to NS). Further, 20 mEq per liter of potassium chloride (20 mEq KCl/L) are usually added to continuous pediatric infusions. Any dextrose and saline combination without potassium should only be used as an intermittent or short-term IV fluid in children. Be wary of isotonic solutions like 5% dextrose in water and 0.9% sodium chloride. They do not contribute enough electrolytes and can quickly lead to water intoxication.

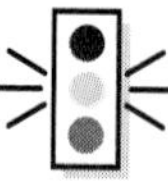

Caution: A *red flag* should go up if either plain 5% dextrose in water or 0.9% sodium chloride (normal saline) are running continuously on an infant or child. Consult the ordering practitioner immediately!

Let's examine the daily rate of maintenance fluids and the hourly flow rate for the children in some examples.

Example 1:

Child who weighs 6 kg

$100 \text{ mL}/\cancel{\text{kg}}/\text{day} \times 6 \cancel{\text{kg}} = 600 \text{ mL/day}$ or per 24 h

$\frac{600 \text{ mL}}{24 \text{ h}} = 25 \text{ mL/h}$

Example 2:

Child who weighs 12 kg

$100 \text{ mL}/\cancel{\text{kg}}/\text{day} \times 10 \cancel{\text{kg}} = 1000 \text{ mL/day}$ (for first 10 kg)

$50 \text{ mL}/\cancel{\text{kg}}/\text{day} \times 2 \cancel{\text{kg}} = 100 \text{ mL/day}$ (for the remaining 2 kg)

Total: 1000 mL/day + 100 mL/day = 1100 mL/day or per 24 h

$\frac{1100 \text{ mL}}{24 \text{ h}} = 45.8$ or 46 mL/h

Example 3:

Child who weighs 24 kg

$100 \text{ mL}/\cancel{\text{kg}}/\text{day} \times 10 \cancel{\text{kg}} = 1000 \text{ mL/day}$ (for first 10 kg)

$50 \text{ mL}/\cancel{\text{kg}}/\text{day} \times 10 \cancel{\text{kg}} = 500 \text{ mL/day}$ (for next 10 kg)

$20 \text{ mL}/\cancel{\text{kg}}/\text{day} \times 4 \cancel{\text{kg}} = 80 \text{ mL/day}$ (for the remaining 4 kg)

Total = 1000 mL/day + 500 mL/day + 80 mL/day = 1580 mL/day or per 24 h

$\frac{1580 \text{ mL}}{24 \text{ h}} = 65.8$ or 66 mL/h

quick review

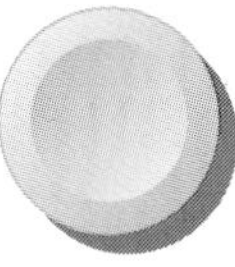

- Minimal and maximal dilution volumes for some IV drugs are recommended to prevent fluid overload and to minimize vein irritation and toxic effects.
- The ratio for recommended dilution equals the ratio for desired drug dilution.
- When mixing IV drug solutions,
  - the *smaller* the added volume, the *stronger or higher* the resulting *concentration* (minimal dilution).
  - the *larger* the added volume, the *weaker (more dilute) or lower* the resulting *concentration* (maximal dilution).
- Daily volume of pediatric maintenance IV fluids based on body weight is:
  - 100 mL/kg/day for first 10 kg.
  - 50 mL/kg/day for next 10 kg.
  - 20 mL/kg/day for each kg above 20 kg.

review set 49

1. If a child is receiving chloramphenicol 400 mg IV q.6h and the maximum concentration is 100 mg/mL, what is the minimum volume of fluid in which the medication can be safely diluted? __________ mL
2. If a child is receiving Gentamicin 25 mg IV q.8h and the minimal concentration is 1 mg/mL, what is the maximum volume of fluid in which the medication can be safely diluted? __________ mL
3. Calculate the hourly IV flow rate for a 25 kg child receiving maintenance IV fluids. __________ mL/h
4. Calculate the hourly IV flow rate for a 13 kg child receiving maintenance IV fluids. __________ mL/h
5. Calculate the hourly IV flow rate for a 77 lb child receiving maintenance fluids. __________ mL/h
6. Calculate the hourly IV flow rate for an 8 lb infant receiving maintenance fluids. __________ mL/h
7. A child is receiving 350 mg IV of a certain medication, and the minimal and maximal dilution range is 30 to 100 mg/mL. What is the minimum volume (maximal concentration) and the maximum volume (minimal concentration) for safe dilution? __________ mL (minimum volume); __________ mL (maximum volume).
8. A child is receiving 52 mg IV of a certain medication, and the minimal and maximal dilution range is 0.8 to 20 mg/mL. What is the minimum volume and the maximum volume of fluid for safe dilution? __________ mL (minimum volume); __________ mL (maximum volume).
9. A child is receiving 175 mg IV of a certain medication, and the minimal and maximal dilution range is 5 to 75 mg/mL. What is the minimum volume and the maximum volume of fluid for safe dilution? __________ mL (minimum volume); __________ mL (maximum volume).
10. Order: *Methicillin sodium 830 mg IV q.6 h.* Child weighs 42 lb. The child's IV of D_5 0.33% NaCl with 20 mEq KCl/L is infusing continuously at 63 mL/h. Drug reference states "IV methicillin sodium: 150–200 mg/kg/day in 4 equally divided doses. Intermittent IV infusion over 15 to 30 minutes at a final concentration not to exceed 20 mg/mL." The safe dosage range for this child is __________ to __________ mg/dose. Is this dosage safe? __________ Supply available: Methicillin sodium 1 g/10 mL. Calculate the amount to be added to the volume control set chamber to infuse over 30 minutes. Add __________ mL medication and __________ mL IV fluid.

After completing these problems, see page 456 and 457 to check your answers.

critical thinking skills

Let's look at an example in which the nurse *prevents* a medication error by calculating the safe dosage of a medication before administering the drug to a child.

error

Dosage that is too high for a child.

possible scenario

Suppose a physician ordered aminophylline 500 mg IV to be diluted in 500 mL of $D_5 \frac{1}{4}$ NS to run at a rate of 22 mL/h. The child weighed 22 lb. The nurse looked up aminophylline in the pediatric reference guide and noted that the safe dosage of aminophylline is 1 mg/kg/h. The nurse converted the child's weight to kilograms and calculated the safe dosage:

$$22 \text{ lb} = \frac{22}{2.2} = 10 \text{ kg}$$

$1 \text{ mg}/\cancel{\text{kg}}/\text{h} \times 10 \text{ kg} = 10 \text{ mg/h}$; the safe dosage for this child.

The nurse calculated that the 10 kg child should receive 10 mL per hour of aminophylline, because if there are 500 mg in 500 mL then there is 1 mg/mL of aminophylline being delivered. At a rate of 22 mL/h, the child would have received 22 mg of aminophylline. It occurred to the nurse that possibly the physician ordered the dosage based on the child's weight in pounds not kilograms. The nurse notified the physician and questioned the order. The physician responded, "Thank you. You are correct. I did order the dosage based on the child's weight in pounds. This was my error. I'm glad you caught it." The physician then decreased the rate of the aminophylline drip to 10 mL/h.

potential outcome

If the nurse had not questioned the order, the child would have received the dosage of 22 mg of aminophylline every hour. The child likely would have developed signs of toxicity beginning with irritability, tachycardia, and progressing to nausea, vomiting, and possibly cardiac arrhythmia and seizures. The severity of the symptoms would be directly related to how long the infusion occurred at double the therapeutic rate.

prevention

This is an instance in which the nurse prevented a medication error by checking the safe dosage and notifying the physician before administering the infusion. Let this be you!

practice problems—chapter 15

Calculate the volume for one dosage. Refer to the West Nomogram on page 349 as needed.

1. Order: *Gentamicin 18 mg IVPB q.8h for a 20 lb child.* The drug reference recommends Gentamicin 2 mg/kg IV.

   Supply: Gentamicin 20 mg/2 mL

   Give: __________ mL

2. The doctor orders Somophyllin 175 mg orally as a loading dosage for a 66 lb child. The drug insert recommends not to exceed 5 mg/kg for the initial loading dosage. Somophyllin is supplied in a dosage strength of 105 mg per 5 mL. Is the dosage ordered safe? __________ What would you do next? ______________________________

3. Order: (Child of normal proportions who weighs 25 pounds) *Mercaptopurine 41 mg p.o. q.d. in AM computed per BSA nomogram*

   Recommended dosage: 80 mg/m^2/day once daily.

   Supply: 50 mg/mL

   Give: __________ mL

4. Order: (1-year-old child, 25 inches tall, weighs 20 pounds) *Sargramostim IV at 10 AM computed per BSA*

   Recommended dosage: 250 mcg/m^2/day once daily.

   The safe dosage the child should receive is __________ mcg.

5. Sargramostim is available in a solution strength of 500 mcg/10 mL. Calculate one dose for the child in #4. __________ mL

6. Use the BSA nomogram to calculate the safe dosage of oral Levodopa for a child who is 35 inches tall and weighs 40 pounds. Recommended dosage: 0.5 g/m^2. Give: __________ mg

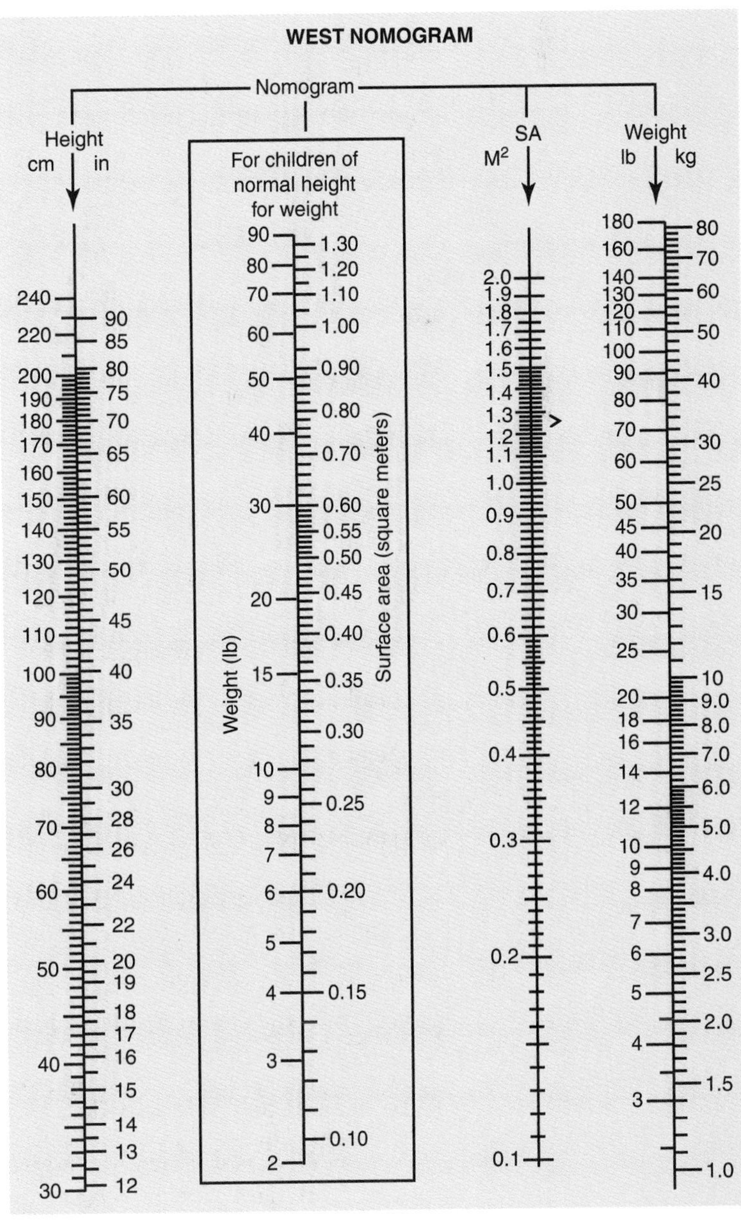

West's Nomogram for Estimation of Body Surface Area. (From *Nelson Textbook of Pediatrics* (15th ed.) by R. E. Behrman, R. M. Kleigman, & A. M. Arvin, 1996, Philadelphia: Saunders. Reprinted with permission.)

7. Levodopa is supplied in 100 mg and 250 mg capsules. Calculate one dose for the child in #6. __________ capsule(s)

8. Determine the safe dosage of IM Oncaspar for a child who is 42 inches tall and weighs 45 pounds. Recommended dosage: 2500 units/m^2/dose. __________ units

9. Oncaspar is reconstituted to 750 units per 1 mL. Calculate one dosage for the child in #8. __________ mL. Should this be given in one injection? __________

10. Order: 55 lb child. *Sandoglobulin 0.2 g/kg IV*

    Supply: Sandoglobulin 6 g/100 mL

    Give: __________ mL

11. Order: 26 lb child. *Ampicillin 50 mg/kg/day IV in equally divided doses q.6h*

    Supply: Ampicillin 125 mg/5 mL

    Give: __________ mL for one dose

12. Order: Child is 55 inches tall and weighs 90 lb. *Adriamycin 20 mg/m^2 IV stat*

    Supply: Adriamycin 2 mg/mL

    Give: __________ mL

For questions #13 through 20, use these formulas to calculate the BSA value. Round BSA to two decimal places.

$$\text{BSA } (\text{m}^2) = \sqrt{\frac{\text{ht (cm)} \times \text{wt (kg) (metric)}}{3600}}$$

$$\text{BSA } (\text{m}^2) = \sqrt{\frac{\text{ht (in)} \times \text{wt (lb) (household)}}{3131}}$$

13. Height: 5 ft 6 in Weight: 136 lb BSA __________ m^2
14. Height: 4 ft Weight: 80 lb BSA __________ m^2
15. Height: 60 cm Weight: 6 kg BSA __________ m^2
16. Height: 68 in Weight: 170 lb BSA __________ m^2
17. Height: 164 cm Weight: 58 kg BSA __________ m^2
18. Height: 100 cm Weight: 17 kg BSA __________ m^2
19. Height: 64 in Weight: 63 kg BSA __________ m^2
20. Height: 85 cm Weight: 11.5 kg BSA __________ m^2
21. What is the safe dosage of one dose of Interferon Alpha-2b required for a child with a BSA of 0.28 m^2, if the recommended dosage is 2 million units/m^2? __________ units

22. What is the safe dosage of Calcium EDTA required for an adult with a BSA of 2.17 m^2, if the recommended dosage is 500 mg/m^2? __________ mg or __________ g

23. What is the total daily dosage range of Mitomycin required for a child with a BSA of 0.19 m^2 if the recommended safe dosage range is 10 to 20 mg/m^2/day? __________ to __________ mg/day

24. What is the total safe daily dosage of Thioplex required for an adult with a BSA of 1.34 m^2, if the recommended safe dosage is 6 mg/m^2/day? __________ mg/day

25. After 5 full days of therapy receiving the recommended dosage, the patient in #24 will have received a total of __________ mg of Thioplex.

26. Order: *Ancef (cefazolin) 0.42 g IV q.12 h in 30 mL D_5NS over 30 min by Buretrol on an infusion controller. Flush with 30 mL.*

    Supply: Cefazolin 500 mg/5 mL

    Flow rate: __________ mL/h Add __________ mL IV fluid to Buretrol

27. After 7 days of IV therapy, the patient referred to in item #26, will have received a total of __________ mL of Ancef.

28. Order: *Clindamycin 285 mg IV q.8h in 45 mL D_5NS over 60 min by Buretrol on an infusion controller. Flush with 25 mL.*

    Supply: Clindamycin 75 mg/0.5 mL

    Flow rate: __________ mL/h Add __________ mL IV fluid to Buretrol

29. After 4 days of Clindamycin therapy, the patient in question #28 will have received a total IV medication volume of __________ mL.

30. Order: *D_5 0.33% NaCl IV at 65 mL/h with Erythromycin 500 mg IV q.h to be infused over 40 min by Buretrol*

    Supply: Erythromycin 50 mg/mL

    Add __________ mL of Erythromycin and __________ mL IV fluid to Buretrol.

31. Order: *D_5 0.45% NaCl IV at 66 mL/h with Fortaz 620 mg IV q.8h to be infused over 40 min by Buretrol*

    Supply: Fortaz 0.5 g/5 mL

    Add __________ mL Fortaz and __________ mL IV fluid to Buretrol.

For questions #32 through 34, calculate the ordered medication for each of the following IV bags to achieve the ordered concentration. Supply: KCl 2 mEq/mL

32. Order: *Add 30 mEq KCl/L of IV fluid.*

    Supply: 360 mL IV solution Add: __________ mEq and __________ mL

33. Order: *Add 20 mEq KCl/L of IV fluid.*

    Supply: 700 mL IV solution Add: __________ mEq and __________ mL

34. Order: *Add 15 mEq KCl/L of IV fluid.*

    Supply: 250 mL IV solution Add: __________ mEq and __________ mL

To calculate the daily volume of pediatric maintenance IV fluids, allow:

100 mL/kg/day for first 10 kg of body weight

50 mL/kg/day for next 10 kg of body weight

20 mL/kg/day for each kg of body weight above 20 kg

35. Calculate the hourly IV flow rate for a 21 kg child receiving maintenance fluids.

    __________ mL/h

36. Calculate the hourly IV flow rate for a 78 lb child receiving maintenance fluids.

    __________ mL/h

37. Calculate the hourly IV flow rate for a 33 lb child receiving maintenance fluids.

    __________ mL/h

38. Calculate the hourly IV flow rate for a 2400 g infant receiving maintenance fluids.

    __________ mL/h

Verify the safety of the following pediatric dosages ordered. If the dosage is safe, calculate one dose and the IV volume to infuse one dose.

Order for a child weighing 15 kg:

D_5 0.45% NaCl IV at 53 mL/h c̄ Ampicillin 275 mg IV q.4h infused over 40 min by Buretrol

Supply: Ampicillin 1 g/10 mL

Recommended dosage: Ampicillin 100–125 mg/kg/day in 6 divided doses

39. Is the ordered dosage safe? __________ If safe, give __________ mL/dose

40. Add __________ mL Ampicillin and __________ mL IV fluid to Buretrol.

Order for a child who weighs 27 lb:

D_5 0.33% NaCl IV at 46 mL/h c̄ Prostaphlin 308 mg IV q.6h to be infused over 30 min by Buretrol

Recommended dosage: Prostaphlin 100 mg/kg/day in 4 divided doses

Supply: Prostaphlin 500 mg/10 mL

41. Is the ordered dosage safe? __________ If safe, give __________ mL Prostaphlin/dose.

42. Add __________ mL Prostaphlin and __________ mL IV fluid to Buretrol.

Order for a child weighing 22 kg:

D_5 0.225% NaCl IV at 50 mL/h c̄ Amikin 165 mg IV q.8h to be infused over 30 min by Buretrol

Recommended dosage: Amikin 15–22.5 mg/kg/day in 3 divided doses q.8h

Supply: Amikin 100 mg/2 mL

43. Is the ordered dosage a safe dose? __________ If safe, give __________ mL/dose

44. Add __________ mL Amikin and __________ mL IV fluid to Buretrol.

Order for a child who weighs 9 kg:

D_5 0.33% NaCl IV at 38 mL/h c̄ Ticar 800 mg IV q.4h to be infused over 40 min by Buretrol

Recommended dosage: Ticar 200–300 mg/kg/day in 6 divided doses every 4 hours

Supply: Ticar 200 mg/mL

45. Is the ordered dosage safe? __________ If safe, give __________ mL/dose.

46. Add __________ mL Ticar and __________ mL IV fluid to Buretrol.

Questions 47–49 refer to the following order for a child who weighs 55 lb:

D_5NS IV at 60 mL/h c̄ Penicillin G potassium 525,000 U q.4h to be infused over 20 min by Buretrol

Recommended dosage: Penicillin G potassium 100,000–250,000 U/kg/day in 6 divided doses q.4h

Supply: Penicillin G potassium 200,000 U/mL

47. Safe dosage range for this child is __________ to __________ U/dose.

48. Is the ordered dosage safe? __________ If safe, give __________ mL/dose.

49. Add __________ mL penicillin G potassium and __________ mL IV fluid to Buretrol.

50. Critical Thinking Skill: Describe the strategy you would implement to prevent this medication error.

possible scenario

Suppose the physician came to the pediatric oncology unit to administer chemotherapy to a critically ill child whose cancer symptoms had recurred suddenly. The nurse assigned to care for the child was floated from the adult oncology unit and was experienced in administering chemotherapy to adults. The physician, recognizing the nurse, said "Oh good, you know how to calculate and prepare chemo. Go draw up 2 mg/m^2 of Oncovin (vincristine) for this child so I can get his chemotherapy started quickly." The nurse consulted the child's chart and saw the following weights written on the assessment sheet: 201.45. No height was recorded.

On the adult unit, that designation means __X__ kg or __Y__ lb. The nurse took the West Nomogram and estimated his BSA based on his weight of 45 lb to be 0.82 m^2. The nurse calculated $2 \text{ mg}/\cancel{m^2} \times 0.82 \cancel{m^2} = 1.64$ mg. Oncovin is supplied as 2 mg/2 mL, so the nurse further calculated 1.6 mL was the dose and drew it up in a 3 mL syringe. As the nurse handed the syringe to the physician, the amount looked wrong. The physician asked the nurse how that amount was obtained. When the nurse told the physician the estimated BSA from the child's weight (45 pounds) is 0.82 m^2, and the dosage is 2 mg/m^2 × 0.82 m^2 = 1.64 mg or 1.6 mL, the physician said "No! This child's *BSA is 0.45 m^2*. I wrote it myself next to his weight—20 pounds." The physician, despite the need to give the medication as soon as possible, took the necessary extra step and examined the amount of medication in the syringe. Though the physician knew and trusted the nurse, the amount of medication in the syringe did not seem right. Perhaps the physician had figured a "ball park" amount of about 1 mL, and the volume the nurse brought in made the physician question what was calculated. The correct dosage of $2 \text{ mg}/\cancel{m^2} \times 0.45 \cancel{m^2} = 0.9$ mg was calculated and 0.9 mL was then drawn up by the nurse and administered.

$$\frac{D}{H} \times Q = \frac{0.9 \cancel{\text{mg}}}{\cancel{2} \cancel{\text{mg}}} \times \cancel{2} \text{ mL} = 0.9 \text{ mL}$$

potential outcome

The child, already critically ill, could have received almost double the amount of medication had the physician rushed to give the dose calculated and prepared by someone else. This excessive amount of medication probably could have caused a fatal overdose. What should have been done to prevent this error?

prevention

____

____

After completing these problems, see pages 457–459 to check your answers.

CHAPTER

16

Advanced Adult Intravenous Calculations

objectives

Upon mastery of Chapter 16, you will be able to perform advanced adult intravenous calculations and apply these skills to patients across the life span. To accomplish this you will also be able to:

- Calculate and assess safe hourly heparin dosage.
- Calculate heparin IV flow rate.
- Calculate the flow rate and assess safe dosages for critical care IV medication administered over a specified time period.
- Calculate the flow rate for primary IV and IVPB solutions for patients with restricted fluid intake requirements.

Nurses are becoming increasingly more responsible for the administration of intravenous (IV) medications in the critical care areas as well as on general nursing units. Patients in life-threatening situations require thorough and timely interventions that frequently involve specialized, potent drugs. This chapter will focus on advanced adult IV calculations with special requirements that can be applied to patients across the life span.

IV Heparin

Heparin is an anticoagulant for the prevention of clot formation. It is measured in USP units (Figure 16-1). Intravenous heparin should be administered by an electronic infusion device. Because of the potential for hemorrhage or clots with incorrect dosage, careful monitoring of patients receiving heparin is a critical nursing skill. The nurse is responsible for administering correct dosage and for ensuring that the dosage is safe.

rule

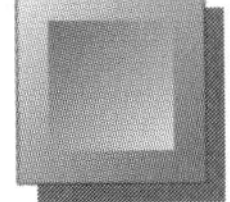

The normal adult heparinizing dosage is 20,000 to 40,000 units IV per 24 hours.

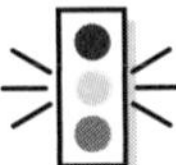

Caution: Heparin order, dosage, vial, and amount to give should be checked by another nurse before administering the dose.

Intravenous heparin is frequently ordered in *units per hour (U/h)*. Based on the normal heparinizing dosage, the nurse must determine if the order is safe and effective.

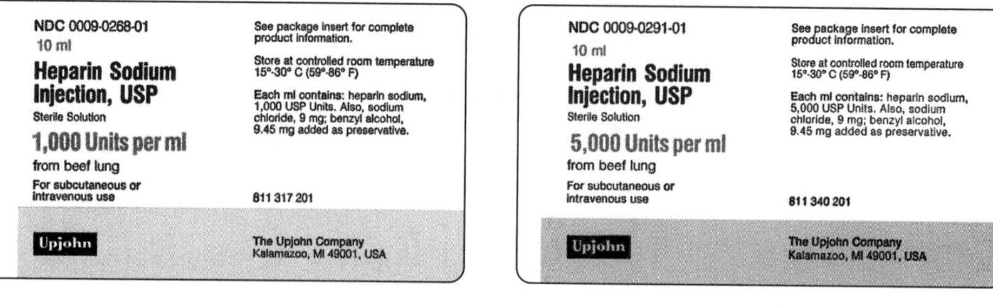

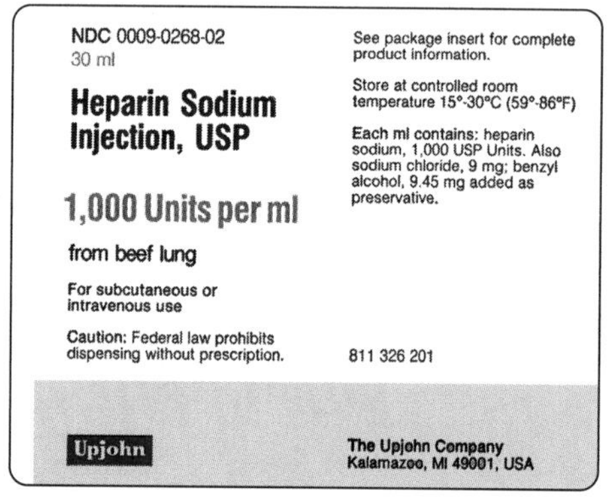

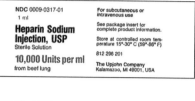

FIGURE 16-1 Various Heparin Dosage Strengths and Container Volumes

Example 1:

Order: *Heparin IV to infuse at 1000 U/h*

Is this dosage safe?

Normal adult range is 20,000–40,000 U/24 h

1,000 U/~~h~~ × 24 ~~h~~ = 24,000 U

Yes, 1000 U/h is safe.

Example 2:

Order: *Heparin IV to infuse at 850 U/h*

Is this dosage safe?

850 U/~~h~~ × 24 ~~h~~ = 20,400 U

Yes, 850 U/h is safe.

Example 3:

Order: *Heparin IV 2000 U/h*

Is this dosage safe?

2000 U/h × 24 ~~h~~ = 48,000 U

No, this dosage is not within the recommended range. Notify the physician.

Calculating Safe IV Heparin Flow Rate

When IV heparin is ordered in U/h, use $\frac{D}{H} \times Q = R$ or ratio-proportion to calculate the flow rate in mL/h.

rule

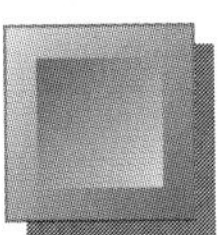

To calculate IV heparin flow rate in mL/h,

$$\frac{\text{D (U/h desired)}}{\text{H (U you have on hand)}} \times \text{Q (mL you have on hand)} = \text{R (mL/h)}$$

Or, ratio of supply dosage is equivalent to ratio of desired dosage rate

Supply, $\frac{\text{U}}{\text{mL}} = \frac{\text{Desired U/h}}{\text{X mL/h}}$

Note: This rule applies to other drugs ordered in mU/h, mg/h, mcg/h, g/h, or mEq/h.

Let's apply the rule to the previous two examples, which we determined are safe orders.

Example 1:

Order: *D_5W 500 mL $\bar{c}$ heparin 25,000 U IV at 1000 U/h*

What is the flow rate in mL/h?

$$\frac{D}{H} \times Q = \frac{1000 \text{ U/h}}{25{,}000 \text{ U}} \times 500 \text{ mL} = \text{R (mL/h)}$$

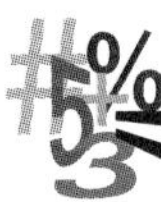

math tip: Units (U) cancel out to leave mL/h in the $\frac{D}{H} \times Q = R$ formula.

$$\frac{1000 \not{U}/h}{\underset{50}{\cancel{25{,}000}} \not{U}} \times \overset{1}{\cancel{500}} \text{ mL} = \frac{1000}{50} = 20 \text{ mL/h}$$

Or, use ratio-proportion to calculate the flow rate in mL/h, which will administer 1000 U/h.

$$\frac{25{,}000 \text{ U}}{500 \text{ mL}} \times \frac{1000 \text{ U/h}}{\text{X mL/h}}$$

$$25{,}000 \text{ X} = 500{,}000$$

$$\frac{25{,}000 \text{ X}}{25{,}000} = \frac{500{,}000}{25{,}000}$$

$$\text{X} = 20 \text{ mL/h}$$

Example 2:

Order: *D_5W 500 mL $\bar{c}$ heparin 25,000 U IV at 850 U/h*

Calculate the flow rate in mL/h.

$$\frac{D}{H} \times Q = \frac{850 \not{U}/h}{\underset{50}{\cancel{25{,}000}} \not{U}} \times \overset{1}{\cancel{500}} \text{ mL} = \frac{850}{50} = 17 \text{ mL/h}$$

Or, use ratio-proportion.

$$\frac{25{,}000 \text{ U}}{500 \text{ mL}} \times \frac{850 \text{ U/h}}{\text{X mL/h}}$$

$$25{,}000 \text{ X} = 425{,}000$$

$$\frac{25{,}000 \text{ X}}{25{,}000} = \frac{425{,}000}{25{,}000}$$

$$\text{X} = 17 \text{ mL/h}$$

Calculating Safe IV Heparin Dosage from Flow Rate

Heparin may also be ordered by the physician to infuse at a predetermined flow rate in milliliters per hour. The nurse must determine the hourly unit dosage to verify that the dosage is within the safe and effective range of 20,000 to 40,000 U/24 h.

Example 1:

Order: *D_5W 1L IV c̄ heparin 40,000 U to infuse at 30 mL/h*

What is the hourly heparin dosage?

$$\frac{40{,}000\ \text{U}}{1000\ \text{mL}} = \frac{X\ \text{U/h}}{30\ \text{mL/h}}$$

$$1000\,X = 1{,}200{,}000$$

$$\frac{1000\,X}{1000} = \frac{1{,}200{,}000}{1000}$$

$$X = 1200\ \text{U/h}$$

Is this hourly dosage safe?

$1200\ \text{U}/\cancel{\text{h}} \times 24\ \cancel{\text{h}} = 28{,}800\ \text{U}$

Yes, it is safe. The dosage is within the normal range.

Example 2:

Order: *D_5W 1000 mL IV c̄ heparin 40,000 U to infuse at 40 mL/h*

What is the hourly heparin dosage?

$$\frac{40{,}000\ \text{U}}{1000\ \text{mL}} = \frac{X\ \text{U/h}}{40\ \text{mL/h}}$$

$$1000\text{U} = 1{,}600{,}000$$

$$\frac{1000X}{1000} = \frac{1{,}600{,}000}{1000}$$

$$X = 1600\ \text{U/h}$$

Is this hourly dosage safe?

$1600\ \text{U}/\cancel{\text{h}} \times 24\ \cancel{\text{h}} = 38{,}400\ \text{U}$

Yes, the dosage is within the normal range.

Example 3:

Order: *D_5NS 500 mL c̄ heparin 5000 U added to infuse at 80 mL/h.*

What is the hourly heparin dosage?

$$\frac{5000\ \text{U}}{500\ \text{mL}} = \frac{X\ \text{U/h}}{80\ \text{mL/h}}$$

$$500X = 400{,}000$$

$$\frac{500X}{500} = \frac{400{,}000}{500}$$

$$X = 800\ \text{U/h}$$

Is this hourly dosage safe?

800 U/~~h~~ × 24 ~~h~~ = 19,200 U

No, this dosage is not within the normal therapeutic range. Therefore, it is not safe to proceed. The physician should be notified and the order should be reviewed.

quick review

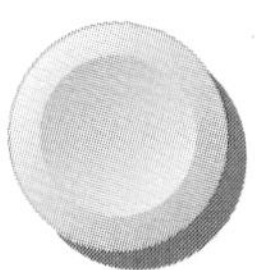

- Normal adult heparinizing dosage is 20,000–40,000 U/24 h.
- Use $\frac{D}{H} \times Q = R$ or ratio-proportion to calculate mL/h when you know U/h and U/mL.
- Use ratio-proportion to calculate U/h when you know mL/h and U/mL.

review set 50

Calculate the flow rate and indicate whether the heparin dosage is safe.

1. Order: *1000 mL 0.45% NS c̄ heparin 25,000 U to infuse at 1000 U/h.*

   Flow rate: 40 mL/h

   Daily heparin dosage: 24000 U/24 h

   Safe? Yes

2. Order: *500 mL D_5W IV c̄ heparin 40,000 U to infuse at 1100 U/h.*

   Flow rate: 13.75 mL/h

   Daily heparin dosage: 26400 U/24 h

   Safe? Yes

3. Order: *500 mL 0.45% NS IV c̄ heparin 25,000 U to infuse at 500 U/h.*

   Flow rate: 10 mL/h

   Daily heparin dosage: 12000 U/24 h

   Safe? no 12,000

4. Order: *500 mL D_5W IV c̄ heparin 40,000 U to infuse at 2500 U/h.*

   On infusion pump with a setting 31 mL/h.

   Daily heparin dosage: 60000 U/24 h

   Is the setting accurate? Yes Is the hourly dosage safe? NO

   If not, what should you do? Call physician

5. Order: *1 L D_5W IV c̄ heparin 25,000 U.* On rounds, you assess the patient and observe that the infusion pump is set at 120 mL/h.

   What is the hourly heparin dosage? 3000 U/h

   What is the daily heparin dosage? 72000 U/24 h

   Is the hourly dosage of heparin safe? no

   If not, what should you do? Wait for physician

6. Order: *500 mL 0.45% NS IV c̄ 30,000 U heparin to infuse at 25 mL/h.*

   Is the hourly dosage safe? 1500 u/hr yes 36000

7. Order: *1 L D_5W IV c̄ heparin 40,000 U to infuse at 80 mL/h.*

   Is the hourly dosage safe? ______

8. Order: *1000 mL D_5W IV c̄ heparin 20,000 U to infuse at 60 mL/h.*

   Is the hourly dosage safe? ______

9. The patient's order is *500 mL D_5W IV c̄ heparin 30,000 U at 96 mL/h.*

   Is the hourly dosage safe? ______

10. Order: *1000 mL $D_5 \frac{1}{2}$ NS IV c̄ heparin 10,000 U at 80 mL/h.*

    Is the hourly dosage safe? ______

The same method can be used to calculate flow rates for other medications ordered at a specified dosage unit per hour. Try the next two problems.

11. Order: *500 mL 0.9% NaCl IV c̄ Humulin N NPH U-100 insulin 500 U to infuse at 10 U/h by electronic infusion pump.*

    Flow rate: ______ mL/h

12. Order: *1 L D_5W IV c̄ KCl 40 mEq to infuse at 2 mEq/h by electronic infusion controller.*

    Set the electronic infusion controller at ______ mL/h.

After completing these problems, see page 459 to check your answers.

Critical Care IV Calculations: Calculating Flow Rate of an IV Medication to be Given Over a Specified Time Period

With increasing frequency, medications are ordered for patients in critical care situations as a prescribed amount to be administered in a specified time period, such as *X mg per minute.* Such medications are usually administered by electronic infusion devices, programmed in mL/h. Careful monitoring of patients receiving life-threatening therapies is a critical nursing skill.

IV Medication Ordered "Per Minute"

rule

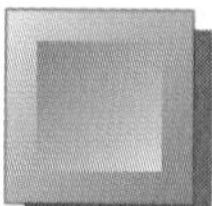

To determine the flow rate (mL/h) for IV medications ordered in mg/min:

STEP 1 Calculate the dosage in mL/min: $\frac{D}{H} \times Q = R$ (mL/min)

STEP 2 Calculate the flow rate of quantity to administer in mL/h:

mL/min × 60 min/h = mL/h

NOTE: The order may also specify mcg/min, g/min, U/min, mU/min, or mEq/min.

In the formula $\frac{D}{H} \times Q = R$ (mL/min),

D = Dosage *desired:* mg/min

H = Dosage you *have* available

Q = *Quantity* of solution you have available

R = Flow *rate:* mL/min

Example 1:

Order: *Lidocaine 2 g IV in 500 mL D_5W at 2 mg/min via infusion pump.* You must prepare and hang 500 mL of D_5W IV solution that has 2 grams of Lidocaine added to it. Then, you must regulate the flow rate so the patient receives 2 milligrams of the Lidocaine every minute. Determine the flow rate in mL/h.

STEP 1 Calculate mL/min.

Apply the formula $\frac{D}{H} \times Q = R$ (mL/min).

D = dosage desired = 2 mg/min

H = dosage you have available = 2 g = 2000 mg

Q = quantity of available solution = 500 mL

$$\frac{D}{H} \times Q = \frac{2 \text{ mg/min}}{2000 \text{ mg}} \times 500 \text{ mL} = R$$

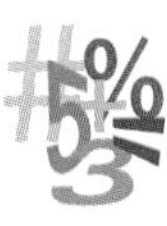

math tip: $\frac{\cancel{\text{mg}}/\text{min}}{\cancel{\text{mg}}} \times \text{mL} = \text{mL/min}$ because mg cancel out.

$$\frac{2 \cancel{\text{mg}}/\text{min}}{\underset{4}{\cancel{2000}} \cancel{\text{mg}}} \times \frac{\overset{1}{\cancel{500}} \text{ mL}}{1} = \frac{2}{4} = 0.5 \text{ mL/min}$$

STEP 2 Determine the flow rate (mL/h).

mL/min × 60 min/h = mL/h

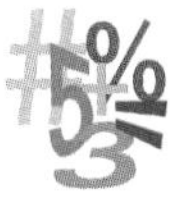

math tip: $\frac{\text{mL}}{\cancel{\text{min}}} \times \frac{\cancel{\text{min}}}{\text{h}} = \text{mL/h}$ because "min" cancel out.

$$\frac{0.5 \text{ mL}}{\cancel{\text{min}}} \times \frac{60 \cancel{\text{min}}}{\text{h}} = 30 \text{ mL/h}$$

Or, you can use ratio-proportion.

$$\frac{0.5 \text{ mL}}{1 \text{ min}} = \frac{X \text{ mL}}{60 \text{ min}}$$

X = 30 mL (per 60 min or 30 mL/h)

Regulate the flow rate to 30 mL/h to deliver 2 mg/min of the drug.

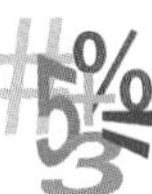

math tip: In the original ratio $\frac{X \text{ mL}}{60 \text{ min}}$ means X mL/60 min or X mL/h. Therefore, the rate is 30 mL/60 min or 30 mL/h.

Set the flow rate to 30 mL/h.

Example 2:

Order: *Nitroglycerin 125 mg IV in 500 mL D_5W to infuse at 42 mcg/min.*

Calculate the flow rate in mL/h to program the infusion pump.

Convert mg to mcg: 1 mg = 1000 mcg; 125 mg = 125 × 1000 = 125,000 mcg

STEP 1 Calculate mL/min.

$$\frac{D}{H} \times Q = \frac{42 \text{ mcg/min}}{125{,}000 \text{ mcg}} \times 500 \text{ mL} = \frac{42}{250} = 0.168 = 0.17 \text{ mL/min}$$

STEP 2 Calculate mL/h. You know that 1 h = 60 min.

mL/min × 60 min/h = mL/h

0.17 mL/min × 60 min/h = 10.2 = 10 mL/h

Or, you can use ratio-proportion.

$$\frac{0.17 \text{ mL}}{1 \text{ min}} \times \frac{X \text{ mL}}{60 \text{ min}}$$

X = 10.2 = 10 mL. Rate is 10 mL/60 min or 10 mL/h

Regulate the flow rate to 10 mL/h to deliver 42 mcg/min of the drug.

IV Medication Ordered "Per Kilogram Per Minute"

The physician may also order the amount of medication in an IV solution that a patient should receive in a specified time period per kilogram of body weight. An electronic infusion device is usually used to administer these orders.

rule

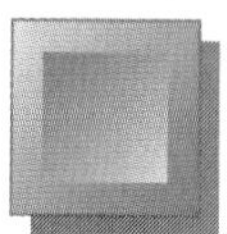

To calculate flow rate (***mL/h***) for IV medications ordered in ***mg/kg/min***:

STEP 1 Convert to like units, such as mg to mcg or lb to kg.

STEP 2 Calculate desired dosage in mg/min.

STEP 3 Calculate the desired dosage in mL/min: $\frac{D}{H} \times Q = R$ (mL/min).

STEP 4 Calculate the flow rate of the quantity to administer in mL/h.

NOTE: The order may also specify mcg/kg/min, g/kg/min, U/kg/min, mU/kg/min, or mEq/kg/min.

Example 1:

Order: *Add 225 mg of a medication to 250 mL of IV solution and administer 3 mcg/kg/min via infusion pump* for a person who weighs 110 lb.

Determine the flow rate (mL/h).

STEP 1 Convert mg to mcg.

1 mg = 1000 mcg

225 mg = 225 × 1000 = 225,000 mcg

Convert lb to kg:

$110 \text{ lb} = \frac{110}{2.2} = 50 \text{ kg}$

STEP 2 Calculate desired mcg/min.

3 mcg/~~kg~~/min × 50 ~~kg~~ = 150 mcg/min

STEP 3 Calculate mL/min.

$$\frac{D}{H} \times Q = \frac{150 \cancel{mcg}/min}{225{,}000 \cancel{mcg}} \times 250 \text{ mL} = 0.166 = 0.17 \text{ mL/min}$$

STEP 4 Calculate mL/h. You know that 1 h = 60 min.

mL/min × 60 min/h = 0.17 mL/min × 60 min/h = 10.2 = 10 mL/h

Or, you can use ratio-proportion.

$$\frac{0.17 \text{ mL}}{1 \text{ min}} \times \frac{X \text{ mL}}{60 \text{ min}}$$

X = 10.2 =10 mL. Rate is 10 mL/60 min or 10 mL/h

Regulate the flow rate to 10 mL/h to deliver 150 mcg/min of the drug.

Titrated IV Drugs

Sometimes IV medications may be ordered to be administered at an initial dosage over a specified time period and then continued at a different dosage and time period. These situations are common in obstetrics. Medications, such as magnesium sulfate, dopamine, Isuprel, and Pitocin, are ordered to be *titrated* or *regulated* to obtain measurable physiologic responses. Dosages will be adjusted until the desired effect is achieved. In some cases, a loading or bolus dose is infused and monitored closely. Most IV medications that require titration usually start at the lowest dosage and are increased or decreased as needed. An upper titration limit is usually set and is not exceeded unless the desired response is not obtained. A new drug order is then required.

Let's look at some of these situations. Apply an alternate method using ratio-proportion rather than the formula method to calculate mL/h.

rule

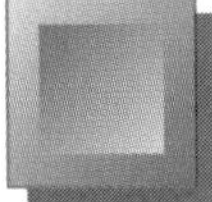

An alternate method to calculate flow rate (mL/h) for IV medications ordered over a specific time period uses ratio-proportion:

STEP 1 Calculate mg/mL.

STEP 2 Calculate mL/h.

NOTE: The order may also specify mcg/min, g/min, U/min, mU/min, or mEq/min.

Example 1:

Order: *Add magnesium sulfate 20 g to RL IV 1000 mL. Start with bolus of 4 g/30 min, then maintain a continuous infusion @ 2 g/h.*

1. What is the flow rate in mL/h for the bolus order?

STEP 1 Calculate the bolus dosage in g/mL.

There are 20 g in 1000 mL. How many mL are necessary to infuse 4 g?

$$\frac{20\text{ g}}{1000\text{ mL}} \times \frac{4\text{ g}}{\text{X mL}}$$

$20\text{X} = 4000$

$$\frac{20\text{X}}{20} = \frac{4000}{20}$$

$\text{X} = 200\text{ mL}$

Therefore, 200 mL contain 4 g, to be administered over 30 min.

STEP 2 Calculate the bolus rate in mL/h.

What is the flow rate in mL/h to infuse 200 mL (which contain 4 g of magnesium sulfate)? Remember 1 h = 60 min.

$$\frac{200\text{ mL}}{30\text{ min}} \times \frac{\text{X mL}}{60\text{ min}}$$

$30\text{X} = 12,000$

$$\frac{30\text{X}}{30} = \frac{12{,}000}{30}$$

$\text{X} = 400\text{ mL}$

Rate is 400 mL/60 min or 400 mL/h.

Set the infusion pump at 400 mL/h to deliver the bolus as ordered at 4 g/30 min.

Now calculate the continuous IV rate in mL/h.

2. What is the flow rate in mL/h for the continuous infusion of magnesium sulfate of 2 g/h? You know from the bolus flow rate calculation that 200 mL contain 4 g. Therefore, you can use ratio-proportion to determine how many mL contain 2 g/h.

$$\frac{4\text{ g}}{200\text{ mL}} \times \frac{2\text{ g/h}}{\text{X mL/h}}$$

$4\text{X} = 400$

$$\frac{4\text{X}}{4} = \frac{400}{4}$$

$\text{X} = 100\text{ mL/h}$

After the bolus has infused in the first 30 min, reset the infusion pump to 100 mL/h to deliver 2 g/h.

Let's look at an example using Pitocin (a drug used to induce labor), measured in units and milliunits.

Example 2:

A drug order is written to induce labor as follows: *Add Pitocin 20 U to LR 1000 mL IV. Begin a continuous infusion IV @ 1 mU/min, increase by 1 mU/min q.15–30 min to a maximum of 20 mU/min.*

1. What is the flow rate in mL/h to deliver 1 mU/min?

In this example, the medication is measured in units (instead of g or mg). Recall that 1 U = 1000 mU.

Convert: 1U = 1000 mU; 20 U = 20 × 1000 = 20,000 mU

STEP 1 Calculate mU/mL.

$$\frac{20{,}000 \text{ mU}}{1000 \text{ mL}} \times \frac{1 \text{ mU}}{X \text{ mL}}$$

$$20{,}000X = 1000$$

$$\frac{20{,}000X}{20{,}000} = \frac{1000}{20{,}000}$$

X = 0.05 mL. Therefore, 0.05 mL contains 1 mU of Pitocin, or there is 1 mU/0.05 mL.

STEP 2 Calculate mL/h.

What is the flow rate in mL/h to infuse 0.05 mL/min (which is 1 mU Pitocin/min)?

$$\frac{0.05 \text{ mL}}{1 \text{ min}} \times \frac{X \text{ mL}}{60 \text{ min}}$$

X = 3 mL. Rate is 3 mL/60 min or 3 mL/h.

Set the infusion pump at 3 mL/h to infuse the order of Pitocin 1 mU/min.

2. What is the maximum flow rate in mL/h that the Pitocin infusion can be set for the titration as ordered? Notice that the standard and the order allow a maximum of 20 mU/min.

   You know that 1 mU/min is infused at 3 mL/h. Use ratio-proportion to calculate the mL/h to infuse 20 mU/min.

$$\frac{3 \text{ mL/h}}{1 \text{ mU/min}} \times \frac{X \text{ mL/h}}{20 \text{ mU/min}}$$

   X = 60 mL/h. Rate of 60 mL/h will deliver 20 mU/min.

Verifying Safe IV Medication Dosage Recommended "Per Minute"

It is also a critical nursing skill to be sure that patients are receiving safe dosages of medications. Therefore, you must also be able to convert critical care IVs with additive medications to **mg/h** or **mg/min** to check safe or normal dosage ranges.

rule

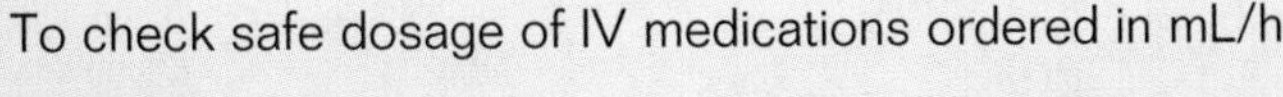

To check safe dosage of IV medications ordered in mL/h:

STEP 1 Calculate mg/h.

STEP 2 Calculate mg/min.

STEP 3 Compare recommended dosage and ordered dosage to decide if the dosage is safe.

Note: The ordered and recommended dosages may also be mcg/min, g/min, U/min, mU/min, or mEg/min.

Example:

The *Hospital Formulary* states that the normal dosage of Lidocaine is 1–4 mg/min. The patient has an order for *500 mL D_5W IV c̄ Lidocaine 1 g to infuse at 30 mL/h*. Is the Lidocaine dosage within the safe normal range?

Convert: 1 g = 1000 mg

STEP 1 Use ratio-proportion to calculate mg/h.

$$\frac{1000 \text{ mg}}{500 \text{ mL}} \times \frac{X \text{ mg/h}}{30 \text{ mL/h}}$$

$$500X = 30,000$$

$$\frac{500X}{500} = \frac{30,000}{500}$$

$$X = 60 \text{ mg/h}$$

60 mg are administered in one hour when the flow rate is 30 mL/h. So 60 mg/h are being infused.

STEP 2 Calculate mg/min. THINK: It is obvious that 60 mg/h is the same as 60 mg/60 min or 1 mg/1 min.

$$\frac{60 \text{ mg}}{60 \text{ min}} \times \frac{X \text{ mg}}{1 \text{ min}}$$

$$60X = 60$$

$$\frac{60X}{60} = \frac{60}{60}$$

X = 1 mg. Rate is 1 mg/min.

STEP 3 Compare ordered and recommended dosages.

1 mg/min is within the normal range of 1 to 4 mg/min. The dosage is safe.

Likewise, IV medications ordered as mL/h and recommended in mg/kg/min require verification of their safety or normal dosage range.

rule

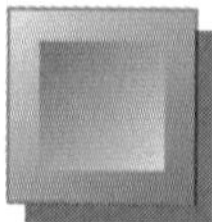

To check safe dosage of IV medications recommended in mg/kg/min and ordered in mL/h:

STEP 1 Convert to like units, such as mg to mcg or lb to kg.

STEP 2 Calculate recommended mg/min.

STEP 3 Calculate ordered mg/h.

STEP 4 Calculate ordered mg/min.

STEP 5 Compare ordered and recommended dosages. Decide if the dosage is safe.

NOTE: The ordered and recommended dosages may also be mcg/kg/min, g/kg/min, U/kg/min, mU/kg/min, or mEq/kg/min.

Example:

The *Pediatric Drug Handbook* states that the normal dosage of Nipride for children and adults starts at 0.3 mcg/kg/min, titrated up to a usual dosage of 3 mcg/kg/min. The patient has an order for *100 mL D_5W IV with Nipride 420 mg to infuse at 1 mL/h.* The patient weighs 154 lb. Is the Nipride dosage within the normal range?

STEP 1 Convert lb to kg. 154 lb = $\frac{154}{2.2}$ = 70 kg

Convert mg to mcg: 420 mg = 420 × 1000 = 420,000 mcg

STEP 2 Calculate recommended mcg/min range.

0.3 mcg/~~kg~~/min × 70 ~~kg~~ = 21 mcg/min *minimum*

3 mcg/~~kg~~/min × 70 ~~kg~~ = 210 mcg/min *maximum*

STEP 3 Calculate ordered mcg/h.

$$\frac{420{,}000 \text{ mcg}}{100 \text{ mL}} \times \frac{X \text{ mcg/h}}{1 \text{ mL/h}}$$

$$100X = 420{,}000$$

$$\frac{100X}{100} = \frac{420{,}000}{100}$$

$$X = 4200 \text{ mcg/h}$$

STEP 4 Calculate ordered mcg/min: 4200 mcg/h = 4200 mcg/60 min

$$\frac{4200 \text{ mcg}}{60 \text{ min}} = 70 \text{ mcg/min}$$

STEP 5 Compare ordered and recommended dosages. Decide if the dosage is safe. 70 mcg/min is within the allowable range of 21 to 210 mcg/min. The ordered dosage is safe.

quick review

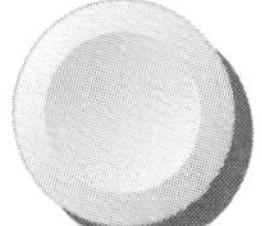

- For IV medications ordered in mg/min, calculate:

  1. $\frac{D}{H} \times Q = R$ (mL/min), and then

  2. mL/h

- Or, calculate:

1. mg/mL, and then
2. mL/h

- To check safe dosages of IV medications recommended in mg/min and ordered in mL/h:

STEP 1 Calculate mg/h.

STEP 2 Calculate mg/min.

STEP 3 Compare recommended and ordered dosages. Decide if the dosage is safe.

- To check safe dosage of IV medications recommended in mg/kg/min and ordered in mL/h:

STEP 1 Convert to like units, such as mg to mcg or lb to kg.

STEP 2 Calculate recommended mg/min.

STEP 3 Calculate ordered mg/h.

STEP 4 Calculate ordered mg/min.

STEP 5 Compare ordered and recommended dosages. Decide if the dosage is safe.

review set 51

Compute the flow rate in mL/h for each of these medications administered by infusion pump.

1. Order: *Lidocaine 2 g IV per 1000 mL D_5W at 4 mg/min*

   Rate: 120 mL/h

2. Order: *Pronestyl 0.5 g IV per 250 mL D_5W at 2 mg/min*

   Rate: 60 mL/h

3. Order: *Isuprel 2 mg IV per 500 cc D_5W at 5 mcg/min*

   Rate: _________ mL/h

4. Order: *Medication "X" 450 mg IV per 500 mL NS at 4 mcg/kg/min*

   Weight: 198 lb

   Rate: _________ mL/h

5. Order: *Dopamine 800 mg in 500 mL NS IV at 15 mcg/kg/min*

   Weight: 70 kg

   Rate: _________ mL/h

Refer to this order for questions 6 through 8.

Order: *500 mL D_5W IV $\bar{c}$ Dobutrex 500 mg to infuse at 15 mL/h.* The patient weighs 125 pounds. Normal range: 2.5–10 mcg/kg/min

6. What mcg/min range of Dobutrex should the patient receive? ____ to ____ mcg/min
7. What mg/min range of Dobutrex should the patient receive? ____ to ____ mg/min
8. Is the Dobutrex as ordered within the safe range? _________

Refer to this order for questions 9 and 10.

Order: *500 mL D_5W IV c̄ Pronestyl 2 g to infuse at 60 mL/h.* Normal range: 2–6 mg/min

9. How many mg/min of Pronestyl is the patient receiving? __________ mg/min

10. Is the dosage of Pronestyl within the normal range? __________

11. Order: *Magnesium sulfate 20 g in 500 mL LR IV. Start with a bolus of 2 g to infuse over 30 min. Then maintain a continuous infusion at 1 g/h.*

    Rate: __________ mL/h for bolus

    __________ mL/h for continuous infusion

12. A drug order is written to induce labor as follows:

    Pitocin 15 U in LR 250 mL. Begin a continuous infusion at the rate of 1 mU/min.

    Rate: __________ mL/h

Refer to this order for questions 13 through 15.

Order: *1000 mL of D_5W IV with Brethine 10 mg to infuse at 150 mL/h.*

Normal dosage range: 10–80 mcg/min

13. How many mg/min of Brethine is the patient receiving? __________ mg/min

14. How many mcg/min of Brethine is the patient receiving? __________ mcg/min

15. Is the dosage of Brethine within the normal range? __________

After completing these problems, see page 460 to check your answers.

Limiting Infusion Volumes

Calculating IV rates to include the IV PB volume is occasionally necessary to limit the total volume of IV fluid a patient receives. In order to do this you must calculate the flow rate for both the regular IV and the piggyback IV. In such instances of restricted fluids, the piggyback IVs are to be included as part of the total prescribed IV volume and time.

rule

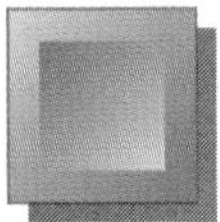

Follow these six steps to calculate the flow rate of an IV, which includes IV PB.
Calculate:

1. *IV PB flow rate:* $\frac{V}{T} \times C = R$

   or, use $\frac{\text{mL/h}}{\text{Drop factor constant}} = R$

2. *Total IV PB time:* *Time* for one dose × # of doses in 24 h

3. *Total IV PB volume:* Volume of one dose × # of doses in 24 h

4. *Total regular IV volume:* Total volume – IV PB volume = Regular IV volume

5. *Total regular IV time:* Total time – IV PB time = Regular IV time

6. *Regular IV flow rate:* $\frac{V}{T} \times C = R$

   or use $\frac{\text{mL/h}}{\text{Drop factor constant}} = R$

Example 1:

Order: *3000 mL 5% dextrose in Lactated Ringer's per 24 h with Kefzol 1 g IV PB/100 mL D_5W q.6h to run 1 hour. Limit total fluids to 3000 mL q.d.*

The drop factor is 10 gtt/mL.

NOTE: The order intends that the patient will receive a maximum of 3000 mL in 24 hours. Remember, when fluids are restricted, the piggybacks are to be *included* in the total 24-hour intake, not in addition to it.

STEP 1 Calculate the flow rate of the IV PB.

$$\frac{V}{T} \times C = \frac{100 \text{ mL}}{\underset{6}{60} \text{ min}} \times \overset{1}{10} \text{ gtt/mL} = \frac{100}{6} = 16.6 = 17 \text{ gtt/min}$$

or, $\frac{\text{mL/h}}{\text{Drop factor constant}} = \text{R}$ (Drop factor constant is 6.)

$$\frac{100}{6} = 16.6 = 17 \text{ gtt/min}$$

Set the flow rate for the IV PB at 17 gtt/min to infuse 1 g Kefzol in 100 mL over 1 hour or 60 min.

STEP 2 Calculate the total time the IV PB will be administered.

q.6 h = 4 times/24 h; 4 × 1 h = 4 h

STEP 3 Calculate the total volume of the IV PB.

100 mL × 4 = 400 mL IV PB per 24 hours.

STEP 4 Calculate the volume of the regular IV fluids to be administered between IV PB. Total volume of regular IV minus total volume of IV PB = 3000 mL – 400 mL = 2600 mL.

STEP 5 Calculate the total regular IV fluid time or the time between IV PB. Total IV time minus total IV PB time = 24 h – 4 h = 20 h

STEP 6 Calculate the flow rate of the regular IV.

$$\text{mL / h} = \frac{2600 \text{ mL}}{20 \text{ h}} = 130 \text{ mL/h}$$

$$\frac{V}{T} \times C = \frac{130 \text{ mL}}{\underset{6}{60} \text{ min}} \times \overset{1}{10} \text{ gtt/mL} = \frac{130}{6} = 21.6 = 22 \text{ gtt/min}$$

or, $\frac{\text{mL/h}}{\text{Drop factor constant}} = \text{R}$ (Drop factor constant is 6.)

$$\frac{130}{6} = 21.6 = 22 \text{ gtt/min}$$

Set the regular IV of D_5LR at the flow rate of 22 gtt/min. Then after 5 hours, switch to the Kefzol IV PB at the flow rate of 17 gtt/min for one hour. Repeat this process 4 times in 24 hours.

Example 2:

Order: *2000 mL NS IV per 24 h with 80 mg gentamycin in 80 mL IV PB q.8h to run for 30 min. Limit fluid intake to 2000 mL q.d.*

Drop factor: 15 gtt/mL

Calculate the flow rate for the regular IV and for the IV PB.

STEP 1 IV PB flow rate:

$$\frac{V}{T} \times C = \frac{80 \not{mL}}{\underset{2}{\not{30}} \text{ min}} \times \overset{1}{\not{15}} \text{ gtt}/\not{mL} = \frac{80}{2} = 40 \text{ gtt/min}$$

STEP 2 Total IV PB time: q.8h = 3 times/24 h; 3×30 min = 90 min = $1\frac{1}{2}$ h

STEP 3 Total IV PB volume: 80 mL $\times$ 3 = 240 mL

STEP 4 Total regular IV volume: 2000 mL – 240 mL = 1760 mL

STEP 5 Total regular IV time: 24 h – $1\frac{1}{2}$ h = $22\frac{1}{2}$ h = 22.5 h

STEP 6 Regular IV flow rate:

$$\text{mL/h} = \frac{1760 \text{ mL}}{22.5 \text{ h}} = 78.2 = 78 \text{ mL/h}$$

$$\frac{V}{T} \times C = \frac{78 \not{mL}}{\underset{4}{\not{60}} \text{ min}} \times \overset{1}{\not{15}} \text{ gtt}/\not{mL} = \frac{78}{4} = 19.5 = 20 \text{ gtt/min}$$

or, $\dfrac{\text{mL/h}}{\text{Drop factor constant}} = R$ (Drop factor constant is 4.)

$\frac{78}{4} = 19.5 = 20$ gtt/min

Set the regular IV of NS at the flow rate of 20 gtt/min. After $7\frac{1}{2}$ hours, switch to the gentamycin IV PB at the flow rate of 40 gtt/min for 30 minutes. Repeat this process 3 times in 24 hours.

Patients receiving a primary IV at a specific rate via an infusion controller or pump may require that the infusion rate be altered when a secondary (piggyback) medication is being administered. To do this, calculate the flow rate of the secondary medication in mL/h as you would for the primary IV, and reset the infusion device.

Some infusion controllers or pumps allow you to set the flow rate for the secondary IV independent of the primary IV. Upon completion of the secondary infusion, the infusion device automatically returns to the original flow rate. If this is not the case, be sure to manually readjust the primary flow rate after the completion of the secondary set.

quick review

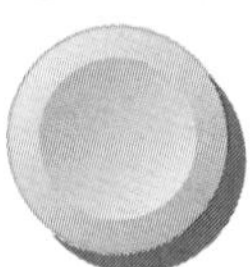

- To calculate the flow rate of a regular IV with an IV PB and restricted fluids, calculate:

STEP 1	IV PB flow rate
STEP 2	Total IV PB time
STEP 3	Total IV PB volume
STEP 4	Total regular IV volume
STEP 5	Total regular IV time
STEP 6	Regular IV flow rate

review set 52

Calculate the flow rates for the IV ordered and the IV PB ordered. These patients are on limited fluid volume (restricted fluids).

1. Order: *3000 mL NS IV for 24 h*

   Penicillin G 1,000,000 U IV PB q.4h in 100 mL NS to run for 30 min

   Drop factor: 10 gtt/mL

   IV PB flow rate: __________ gtt/min

   IV flow rate: __________ gtt/min

2. Order: *1000 mL D_5W IV for 24 h*

   Garamycin 40 mg q.i.d. in 40 mL IV PB to run 1 h

   Drop factor: 60 gtt/mL

   IV PB flow rate: __________ gtt/min

   IV flow rate: __________ gtt/min

3. Order: *3000 mL D_5 LR IV for 24 h*

   Ampicillin 0.5 g q.6h IV PB in 50 mL D_5W to run 30 min

   Drop factor: 15 gtt/mL

   IV PB flow rate: __________ gtt/min

   IV flow rate: __________ gtt/min

4. Order: *2000 mL $\frac{1}{2}$ NS IV for 24 h*

   Chloromycetin 500 mg/50 mL NS IV PB q.6h to run 1 h

   Drop factor: 60 gtt/mL

   IV PB flow rate: __________ gtt/min

   IV flow rate: __________ gtt/min

5. Order: *1000 mL LR IV for 24 h*

   Kefzol 250 mg IV PB/50 mL D_5W q.8h to run 1 h

   Drop factor: 60 gtt/mL

   IV PB flow rate: __________ gtt/min

   IV flow rate: __________ gtt/min

6. Order: *2400 cc of D_5 LR for 24 h*

   Ancef 1 g IV PB q.6h in 50 cc D_5W to run in over 30 min

   Drop factor: On infusion pump

   IV PB flow rate: __________ mL/h

   IV flow rate: __________ mL/h

7. Order: *2000 cc NS for 24 h*

   Garamycin 100 mg IV PB q.8h in 100 cc D_5W to run in over 30 min

   Drop factor: On infusion controller

   IV PB flow rate: __________ mL/h

   IV flow rate: __________ mL/h

8. Order; *3000 cc D_5 0.45% NS to run over 24 h*

   Zantac 50 mg q.6h in 50 cc D_5W to infuse over 15 min

   Drop factor: On infusion controller

   IV PB flow rate: __________ mL/h

   IV flow rate: __________ mL/h

9. Order: *1500 c D_5 NS to run over 24 h*

   Kefzol 500 mg IV PB/50 mL D_5W q.8 h to run 1 h

   Drop factor: 20 gtt/mL

   IV PB flow rate: __________ gtt/min

   IV flow rate: __________ gtt/min

10. Order: *2700 cc NS IV for 24 h*

    Gentamycin 60 mg in 60 mL D_5W IV PB q.8h to run for 30 min

    Drop factor: On infusion pump

    IV PB flow rate: __________ mL/h

    IV flow rate: __________ mL/h

After completing these problems, see pages 460–462 to check your answers.

critical thinking skills

The importance of knowing the therapeutic dosage of a given medication is a critical nursing skill. Let's look at an example in which the order was unclear, and the nurse did not verify the safe dosage.

error

Failing to clarify an order and failing to recognize a dosage that was unsafe.

possible scenario

Suppose the physician ordered a heparin drip for a patient with thrombophlebitis. The order was written this way:

Heparin 20,000 units in 500 mL of D_5W at 30 mL/h

The nurse, unsure if the order was for 30 mL/h or 80 mL/h, asked a co-worker what the order meant. The co-worker stated, "It looks like 80 mL/h to me, but I'm not sure." The nurse set up the heparin drip and decided to run the rate at 80 mL/h as the co-worker suggested. The patient received the heparin for 24 hours when he began to bleed from his IV site, had blood in his urine, and developed tachycardia and hypotension. When notified, the physician asked, "What is the rate of the heparin drip?" The nurse replied, "80 milliliters per hour," to which the physician stated, "I ordered the drip at 30 mL/h not 80 mL/h; 80 mL/h is an unsafe dosage."

potential outcome

The physician would likely have discontinued the heparin, ordered a stat PTT to evaluate the patient's clotting times, and ordered protamine sulfate, the antidote for heparin. Whether the interventions would have occurred in time to help this patient are unknown.

prevention

The nurse had several opportunities to correct this potentially fatal error. First, had the nurse clarified the unclear order with the physician who ordered the medication, this error would not have occurred. Second, had the nurse calculated the hourly dosage of heparin at 80 mL/h, the unsafe dosage would have been discovered. The nurse would have known to question the order. Let's look at the calculations. First, the nurse gave the following:

$$\frac{20{,}000\text{ U}}{500\text{ mL}} \times \frac{X\text{ U}}{80\text{ mL}}$$

$$500X = 1,600,000$$

$$\frac{500X}{500} = \frac{1{,}600{,}000}{500}$$

X = 3200 units of heparin per hour

3200 × 24 = 76,800 units in 24 hours

This dosage (76,800 U/24 h) exceeds the recommended daily dose by almost two times. You recall that the therapeutic dose of heparin is 20,000 to 40,000 units per 24 hours. Now let's look at what the physician intended for the patient to receive.

$$\frac{20{,}000\text{ U}}{500\text{ mL}} \times \frac{X\text{ U}}{30\text{ mL}}$$

$$500X = 600,000$$

$$\frac{500X}{500} = \frac{600{,}000}{500}$$

X = 1200 units per hour

1200 × 24 = 28,800 units in 24 hours, a safe dosage.

The nurse had two opportunities to prevent this error. Whenever an order is unclear, clarify with the writer. Also, as part of the professional staff we are accountable for our actions and inactions. The nurse should have calculated the hourly heparin dosage to verify what dosage to administer to the patient and to determine its safety.

practice problems—chapter 16

You are working on the day shift 0700–1500 hours. You observe that one of the patients assigned to you has an intravenous infusion with a Buretrol volume control set. His orders include:

D_5W IV @ 50 mL/h for continuous infusion

Pipracil 1 g IV q.6h

The pharmacy supplies the Pipracil in a prefilled syringe labeled *1 g per 5 mL* with instructions to "add Pipracil to Buretrol, and infuse over 30 minutes." Answer questions 1 through 5.

1. What is the drop factor of the Buretrol? __________ gtt/mL
2. What amount of Pipracil will you add to the Buretrol? __________ mL
3. How much D_5W IV fluid will you add to the Buretrol with the Pipracil? __________ mL
4. To maintain the flow rate at 50 mL/h, you will time the IV Pipracil to infuse at __________ gtt/min.
5. The medication administration record indicates that the patient received his last dose of IV Pipracil at 0600. How many doses of Pipracil will you administer during your shift?

   ____

6. Order: *Heparin 25,000 U in 250 mL 0.45% NS to infuse at 1200 U/h*

   Drop Factor: On infusion controller

   Flow rate: 12 mL/h. The patient is receiving 28,800 U/24 h of heparin.

   Is this order safe? Yes

7. Order: *Aminophylline 0.5 g in 250 mL D_5W IV to infuse at 30 mg/h*

   Drop factor: On infusion pump

   Flow rate: 15 mL/h

8. Order: *Magnesium sulfate 4 g in 500 mL D_5W at 500 mg/h*

   Drop factor: On infusion pump

   Flow rate: 62.5 mL/h 63

9. You monitor a patient's IV of 1 L D_5W with 40,000 U heparin infusing at 100 mL/h on an infusion pump. The patient is receiving __________ U/h of heparin. Is the hourly heparin dosage safe? __________
10. At the rate of 4 cc/min, how long will it take to administer 1.5 L of IV fluid? __________ h __________ min
11. Order: *Lidocaine drip IV to run @ 4 mg/min*

    Supply: 500 mL D_5W with Lidocaine 2 g added

    Drop factor: On infusion pump

    Flow rate: __________ mL/h

12. Order: *Xylocaine 1 g IV in 250 mL D_5W at 3 mg/min*

    Drop factor: On infusion controller

    Flow rate: __________ mL/h

13. Order: *Procainamide 1 g in 500 cc D_5W to infuse at 2 mg/min*

    Drop factor: On infusion pump

    Flow rate: __________ mL/h

14. Order: *Dobutamine 250 mg in 250 cc D_5W to infuse at 5 mcg/kg/min*

    Weight: 80 kg

    Drop factor: On infusion controller

    Flow rate: __________ mL/h

15. Your patient has *1 L D_5W with 2 g Lidocaine added infusing at 75 mL/h.* The normal continuous IV dosage of Lidocaine is 1–4 mg/min. Is this dosage safe? __________

16. Order: *Restricted fluids: 3000 mL D_5 NS IV for 24 h*

    Chloromycetin 1 g IV PB in 100 mL NS q.6h to run 1 h

    Drop factor: 10 gtt/mL

    Flow rate: __________ gtt/min IV PB and __________ gtt/min primary IV

17. Order: *Restricted fluids: 3000 mL D_5W IV for 24 h*

    Ampicillin 500 mg in 50 mL D_5W IV PB q.i.d. for 30 min

    Drop factor: On infusion pump

    Flow rate: __________ mL/h IV PB and __________ mL/h primary IV

18. Order: *50 mg Nitropress IV in 500 mL D_5W to infuse at 3 mcg/kg/min*

    Weight: 125 lb

    Drop factor: On infusion pump

    Flow rate: __________ mL/h

19. Order: *KCl 40 mEq to each liter IV fluid*

    Situation: IV discontinued with 800 mL remaining

    How much KCl infused? __________

20. A patient's infusion rate is 125 mL/h. The rate is equivalent to __________ mL/min

21. A patient has 250 mL of IV fluid remaining. The flow rate is 25 gtt/min. The drop factor is 10 gtt/mL. Calculate the time remaining. __________ h and __________ min

22. The time is 1630, and you find 100 mL of an IV running at a flow rate of 33 gtt/min. The drop factor is 60 gtt/mL. At what time will this 100 mL be completed? __________

23. An IV has a flow rate of 48 gtt/min. The infusion set has a drop factor of 15 gtt/mL. How much IV fluid will be infused in 8 hours? __________ mL

24. Order: *1500 mL $\frac{1}{2}$ NS to run at 100 mL/h.* Calculate the infusion time. __________ h

Use the infusion set that follows to calculate the information requested for items 25 and 26.

Baxter Continu-Flo® Set 2.7 m (108") long 3 Inj Sites Luer Lock 60 drops/mL To Open Tear Here recyclable

25. Order: *KCl 40 mEq/L D_5W IV to infuse at 2 mEq/h*

    Rate: __________ mL/h

    Rate: __________ gtt/min

26. Order: *Heparin 50,000 U/L D_5W to infuse at 3750 U/h*

    Rate: __________ mL/h

    Is this dosage safe? __________

27. If the minimal dilution for Tobramycin is 5 mg/mL and you are giving 37 mg, what is the least amount of fluid in which you could safely dilute the dosage? __________ mL

28. Order; *Oxytocin 10 U IV in 500 mL NS. Infuse 4 mU/min for 20 min, followed by 6 mU/min for 20 min. Use electronic infusion pump.*

    Rate: __________ mL/h for first 20 min

    Rate: __________ mL/h for next 20 min

29. Order: *Magnesium sulfate 20 g IV in 500 mL of LR solution. Start with a bolus of 3 g to infuse over 30 min. Then maintain a continuous infusion at 2 g/h.*

    You will use an electronic infusion pump.

    Rate: __________ mL/h for bolus

    Rate: __________ mL/h for continuous infusion

30. Order: *Pitocin 15 U in 500 mL of LR solution. Infuse @ 1 mU/min.*

    You will use an electronic infusion pump.

    Rate: __________ mL/h

31. Order: *Heparin drip 40,000 U/L D_5W to infuse at 1,400 U/h*

    Drop factor: On infusion pump

    Flow rate: __________ mL/h

    Is this order safe? __________

32. Order: *Heparin drip 20,000 U in 500 mL D_5W at 37.5 mL/h*

    The IV is on an infusion pump. The patient is receiving __________ U/h of heparin. Is the hourly order safe? __________

Refer to this order for questions 33 and 34.

Order: *Magnesium sulfate 4 g in 500 mL D_5W at 500 mg/h on an infusion pump.*

33. What is the solution concentration? __________ mg/mL

34. What is the hourly flow rate? __________ mL/h

Calculate the concentration of the following IV solutions as requested

35. A solution containing 80 U of oxytocin (Pitocin) in 1000 mL of D_5W: ________ mU/mL

36. A solution containing 200 mg of nitroglycerin in 500 mL of D_5W: ________ mg/mL

37. A solution containing 4 mg of Isuprel in 1000 mL of D_5W: ________ mcg/mL

38. A solution containing 2 g of Lidocaine in 500 mL of D_5W: ________ mg/mL

39. A solution containing 200 mg of Yutopar in 1000 mL of D_5W: ________ mcg/mL

Refer to this order for questions 40 through 42.

Order: *Norcuron IV l mg/kg/min to control respirations for a ventilated patient.*

40. The patient weighs 220 pounds, which is equal to __________ kg.

41. The available Norcuron 20 mg is dissolved in 100 mL NS. This available solution concentration is __________ mg/mL, which is equivalent to __________ mcg/mL.

42. The IV is infusing at the rate of 1 mcg/kg/min on an infusion pump. The hourly rate is __________ mL/h.

Refer to this order for questions 43 through 48.

Order: *Restricted fluids: 3000 mL total for 24 h. Primary IV of D_5LR running via infusion pump. Ampicillin 3 g IV PB q.6h in 100 mL of D_5W over 30 min and Gentamycin 170 mg IV PB q.8h in 50 mL of D_5W in 1 h.*

43. Calculate the IV PB flow rates. Ampicillin: ________ mL/h; Gentamycin: ________ mL/h
44. Calculate the total IV PB time. ________ h
45. Calculate the total IV PB volume. ________ mL
46. Calculate the total regular IV volume. ________ mL
47. Calculate the total regular IV time. ________ h
48. Calculate the regular IV flow rate. ________ mL/h
49. A 190 pound patient in renal failure receives *Dopamine 800 mg in 500 mL of D_5W IV at 4 mcg/kg/min.* As the patient's blood pressure drops, the nurse titrates the IV drip to *12 mcg/kg/min* as ordered.

    What is the initial flow rate? ________ mL/h

    After titration, what is the flow rate? ________ mL/h
50. Critical Thinking Skill: Describe the strategy you would implement to prevent this medication error.

    possible scenario

    Suppose the physician writes an order to induce labor, as follows: *Pitocin 20 units added to 1 liter of LR beginning at 1 mU/min, then increase by 1 mU/min q 15–30 min to a maximum of 20 mU/min until adequate labor is reached.* The labor and delivery unit stocks Pitocin ampules 20 U mL in boxes of 50 ampules. The nurse preparing the IV solution misread the order as "20 mL of Pitocin added to 1 liter of lactated Ringer's . . ." and pulled 20 ampules of Pitocin from the supply shelf. Another nurse, seeing this nurse drawing up medication from several ampules, asked what the nurse was preparing. When the nurse described the IV solution being prepared, the nurse suddenly realized the order was misread.

    potential outcome

    The amount of Pitocin that was being drawn up (20 mL) to be added to the IV solution would have been 10 U/mL × 20 mL = 200 U of Pitocin, 10 times the ordered amount of 20 U. Starting this Pitocin solution even at the usual slow rate would have delivered an excessively high amount of Pitocin that could have led to fatal consequences for both the fetus and laboring mother. What should the nurse have done to avoid this type of error?

    prevention

    ____

    ____

After completing these problems, see pages 462–465 to check your answers.

Section 4 Self-Evaluation

Chapter 13: Reconstitution of Noninjectable Solutions

Use the following information to answer questions 1 and 2. You will prepare *360 mL of $\frac{1}{3}$ strength hydrogen peroxide* diluted with normal saline to irrigate a wound.

1. Add __________ mL solute.
2. Add __________ mL solvent.
3. You will prepare a *$\frac{3}{4}$ strength solution of hydrogen peroxide* diluted with normal saline. You use 60 mL of stock hydrogen peroxide. Add __________ mL of normal saline as the solvent.

Refer to this order for questions 4 and 5.

Order: *Give $\frac{2}{3}$ strength Ensure 240 mL via NG tube q.3h.*

Supply: Ready-to-use Ensure 8 ounce can and sterile water.

4. How much water would you add to the 8 ounce can of Ensure? __________ mL
5. How many feedings would this make? __________ feedings

Refer to this order for questions 6 and 7.

Order: *$\frac{3}{8}$ strength Enfamil 26 mL via NG tube q.h × 8 feedings.*

Supply: Ready-to-use Enfamil 3 ounce bottles and sterile water.

6. How any bottles of Enfamil would be needed to prepare all 8 feedings? __________ bottle(s)
7. How much unused reconstituted formula would remain after the eighth feeding? __________ mL

Use the following information to answer questions 8 and 9.

You will prepare formula to feed 9 infants in the nursery. Each infant has an order for *4 ounces of $\frac{1}{2}$ strength Isomil formula q.3h.* You have 8 ounce cans of ready-to-use Isomil and sterile water.

8. How many cans of formula will you need to open to prepare the reconstituted formula for all 9 infants for one feeding each? __________ can(s)
9. How many mL of water will you add to the Isomil to reconstitute the formula for one feeding for all 9 infants? __________ mL
10. Your patient needs home care instructions to prepare an irrigant of *500 mL of warm NS*. The patient will have table salt, sterile water, and household measuring devices available. State your home care instructions. ______________________________

____

Chapter 14: Intravenous Solutions, Equipment, and Calculations

Classify the following IV solutions as *hypotonic, isotonic,* or *hypertonic.*

11. 0.9% sodium chloride (308 mOsm/L) __________
12. D_5 and 0.45% NaCl (405 mOsm/L) __________
13. 0.45% sodium chloride (154 mOsm/L) __________

Use the following information to answer questions 14 and 15.

Order: *1000 mL of D_5 0.33% NaCl IV*

14. The IV solution contains __________ g dextrose.
15. The IV solution contains __________ g sodium chloride.
16. An order specifies *500 mL 0.45% NS IV.* The IV solution contains __________ g sodium chloride.

Refer to this order for questions 17 through 19.

Order: *750 mL D_{10} 0.9% NaCl IV.*

17. The IV solution contains __________ g dextrose.
18. The IV solution contains __________ g sodium chloride.
19. Are most electronic infusion devices calibrated in gtt/min, mL/h, mL/min, or gtt/mL? __________

Use the following information to answer questions 20 and 21.

Mrs. Wilson has an order to receive *2000 mL of IV fluids over 24 h.* The IV tubing is calibrated for a drop factor of 15 gtt/mL.

20. Calculate the "watch count" flow rate for Mrs. Wilson's IV. __________ gtt/min
21. An infusion controller becomes available, and you decide to use it to regulate Mrs. Wilson's IV. Set the controller at __________ mL/h.
22. Mrs. Hawkins returns from the delivery room at 1530 with 400 mL D_5LR infusing at 24 gtt/min with your hospital's standard macrodrop infusion control set calibrated at 15 gtt/mL. You anticipate that Mrs. Hawkins' IV will be complete at __________ (hours).
23. You start your shift at 3:00 PM. On your nursing assessment rounds you find that Mr. Johnson has an IV of $D_5 \frac{1}{2}$ NS infusing at 32 gtt/min. The tubing is calibrated for 10 gtt/mL. Mr. Johnson will receive __________ mL during your 8 hour shift.

Use the following information to answer questions 24 through 26.

As you continue on your rounds you find Mr. Boyd with an infiltrated IV and decide to restart it and regulate it on an electronic infusion pump. The order specifies: *1000 mL NS IV $\bar{c}$ 20 mEq KCl q.8h, & Kefzol 250 mg IV PB/100 mL NS q.8h over 30 min. Limit IV fluids to 3000 mL q.d.*

24. Interpret Mr. Boyd's IV and medication order. __________
25. Regulate the electronic infusion pump for Mr. Boyd's standard IV at __________ mL/h.
26. Regulate the electronic infusion pump for Mr. Boyd's IV PB at __________ mL/h.
27. Order: *D_5LR 1200 mL IV @ 100 mL/h.* You start this IV at 1530 and regularly observe the IV and the patient. The IV has been infusing as scheduled, but during your nursing assessment at 2200, you find 650 mL remaining. The flow rate is 100 gtt/min using a microdrip infusion set. Describe your action now. __________

Chapter 15: Advanced Pediatric Calculations

28. Order: *20 mEq KCl/L D_5NS IV continuous infusion at 20 mL/h.*

    Supply: Because this is a child, you choose a 250 mL IV bag of D_5W. The KCl is available in a solution strength of 2 mEq/mL. Add __________ mL KCl to the 250 mL bag of D_5W.

Calculate the hourly maintenance IV rate for the children described in questions 29 and 30. Use the following recommendations:

First 10 kg of body weight: 100 mL/kg/day

Second 10 kg of body weight: 50 mL/kg/day

Each additional kg over 20 kg of body weight: 20 mL/kg/day

29. 40 lb child has a rate of __________ mL/h.
30. 1185 g infant has a rate of __________ mL/h.

Use the following formulas to calculate the BSA (m^2) for the following patients described in questions 31 and 32.

$$\text{BSA } (m^2) = \sqrt{\frac{\text{ht (cm)} \times \text{wt (kg)}}{3600}} \qquad \text{BSA } (m^2) = \sqrt{\frac{\text{ht (in)} \times \text{wt (lb)}}{3131}}$$

31. Height: 30 in Weight: 24 lb BSA: __________ m^2
32. Height: 155 cm Weight: 39 kg BSA: __________ m^2

Use the West Nomogram and the following information to answer questions 33 through 37.

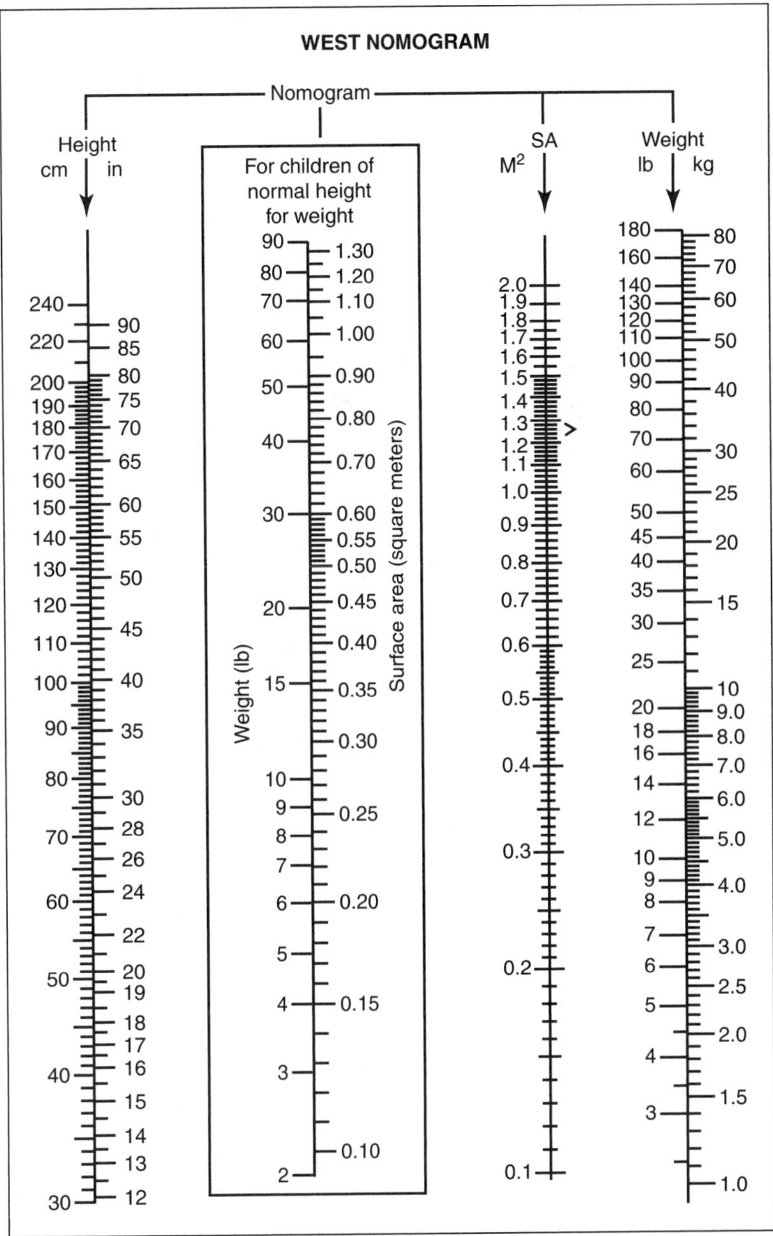

West's Nomogram for Estimation of Body Surface Area. (From *Nelson Textbook of Pediatrics* (15th ed.) by R. E. Behrman, R. M. Kleigman, & A. M. Arvin, 1996, Philadelphia: Saunders. Reprinted with permission.)

A child who is 28 inches tall and weighs 25 lb is to receive one dose of Cisplatin IV. The recommended dosage is 37 to 75 mg/m^2 once every 2 to 3 weeks. The order reads *Cisplatin 18.5 mg IV @ 1 mg/min today at 1500 hours.* You have available a 50 mg vial of Cisplatin. Reconstitution directions state to add 50 mL of sterile water to yield 1 mg/mL. Minimal dilution instructions require 2 mL of IV solution for every 1 mg of Cisplatin.

33. The child's BSA is __________ m^2.

34. The safe dosage range for this child is __________ to __________ mg.

35. Is the dosage ordered safe? __________. If safe, you will prepare __________ mL.

36. Given the ordered rate of 1 mg/min, set the infusion pump at __________ mL/h.

37. How long will this infusion take? __________ min

38. Order: *Oncovin 1.6 mg IV stat.* The child is of normal height and weighs 44 lb. The West Nomogram you have available is on page 381. The following label represents the Oncovin solution you have available. The recommended dosage of Oncovin is 2 mg/m^2 q.d. Is the dosage ordered safe? __________. If it is safe, you will add __________ mL Oncovin to the IV.

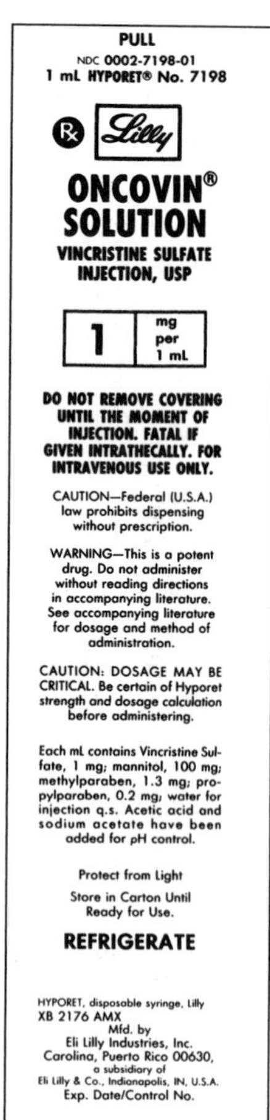

39. Order: *NS IV for continuous infusion at 40 mL/h c̄ Ancef 250 mg IV q.8h over 30 min by Buretrol.*

Available: Ancef 125 mg/mL

Add __________ mL NS and __________ mL Ancef to the Buretrol to infuse at 40 mL/h.

40. Order: *Ticarcillin 750 mg IV q.6h. Recommended minimal dilution (maximal concentration) is 100 mg/mL.* Calculate the number of mL of IV solution to be used for minimal dilution of the Ticarcillin as ordered. __________ mL

Chapter 16: Advanced Adult Intravenous Calculations

41. Mr. Black has a new order for *10,000 U heparin in 500 mL NS IV at 750 U/h.* Is Mr. Black's order safe? __________

Use the following information to answer questions 42 through 44.

Mr. Smith is on restricted fluids. Order: *1500 mL NS IV/24 h c̄ 300,000 U penicillin G potassium IV PB 100 mL NS q.4h over 30 min.* The infusion set is calibrated at 60 gtt/mL.

42. Set Mr. Smith's regular IV at __________ gtt/min.

43. Set Mr. Smith's IV PB at __________ gtt/min.

44. Later during your shift, an electronic infusion pump becomes available. You decide to use it to regulate Mr. Smith's IVs. Regulate Mr. Smith's regular IV at __________ mL/h. Regulate Mr. Smith's IV PB at __________ mL/h.

45. Order: *KCl 40 mEq/L D_5W IV @ 2 mEq/h.*

    Regulate the infusion pump at __________ mL/h.

46. Order: *Nitroglycerin 25 mg/L D_5W IV @ 5 mcg/min*

    Regulate the infusion pump at __________ mL/h.

Refer to this order for questions 47 and 48.

Order: *Induce labor c̄ Pitocin 15 U/L LR IV continuous infusion @ 2 mU/min; increase by 1 mU/min q.30 min to a maximum of 20 mU/min*

47. Regulate the electronic infusion pump at __________ mL/h to initiate the order.

48. The infusion pump will be regulated at a maximum of __________ mL/h to infuse the maximum of 20 mU/min.

Use the following information to answer questions 49 and 50.

Order for Ms. Hill, who weighs 150 lb: *Dopamine 600 mg/0.5 L D_5W at 4 mcg/kg/min titrated to 12 mcg/kg/min to stabilize blood pressure*

49. Regulate the electronic infusion pump for Ms. Hill's IV at __________ mL/h to initiate the order.

50. Anticipate that the maximum flow rate for Ms. Hill's IV to achieve the maximum safe titration would be __________ mL/h.

After completing these problems, refer to pages 465–468 to check your answers.

Perfect Score = 100% My score = __________

Minimum mastery score = 86% (43 correct)

Essential Skills Evaluation

This evaluation is designed to assess your mastery of essential dosage calculation skills. It is similar to the type of entry-level test given by hospitals and health care agencies during orientation for new graduates and new employees. It excludes the advanced calculation skills presented in Chapters 13, 15, and 16.

You are assigned to give "Team Medications" on a busy Adult Medical Unit. The following labels represent the medications available in your medication cart. Calculate the amount you will administer for one dose. Assume all tablets are scored. Draw an arrow on the appropriate syringe to indicate how much you will prepare for parenteral medications.

1. Order: *Dilantin 50 mg IV q.8h*

   Give: __________ mL

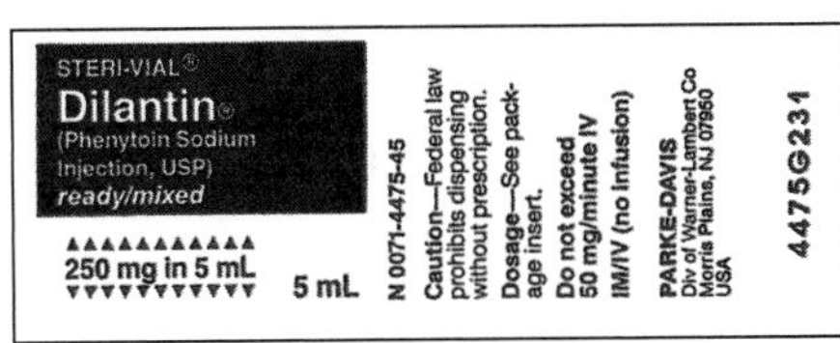

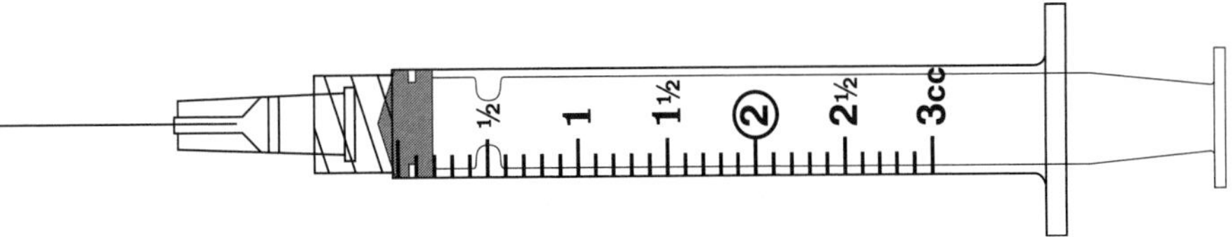

2. Order: *Phenergan 12.5 mg IM q.3–4h p.r.n. nausea*

   Give: __________ mL

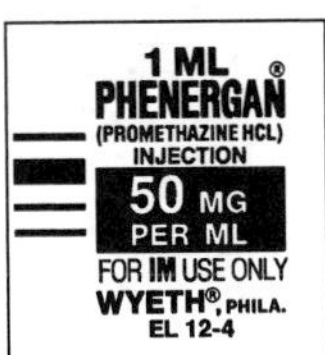

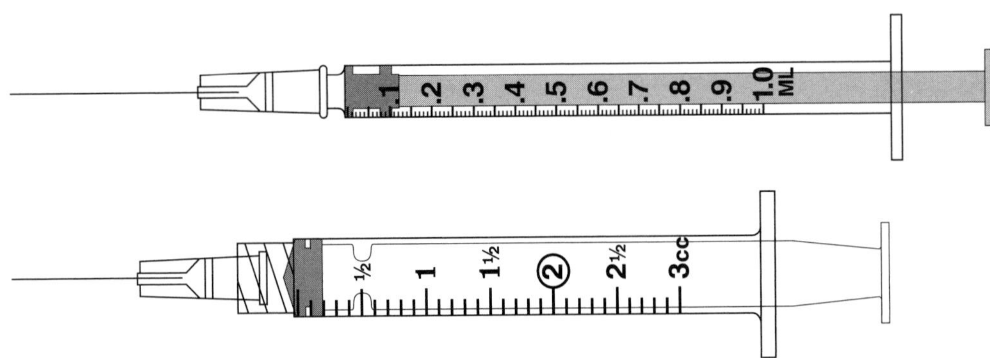

3. Order: *Thorazine 35 mg IM stat*

   Give: __________ mL

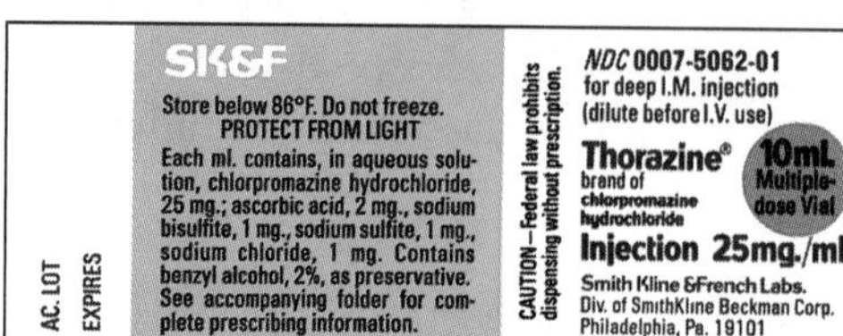

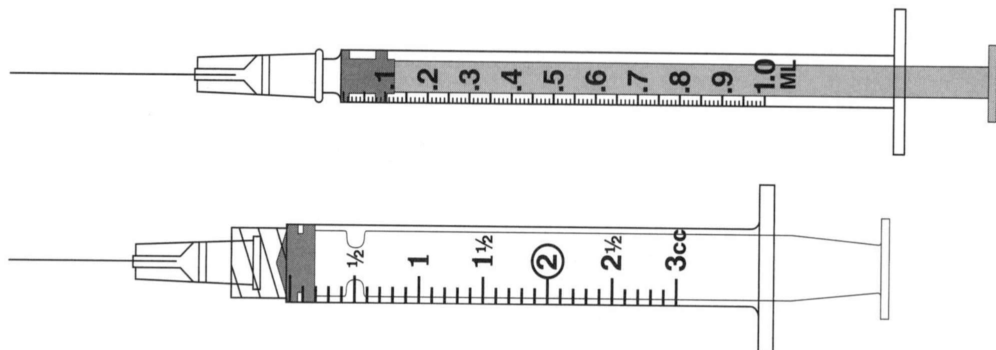

4. Order: *Tagamet 400 mg p.o. h.s.*

   Give: __________ tablet(s)

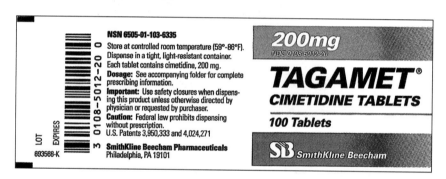

5. Order: *Lortab 7.5 mg p.o. p.r.n. q.3h*

   Give: __________ tablet(s)

PHARMACIST:
Dispense in a tight, light-resistant container as defined in the USP.

STORAGE:
Store at controlled room temperature, 15°-30°C (59°-86°F).

Lot No.:
Exp. Date:

Manufactured by
D.M. GRAHAM Laboratories, Inc.
Hobart, NY 13788

RUSS® CIII
NDC 50474-902-01
LORTAB® 5 mg
HYDROCODONE BITARTRATE AND ACETAMINOPHEN TABLETS
Each scored white with blue specks tablet contains:
Hydrocodone Bitartrate* ...... 5 mg
***WARNING: May be habit forming.**
Acetaminophen .... 500 mg
CAUTION: Federal law prohibits dispensing without prescription.
100 TABLETS

DOSAGE:
The usual adult dosage is one or two tablets every four to six hours as needed for pain. The total 24 hour dose should not exceed 8 tablets.

See package insert for full prescribing information.

KEEP THIS AND ALL MEDICATIONS OUT OF THE REACH OF CHILDREN.

Rev. 10/89

Manufactured for
RUSS Pharmaceuticals, Inc.
Birmingham, AL 35242

6. Order: *Lanoxin 0.125 mg IV q. AM*

   Give: __________ mL

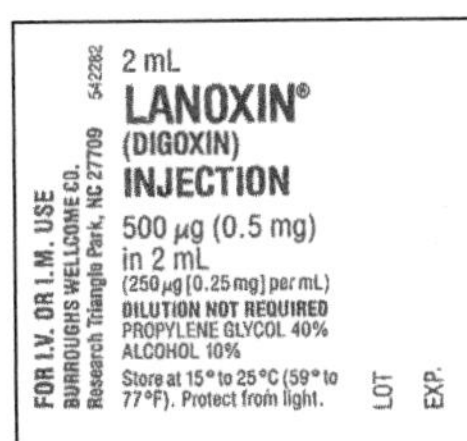

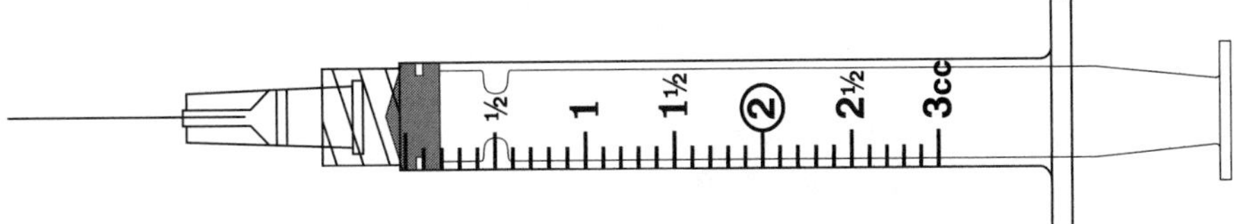

7. Order: *Phenobarbital gr $\frac{1}{8}$ p.o. q.i.d.*

   Give: __________ tablet(s)

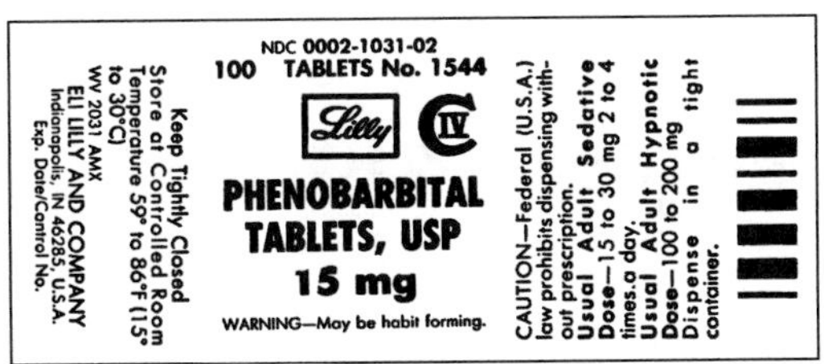

8. Order: *Kantrex 350 mg IM b.i.d.*

   Give: __________ mL

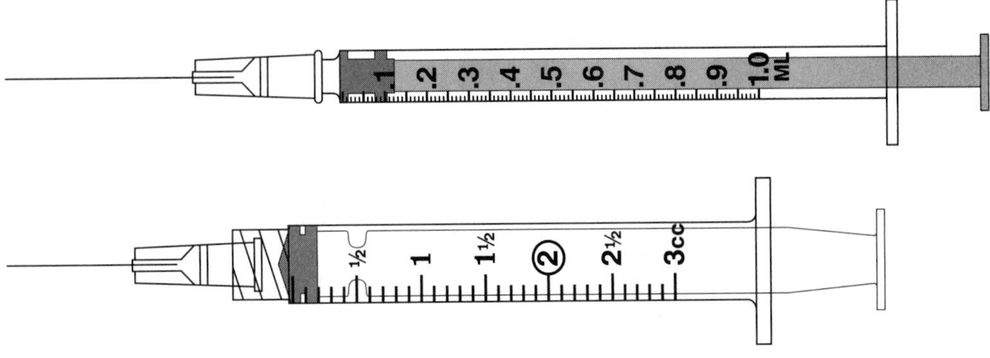

9. Order: *Novolin L Lente human U-100 insulin 46 U c̄ Novolin R regular human U-100 insulin 22 U SC stat.*

You will give __________ U total.

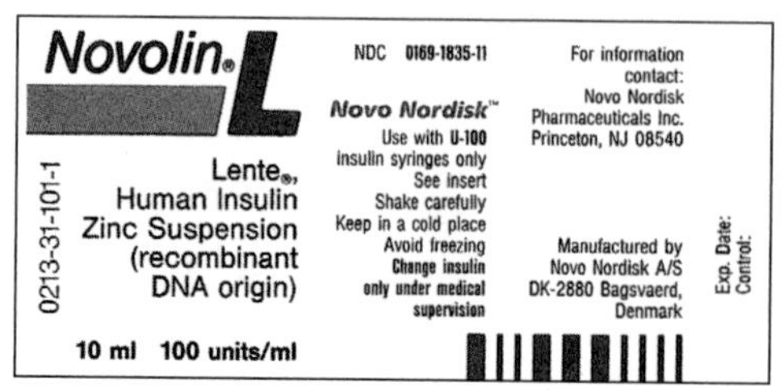

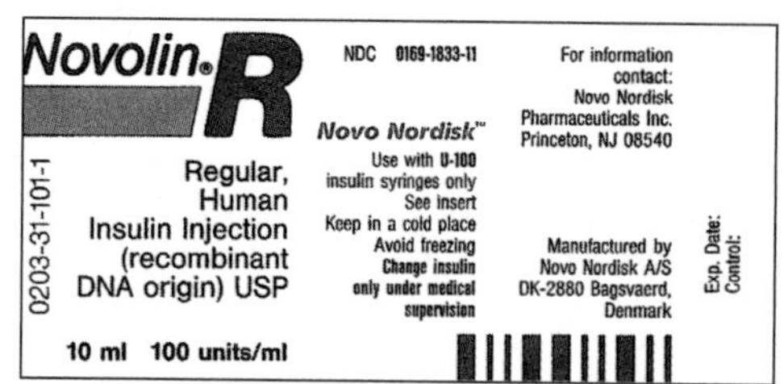

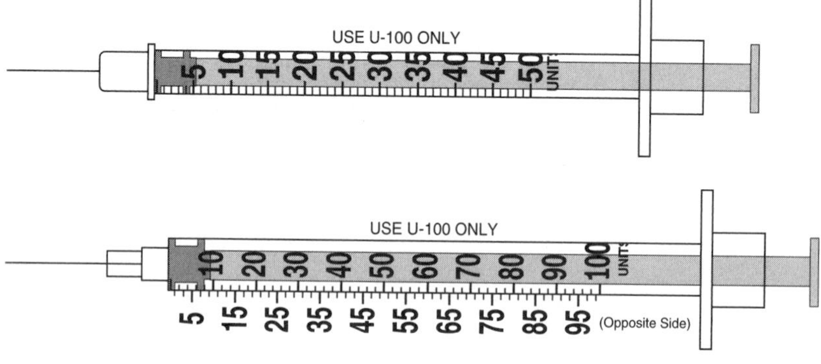

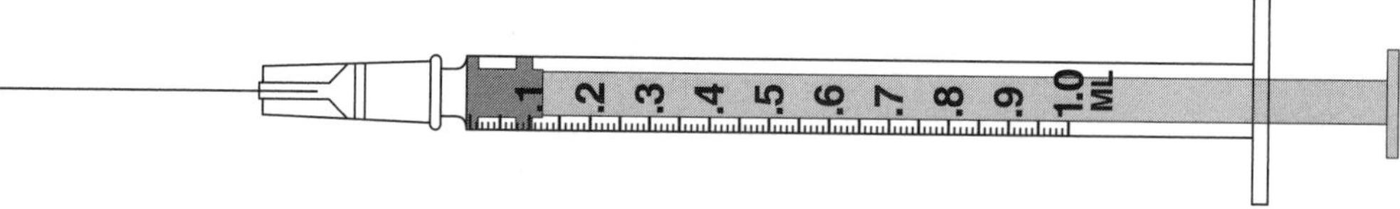

10. Order: *Synthroid 0.05 mg p.o. q. AM*

Give: __________ tablet(s)

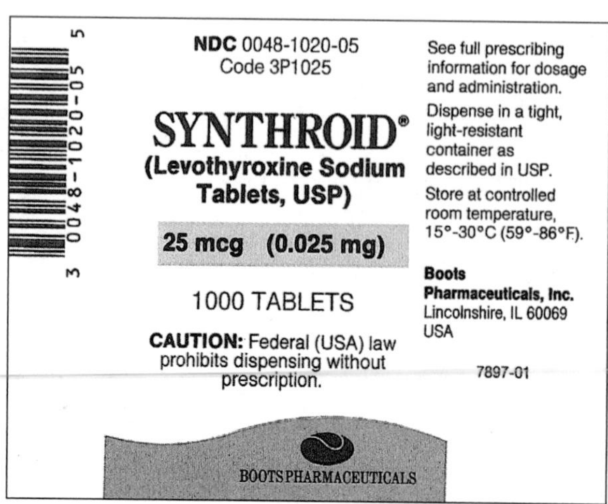

11. Order: *Calan 40 mg p.o. t.i.d.*

    Give: __________ tablet(s)

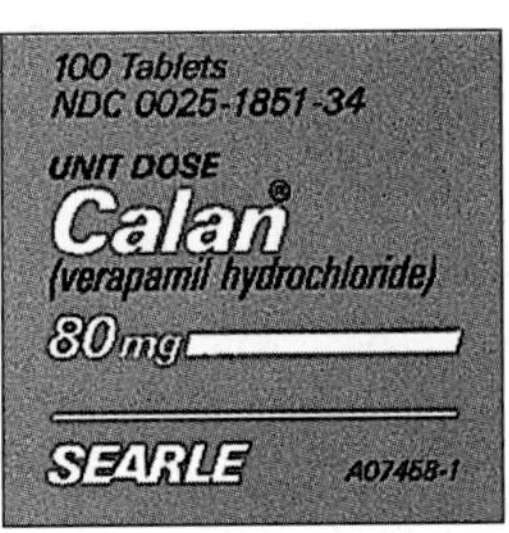

12. Order: *Naprosyn 375 mg p.o. b.i.d.*

    Give: __________ tablet(s)

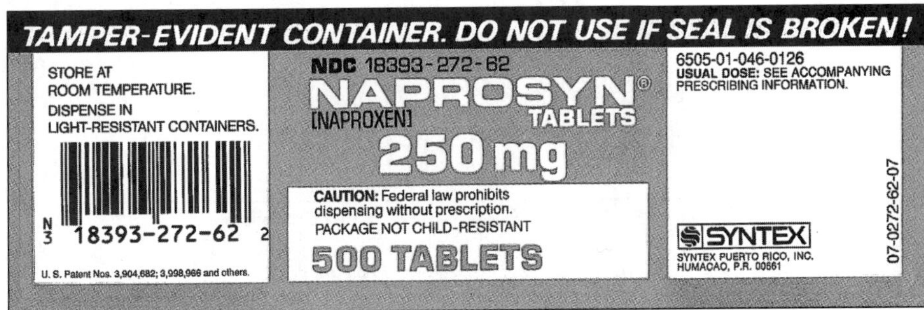

13. Order: *Phenergan 40 mg IM stat*

    Give: __________ mL

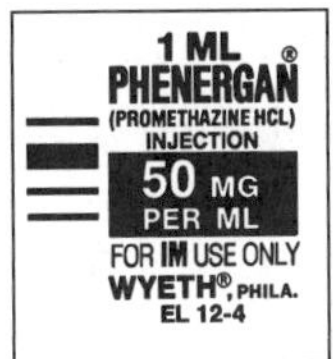

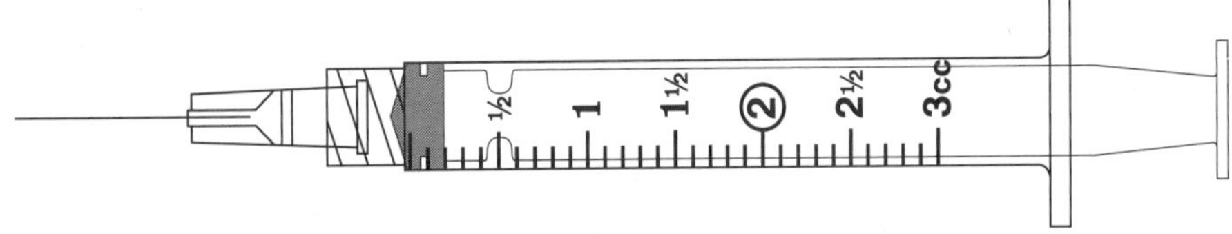

14. Order: *Stadol 3 mg IM stat*

    Give: __________ mL

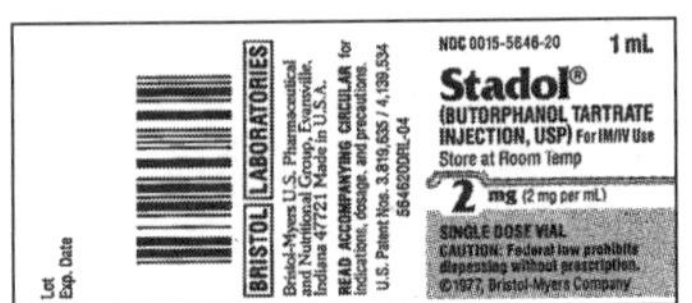

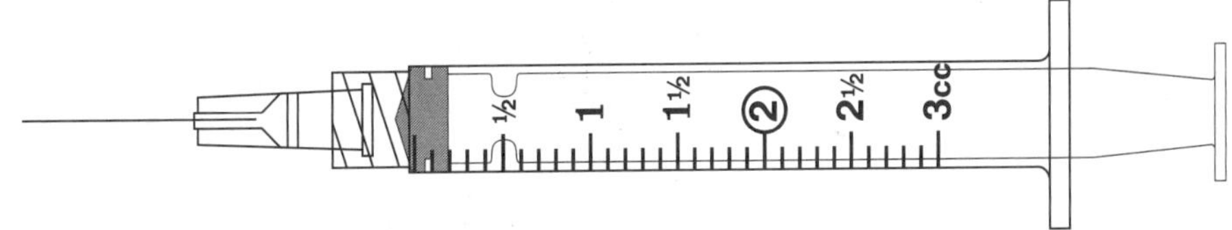

15. Order: *Betapen-VK 100 mg p.o. q.6h*

    Give: __________ mL

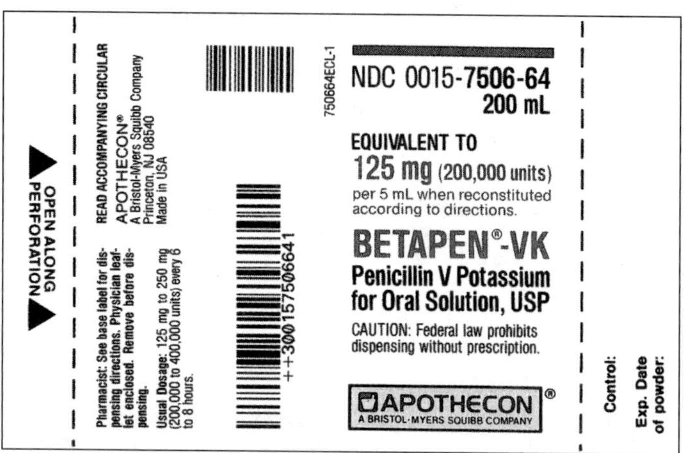

16. Order: *Atropine gr $\frac{1}{100}$ IM stat*

    Give: __________ mL

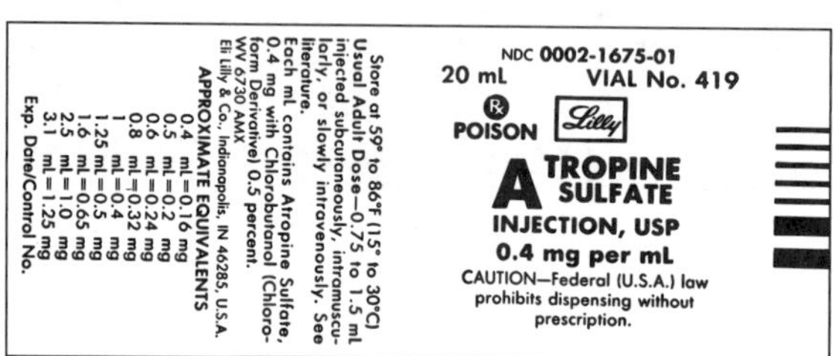

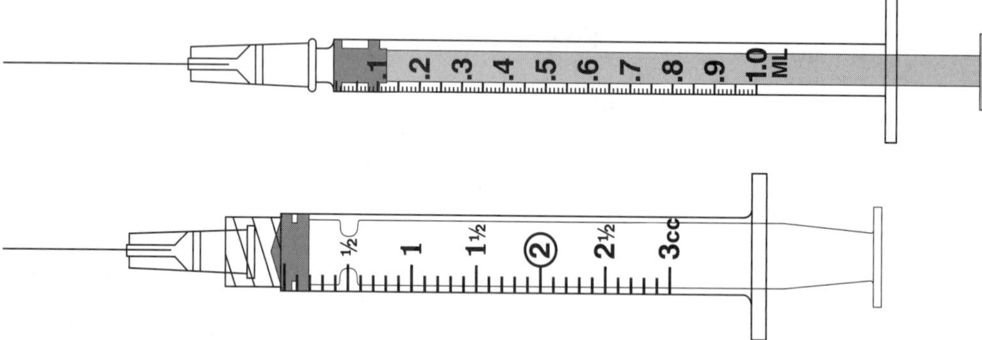

17. Order: *Ampicillin 0.5 g in 50 mL normal saline IV PB over 30 min.*

    Add __________ mL ampicillin to the normal saline, and set the flow rate to __________ gtt/min.

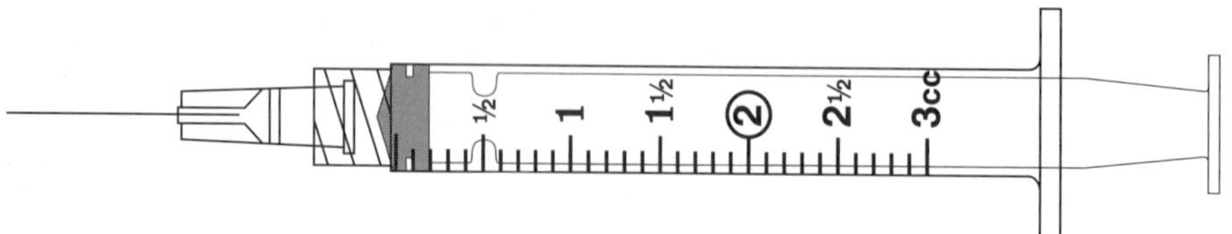

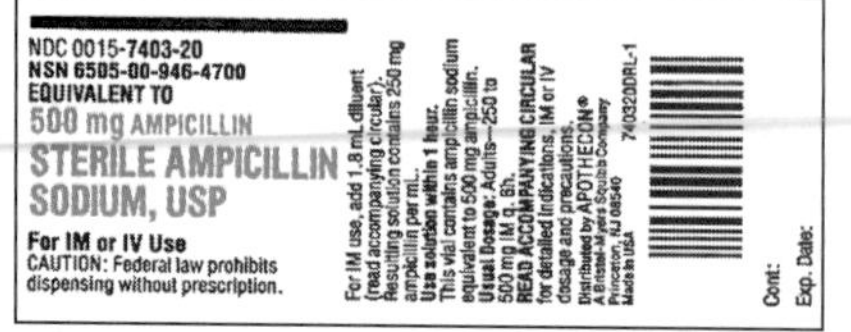

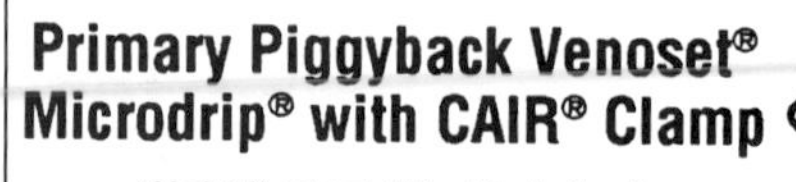

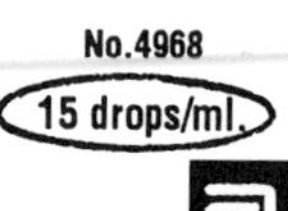

Refer to the following MAR to answer questions 18 through 22.

09/11/xx
06:26 PM
CHECKED BY: ————————————

MEDICATION ADMINISTRATION RECORD

PAGE: 1
REPT: PHR20B

2ND 241
217A 532729
Smedley, Betty

DIAGNOSIS: 71590
ALLERGIES: NKA
NOTES:

DIET: Regular
ADMIT: 09/11/xx
WT: 154 lbs.

DX: OSTEOARTHROS NOS-UNSPEC

ADMINISTRATION PERIOD: 07:30 09/12/xx TO 07:29 09/13/xx

ORDER # DRUG NAME, STRENGTH, DOSAGE FORM DOSE RATE ROUTE SCHEDULE	START	STOP	TIME PERIOD 07:30 TO 15:29	TIME PERIOD 15:30 TO 23:29	TIME PERIOD 23:30 TO 07:29
NURSE:					
• • • PRN's FOLLOW • • •			• • • PRN's FOLLOW • • •		
264077 TYLENOL 325MG TABLET PRN **2 TABS** ORAL Q4H/PRN FOR TEMP > 101 F	09:30 09/11/xx				
264147 TORADOL 60MG SYRINGE PRN **60 MG** IM PRN GIVE 60MG FOR BREAKTHROUGH PAIN X1 DOSE THEN 30MG Q6H/PRN	15:00 09/11/xx				
264148 TORADOL 60MG SYRINGE PRN **30 MG** IM Q6H/PRN GIVE 6 HOURS AFTER 60MG DOSE FOR BREAK-THROUGH PAIN.	15:00 09/11/xx				
264151 INAPSINE 2.5MG/ML AMPULE PRN **SEE NOTE** IV Q6H/PRN SAME AS DROPERIDOL; DOSE IS 0.625MG TO 1.25MG (0.5-1.0 ML) FOR NAUSEA	15:00 09/11/xx				
264152 NUBAIN 10MG/ML AMPULE PRN **2 MG** IV Q4H/PRN FOR ITCHING	15:00 09/11/xx				
264153 NARCAN 0.4MG/ML AMPULE PRN **0.4 MG** IV PRN FOR RR< 8 AND IF PT. IS UNAROUSABLE	15:00 09/11/xx				
NURSE:					
NURSE:					

INITIALS	SIGNATURE	INITIALS	SIGNATURE	NOTES	

1500 0100

PHYSICIAN: J. Physician, MD

217A Betty Smedley AGE: 73 SEX: F

Mrs. Betty Smedley in Room 217A is assigned to your team. She is hospitalized with osteoarthritis. The medications available from the pharmacy are noted on the MAR on page 391.

18. Mrs. Smedley had her last dose of Tylenol at 2110 hours. It is now 0215 hours, and her temperature is 39°C. Is Tylenol indicated? ______________________

    Explain: ______________________

    ____

19. How many tablets of Tylenol should she receive for each dose? __________ tablet(s)

    Each dose is equivalent to __________ mg Tylenol.

20. Mrs. Smedley had 60 mg of Toradol at 1500 hours. At 2130 hours she is complaining of severe pain again. How much Toradol in the prefilled syringe will you give her now? Give __________ of the syringe amount.

21. Mrs. Smedley is complaining of itching. What p.r.n. medication would you select, and how much will you administer? Select __________, and give __________ mL. Draw an arrow on the appropriate syringe to indicate how much you will give.

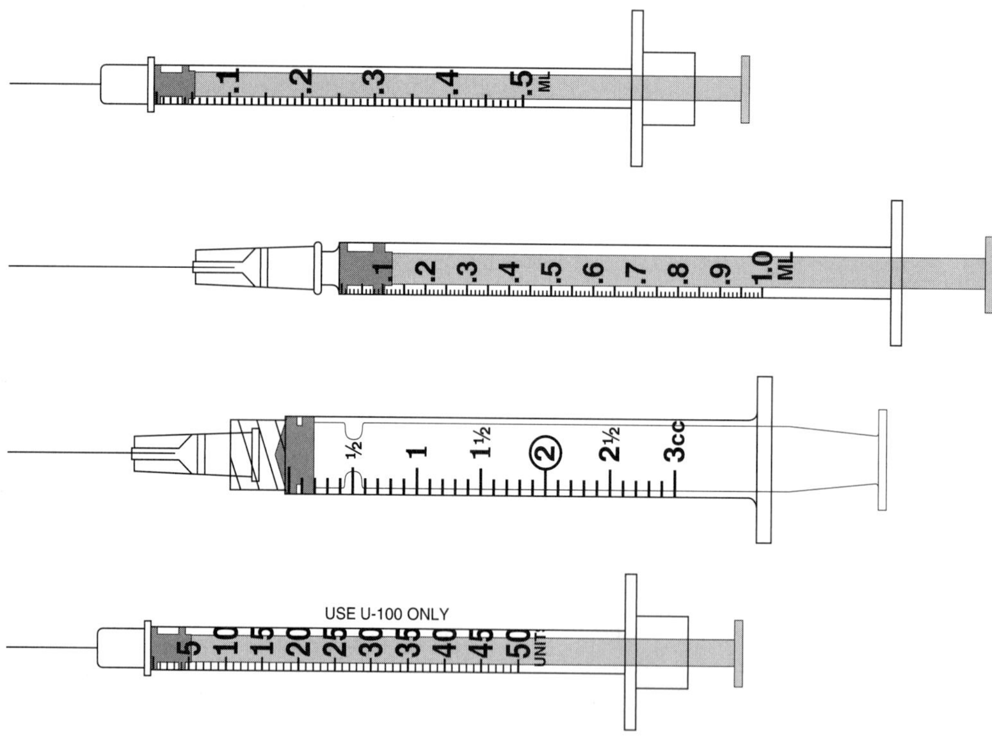

22. Mrs. Smedley's respiratory rate (R.R.) is 7, and she is difficult to arouse. What medication is indicated? __________ Give __________ mL. Draw an arrow on the syringe to indicate how much of this medication you will give.

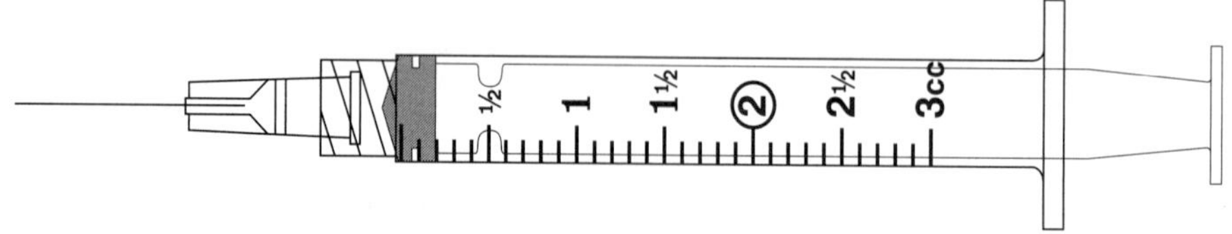

Refer to the following MAR to answer questions 23 through 27.

PAGE ____ of ____

MEDICATION ADMINISTRATION RECORD

ORIGINAL ORDER DATE	DATE STARTED / RENEWED	MEDICATION - DOSAGE	ROUTE	SCHEDULE 11-7	SCHEDULE 7-3	SCHEDULE 3-11	DATE 3-10-xx 11-7	7-3	3-11	DATE 3-11-xx 11-7	7-3	3-11	DATE 3-12-xx 11-7	7-3	3-11	DATE 3-14 11-7	7-3	3-11
3-10 XX	3-10	Aminophylline 150 mg in 50 ml D_5W x 30 min q.6h	IV PB	12 6	12	6		GP 12	MS 6	JJ12 JJ6								
3-10 XX	3-10	Solu-Medrol 125 mg q.6h	IV	12 6	12	6		GP 12	MS 6	JJ12 JJ6								
3-10 XX	3-10	Carafate 1 g 15 min ac & hs	PO	7:45	11:45	5:45 10:00		GP 11:45	MS5:45 MS9:45	JJ6:45								
3-10 XX	3-10	Novulin R Regular U-100 insulin 30 min ac per sliding scale:	SC					GP7:30 GP11:30	MS5:30									
		Blood sugar Units																
		0-150 0 U																
		151-250 8 U																
		251-350 13 U																
		351-400 18 U																
		>400 Call M.D.																

PRN

INJECTION SITES

B - RIGHT ARM
C - RIGHT ABDOMEN
D - RIGHT ANTERIOR THIGH
G - LEFT ARM
H - LEFT ABDOMEN
J - LEFT ANTERIOR THIGH
L - LEFT BUTTOCKS
M - RIGHT BUTTOCKS

DATE GIVEN	TIME	INT.	ONE - TIME MEDICATION - DOSAGE	RT.

SIGNATURE OF NURSE ADMINISTERING MEDICATIONS	DATE	DATE	DATE	DATE
11-7	GP. G.Pickar,RN	JJ J.Jones LPN		
7-3				
3-11	MS. M.Smith,RN			

DATE GIVEN	TIME	INT.	MEDICATION-DOSAGE-CONT.	RT.
			RECOPIED BY:	
			CHECKED BY:	

Beck, John
ID #76834-21

ALLERGIES:

602-31 (7-xx) (MPC# 1355)

1 ORIGINAL COPY

LITHO IN U.S.A. K6509 (7-92) D395538

PRINTED BY STANDARD REGISTER U.S.A. ZIPSET ®

John Beck, 19 years old, is diabetic. He is admitted to the medical unit with asthma. You are administering his medications. The MAR on page 393 is in the medication notebook on your medication cart. The labels represent the infusion set available and the medications in his medication cart drawer. Questions 23 through 27 refer to John.

23. Aminophylline is available in a solution strength of 250 mg/10 mL. There will be __________ mL aminophylline in the IV PB. Set the flow rate at __________ gtt/min.

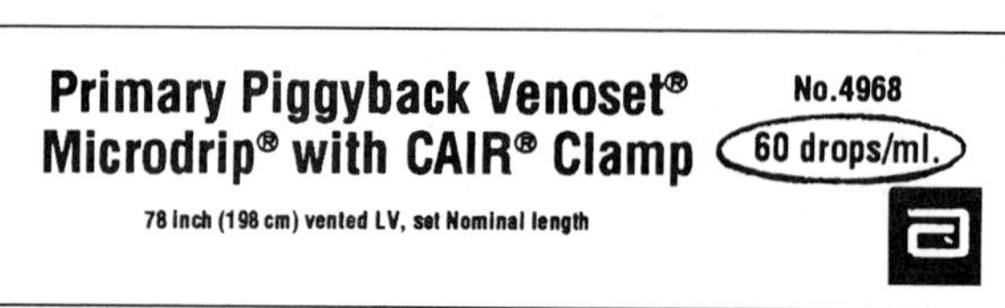

24. An infusion pump becomes available, and you decide to use it for John's IV. It is calibrated in mL/h. To administer the aminophylline by infusion pump, set the pump at __________ mL/h.

25. Reconstitute the Solu-Medrol with __________ mL diluent, and give __________ mL.

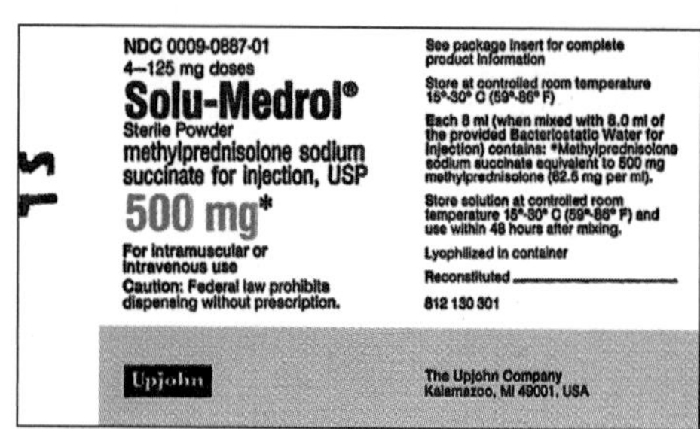

26. Mealtimes and bedtime are 8 AM, 12 N, 6 PM, and 10 PM. Using international time, give __________ tablet(s) of Carafate per dose each day at __________, __________, __________, and __________ hours.

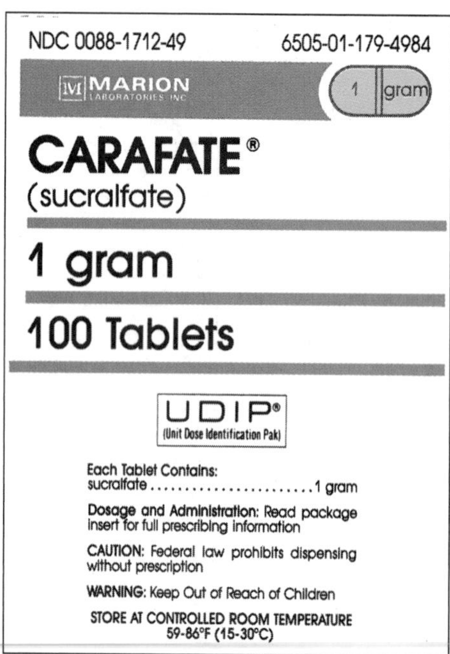

27. At 0730 John's blood sugar is 360. You will give him __________ U of insulin by the __________ route. Draw an arrow on the appropriate syringe to indicate the correct dosage.

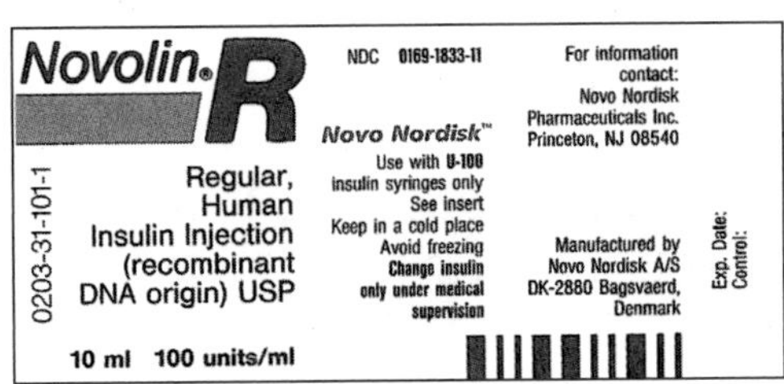

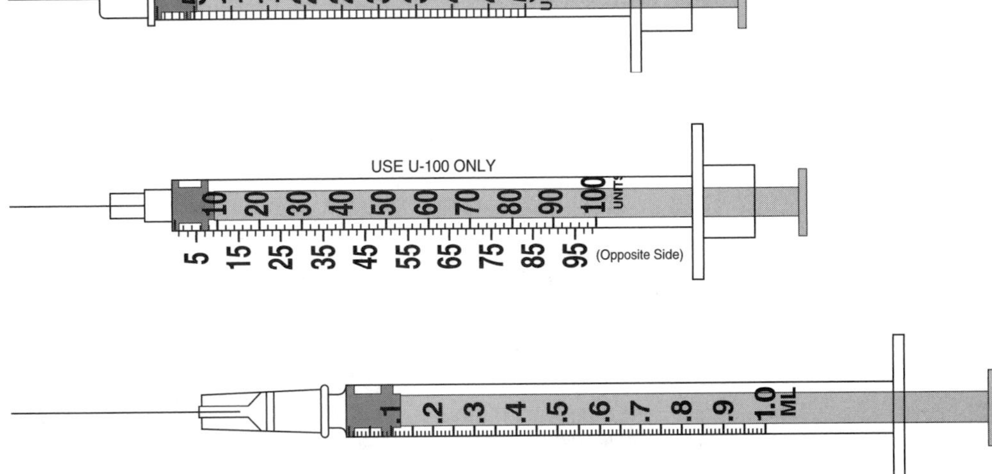

Jimmy Bryan is brought to the pediatric clinic by his mother. He is a 15 pound baby with an ear infection. Questions 28 through 31 refer to Jimmy.

28. The physician orders *amoxicillin 50 mg p.o. q.8h* for Jimmy. To reconstitute the amoxicillin, add __________ mL water.

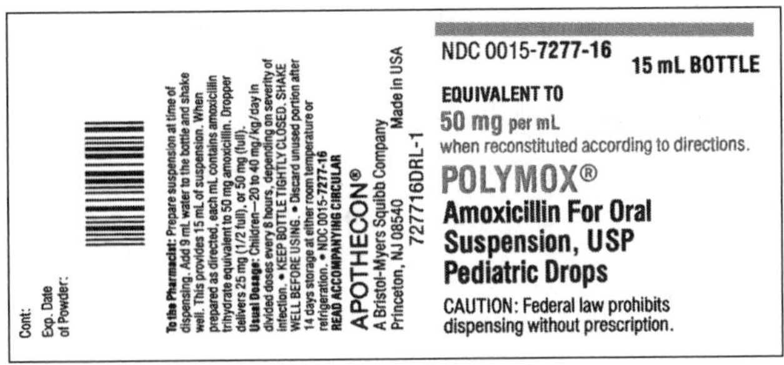

29. Is Jimmy's amoxicillin order safe and reasonable? __________.

Explain: ____

____

30. The physician asks you to give Jimmy one dose of the amoxicillin stat. You will give Jimmy __________ mL.

31. The physician also asks you to instruct Jimmy's mother about administering the medication at home. Tell Jimmy's mother to give the baby __________ droppersful for each dose. How often? __________

32. Jill Jones is a 16-year-old, 110-pound teenager with a duodenal ulcer and abdominal pain. She has an order for *cimetidine 250 mg q.6h in 50 mL D_5W IV PB to be infused in 20 min* The recommended cimetidine dosage is 20 to 40 mg/kg/day in 4 divided doses. Available is cimetidine for injection, 300 mg/2 mL. The label represents the infusion set available. Is this ordered dosage safe? __________.
If safe, add __________ mL cimetidine, and set the flow rate at __________ gtt/min.

Baxter Continu-Flo® Set 2.7 m (105") long 3 Inj Sites Luer Lock 10 drops/mL

33. The doctor writes a new order for strict intake and output assessment for a child. During your eight-hour shift, in addition to his IV fluids of 200 mL D_5Ns, he consumed the following oral fluids:

gelatin—℥ iv

water—℥ iii × 2

apple juice—pt i

What is his total fluid intake during your shift? __________ mL

Use the following information to answer questions 34 through 36.

Order for child with severe otitis media (inner ear infection) who weighs 40 lb: *Augmentin 240 mg p.o. q.8h.* The following Augmentin label represents the dosage you have available. Recommended Augmentin dosage is 40 mg/kg/day q.8h in divided doses.

AUGMENTIN® 250mg/5mL
NSN 6505-01-207-8205
Directions for mixing: Tap bottle until all powder flows freely. Add approximately 2/3 of total water for reconstitution (total = 65 mL); shake vigorously to wet powder. Add remaining water; again shake vigorously.
Dosage: See accompanying prescribing information.
Keep tightly closed. Shake well before using. Must be refrigerated. Discard after 10 days.

250mg/5mL
NDC 0029-6090-39
AUGMENTIN®
AMOXICILLIN/ CLAVULANATE POTASSIUM FOR ORAL SUSPENSION
When reconstituted, each 5 mL contains: AMOXICILLIN, 250 MG, as the trihydrate CLAVULANIC ACID, 62.5 MG, as clavulanate potassium
75mL (when reconstituted)
SB SmithKline Beecham

Use only if inner seal is intact. **Net contents:** Equivalent to 3.75 g amoxicillin and 0.938 g clavulanic acid. Store dry powder at room temperature. **Caution:** Federal law prohibits dispensing without prescription. **SmithKline Beecham Pharmaceuticals** Philadelphia, PA 19101
LOT
EXP.
9405844-F
3 0029-6090-39 7

34. Is the ordered dosage safe? __________

35. If it is safe, how much would you administer to the child? __________ mL per dose.
If it is not safe, what would you do next? __________

36. The physician has ordered *washed, packed red blood cells 2 units (600 mL) IV to infuse in 4 h.* The IV tubing has a drop factor of 15 gtt/mL. You will regulate the IV flow rate at __________ gtt/min.

Use the following information to answer questions 37 and 38.

A child who weighs 61 lb 8 oz has an elevated temperature. For hyperthermia in children the recommended dosage of acetaminophen is 10 to 15 mg/kg p.o. q.4–6 h, not to exceed 5 doses per day.

37. What is the safe dosage range of acetaminophen for this child? __________ to __________ mg

38. If the physician orders the maximum safe dosage and acetaminophen is available as a suspension of 80 mg/2.5 mL, how many mL will you give per dose? __________ mL

Classify the following IV solutions in questions 39 and 40 as *hypotonic*, *isotonic*, or *hypertonic*.

39. D_5LR IV solution (525 mOsm/L) __________

40. Lactated Ringer's solution (273 mOsm/L) __________

Use the following information to answer questions 41 and 42 for a child weighing 52 lb.

Order: *Benadryl 25 mg IV q.6h*

Supply: Benadryl 10 mg/mL

Recommended dosage: 5 mg/kg/day in 4 divided doses

41. A safe dosage for this child is __________ mg/dose. Is the order safe? __________

42. If safe, administer __________ mL. If not safe, what should you do? __________

Use the following information to answer questions 43 through 47.

At 1430, a patient is started on *Demerol PCA IV pump at 10 mg q.10 min*. The Demerol syringe in the pump contains 300 mg/30 mL.

43. The patient can receive __________ mL every 10 minutes.

44. If the patient attempts 5 doses this hour, he would receive __________ mg and __________ mL of Demerol.

45. Based on the amount of Demerol in the syringe in the PCA pump, how many total doses can the patient receive? __________ dose(s)

46. If the patient receives 5 doses every hour, the Demerol will be empty at __________ hours. Convert this time to traditional AM/PM time. __________

47. Order: *Aldomet 250 mg in 100 mL D_5W IV PB, infuse over 30 min*

    Regulate the electronic infusion pump at __________ mL/h.

Use the following information to answer questions 48 and 49.

Order: *Ancef 0.5 g IM q.8h.* The following label represents the Ancef you have available. You reconstitute the drug at 1400 on 1/30/XX.

EXPIRES
LOT

equivalent to
1gram cefazolin
NDC 0007-3130-01

ANCEF®
STERILE CEFAZOLIN SODIUM (LYOPHILIZED)

SB SmithKline Beecham

For I.V. or I.M. use.
Before reconstitution protect from light and store at controlled room temperature 15°-30°C (59°-86°F).
Usual Adult Dose: 250 mg to 1 gram every six to eight hours. See literature.
For I.M. use, add 2.5 mL Sterile Water for Injection and shake. Provides an approximate volume of 3.0 mL (330 mg/mL).
For I.V. use see accompanying literature.
Reconstituted *Ancef* is stable 24 hours at room temperature or 96 hours if refrigerated.
Caution: Federal law prohibits dispensing without prescription. U.S. Pat. 3,516,997
SmithKline Beecham Pharmaceuticals
Philadelphia, PA 19101 693820-U

48. The total volume of Ancef after reconstitution is __________ mL with a resulting dosage strength of __________ mg per __________ mL.

49. Give __________ mL of Ancef.

50. Prepare a reconstitution label for the Ancef.

____

____

After completing these problems, see pages 468–471 to check your answers.

Perfect Score = 100   Minimum mastery score = 90% (45 correct)

My score = __________

Comprehensive Skills Evaluation

This evaluation is a comprehensive assessment of your mastery of the concepts presented in all sixteen chapters of *Dosage Calculations*.

Donna Smith, a 46-year-old patient of Dr. J. Physician, has been admitted to the Progressive Care Unit (PCU) with complaints of an irregular heartbeat, shortness of breath, and chest pain relieved by nitroglycerin. Questions #1 through 14 refer to the admitting orders on page 400 for Mrs. Smith. The labels shown represent available medications and infusion set.

1. How much Lasix will you give Mrs. Smith for her first dose? Draw an arrow on the appropriate syringe to indicate how much you will prepare.

   Give: __________ mL

   Lasix® (furosemide) Injection IM/IV
   For Single Use Only
   4 mL Vial
   4 mL = 40 mg (10 mg/mL)
   Caution: Federal law prohibits dispensing without prescription.
   Manufactured for: HOECHST-ROUSSEL Pharmaceuticals Inc. Somerville, N.J. 08876
   65604285
   Store at controlled room temperature (59°-86°F). Do not use if solution is discolored.

2. After the initial dose of Lasix, how much will you administer for the subsequent doses?

   Give: __________ tablet(s)

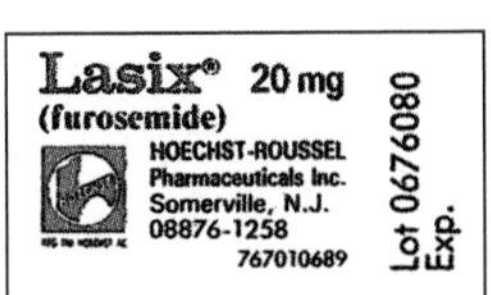

3. How many capsules of Nitro-Bid will you give Mrs. Smith?

   Give: __________ capsules

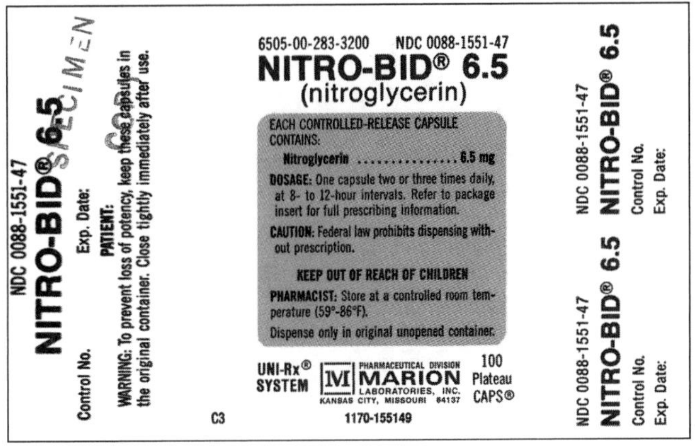

ENTERED	FILLED	CHECKED	VERIFIED
			—

NOTE: A NON-PROPRIETARY DRUG OF EQUAL QUALITY MAY BE DISPENSED - IF THIS COLUMN IS NOT CHECKED!

DATE	TIME WRITTEN	PLEASE USE BALL POINT - PRESS FIRMLY	✓	TIME NOTED	NURSES SIGNATURE
9/3/xx	1600	Admit to PCU, monitored bed	✓		
		Bedrest c̄ bathroom privileges	✓		
		Nitro-Bid 13 mg p.o. q.8h	✓		
		Lasix 20 mg IV stat, then 20 mg p.o. b.i.d.	✓		
		Digoxin 0.25 mg IV stat, repeat in 4 hours,	✓	1610	GP
		then 0.125 mg p.o. q.d.			
		KCl 10 mEq per L D_5 1/2 NS IV @ 80 cc/h	✓		
		Acetaminophen 650 mg p.r.n headache	✓		
		Labwork: Electrolytes and CBC in am	✓		
		Soft diet, advance as tolerated	✓		
		Dr. J. Physician			

AUTO STOP ORDERS: UNLESS REORDERED, FOLLOWING WILL BE D/C'D AT 0800 ON:

DATE	ORDER		
		☐ CONT ☐ D/C	PHYSICIAN SIGNATURE
		☐ CONT ☐ D/C	PHYSICIAN SIGNATURE
		☐ CONT ☐ D/C	PHYSICIAN SIGNATURE

CHECK WHEN ANTIBIOTICS ORDERED ☐ Prophylactic ☐ Empiric ☐ Therapeutic

Allergies: None Known

Chest Pain
PATIENT DIAGNOSIS

HEIGHT 5' 6" WEIGHT 110 lb

Smith, Donna
ID #257-226-3

FORM 959-708 (8xx) **PHYSICIANS ORDER** Reynolds + Reynolds LITHO IN U.S.A. K41814 (7-90) D339380

1

4. Sometimes Nitro-Bid is ordered by the SL route. "SL" is the medical abbreviation for ______________________. Explain: ____

____

5. How much IV Lanoxin will you give on admission? Draw an arrow on the syringe to indicate how much you will prepare.

Give: __________ mL

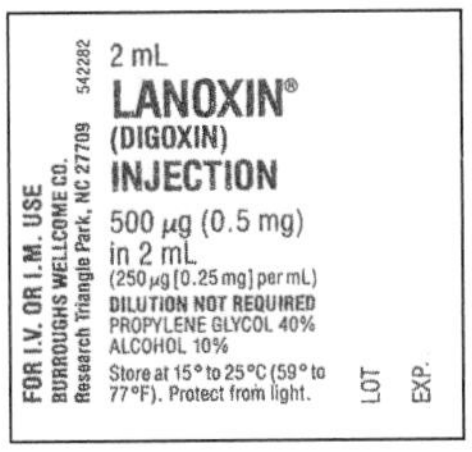
2 mL
LANOXIN®
(DIGOXIN)
INJECTION
500 μg (0.5 mg)
in 2 mL
(250 μg [0.25 mg] per mL)
DILUTION NOT REQUIRED
PROPYLENE GLYCOL 40%
ALCOHOL 10%
Store at 15° to 25°C (59° to 77°F). Protect from light.
FOR I.V. OR I.M. USE
BURROUGHS WELLCOME CO.
Research Triangle Park, NC 27709
542282
LOT
EXP.

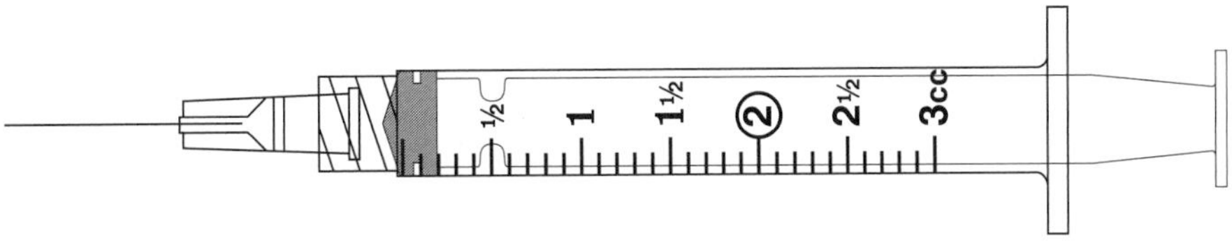
½
1
1½
2
2½
3cc

6. How many Lanoxin tablets will you need for a 24 hour supply for the p.o. order?
__________ tablet(s)

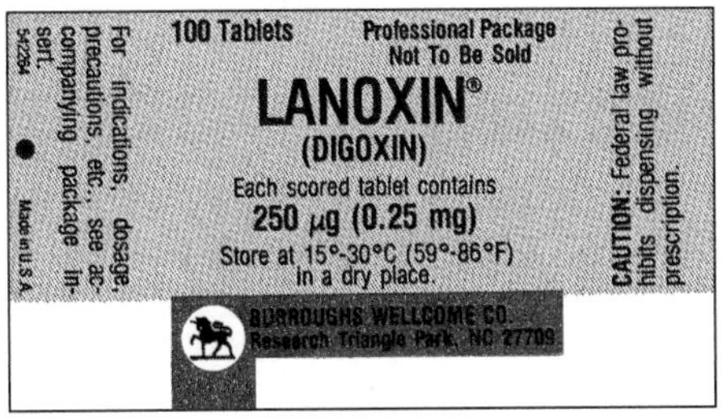
100 Tablets
Professional Package Not To Be Sold
LANOXIN®
(DIGOXIN)
Each scored tablet contains
250 μg (0.25 mg)
Store at 15°-30°C (59°-86°F) in a dry place.
BURROUGHS WELLCOME CO.
Research Triangle Park, NC 27709
For indications, dosage, precautions, etc., see accompanying package insert.
Made in U.S.A.
CAUTION: Federal law prohibits dispensing without prescription.

7. Calculate the "watch count" flow rate for the IV fluid ordered. __________ gtt/min

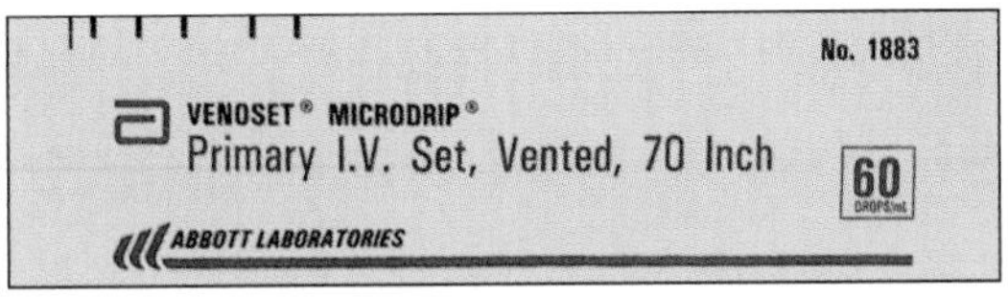
No. 1883
VENOSET® MICRODRIP®
Primary I.V. Set, Vented, 70 Inch
60
ABBOTT LABORATORIES

8. The KCl is available in a solution strength of 30 mEq per 15 mL. How much KCl will you add to the IV? Draw an arrow on the appropriate syringe to indicate the amount.
Add: __________ mL

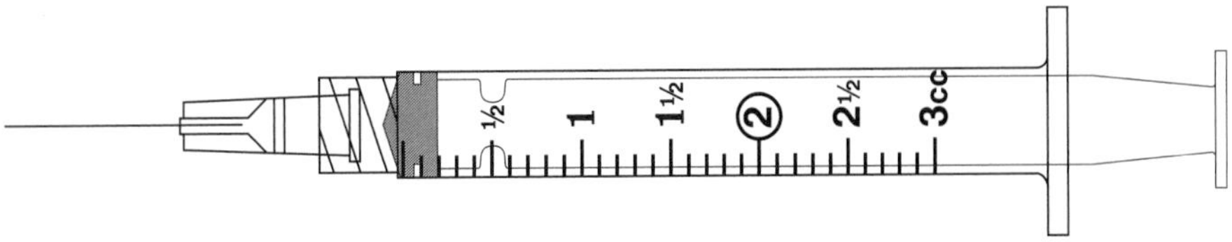
½
1
1½
2
2½
3cc

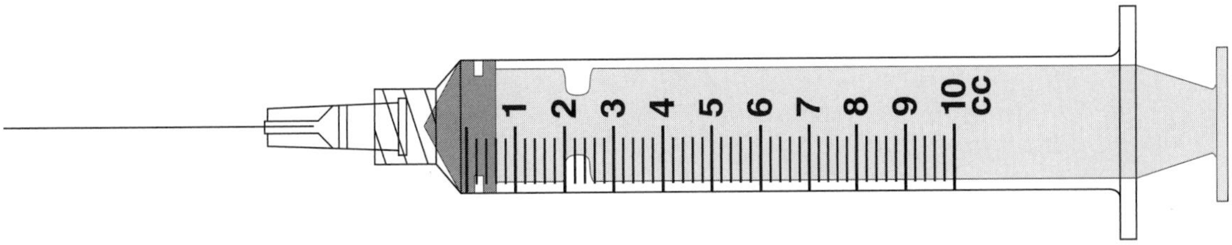
1
2
3
4
5
6
7
8
9
10
cc

9. How many mEq KCl will Mrs. Smith receive per hour? __________ mEq/h

10. At the present infusion rate, how much $D_5\frac{1}{2}$NS will Mrs. Smith receive in a 24 hour period? __________ mL

11. The IV is started at 1630. Estimate the time and date that you should plan to hang the next liter of $D_5\frac{1}{2}$NS. __________ hours __________ date

12. Mrs. Smith has a headache. How much acetaminophen will you give her?

    Give: __________ tablet(s)

See New Label
REGULAR STRENGTH
TYLENOL®
Safe Pain Relief
Contains No Aspirin
Tablets
acetaminophen
24 TABLETS – 325 MG EACH

13. You have located an infusion controller for Mrs. Smith's IV. At what rate will you set the controller? __________ mL/hr

14. Which of Mrs. Smith's medications are ordered by their generic or chemical names?

    ____

Despite your excellent care, Mrs. Smith's condition worsens. She is transferred into the coronary care unit (CCU) with the medical orders noted on page 403. Questions #15 through 20 refer to these orders. She weighs 110 pounds.

15. How much lidocaine will you give for the bolus? You have lidocaine 10 mg/mL available. Draw an arrow on the appropriate syringe to indicate the amount you will give.

    Give: __________ mL

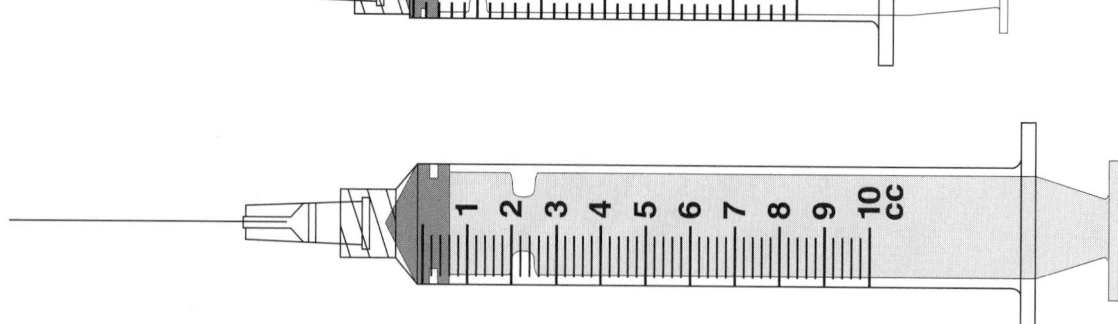

16. The infusion pump is calibrated to administer mL/h. At what rate will you initially set the infusion pump for the lidocaine drip? __________ mL/h

ENTERED	FILLED	CHECKED	VERIFIED
			–

NOTE: A NON-PROPRIETARY DRUG OF EQUAL QUALITY MAY BE DISPENSED - IF THIS COLUMN IS NOT CHECKED!

DATE	TIME WRITTEN	PLEASE USE BALL POINT - PRESS FIRMLY	✓	TIME NOTED	NURSES SIGNATURE
9/4/xx	2230	Transfer to CCU	✓		
		NPO	✓		
		Discontinue Nitro-Bid	✓		
		Lidocaine bolus 50 mg IV stat, then begin	✓		
		lidocaine drip 2 g in 500 cc D_5W			
		@ 2 mg/min by infusion pump			
		Increase lidocaine to 4 mg/min if PVCs	✓		
		(premature ventricular contractions)			
		persist		2235	MS
		Dopamine 400 mg IV PB in 250 cc D_5W	✓		
		@ 10 mcg/kg/min by infusion pump			
		Increase KCl to 20 mEq per L D_5W	✓		
		1/2 NS IV @ 50 cc/h			
		Increase Lasix to 40 mg IV q. 12h	✓		
		O_2 @ 30% p̄ ABGs (arterial blood gases)	✓		
		Labwork: Electrolytes stat and in am and	✓		
		ABGs stat & p.r.n.			
		Dr. J. Physician			

AUTO STOP ORDERS: UNLESS REORDERED, FOLLOWING WILL BE D/C'D AT 0800 ON:

DATE	ORDER		PHYSICIAN SIGNATURE
		☐ CONT ☐ D/C	PHYSICIAN SIGNATURE
		☐ CONT ☐ D/C	PHYSICIAN SIGNATURE
		☐ CONT ☐ D/C	PHYSICIAN SIGNATURE

CHECK WHEN ANTIBIOTICS ORDERED ☐ Prophylactic ☐ Empiric ☐ Therapeutic

Allergies: None Known

Chest Pain
PATIENT DIAGNOSIS

HEIGHT 5' 6" WEIGHT 110 lb

Smith, Donna
ID #257-226-3

FORM 959-708 (8-xx) **PHYSICIAN'S ORDER** Reynolds + Reynolds LITHO IN U.S.A. K41814 (7-90) D339366

1

17. How much dopamine will you add to mix the dopamine drip? You have dopamine 80 mg/mL available. Draw an arrow on the appropriate syringe to indicate the amount you will add. Add: __________ mL

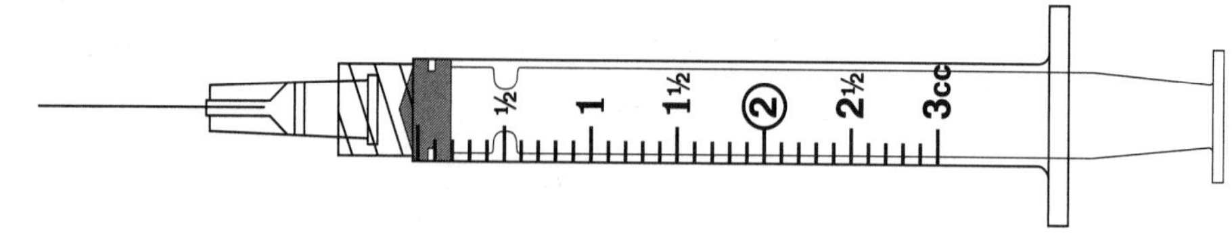

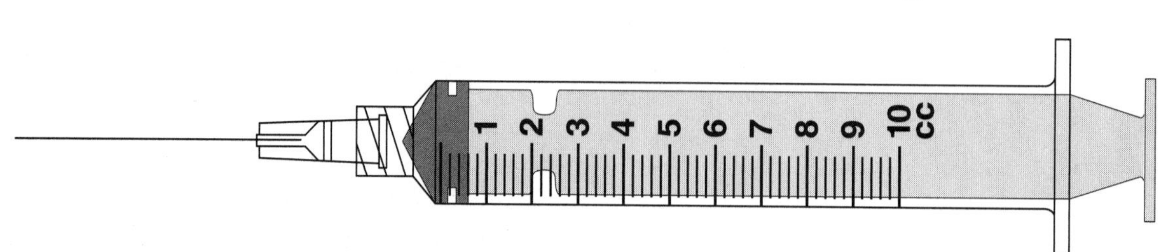

18. Calculate the rate for the infusion pump for the dopamine drip. __________ mL/h

19. How many mEq KCl will Mrs. Smith now receive per hour? __________ mEq/h

20. Mrs. Smith is having increasing amounts of PVCs. To increase her lidocaine drip to 4 mg/min you will now change your IV infusion pump setting to __________ mL/hr.

21. Julie Thomas is a six-year-old pediatric patient who weights 33 pounds. She is in the hospital for fever of unknown origin. Julie complains of burning on urination and her urinalysis shows *E. coli* bacterial infection. The doctor prescribes Kantrex 75 mg IV q.8h to be administered by Buretrol on an infusion pump in 25 mL $D_5W\frac{1}{2}$ NS followed by 15 mL flush over 1 hour. The maximum recommended dose of Kantrex is 15 mg/kg/day IV in three doses. Is the order safe? __________ If safe, calculate one dose of and the flow rate for Julie's Kantrex. Add __________ mL Kantrex and __________ mL D_5W to the Buretrol, and set the flow rate for __________ mL/h.

Jane Short is a 10-year-old with asthma. She weighs 55 pounds. Questions #22 and 23 refer to Jane.

Order: *D_5W 250 mL $\bar{c}$ aminophylline 250 mg at 25 mg/h.* You are using an IV pump.

22. The recommended maintenance dosage of aminophylline is 1 mg/kg/h. Is Jane's order safe and reasonable? __________

23. If safe, set the IV pump to deliver __________ mL/h.

Jamie Smith is hospitalized with a staphylococcal bone infection. He weighs 66 pounds. Questions 24 through 27 refer to Jamie.

Orders: *$D_5\frac{1}{2}$ NS IV @ 50 mL/h for continuous infusion.*

Vancocin 300 mg IV q.6h.

Supply: Vancocin 500 mg/10 mL with instructions to "add to Buretrol and infuse over 60 min"

Recommended dosage: Vancomycin 40 mg/kg/day IV in 4 equally divided doses.

24. Is this drug order safe? __________. Explain ______________________________

25. If safe, how much Vancocin will you add to the Buretrol? __________ mL

26. How much IV fluid will you add to the Buretrol with the Vancocin? __________ mL

27. How much IV fluid will Jamie receive in 24 hours? __________ mL

Questions #28 and 29 refer to the following situation.

You are preparing IV fluids for a young child according to the following order:

$D_5\frac{1}{2}$ NS $\bar{c}$ KCl 20 mEq/L IV at 30 cc/h

28. You have chosen to use a 250 mL bag of $D_5\frac{1}{2}$NS. How many mEq KCl will you add? __________ mEq

29. Your supply of KCl is 2 mEq/mL. How much KCl will you add to the 250 mL bag? __________ mL

Use the related orders and labels to answer questions 30 through 35. Select and mark the dose volume on the appropriate syringe; as indicated.

Order: *Prostaphlin 500 mg IV q.6h in 50 mL D_5W IV by Buretrol over 60 min. Follow with 15 mL IV flush.*

30. Reconstitute with __________ mL diluent.

31. Add __________ mL Prostaphlin and __________ mL D_5W to Buretrol.

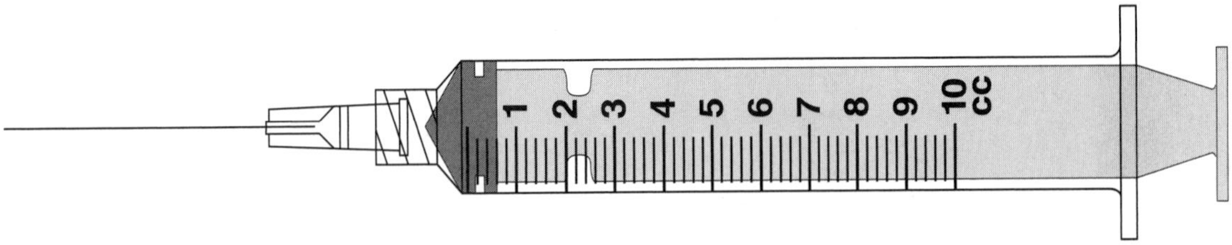

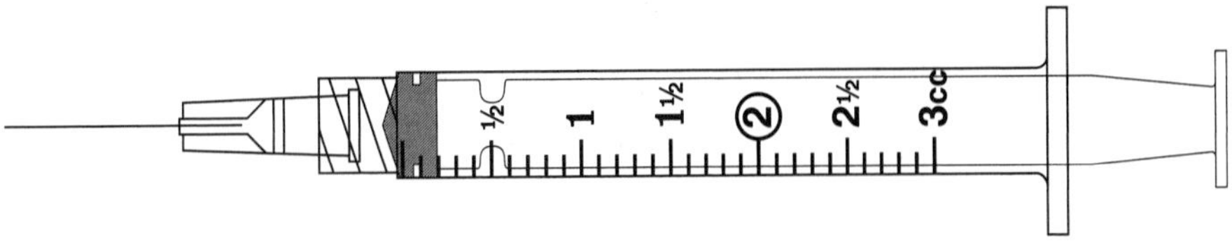

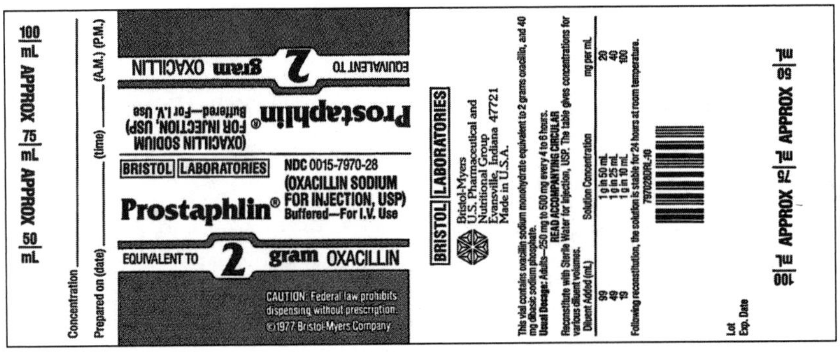

32. The IV is regulated on an infusion pump. Set the Buretrol flow rate at __________ mL/h.

33. Order: *Heparin 10,000 U IV in 500 cc D_5W to infuse @ 1200 U/h.*

Is this order safe? __________ . If safe, add __________ mL heparin to the IV solution. Set the flow rate to __________ mL/h on an IV infusion pump. If it is not safe, describe your action.

____

____

NDC 0009-0291-01
10 ml
Heparin Sodium Injection, USP
Sterile Solution
5,000 Units per ml
from beef lung
For subcutaneous or intravenous use
See package insert for complete product information.
Store at controlled room temperature 15°-30° C (59°-86° F)
Each ml contains: heparin sodium, 5,000 USP Units. Also, sodium chloride, 9 mg; benzyl alcohol, 9.45 mg added as preservative.
811 340 201
Upjohn
The Upjohn Company
Kalamazoo, MI 49001, USA

34. Order: *Novolin R Regular U-100 insulin SC ac per sliding scale and blood sugar (BS) level. The patient's blood sugar at 1730 hours is 238.*

Sliding Scale		Insulin Dosage
BS:	0–150	0 U
BS:	151–250	8 U
BS:	251–350	13 U
BS:	351–400	18 U
BS:	>400	Call M.D.

Give: __________ U, which equals __________ mL.

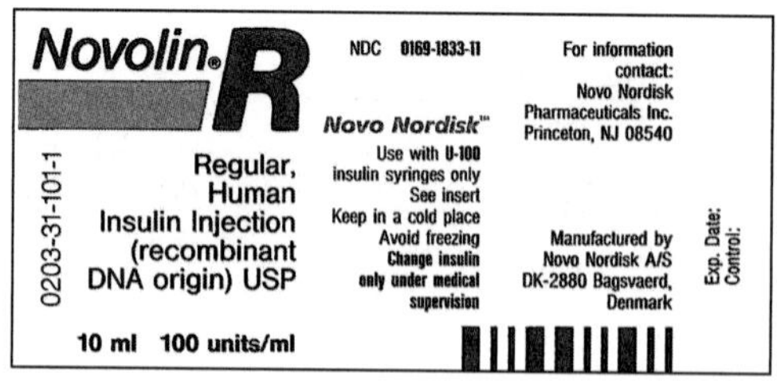

Novolin® R
Regular, Human Insulin Injection (recombinant DNA origin) USP
10 ml 100 units/ml
0203-31-101-1
NDC 0169-1833-11
Novo Nordisk™
Use with U-100 insulin syringes only
See insert
Keep in a cold place
Avoid freezing
Change insulin only under medical supervision
For information contact:
Novo Nordisk Pharmaceuticals Inc.
Princeton, NJ 08540
Manufactured by Novo Nordisk A/S
DK-2880 Bagsvaerd, Denmark
Exp. Date:
Control:

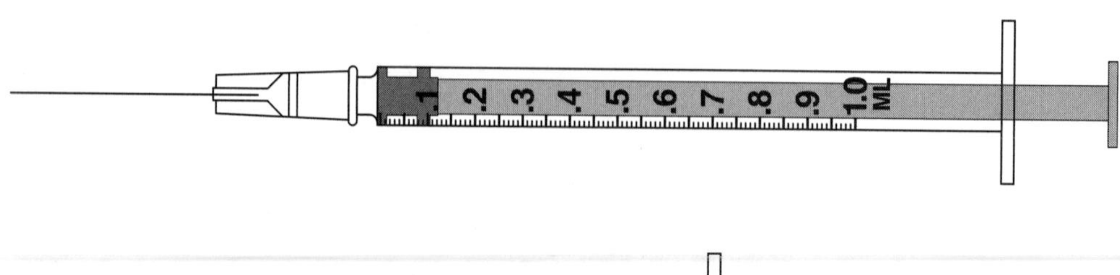

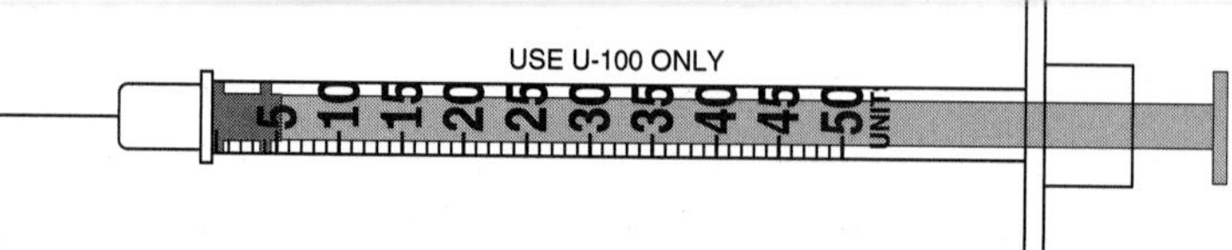

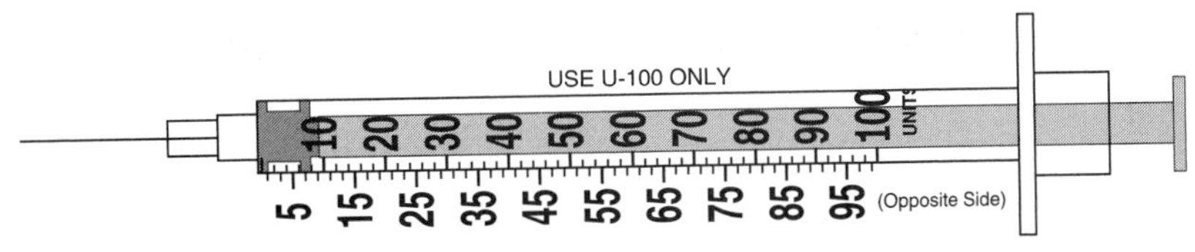

35. Order: *Humulin R Regular U-100 insulin 15 U c̄ Humulin N NPH U-100 insulin 45 U SC at 0730*

You will give a total of __________ U insulin.

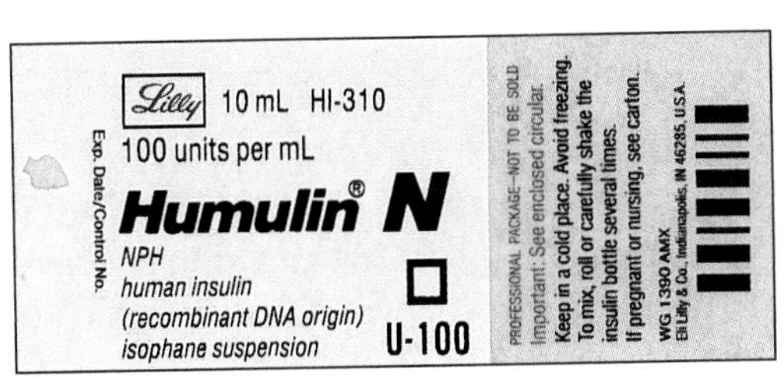

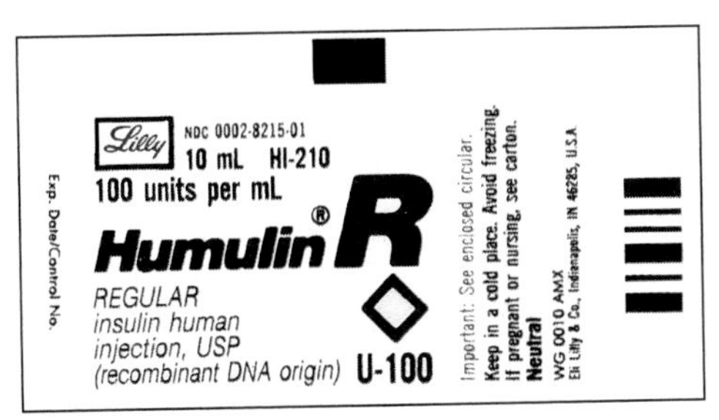

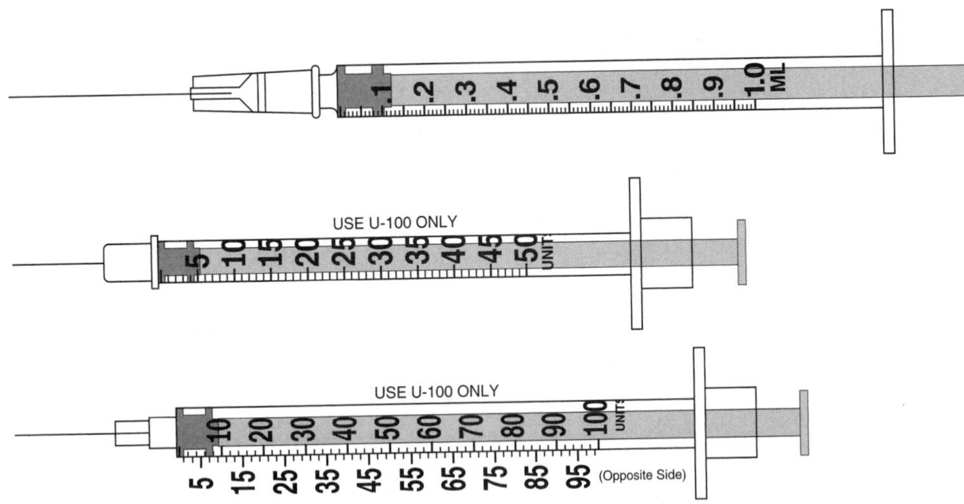

36. A diabetic patient is receiving an insulin drip of 300 U of Humulin R regular U-100 insulin in 150 mL NS infusing at 10 mL/h. How many U/h of insulin is this patient receiving? __________ U/h

Joshua weighs 16 pounds and is admitted to the pediatric unit with vomiting and diarrhea of 3 days' duration.

Questions 37 through 40 refer to Joshua.

Order: *$\frac{1}{4}$ strength Isomil 80 cc q.3h for 4 feedings; if tolerated, increase Isomil to $\frac{1}{2}$ strength 80 cc q.3h for 4 feedings*

Supply: Isomil Ready-to-Feed formula in 8 ounce cans

37. To reconstitute a full 8 ounce can of Isomil ready-to-feed to $\frac{1}{4}$ strength, you would add __________ mL water to mix a total of __________ mL $\frac{1}{4}$ strength reconstituted Isomil.

38. After the 4 ordered feedings are given, how many mL of reconstituted $\frac{1}{4}$ strength formula will remain? __________ mL

39. The child is not tolerating the oral feedings. Calculate this child's allowable daily IV maintenance fluids using the following recommendation. __________ mL/day.

    Daily rate of pediatric maintenance IV fluids:

    100 mL/kg for first 10 kg of body weight

    50 mL/kg for next 10 kg of body weight

    20 mL/kg for each kg above 20 Kg of body weight

40. The child's hourly IV rate would be __________ mL/h.

41. A patient has *1 L NS with 10 mEq KCl IV continuous infusion.* The doctor calls to change the IV order to *NS with 40 mEq KCl/L* because of a drop in the patient's potassium level. KCl is supplied as 40 mEq in a 20 mL ampule. There are 800 mL left in the current IV bag. How many mL KCl will you add to the 800 mL remaining? __________ mL

Use the following information to answer questions 42 through 48.

A child has a BSA of 0.6 m^2 determined by the West Nomogram. He is of average height and weight. Use the nomogram to find the child's weight.

WEST NOMOGRAM

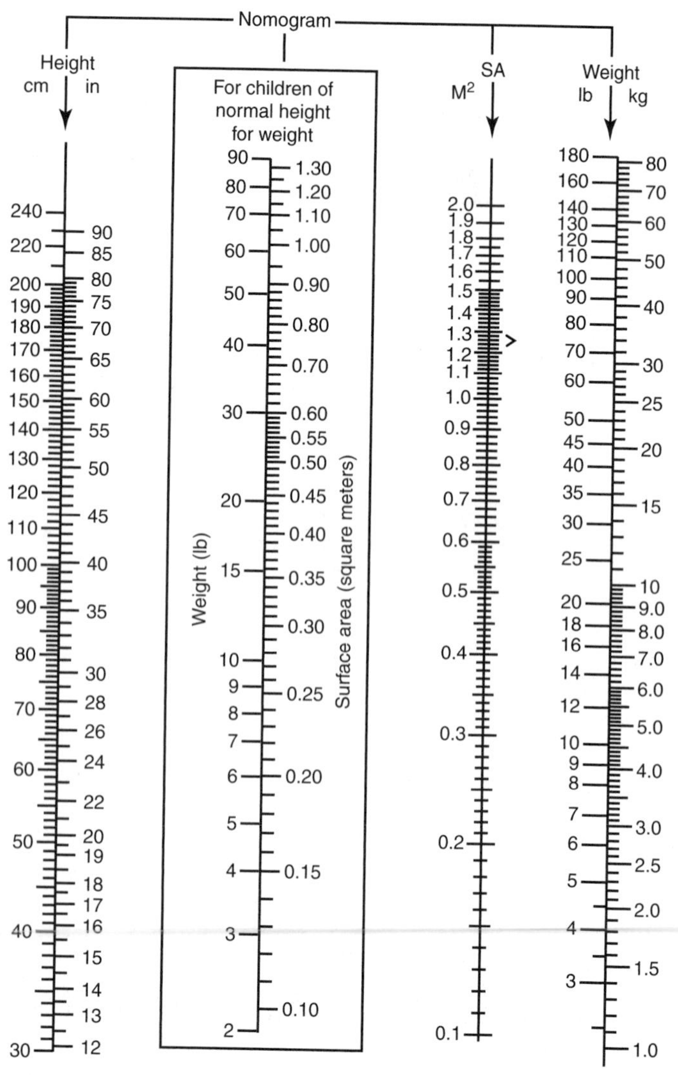

West's Nomogram for Estimation of Body Surface Area. (From *Nelson Textbook of Pediatrics* (15th ed.) by R. E. Behrman, R. M. Kleigman, & A. M. Arvin, 1996, Philadelphia: Saunders. Reprinted with permission.)

42. The child weighs __________ lb. Use the pediatric daily maintenance IV fluid recommendation in question 39 to determine this child's total daily maintenance fluid need. __________ mL/day

43. Based on his maintenance need, calculate the continuous IV flow rate. __________ mL/h

44. The child's IV is *1 L D_5 0.33% NaCl*. Calculate the amount of solute in this IV solution. __________ g dextrose and __________ g NaCl.

45. The order says to *add 20 mEq KCl/L after first void*. KCl is available as 40 mEq/20 mL. When it is time to add the KCl, there are 400 mL left in the IV bag. How many mEq of KCl will you add? __________ mEq How much KCl will you add? __________ mL

This new order is written for this same child: *Nafcillin 540 mg IV q.6h in IV fluid for total volume of 50 mL to infuse over 1 h*

NDC 0015-7225-20
EQUIVALENT TO
1 gram NAFCILLIN
NAFCILLIN SODIUM FOR INJECTION, USP
Buffered-For IM or IV Use
CAUTION: Federal law prohibits dispensing without prescription.
APOTHECON
A BRISTOL-MYERS SQUIBB COMPANY

When reconstituted with 3.4 mL diluent, (SEE INSERT-INTRAMUSCULAR ROUTE), each vial contains 4 mL solution. Each mL of solution contains nafcillin sodium, as the monohydrate, equivalent to 250 mg nafcillin, buffered with 10 mg sodium citrate. Read accompanying circular for complete stability data.
Usual Dosage: Adults—500 mg every 4 to 6 hours. Read accompanying circular for directions for IM or IV use.

Distributed by APOTHECON®
A Bristol-Myers Squibb Company
Princeton, NJ 08540
Made in USA
722520DRL-1

Cont:
Exp. Date:

46. Add __________ mL Nafcillin into the Buretrol.

47. Add __________ mL IV fluid to the IV med in the Buretrol.

48. The minimal dilution (maximal concentration) of Nafcillin is 40 mg/mL. Is the ordered amount of IV fluid sufficient to safely dilute the Nafcillin? __________. Explain __________

____

Use the following information to answer questions 49 and 50.

Order: *Penicillin G potassium 400,000 U IV PB q.4h* for a child who weighs 10 kg

Supply: Penicillin G potassium reconstituted to 200,000 U/mL

Recommended administration from package insert: Give Penicillin G potassium 100,000–250,000 U/kg/day in divided doses q.4h; dilute with 50,000 U/mL of D_5W or NS; infuse over 20 minutes.

NDC 0002-1406-01
VIAL No. 526
Lilly
PENICILLIN G POTASSIUM FOR INJECTION USP
(BUFFERED)
1,000,000 Units

CAUTION—Federal (U.S.A.) law prohibits dispensing without prescription.
Sterile solution may be kept in refrigerator for 7 days without significant loss of potency.

Add diluent	Conc. of Solution
9.6 ml	100,000 Units/ml
4.6 ml	200,000 Units/ml
1.6 ml	500,000 Units/ml

Usual Adult Dose—Intramuscularly, 400,000 units 4 times a day. Intravenously, 10,000,000 units a day. See literature. Contains sodium citrate-citric acid buffer.
YA 3175 AMX
Eli Lilly & Co., Indianapolis, IN 46285, U.S.A.

Exp. Date/Control No.

49. How many U/kg/day of Penicillin G is this child ordered to receive? __________ U/kg/day. Is the ordered dosage safe? __________

50. The child's IV is infusing on an electronic infusion pump and the IV tubing requires a 15 mL flush. If the dosage is safe, what is the IV flow rate to safely administer the order? __________ mL/h

After completing these problems, see pages 472–475 to check your answers.

Perfect Score = 100%   Minimum mastery score = 90% (45 correct)

My score = __________

Mathematics Diagnostic Evaluation from pages 3–5

1) 1517.63 **2)** 27 **3)** 100.66 **4)** \$323.72 **5)** 46.11 **6)** 754.5 **7)** VIII **8)** 19,494.7 **9)** \$173.04 **10)** 403.26 **11)** 36 **12)** 2500 **13)** XI **14)** 6.25 **15)** $\frac{4}{5}$ **16)** 40% **17)** 0.4% **18)** 0.05 **19)** 1:3 **20)** 0.02 **21)** $1\frac{1}{4}$ **22)** $6\frac{13}{24}$ **23)** $1\frac{11}{18}$ **24)** $\frac{3}{5}$ **25)** $14\frac{7}{8}$ **26)** $\frac{1}{100}$ **27)** 0.009 **28)** 320 **29)** 3 **30)** 0.05 **31)** 4 **32)** 0.09 **33)** 0.22 **34)** 25 **35)** 4 **36)** 0.75 **37)** 3 **38)** 500 **39)** 18.24 **40)** 2.4 **41)** $\frac{1}{5}$ **42)** 1:50 **43)** 5 tablets **44)** $\frac{1}{4}$ pound **45)** 30 kilograms **46)** 3.3 pounds **47)** $6\frac{2}{3} = 6.67$ centimeters **48)** 5 quarters **49)** 90% **50)** 5:1

Solutions—Mathematics Diagnostic Evaluation

3)
$$\begin{array}{r} 9.50 \\ 17.06 \\ 32.00 \\ 41.11 \\ \underline{0.99} \\ 100.66 \end{array}$$

6)
$$\begin{array}{r} 1005.0 \\ \underline{-\ 250.5} \\ 754.5 \end{array}$$

10)
$$\begin{array}{r} 17.16 \\ \underline{23.5} \\ 8580 \\ 5148 \\ \underline{3432} \\ 403.260 \end{array} = 403.26$$

12) $0.001\overline{)2.500.}$ = 2500 (quotient 2500.)

19) $\dfrac{33\frac{1}{3}}{100} = \dfrac{\frac{100}{3}}{100} = \dfrac{100}{3} \div \dfrac{100}{1} = \dfrac{\cancel{100}}{3} \times \dfrac{1}{\cancel{100}} = \dfrac{1}{3} = 1:3$

23)
$$\begin{array}{rl} 1\frac{5}{6} = & 1\frac{15}{18} \\ -\frac{2}{9} = & \frac{4}{18} \\ \hline & 1\frac{11}{18} \end{array}$$

25) $4\frac{1}{4} \times 3\frac{1}{2} = \frac{17}{4} \times \frac{7}{2} = \frac{119}{8} = 14\frac{7}{8}$

29) $\dfrac{0.02 + 0.16}{0.4 - 0.34}$

$$\begin{array}{r} 0.02 \\ \underline{+0.16} \\ 0.18 \end{array} \qquad \begin{array}{r} 0.40 \\ \underline{-0.34} \\ 0.06 \end{array}$$

$\dfrac{0.18}{0.06} = 0.06.\overline{)0.18.}$ = 3 (quotient 3.)

32) $\frac{1}{2}\% = 0.5\% = 0.005$

$$\begin{array}{r} 18 \\ \underline{\times\ 0.005} \\ 0.090 \end{array} = 0.09$$

34) $\dfrac{\frac{1}{1000}}{\frac{1}{100}} \times 250 = \dfrac{1}{\cancel{1000}_{10}} \times \dfrac{\cancel{100}^{1}}{1} \times \dfrac{250}{1} = \dfrac{250}{10} = 25$

45) 66 pounds = $\dfrac{66}{2.2}$ = 30 kilograms or

$\dfrac{2.2 \text{ pounds}}{1 \text{ kilogram}} = \dfrac{66 \text{ pounds}}{X \text{ kilograms}}$

2.2X = 66

$\dfrac{2.2\,X}{2.2} = \dfrac{66}{2.2}$

X = 30 kilograms

49)
$$\begin{array}{r} 50 \\ \underline{-5} \\ 45 \end{array} \qquad \frac{45}{50} = \frac{9}{10} = 90\%$$

Review Set 1 from pages 9 and 10.

1) XXVIII **2)** XIII **3)** XVII **4)** XV **5)** IX **6)** XII **7)** 30 **8)** 23 **9)** 5 **10)** 24 **11)** 4 **12)** 12 **13)** XX **14)** XXX **15)** IV **16)** XII **17)** V **18)** XXIV **19)** IX **20)** VII

Review Set 2 from pages 15 and 16.

1) $\frac{6}{6}, \frac{7}{5}$

2) $\dfrac{\frac{1}{100}}{\frac{1}{150}}$

3) $\frac{1}{4}, \frac{1}{14}$

4) $1\frac{2}{9}, 1\frac{1}{4}, 5\frac{7}{8}$

5) $\frac{3}{4} = \frac{6}{8}, \frac{1}{5} = \frac{2}{10}, \frac{3}{9} = \frac{1}{3}$

6) $\frac{13}{2}$ **7)** $\frac{6}{5}$ **8)** $\frac{32}{3}$ **9)** $\frac{47}{6}$ **10)** $\frac{411}{4}$ **11)** 2 **12)** 1 **13)** $3\frac{1}{3}$ **14)** $1\frac{1}{3}$ **15)** $2\frac{3}{4}$ **16)** $\frac{6}{8}$ **17)** $\frac{4}{16}$ **18)** $\frac{8}{12}$ **19)** $\frac{4}{10}$ **20)** $\frac{6}{9}$ **21)** $\frac{1}{100}$ **22)** $\frac{1}{10,000}$ **23)** $\frac{5}{9}$ **24)** $\frac{3}{10}$ **25)** $\frac{1}{8}$ **26)** $1\frac{1}{2}$ bottles **27)** $\frac{1}{20}$ **28)** $\frac{9}{10}$ **29)** $\frac{1}{2}$ dose **30)** $\frac{1}{2}$ teaspoon

Solutions—Review Set 2

8) $10\frac{2}{3} = \frac{(3\times10)+2}{3} = \frac{32}{3}$

14) $\frac{100}{75} = 1\frac{25}{75} = 1\frac{1}{3}$

18) $\frac{2}{3} \times \frac{4}{4} = \frac{8}{12}$

25)

child
child
adult
adult
adult

$\frac{1}{2}$ of $\frac{1}{4} = \frac{1}{2} \times \frac{1}{4} = \frac{1}{8}$

27)
$$\begin{array}{r} 57 \\ +\ 3 \\ \hline 60 \end{array}$$
people in class

The men represent $\frac{3}{60}$ or $\frac{1}{20}$ of the class.

29) $\frac{80}{160} = \frac{1}{2}$ of a dose

30) $\frac{1}{2}$ of 1 teaspoon = $\frac{1}{2}$ teaspoon

Review Set 3 from pages 18 and 19.

1) $8\frac{7}{15}$ **2)** $1\frac{5}{12}$ **3)** $17\frac{5}{24}$ **4)** $1\frac{1}{24}$ **5)** $32\frac{5}{6}$ **6)** $5\frac{7}{12}$ **7)** $1\frac{34}{385}$ **8)** $5\frac{53}{72}$ **9)** 43 **10)** $5\frac{118}{119}$ **11)** $2\frac{8}{15}$ **12)** $\frac{53}{132}$ **13)** $\frac{1}{2}$ **14)** $4\frac{5}{6}$ **15)** $\frac{1}{24}$ **16)** $63\frac{2}{3}$ **17)** $299\frac{4}{5}$ **18)** $\frac{1}{6}$ **19)** $1\frac{2}{5}$ **20)** $7\frac{1}{16}$ **21)** $76\frac{2}{9}$ **22)** $1\frac{1}{4}$ **23)** $241\frac{6}{11}$ **24)** $\frac{7}{12}$ **25)** $\frac{2}{3}$ **26)** $\frac{7}{12}$ ounce **27)** $1\frac{1}{8}$ inches **28)** 8 inches **29)** $21\frac{1}{2}$ pints **30)** $20\frac{1}{16}$ pounds

Solutions—Review Set 3

1) $7\frac{4}{5} + \frac{2}{3} = 7\frac{12}{15}$
$$\begin{array}{r} 7\frac{12}{15} \\ +\frac{10}{15} \\ \hline 7\frac{22}{15} \end{array} = 8\frac{7}{15}$$

3) $4\frac{2}{3} + 5\frac{1}{24} + 7\frac{1}{2} = 4\frac{16}{24}$
$$\begin{array}{r} 4\frac{16}{24} \\ 5\frac{1}{24} \\ +\ 7\frac{12}{24} \\ \hline 16\frac{29}{24} \end{array} = 17\frac{5}{24}$$

4) $\frac{3}{4} + \frac{1}{8} + \frac{1}{6} = \frac{18}{24} + \frac{3}{24} + \frac{4}{24} = \frac{18+3+4}{24} = \frac{25}{24} = 1\frac{1}{24}$

14) $8\frac{1}{12} - 3\frac{1}{4} = 8\frac{1}{12} - 3\frac{3}{12} = 7\frac{13}{12}$
$$\begin{array}{r} 7\frac{13}{12} \\ -3\frac{3}{12} \\ \hline 4\frac{10}{12} \end{array} = 4\frac{5}{6}$$

21) $256 - 179\frac{7}{9} = 255\frac{9}{9}$
$$\begin{array}{r} 255\frac{9}{9} \\ -\ 179\frac{7}{9} \\ \hline 76\frac{2}{9} \end{array}$$

25) $12 - 4 = 8$

$\frac{8}{12} = \frac{2}{3}$

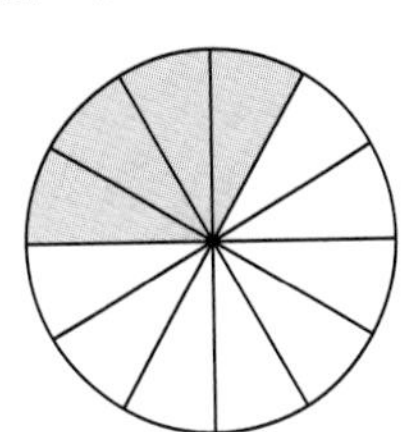

29) $56 - 34\frac{1}{2} = 55\frac{2}{2}$
$$\begin{array}{r} 55\frac{2}{2} \\ -\ 34\frac{1}{2} \\ \hline 21\frac{1}{2} \end{array}$$
pints

30) $30\frac{1}{8} - 10\frac{1}{16} = 30\frac{2}{16}$
$$\begin{array}{r} 30\frac{2}{16} \\ -\ 10\frac{1}{16} \\ \hline 20\frac{1}{16} \end{array}$$
pounds

Review Set 4 from pages 23 and 24.

1) $\frac{1}{40}$ **2)** $\frac{36}{125}$ **3)** $\frac{35}{48}$ **4)** $\frac{3}{100}$ **5)** 3 **6)** $1\frac{2}{3}$ **7)** $\frac{4}{5}$ **8)** $6\frac{8}{15}$ **9)** $\frac{1}{2}$ **10)** $23\frac{19}{36}$ **11)** $\frac{3}{32}$ **12)** $254\frac{1}{6}$ **13)** 3 **14)** $1\frac{34}{39}$ **15)** $\frac{3}{14}$ **16)** $\frac{1}{11}$ **17)** $\frac{1}{2}$ **18)** $\frac{1}{30}$ **19)** $3\frac{1}{3}$ **20)** $\frac{3}{20}$ **21)** $\frac{1}{3}$ **22)** $1\frac{1}{3}$ **23)** $1\frac{1}{9}$ **24)** 60 calories **25)** 560 seconds **26)** 40 doses **27)** $31\frac{1}{2}$ tablets **28)** 1275 milliliters **29)** $52\frac{1}{2}$ ounces **30)** 6 full days

Answers

Solutions—Review Set 4

3) $\frac{5}{8} \times 1\frac{1}{6} = \frac{5}{8} \times \frac{7}{6} = \frac{35}{48}$

5) $\dfrac{\frac{1}{6}}{\frac{1}{4}} \times \dfrac{3}{\frac{2}{3}} = \left(\frac{1}{6} \times \frac{4}{1}\right) \times \left(\frac{3}{1} \times \frac{3}{2}\right) = \frac{\overset{2}{\cancel{4}}}{\underset{3}{\cancel{6}}} \times \frac{9}{2} = \frac{\overset{1}{\cancel{2}}}{\underset{1}{\cancel{3}}} \times \frac{\overset{3}{\cancel{9}}}{\underset{1}{\cancel{2}}} = 3$

16) $\frac{1}{33} \div \frac{1}{3} = \frac{1}{33} \times \frac{3}{1} = \frac{3}{33} = \frac{1}{11}$

19) $2\frac{1}{2} \div \frac{3}{4} = \frac{5}{2} \div \frac{3}{4} = \frac{5}{\underset{1}{\cancel{2}}} \times \frac{\overset{2}{\cancel{4}}}{3} = \frac{10}{3} = 3\frac{1}{3}$

22) $\dfrac{\frac{3}{4}}{\frac{7}{8}} \div \dfrac{1\frac{1}{2}}{2\frac{1}{3}} = \left(\frac{3}{\underset{1}{\cancel{4}}} \times \frac{\overset{2}{\cancel{8}}}{7}\right) \div \left(\frac{3}{2} \times \frac{3}{7}\right) = \frac{6}{7} \div \frac{9}{14} = \frac{\overset{2}{\cancel{6}}}{\underset{1}{\cancel{7}}} \times \frac{\overset{2}{\cancel{14}}}{\underset{3}{\cancel{9}}} = \frac{4}{3} = 1\frac{1}{3}$

27) $3 \times 7 = 21$ doses

$21 \times 1\frac{1}{2} = 21 \times \frac{3}{2} = \frac{63}{2} = 31\frac{1}{2}$ tablets

28) $850 \div \frac{2}{3} = \frac{\overset{425}{\cancel{850}}}{1} \times \frac{3}{\underset{1}{\cancel{2}}} = 1275$ milliliters

30)

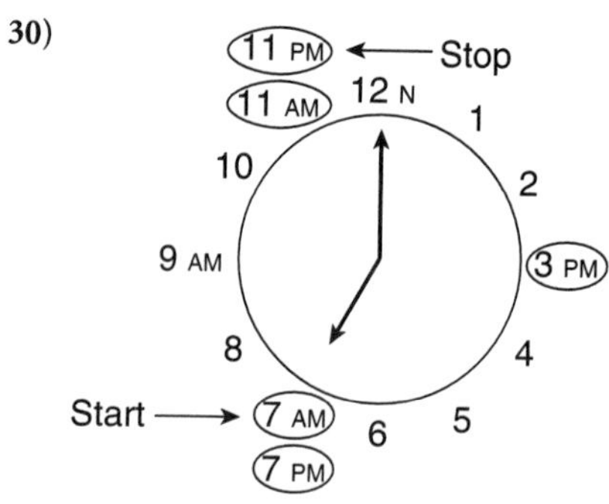

Daily doses would be taken at: 7 AM, 11 AM, 3 PM, 7 PM, and 11 PM for 5 doses/day.

5 doses/day $\times \frac{1}{2}$ ounce/dose $= \frac{5}{2} = 2\frac{1}{2}$ ounces/day

16 ounces $\div 2\frac{1}{2}$ ounces/day $= \frac{16}{1} \div \frac{5}{2} = \frac{16}{1} \times \frac{2}{5} = \frac{32}{5} = 6\frac{2}{5}$ days or 6 full days

Review Set 5 from pages 29 and 30.

1) 0.2, two tenths **2)** $\frac{17}{20}$, 0.85 **3)** $1\frac{1}{20}$, one and five hundredths **4)** $\frac{3}{500}$, six thousandths **5)** 10.015, ten and fifteen thousandths **6)** $1\frac{9}{10}$, one and nine tenths **7)** $5\frac{1}{10}$, 5.1 **8)** 0.8, eight tenths **9)** $250\frac{1}{2}$, two hundred fifty and five tenths **10)** 33.03, thirty-three and three hundredths **11)** $\frac{19}{20}$, ninety-five hundredths **12)** 2.75, two and seventy-five hundredths **13)** $7\frac{1}{200}$, 7.005 **14)** 0.084, eighty-four thousandths **15)** $12\frac{1}{8}$, twelve and one hundred twenty-five thousandths **16)** $20\frac{9}{100}$, twenty and nine hundredths **17)** $22\frac{11}{500}$, 22.022 **18)** $\frac{3}{20}$, fifteen hundredths **19)** 1000.005, one thousand and five thousandths **20)** $4085\frac{3}{40}$, 4085.075 **21)** 0.0170 **22)** 0.25 **23)** 0.75 **24)** $\frac{9}{200}$ **25)** 0.120 **26)** 0.063 **27)** False **28)** False **29)** True **30)** 0.8 gram and 1.25 grams

Solutions—Review Set 5

4) $0.006 = \frac{6}{1000} = \frac{3}{500}$

8) $\frac{4}{5} = 5\overline{)4.0}$ = 0.8

14) $\frac{21}{250} = 250\overline{)21.000}$ = 0.084

$$\begin{array}{r} 0.084 \\ 250\overline{)21.000} \\ 20\ 00 \\ \hline 1\ 000 \\ 1\ 000 \\ \hline \end{array}$$

15) $12.125 = 12\frac{125}{1000} = 12\frac{1}{8}$

18) $0.15 = \frac{15}{100} = \frac{3}{20}$

30) 0.5 gram $\leq$ safe dose $\leq$ 2 grams Safe doses: 0.8 grams and 1.25 grams

Note: "$\leq$" means "less than or equal to"

Review Set 6 from pages 31 and 32.

1) 22.585 **2)** 44.177 **3)** 12.309 **4)** 11.3 **5)** 175.199 **6)** 25.007 **7)** 0.518 **8)** \$9.48 **9)** \$18.91 **10)** \$22.71 **11)** 6.403 **12)** 0.27 **13)** 4.15 **14)** 1.51 **15)** 10.25 **16)** 2.517 **17)** 374.35 **18)** 604.42 **19)** 27.449 **20)** 23.619 **21)** 0.697 gram **22)** 18.55 ounces **23)** \$2,058.06 **24)** 12.3 grams **25)** 8.1 hours

Solutions—Review Set 6

2)
$$\begin{array}{r} 7.517 \\ 3.200 \\ 0.160 \\ 33.300 \\ \hline 44.177 \end{array}$$

9)
$$\begin{array}{r} 8\ 9\ 10 \\ \$1\cancel{9}.\cancel{0}\cancel{0} \\ -\ 0.09 \\ \hline \$18.91 \end{array}$$

25) 3 h 20 min
40 min
3 h 30 min
24 min
12 min

6 h 126 min = 8 h 6 min (60 minutes/hour)

$= 8\frac{6}{60} = 8\frac{1}{10} = 8.1$ hours

Review Set 7 from pages 36 and 37.

1) 5.83 **2)** 2.20 **3)** 42.75 **4)** 0.15 **5)** 403.14 **6)** 75,100.75 **7)** 32.86 **8)** 2.78 **9)** 348.58 **10)** 0.02 **11)** 400 **12)** 3.74 **13)** 5 **14)** 2.98 **15)** 4120 **16)** 5.45 **17)** 272.67 **18)** 1.5 **19)** 50,020 **20)** 300 **21)** 562.50. = 56,250 **22)** 16.0. = 160 **23)** .025. = 0.025 **24)** .032.005 = 0.032005 **25)** .00.125 = 0.00125 **26)** 23.2.5 = 232.5 **27)** 71.7.717 = 71.7717 **28)** 83.1.6 = 831.6 **29)** 0.33. = 33 **30)** 14.106. = 14,106

Solutions—Review Set 7

10) $1.14 \times 0.014 = 0.01596 = 0.02$

14) $45.5 \div 15.25 = 2.983 = 2.98$

Practice Problems—Chapter 1 from pages 37 and 38.

1) V **2)** XXV **3)** XXII **4)** XVI **5)** XVIII **6)** XIII **7)** XI **8)** III **9)** IV **10)** XVII **11)** 30 **12)** 9 **13)** 16 **14)** 14 **15)** 21 **16)** 23 **17)** 7 **18)** 16 **19)** 20 **20)** 19 **21)** $3\frac{7}{15}$ **22)** $7\frac{29}{60}$ **23)** $\frac{1}{2}$ **24)** $2\frac{7}{24}$ **25)** $\frac{7}{27}$ **26)** $10\frac{1}{8}$ **27)** $4\frac{4}{17}$ **28)** $5\frac{1}{55}$ **29)** $5\frac{5}{18}$ **30)** $2\frac{86}{87}$ **31)** $\frac{3}{20}$ **32)** $\frac{1}{3125}$ **33)** $\frac{1}{4}$ **34)** $1\frac{5}{7}$ **35)** 60.27 **36)** 66.74 **37)** 42.98 **38)** 4833.92 **39)** 190.80 **40)** 19.17 **41)** 12,930.43 **42)** 3200.63 **43)** 2 **44)** 150.96 **45)** 147 ounces **46)** 138 nurses; 46 maintenance cleaners; 92 technicians, 92 others **47)** False **48)** $915.08 **49)** $1.46 **50)** 0.31 gram

Solutions—Practice Problems—Chapter 1

45) $3\frac{1}{2}$ ounces/feeding × 6 feedings/day =
21 ounces/day and, 21 ounces/day × 7 days/week =
147 ounces in one week

46) $\frac{3}{8} \times 368 = 138$ nurses

$\frac{1}{8} \times 368 = 46$ maintenance cleaners

$\frac{1}{4} \times 368 = 92$ technicians and 92 others

47) $1\frac{2}{32} = 1.0625$; False, it's greater than normal.

48) 40 hours × $17.43/hour = $697.20
6.25 hours overtime × $34.86 = + 217.88
(Overtime rate = $17.43 × 2 = $34.86) $915.08

49) A case of 12 boxes with 12 catheters/box = 144 catheters
By case: $975 ÷ 144 = $6.77/catheter
By box: $98.76 ÷ 12 = $8.23/catheter
$8.23
−6.77
$ 1.46 savings/catheter

50) 0.065 gram/ounce × 4.75 ounces = 0.31 gram

Review Set 8 from page 43.

1) $\frac{1}{50}$ **2)** $\frac{3}{5}$ **3)** $\frac{1}{3}$ **4)** $\frac{4}{7}$ **5)** $\frac{3}{4}$ **6)** 0.5 **7)** 0.15 **8)** 0.14 **9)** 0.07 **10)** 0.24 **11)** 25% **12)** 40% **13)** 12.5% **14)** 70% **15)** 50% **16)** $\frac{9}{20}$ **17)** $\frac{3}{5}$ **18)** $\frac{1}{200}$ **19)** $\frac{1}{100}$ **20)** $\frac{2}{3}$ **21)** 0.03 **22)** 0.05 **23)** 0.06 **24)** 0.33 **25)** 0.01 **26)** 4:25 **27)** 1:4 **28)** 1:2 **29)** 9:20 **30)** 3:50 **31)** 0.9 **32)** $\frac{1}{5}$ **33)** 0.25% **34)** 0.5 **35)** $\frac{1}{100}$

Solutions—Review Set 8

1) $\frac{3}{150} = \frac{\overset{1}{\cancel{3}}}{\underset{50}{\cancel{150}}} = \frac{1}{50}$

3) $\frac{\overset{1}{\cancel{0.05}}}{\underset{3}{\cancel{0.15}}} = \frac{1}{3}$

7) $\frac{\frac{1}{1000}}{\frac{1}{150}} = \frac{1}{\underset{100}{\cancel{1000}}} \times \frac{\overset{15}{\cancel{150}}}{1} = \frac{15}{100} = 0.15. = 0.15$

12) $2{:}5 = \frac{2}{5} = 0.4;\ 0.4 = \frac{4}{10} = \frac{40}{100} = 40\%$

13) $0.08 : 0.64 = \frac{0.08}{0.64} = \frac{1}{8} = 0.125;$

$0.125 = \frac{125}{1000} = \frac{12.5}{100} = 12.5\%$

17) $60\% = \frac{60}{100} = \frac{3}{5}$

18) $0.5\% = \frac{0.5}{100} = 0.5 \div 100 = 0.00.5 = 0.005 = \frac{5}{1000} = \frac{1}{200}$

21) $2.94\% = \frac{2.94}{100} = 2.94 \div 100 = 0.02.94 = 0.029 = 0.03$

30) $6\% = \frac{6}{100} = \frac{3}{50} = 3{:}50$

31) Convert to decimals and compare:

0.9% = 0.009
0.9 = 0.900 (largest)
1:9 = 0.111
1:90 = 0.011

Review Set 9 from pages 46 and 47.

1) 3 **2)** 3.3 **3)** 1.25 **4)** 5.33 **5)** 0.56 **6)** 1.8 **7)** 0.64 **8)** 12.6 **9)** 40 **10)** 0.48 **11)** 1 **12)** 0.96 **13)** 4.5 **14)** 0.94 **15)** 10 **16)** 0.4 **17)** 1.5 **18)** 10 **19)** 20 **20)** 1.8

Solutions—Review Set 9

2) $\frac{\frac{3}{4}}{\frac{1}{2}} \times 2.2 = X$

$\frac{3}{4} \div \frac{1}{2} \times \frac{2.2}{1} = X$

$\frac{3}{\not{4}_{2}} \times \frac{\not{2}^{1}}{1} \times \frac{2.2}{1} = X$

$\frac{6.6}{2} = X$

$X = 3.3$

4) $\frac{40\%}{60\%} \times 8 = X$

$\frac{\not{0.4}^{2}}{\not{0.6}_{3}} \times 8 = X$

$\frac{2}{3} \times \frac{8}{1} = X$

$\frac{16}{3} = X$

$X = 5.333$

$X = 5.33$

6) $\frac{0.15}{0.1} \times 1.2 = X$

$\frac{\not{0.15}^{3}}{\not{0.10}_{2}} \times \frac{1.2}{1} = X$

$\frac{3}{2} \times \frac{1.2}{1} = X$

$\frac{3.6}{2} = X$

$X = 1.8$

8) $\frac{\not{1{,}200{,}000}^{3}}{\not{400{,}000}_{1}} \times 4.2 = X$

$\frac{3}{1} \times \frac{4.2}{1} = X$

$\frac{12.6}{1} = X$

$X = 12.6$

10) $\frac{\not{30}^{3}}{\not{50}_{5}} \times 0.8 = X$

$\frac{3}{5} \times \frac{0.8}{1} = X$

$\frac{2.4}{5} = X$

$X = 0.48$

14) $\frac{\not{250{,}000}^{1}}{\not{2{,}000{,}000}_{8}} \times 7.5 = X$

$\frac{1}{8} \times \frac{7.5}{1} = X$

$\frac{7.5}{8} = X$

$X = 0.937$

$X = 0.94$

20) $\frac{\frac{1}{100}}{\frac{1}{150}} \times 1.2 = X$

$\frac{1}{100} \div \frac{1}{150} \times \frac{1.2}{1} = X$

$\frac{1}{\not{100}_{2}} \times \frac{\not{150}^{3}}{1} \times \frac{1.2}{1} = X$

$\frac{1}{2} \times \frac{3}{1} \times \frac{1.2}{1} = X$

$\frac{3.6}{2} = X$

$X = 1.8$

Review Set 10 from page 51.

1) 0.25 **2)** 1 **3)** 0.56 **4)** 1000 **5)** 0.7 **6)** 514.29 **7)** 2142.86 **8)** 500 **9)** 200 **10)** 10.5 **11)** 3 **12)** 0.63 **13)** 10 **14)** 0.67 **15)** 1.25 **16)** 31.25 **17)** 16.67 **18)** 240 **19)** 0.75 **20)** 2.27 **21)** 1 **22)** 6 **23)** 108 nurses **24)** 72 calories **25)** 81.82 milligrams/hour

Solutions—Review Set 10

4) $\frac{0.5}{2} = \frac{250}{X}$

$0.5X = 500$

$\frac{0.5X}{0.5} = \frac{500}{0.5}$

$X = 1000$

6) $\frac{1200}{X} \times 12 = 28$

$\frac{1200}{X} \times \frac{12}{1} = 28$

$\frac{14{,}400}{X} = \frac{28}{1}$

$28X = 14{,}400$

$\frac{28X}{28} = \frac{14{,}400}{28}$

$X = 514.285$

$X = 514.29$

9) $\frac{15}{500} \times X = 6$

$\frac{15X}{500} = \frac{6}{1}$

$15X = 3000$

$\frac{15X}{15} = \frac{3000}{15}$

$X = 200$

10) $\frac{5}{X} = \frac{10}{21}$

$10X = 105$

$\frac{10X}{10} = \frac{105}{10}$

$X = 10.5$

11) $\frac{250}{1} = \frac{750}{X}$

$250X = 750$

$\frac{250X}{250} = \frac{750}{250}$

$X = 3$

14) $\frac{\frac{1}{100}}{1} = \frac{\frac{1}{150}}{X}$

$\frac{1}{100} X = \frac{1}{150}$

$\frac{\frac{1}{100} X}{\frac{1}{100}} = \frac{\frac{1}{150}}{\frac{1}{100}}$

$X = \frac{1}{150} \div \frac{1}{100}$

$X = \frac{1}{\cancel{150}_{3}} \times \frac{\cancel{100}^{2}}{1}$

$X = \frac{2}{3} = 0.666 = 0.67$

22) $\frac{25\%}{30\%} = \frac{5}{X}$

$\frac{0.25}{0.3} = \frac{5}{X}$

$0.25X = 1.5$

$\frac{0.25X}{0.25} = \frac{1.5}{0.25}$

$X = 6$

23) $\frac{45}{100} = \frac{X}{240}$

$100X = 10{,}800$

$\frac{100X}{100} = \frac{10{,}800}{100}$

$X = 108$

Review Set 11 from pages 53 and 54.

1) 1.3 **2)** 4.75 **3)** 56 **4)** 0.43 **5)** 26.67 **6)** 8.4% **7)** 3% **8)** 23.53% **9)** 22.22% **10)** 4.35% **11)** 12.5 ounces **12)** 120 cups **13)** 25 tsp **14)** 1.92 quarts **15)** 1000 pills **16)** 5120 patients **17)** A. 11.65% B. 18.45% **18)** $3,530.21 **19)** 7.2 ounces **20)** 19%

Solutions—Review Set 11

1) $X = 0.0025 \times 520 = 1.3$

6) $6.3 = X \times 75$

$75X = 6.3$

$\frac{75X}{75} = \frac{6.3}{75}$

$X = 0.084 = 8.4\%$

11) $8 = 0.64 \times X$

$0.64X = 8$

$\frac{0.64X}{0.64} = \frac{8}{0.64}$

$X = 12.5$ oz

12) $12 = 0.1 \times X$

$0.1X = 12$

$\frac{0.1X}{0.1} = \frac{12}{0.1}$

$X = 120$ cups

16) $2048 = 0.4 \times X$

$0.4X = 2048$

$\frac{0.4X}{0.4} = \frac{2048}{0.4}$

$X = 5120$ patients

17) A. $24 = 206 \times X$

$206X = 24$

$\frac{206X}{206} = \frac{24}{206}$

$X = 0.1165 = 11.65\%$

B. $38 = 206 \times X$

$206X = 38$

$\frac{206X}{206} = \frac{38}{206}$

$X = 0.1845 = 18.45\%$

18) 80% of \$17,651.07 = 0.8 × \$17,651.07 = \$14,120.86

\$17,651.07	total bill
−14,120.86	paid by insurance co.
\$ 3,530.21	paid by patient

19) $X = 0.4 \times 18$

$X = 7.2$ ounces

20)

$$675 = X \times 3500$$
$$3500X = 675$$
$$\frac{3500X}{3500} = \frac{675}{3500}$$
$$X = 0.19 = 19\%$$

Practice Problems—Chapter 2 from pages 54–56.

1) 0.4, 40%, 2:5 **2)** $\frac{1}{20}$, 5%, 1:20 **3)** 0.17, $\frac{17}{100}$, 17:100 **4)** 0.25, $\frac{1}{4}$, 25% **5)** 0.06, $\frac{3}{50}$, 3:50 **6)** 0.17, 17%, 1:6 **7)** 0.5, $\frac{1}{2}$, 1:2 **8)** 0.01, $\frac{1}{100}$, 1% **9)** $\frac{9}{100}$, 9%, 9:100 **10)** 0.38, 38%, 3:8 **11)** 0.67, $\frac{2}{3}$, 67% **12)** 0.33, 33%, 1:3 **13)** $\frac{13}{25}$, 52%, 13:25 **14)** 0.45, $\frac{9}{20}$, 45% **15)** 0.86, 86%, 6:7 **16)** 0.3, $\frac{3}{10}$, 30% **17)** 0.02, 2%, 1:50 **18)** $\frac{3}{5}$, 60%, 3:5 **19)** $\frac{1}{25}$, 4%, 1:25 **20)** 0.1, $\frac{1}{10}$, 1:10 **21)** 0.04 **22)** 1:40 **23)** 7.5% **24)** $\frac{1}{2}$ **25)** 3:4 **26)** 262.5 **27)** 3.64 **28)** 1.97 **29)** 25% **30)** 19% **31)** 84 **32)** 90,000 **33)** 1 **34)** 1.1 **35)** 100 **36)** 2.5 **37)** 0.75 **38)** 21 **39)** 17.29 **40)** 248.4 **41)** A. 20% B. 4.8% **42)** 87.33% **43)** 60 minutes **44)** 48% **45)** 2% **46)** 5.4 grams **47)** 283.5 milligrams **48)** 8% **49)** \$10.42 **50)** 6 total doses

Solutions—Practice Problems—Chapter 2

36)

$$\frac{\frac{1}{200}}{\frac{1}{4}} \times 125 = X$$
$$\frac{1}{200} \div \frac{1}{4} \times \frac{125}{1} = X$$
$$\frac{1}{\cancel{200}_{50}} \times \frac{\cancel{4}^{1}}{1} \times \frac{125}{1} = X$$
$$X = \frac{125}{50}$$
$$X = 2.5$$

41) A. Percentage (part) = Percent × Whole Quantity

$$25 = X \times 125$$
$$125X = 25$$
$$\frac{125X}{125} = \frac{25}{125}$$
$$X = 0.2 = 20\%$$

B. Percentage (part) = Percent × Whole Quantity

$$6 = X \times 125$$
$$125X = 6$$
$$\frac{125X}{125} = \frac{6}{125}$$
$$X = 0.048 = 4.8\%$$

42) Percentage (part) = Percent × Whole Quantity

$$131 = X \times 150$$
$$150X = 131$$
$$\frac{150X}{150} = \frac{131}{150}$$
$$X = 0.8733 = 87.33\%$$

43)

$$\frac{90}{27} = \frac{200}{X}$$
$$90X = 5400$$
$$\frac{90X}{90} = \frac{5400}{90}$$
$$X = 60$$

44) Percentage (part) = Percent × Whole Quantity

$$28.75 = X \times 60$$
$$60X = 28.75$$
$$\frac{60X}{60} = \frac{28.75}{60}$$
$$X = 0.479 = 48\%$$

46)

$$\frac{2.7}{0.75} = \frac{X}{1.5}$$
$$0.75X = 4.05$$
$$\frac{0.75X}{0.75} = \frac{4.05}{0.75}$$
$$X = 5.4$$

47)

$$\frac{6.75}{1} = \frac{X}{42}$$
$$X = 283.5$$

48) Percentage (part) = Percent × Whole Quantity

$$0.5 = X \times 6.5$$
$$6.5X = 0.5$$
$$\frac{6.5X}{6.5} = \frac{0.5}{6.5}$$
$$X = \frac{0.5}{6.5} = 0.076 = 0.08 = 8\%$$

49) $X = 0.17 \times \$12.56 = 2.14$; \$12.56 − 2.14 = \$10.42

50) 10% of 150 = 0.10 × 150 = 15;

150 mg	first dose
−15	
135 mg	second dose
−15	
120 mg	third dose
−15	
105 mg	fourth dose
−15	
90 mg	fifth dose
−15	
75 mg	sixth dose
	6 total doses

Section 1—Self-Evaluation from pages 57 and 58.

1) XIV **2)** XXV **3)** VIII **4)** XX **5)** 7 **6)** 24 **7)** 19 **8)** 30 **9)** $\frac{11}{12}$ **10)** $\frac{47}{63}$ **11)** 1 **12)** $\frac{1}{2}$ **13)** 45.78 **14)** 59.24 **15)** 0.09 **16)** 12 **17)** $\frac{2}{3}$ **18)** $\frac{1}{2}$ **19)** 0.02 **20)** 0.64 **21)** $\frac{1}{10}, \frac{1}{6}, \frac{1}{5}, \frac{1}{3}, \frac{1}{2}$ **22)** $\frac{2}{3}, \frac{3}{4}, \frac{5}{6}, \frac{7}{8}, \frac{9}{10}$ **23)** 0.009, 0.125, 0.1909, 0.25, 0.3 **24)** $\frac{1}{2}$%, 0.9%, 50%, 100%, 500% **25)** 0.01 **26)** 0.04 **27)** 0.9% **28)** $\frac{1}{3}$ **29)** 5:9 **30)** $\frac{1}{20}$ **31)** 1:200 **32)** $\frac{2}{3}$ **33)** 75% **34)** 40% **35)** 0.17 **36)** 1.21 **37)** 1.3 **38)** 2.5 **39)** 0.67 **40)** 100 **41)** 4 **42)** 20,000 **43)** 3.3 **44)** 300 **45)** 8.33 **46)** 20% **47)** 11 dimes **48)** \$2.42 **49)** 12 cans of water **50)** 8 centimeters

Solutions—Section 1—Self-Evaluation

17) $\frac{1}{150} \div \frac{1}{100} = \frac{1}{150} \times \frac{100}{1} = \frac{\cancel{100}^{2}}{\cancel{150}_{3}} = \frac{2}{3}$

20) $\frac{16\%}{\frac{1}{4}} = 16\% \times \frac{4}{1} = 0.16 \times 4 = 0.64$

33) $3:4 = \frac{3}{4} = 4\overline{)3.0}$ with quotient 0.75 $= 75\%$

37) $\frac{0.3}{.62} \times \frac{0.15}{X}$

$0.3X = 2.6 \times 0.15$

$0.3X = 0.39$

$\frac{0.3X}{0.3} = \frac{0.39}{0.3}$

$X = 1.3$

42) $\frac{10\%}{\frac{1}{2}\%} \times 1000 = X$

$\frac{0.1}{0.005} \times \frac{1000}{1} = X$

$\frac{100}{0.005} = X$

$X = 20,000$

46) Percentage (part) = Percent × Whole Quantity

$6 = X \times 30$

$6 = 30X$

$30X = 6$

$\frac{30X}{30} = \frac{6}{30}$

$X = 0.2 = 20\%$

Review Set 12 from pages 64 and 65.

1) metric **2)** volume **3)** weight **4)** length **5)** $\frac{1}{1000}$ or 0.001 **6)** 1000 **7)** 10 **8)** kilogram **9)** milligram **10)** 1000 **11)** 1 **12)** 1000 **13)** 10 **14)** 0.3 g **15)** 1.33 mL **16)** 5 kg **17)** 1.5 mm **18)** 10 mg **19)** microgram **20)** milliliter **21)** cubic centimeter **22)** gram **23)** millimeter **24)** kilogram **25)** centimeter

Review Set 13 from pages 66 and 67.

1) dram **2)** ounce **3)** minim **4)** one-half **5)** grain **6)** ℥ ss **7)** gr $\frac{1}{6}$ **8)** ℥ iv **9)** pt ii **10)** qt i$\frac{1}{4}$ **11)** gr x **12)** ℥ viiiss **13)** gr ii **14)** pt 16 **15)** gr iii **16)** ℥ 32 **17)** gr viiss **18)** 32 **19)** i **20)** ii

Review Set 14 from page 69.

1) twenty drops **2)** one thousand units **3)** ten milliequivalents **4)** four teaspoons **5)** ten tablespoons **6)** 4 gtt **7)** 30 mEq **8)** 5 T **9)** 1500 U **10)** 10 t **11)** False **12)** False **13)** units, U **14)** 3 **15)** 9 **16)** 2 **17)** 2 **18)** 12 **19)** 5 **20)** international unit, IU

Practice Problems—Chapter 3 from pages 71 and 72.

1) milli **2)** micro **3)** centi **4)** kilo **5)** 1 milligram **6)** 1 kilogram **7)** 1 microgram **8)** 1 centimeter **9)** meter **10)** gram **11)** liter **12)** drop **13)** ounce **14)** ounce **15)** grain **16)** milligram **17)** microgram **18)** unit **19)** milliequivalent **20)** teaspoon **21)** milliunit **22)** milliliter **23)** cubic centimeter **24)** pint **25)** tablespoon **26)** millimeter **27)** gram **28)** centimeter **29)** liter **30)** meter **31)** kilogram **32)** international unit **33)** gr ss **34)** 2 t **35)** ℥ $\frac{1}{3}$ **36)** 500 mg **37)** 0.5 L **38)** ℥ $\frac{1}{4}$ **39)** gr $\frac{1}{200}$ **40)** 0.05 mg **41)** eight and one-quarter ounces **42)** three hundred seventy-five international units **43)** one one-hundred twenty-fifths of a grain **44)** two and six tenths milliliters **45)** twenty milliequivalents **46)** four tenths of a liter **47)** four and one-half grains **48)** seventeen hundredths of a milligram **49)** Critical Thinking Skill: Prevention. This type of error can be prevented by avoiding the use of a decimal point or extra zero when not necessary. In this instance the decimal point and zero serve no purpose and can easily be misinterpreted, especially if the decimal point is difficult to see. Question any order that is unclear or unreasonable. **50)** Critical Thinking Skill: Prevention. This is both an error in notation and transcription. One grain should have been written *gr i*. Health care facilities would be wise to require the use of metric notation, especially for narcotics. The nurse's knowledge of correct notation as well as common dosages for pain medication should signal a problem. Question any order that is unclear or unreasonable.

Answers

Review Set 15 from page 76.

1) divide **2)** multiply **3)** 3 **4)** 3 **5)** $3\frac{1}{2}$ **6)** 16 **7)** 72 **8)** $1\frac{1}{2}$ **9)** $\frac{2}{3}$ **10)** 52 **11)** $\frac{1}{4}$ **12)** 30 **13)** $3\frac{1}{3}$ **14)** 14 **15)** $\frac{3}{4}$ **16)** $\frac{1}{12}$ **17)** $\frac{2}{3}$ **18)** $\frac{1}{4}$ **19)** 40 **20)** $3\frac{1}{2}$ **21)** 20 servings **22)** 8 quarts **23)** 64¢ **24)** 19.5¢ **25)** 23.5¢

Solutions—Review Set 15

6) $32 \div 2 = 16$

8) $\frac{1}{2} \times 3 = \frac{3}{2} = 1\frac{1}{2}$

19) $2\frac{1}{2} \times 16 = \frac{5}{\cancel{2}_{1}} \times \frac{\cancel{16}^{8}}{1} = 40$

20) $\frac{126}{36} = 3\frac{18}{36} = 3\frac{1}{2}$

21)
2 quarts = 8 cups
$\frac{1}{2}$ gallon = 8 cups
+ 4 cups
20 cups or 20 1-cup servings

23)
Store A: $1.56 × 2 = $3.12/gallon
Store B: $0.94 × 4 = $3.76/gallon
− 3.12
$0.64 savings at Store A

24) $1.56 ÷ 8 = $0.195 or 19.5¢/cup

25) $0.94 ÷ 4 = $0.235 or 23.5¢/cup

Review Set 16 from pages 79 and 80.

1) 0.5 **2)** 15 **3)** 0.008 **4)** 0.01 **5)** 0.06 **6)** 0.3 **7)** 0.0002 **8)** 1200 **9)** 2.5 **10)** 65 **11)** 5 **12)** 1500 **13)** 2 **14)** 0.25 **15)** 2000 **16)** 56.08 **17)** 79.2 **18)** 1000 **19)** 1000 **20)** 0.001 **21)** 0.023 **22)** 0.00105 **23)** 0.018 **24)** 400 **25)** 0.025 **26)** 0.5 **27)** 10,000 **28)** 0.45 **29)** 0.005 **30)** 30,000

Solutions—Review Set 16

2) 0.015. g = 15 mg; g is larger than mg. To convert from larger to smaller unit, multiply. It takes more of mg (smaller) unit to make equivalent amount of g (larger) unit. Equivalent: 1 g = 1000 mg. Therefore, multiply by 1000 or move decimal point three places to right.

3) .008. mg = 0.008 g; mg is smaller unit than g. To convert from smaller to larger unit, divide. It takes fewer of g (larger) unit to make equivalent amount of mg (smaller) unit. Therefore, divide by 1000 or move decimal point three places to left.

7) .0000.2 mg = 0.0002 g **9)** 0.002.5 kg = 2.5 g **17)** 79.200. mL = 79.2 L **20)** .001. mL = 0.001 L **23)** .018. mcg = 0.018 mg

Review Set 17 from pages 84 and 85.

1) 30, gr i = 60 mg **2)** 45, gr i = 60 mg **3)** $\frac{9}{20}$, 1 g = gr 15 **4)** 0.4, gr i = 60 mg **5)** 0.5, 1 g = gr 15 **6)** $\frac{1}{4}$, gr i = 60 mg **7)** 65, 1 t = 5 cc **8)** ss, ℥ i = 30 cc **9)** 75, ℥ i = 30 mL **10)** iss, pt i = 500 mL **11)** 4, 1t = 5 mL **12)** 60, 1 T = 15 cc **13)** 19.8, 1 kg = 2.2 lb **14)** 8, qt i = pt ii **15)** 96, 1 L = ℥ 32 **16)** 121, 1 kg = 2.2 lb **17)** 30, 1 in = 2.5 cm **18)** 2, qt i = 1 L **19)** 15, 1 t = 5 mL **20)** 45, 1 kg = 2.2 lb **21)** $\frac{1}{150}$, gr i = 60 mg **22)** $\frac{1}{100}$, gr i = 60 mg **23)** 500, pt i = 500 mL **24)** 600, gr i = 60 mg **25)** v, gr i = 60 mg **26)** 12, 1 in = 2.5 cm **27)** iss, gr i = 60 mg **28)** ii, ℥ i = 30 mL **29)** 10, gr i = 60 mg **30)** ss, gr i = 60 mg **31)** 80, 1 in = 2.5 cm **32)** 14, 1 in = 2.5 cm **33)** 3, 1 in = 2.5 cm, 1 cm = 10 mm **34)** 50, 1 in = 2.5 cm, 1 cm = 10 mm **35)** 88, 1 kg = 2.2 lb **36)** 7160, 1 kg = 1000 g **37)** 50, 1 kg = 2.2 lb **38)** 7.7, 1 kg = 2.2 lb **39)** 28.64, 1 kg = 2.2 lb **40)** 53.75 **41)** 4, $\frac{1}{2}$ **42)** 3.75 **43)** 2430 **44)** 1.25 **45)** 10 **46)** Dissolve 4 tablespoons or 2 ounces of Epsom Salts in 1 quart of water. **47)** 2 **48)** 3 **49)** 16 **50)** 93.64

Solutions—Review Set 17

2) gr → mg; larger → smaller: (×)

$\text{gr } \frac{3}{4} = \frac{3}{\cancel{4}_{1}} \times \frac{\cancel{60}^{15}}{1} = 45 \text{ mg}$

3) g → gr; larger → smaller: (×)

$0.03 \text{ g} = \frac{3}{\cancel{100}_{20}} \times \frac{\cancel{15}^{3}}{1} = \text{gr } \frac{9}{20}$

4) gr → mg; larger → smaller: (×)

$\text{gr } \frac{1}{150} = \frac{1}{\cancel{150}_{5}} \times \frac{\cancel{60}^{2}}{1} = \frac{2}{5} = 0.4 \text{ mg}$

5) gr → g; smaller → larger unit: (÷)

gr viiss = gr $7\frac{1}{2}$ = 7.5 ÷ 15 = 0.5 g

6) mg → gr; smaller → larger: (÷)

15 mg = 15 ÷ 60 = gr $\frac{1}{4}$

9) ℥ → mL; larger → smaller: (×)

℥ iss = ℥ $2\frac{1}{2}$ = 2.5 × 30 = 75 mL

11) mL → t; smaller → larger: (÷)

20 mL = 20 ÷ 5 = 4 t

16) kg → lb; larger → smaller: (×)

55 kg = 55 × 2.2 = 121 lb

20) lb → kg; smaller → larger: (÷)

99 lb = 99 ÷ 2.2 = 45 kg

24) gr → mg; larger → smaller: (×)

gr x = gr 10 = 10 × 60 = 600 mg

28) mL → ℥; smaller → larger: (÷)

60 mL = 60 ÷ 30 = 2 = ℥ ii

34) in → mm; larger → smaller: (×)

2 in = 2 × 2.5 cm = 5 cm

cm → mm; larger → smaller: (×)

5 cm = 5 × 10 = 50 mm

41) mL → oz; smaller → larger: (÷)

120 mL = 120 ÷ 30 = 4 = ℥ iv

℥ → cups; smaller to larger: (÷)

℥ iv = ℥4 = 4 ÷ 8 = $\frac{1}{2}$ cup

42) m → km; smaller to larger: (÷)

500 m = 500 ÷ 1000 = 0.5 km

0.75	Day 1
+ .50	
1.25	Day 2
+ .50	
1.75	Day 3
+ .50	
2.25	Day 4
+ .50	
2.75	Day 5
+ .50	
3.25	Day 6
+ .50	
3.75	Day 7

43) Add up the ounces: 81 ounces

℥ → mL; larger → smaller: (×)

℥ 81 = 81 × 30 = 2430 mL

44) lb → kg; smaller → larger: (÷)

55 kg = 55 ÷ 2.2 = 25 kg

0.05 mg/kg = 0.05 mg/kg × 25 kg = 1.25 mg

45) Find the total number of mL per day and the total number of mL per bottle.

Per day: 12 mL × 4 = 48 mL

Per bottle: 16 ounces × 30 mL/ounce = 480 mL

480 ~~mL~~ ÷ 48 ~~mL~~/day = 10 days

46) mL → t; smaller → larger: (÷)

60 mL = 60 ÷ 5 = 12 t or

mL → ℥, smaller → larger: (÷)

60 mL = 60 ÷ 30 = ℥ ii Epsom Salts

t → T; smaller → larger: (÷)

12 t = 12 ÷ 3 = 4 T Epsom Salts

1 L (1000 mL) = qt i water

48) qt i = ℥ 32 per container

4 oz/~~feeding~~ × 8 ~~feedings~~/day = ℥ 32 per day

Need 3 containers for 3 days.

Review Set 18 from pages 87 and 88.

1) 0.05, 1 L = 1000 mL **2)** 45, 1 g = gr 15 **3)** 38.18, 1 kg = 2.2 lb **4)** 1.33, 1 g = gr 15 **5)** 7.5, gr i = 60 mg **6)** iiss, ℥ i = 30 mL **7)** iss, pt i = 500 mL **8)** 45, ℥ i = 30 mL **9)** $\frac{1}{4}$, gr i = 60 mg **10)** 0.625, 1 mg = 1000 mcg **11)** $\frac{1}{2}$, 1 t = 5 mL **12)** 30, gr i = 60 mg, **13)** $\frac{1}{8}$, gr i = 60 mg **14)** $\frac{1}{100}$, gr i = 60 mg **15)** 3, 1 in = 2.5 cm **16)** 16,000, 1 g = 1000 mg **17)** ss, ℥ i = 30 mL **18)** ss, qt i = ℥ 32 **19)** 2, qt i = 1 L **20)** ss, qt i = pt ii **21)** 5, ℥ i = 30 mL **22)** 1, 1t = 5 mL **23)** 8, 1 L = 1000 mL, 1 L = qt i, qt i = ℥ 32 **24)** 3; 1 t = 5 mL **25)** 15, gr i = 60 mg

Solutions—Review Set 18

3) $\frac{1 \text{ kg}}{2.2 \text{ lb}} = \frac{X \text{ kg}}{84 \text{ lb}}$

$2.2X = 84$

$\frac{2.2X}{2.2} = \frac{84}{2.2}$

$X = 38.18$ kg

5) $\frac{\text{gr i}}{60 \text{ mg}} = \frac{\text{gr } \frac{1}{8}}{X \text{ mg}}$

$X = 60 \times \frac{1}{8}$

$X = \frac{60}{8} = 7.5$ mg

7) $\frac{500\text{ mL}}{\text{pt i}} = \frac{750\text{ mL}}{X}$

500X = 750

$\frac{500X}{500} = \frac{750}{500}$

X = $1\frac{1}{2}$

X = pt iss

14) $\frac{\text{gr i}}{60\text{ mg}} = \frac{X\text{ gr}}{0.6\text{ mg}}$

60X = 0.6

$\frac{60\,X}{60} = \frac{0.6}{60}$

X = 0.01 = gr $\frac{1}{100}$

23) 2000 mL = 2 L

2 L = qt ii = 64 ounces

$\frac{\text{ʒ}8}{1\text{ cup}} = \frac{\text{ʒ}64}{X\text{ cup}}$

8X = 64

$\frac{8X}{8} = \frac{64}{8}$

X = 8 cups or 8 8-oz glasses

Practice Problems—Chapter 4 from pages 89 and 90.

1) 500 **2)** 10 **3)** 7.5 **4)** 3 **5)** 0.004 **6)** 0.5 **7)** ss **8)** 0.3 **9)** 70 **10)** 149.6 **11)** 180 **12)** 105 **13)** 0.3 **14)** 15 **15)** 6 **16)** 90 **17)** 32.05 **18)** 7.99 **19)** 0.008 **20)** 2 **21)** 95 **22)** viiss **23)** $\frac{1}{100}$ **24)** 0.67 **25)** 68.18 **26)** i **27)** 1 **28)** 500 **29)** 2 **30)** iii **31)** 30 **32)** 30 **33)** 1 **34)** 1 **35)** 1 **36)** 1500 **37)** 45 **38)** iss **39)** $\frac{1}{6}$ **40)** 0.025 **41)** 4300 **42)** 0.06 **43)** 15 **44)** 45 **45)** 0.8 **46)** 9 **47)** 8 **48)** 840 **49)** 100%; all of it **50)** Critical Thinking Skill: Prevention The nurse didn't use the conversion rules correctly. The nurse divided instead of multiplying. Further, the conversion factor is 1000 not 2. This type of medication error is avoided by double checking your dosage calculations and asking yourself, "Is this dosage reasonable?" Certainly you know if there are 1000 mg in 1 g, and you want to give 2 g, then you need *more* than 1000 milligrams, not less. Remember: To convert from a larger unit (g) to a smaller unit (mg), *multiply* by the conversion factor. Larger → Smaller: (×).

Solutions—Practice Problems—Chapter 4

46) ʒ iv per bottle = 4 × 30 = 120 mL/bottle (ʒ i = 30 mL)

Each dose = $2\frac{1}{2}$ t = $2\frac{1}{2} \times 5$ = 12.5 mL (1 t = 5 mL)

Bottle holds 120 mL; each dose is 12.5 mL.

120 mL ÷ 12.5 mL/dose = 9.6 doses or 9 *full* doses.

47) 120 mL ÷ 15 mL/dose = 8 doses (1T = 15 mL)

48) 4 + 8 + 6 + 10 = 28 ounces = 28 ~~oz~~ × 30 mL/~~oz~~ = 840 mL (ʒ i = 30 mL)

49) gr $\frac{1}{6} = \frac{1}{6} \times \frac{60}{1} = \frac{60}{6}$ = 10 mg ordered (gr i = 60 mg)

The ampule contains 10 mg, and the doctor orders gr $\frac{1}{6}$ or 10 mg; therefore, the patient should receive all of the solution in the ampule.

Review Set 19 from page 94.

1) 12:32 AM **2)** 7:30 AM **3)** 4:40 PM **4)** 9:21 PM **5)** 11:59 PM **6)** 12:15 PM **7)** 2:20 AM **8)** 10:10 AM **9)** 1:15 PM **10)** 6:25 PM **11)** 1330 **12)** 0004 **13)** 2145 **14)** 1200 **15)** 2315 **16)** 0345 **17)** 2400 **18)** 1530 **19)** 0620 **20)** 1745 **21)** "zero-six-twenty-three" **22)** "zero-zero-forty-one" **23)** "nineteen-zero-three" **24)** "twenty-three-eleven" **25)** "zero-three hundred"

Review Set 20 from pages 96 and 97.

1) −17.8 **2)** 185 **3)** 212 **4)** 89.6 **5)** 22.2 **6)** 37.2 **7)** 39.8 **8)** 104 **9)** 176 **10)** 97.5 **11)** 37.8 **12)** 66.2 **13)** 39.2 **14)** 34.6 **15)** 39.3 **16)** 35.3 **17)** 44.6 **18)** 31.1 **19)** 98.6 **20)** 39.7

Solutions—Review Set 20

1) $°C = \frac{°F - 32}{1.8}$

$°C = \frac{0 - 32}{1.8}$

$°C = \frac{-32}{1.8}$

°C = −17.8°

2) °F = 1.8 °C + 32

°F = (1.8 × 85) + 32

°F = 153 + 32

°F = 185°

Practice Problems—Chapter 5 from pages 97 and 98.

1) 2:57 AM **2)** 0310 **3)** 1622 **4)** 8:01 PM **5)** 11:02 AM **6)** 0033 **7)** 0216 **8)** 4:42 PM **9)** 11:56 PM **10)** 0420 **11)** 1931 **12)** 2400 or 0000 **13)** 0645 **14)** 9:15 AM **15)** 9:07 PM **16)** 6:23 PM **17)** 5:40 AM **18)** 1155 **19)** 2212 **20)** 2106 **21)** 4 h **22)** 7 h **23)** 8 h 30 min **24)** 12 h 15 min **25)** 14 h 50 min **26)** 4 h 12 min **27)** 4 h 48 min **28)** 3 h 41 min **29)** 6 h 30 min **30)** 16 h 38 min **31)** False **32)** a. AM; b. PM; c. AM; d. PM **33)** 37.6 **34)** 97.7 **35)** 102.6 **36)** 37.9 **37)** 36.7 **38)** 99.3 **39)** 32 **40)** 40 **41)** 36.6 **42)** 95.7 **43)** 39.7 **44)** 77 **45)** 212 **46)** 5.6 **47)** –7.8 **48)** 105.8 **49)** 37.2, 99 (98.96° rounds to 99.0°F) **50)** True

Solutions—Practice Problems—Chapter 5

24)
$$\begin{array}{r} 2150 \\ -0935 \\ \hline 1215 \end{array} = 12 \text{ h } 15 \text{ min}$$

26) 2316 = 11:16 PM, 0328 = 3:28 AM

11:16 PM → 3:16 AM = 4 h
3:16 AM → 3:28 AM = 12 minutes
4 h 12 min

28) 4:35 pm → 7:35 pm = 3 h
7:35 pm → 8:16 pm = 41 min
3 h 41 min

49) $\frac{37.6 + 35.5 + 38.1 + 37.6}{4} = \frac{148.8}{4} =$

37.2°C (average temp);

°F = 1.8(37.2) + 32 = 99°

Review Set 21 from pages 108 and 109.

1) tuberculin **2)** a. yes; b. Round 1.25 to 1.3 and measure on the cc scale as 1.3 cc. **3)** No **4)** 0.5 cc **5)** a. False b. The size of the drop varies according to the diameter of the tip of the dropper. **6)** No **7)** Measure the oral liquid in a 3 cc syringe, which is not intended for injections. **8)** 5 **9)** Discard the excess prior to injecting the patient. **10)** To prevent needlestick injury.

11)

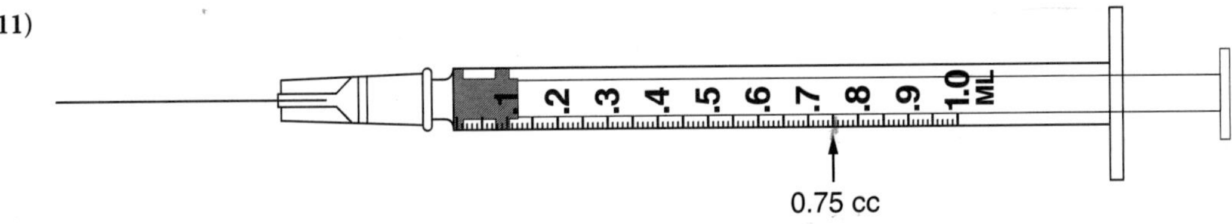

12)

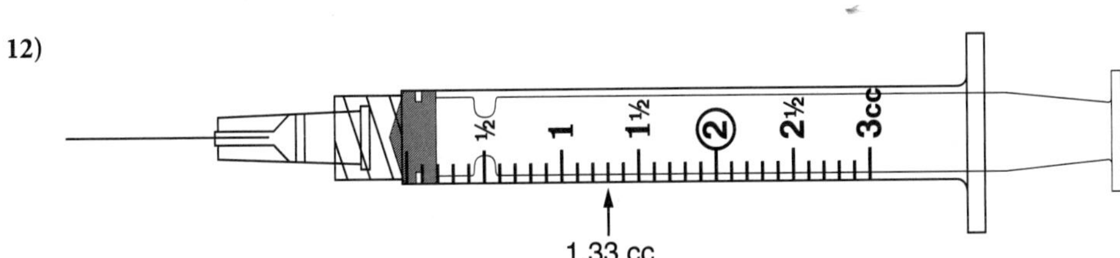

13)

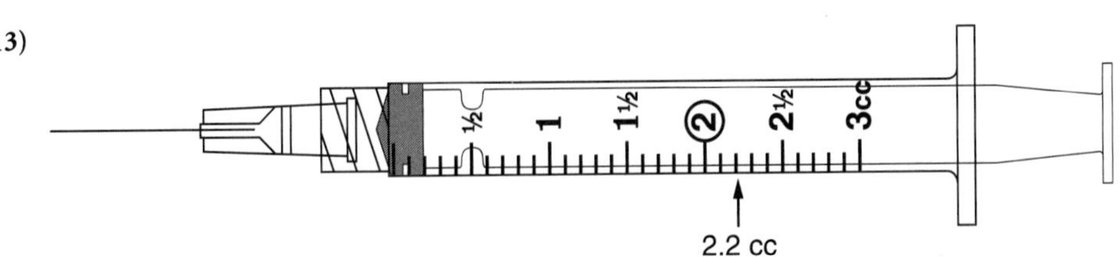

14)

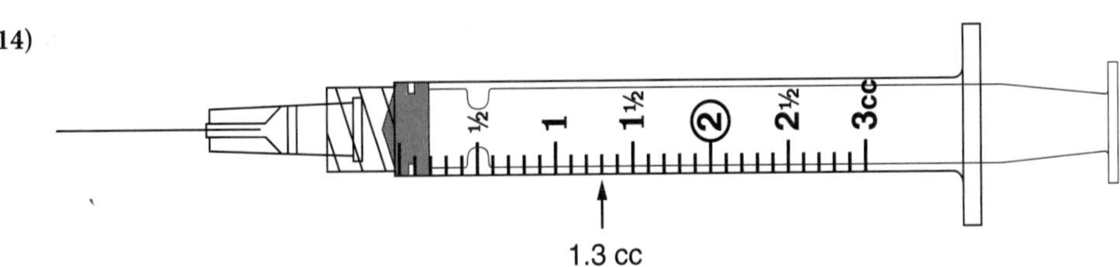

15)

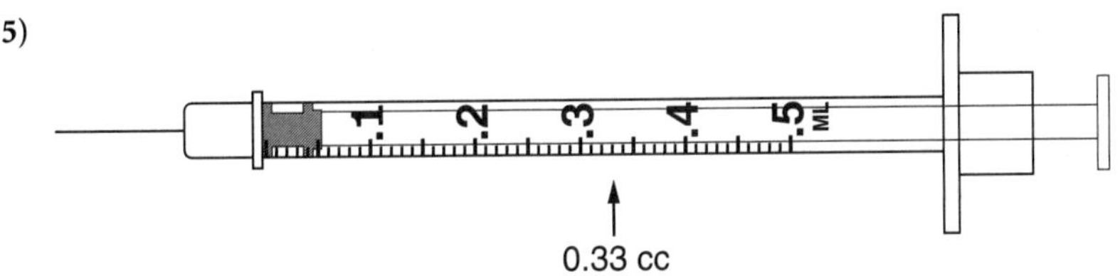

16)

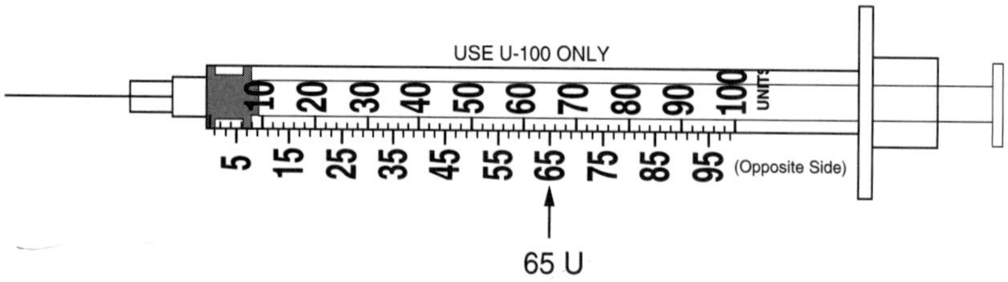

USE U-100 ONLY
(Opposite Side)
65 U

17)

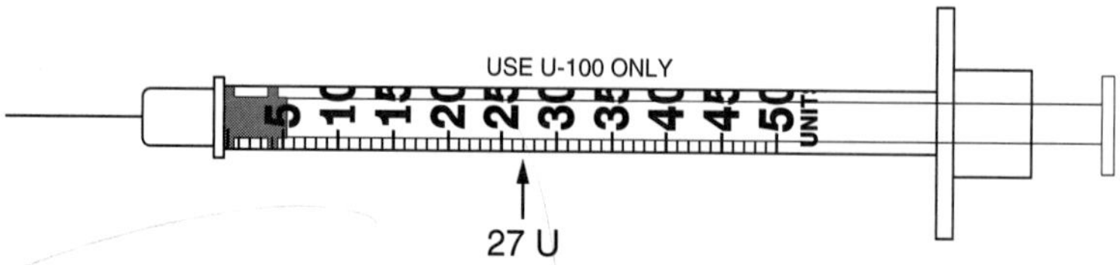

USE U-100 ONLY
27 U

18)

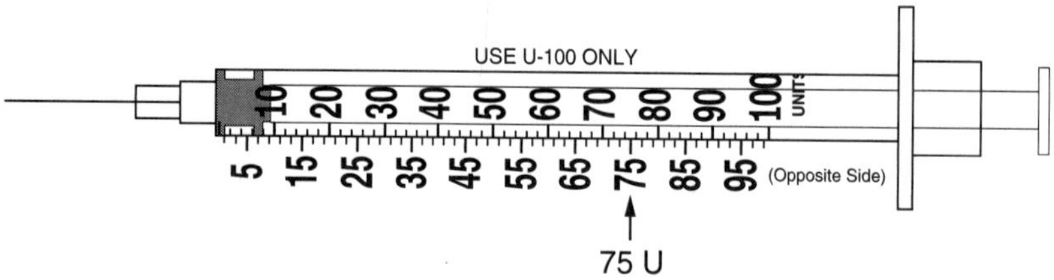

USE U-100 ONLY
(Opposite Side)
75 U

19)

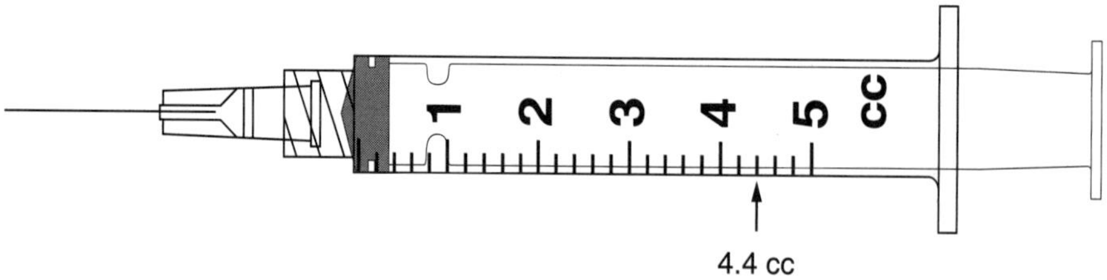

4.4 cc

20)

16 cc

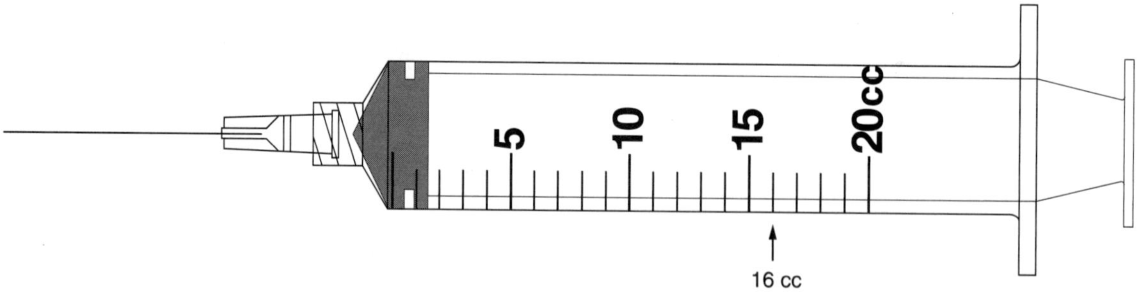

Practice Problems—Chapter 6 from pages 110–112.

1) 1 **2)** hundredths or 0.01 **3)** No. The tuberculin syringe has a maximum capacity of 1 mL. **4)** Round to 1.3 mL and measure at 1.3 mL. **5)** 30 mL or 1 oz **6)** 1 mL tuberculin **7)** 0.75 **8)** False **9)** False **10)** True **11)** To prevent accidental needlesticks during intravenous administration. **12)** top ring **13)** 10 **14)** minim **15)** standard 3 cc, tuberculin, and insulin

16)

0.45 mL

17)

USE U-100 ONLY
(Opposite Side)
80 U

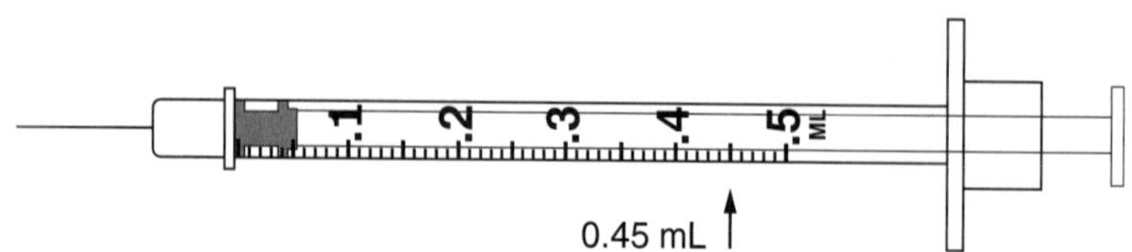

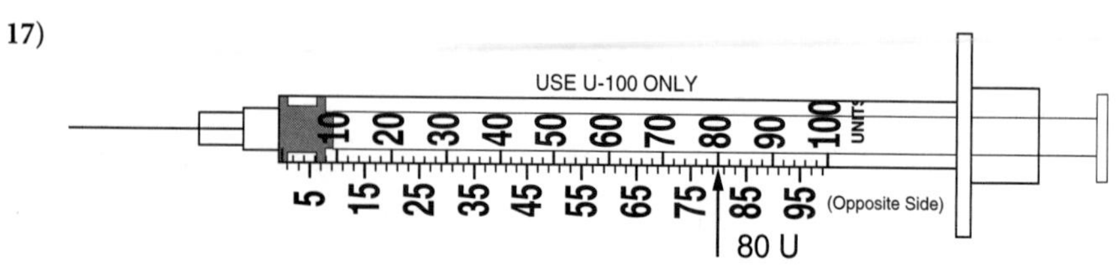

18)

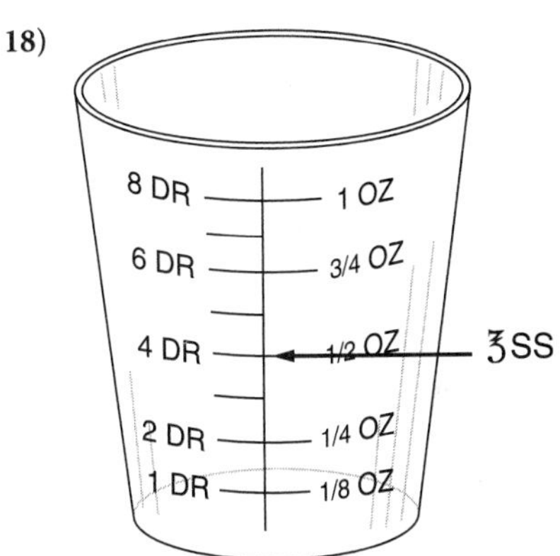

19)

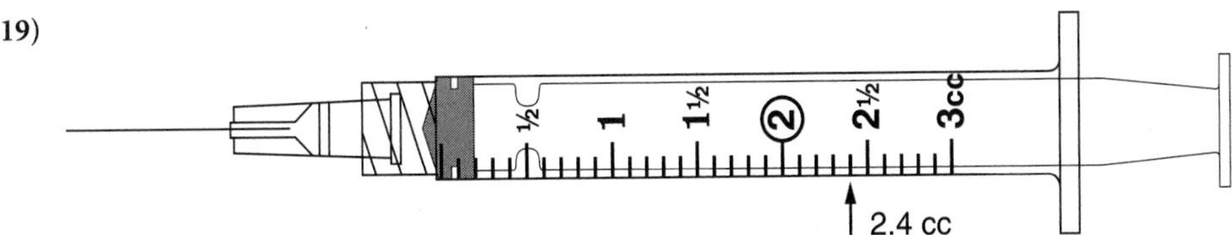

20)

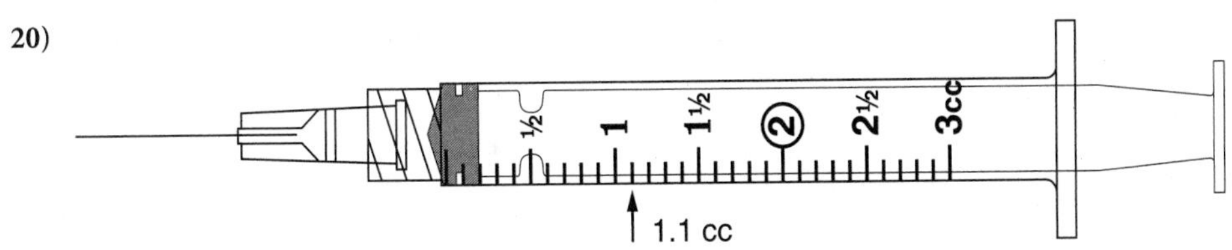

21)

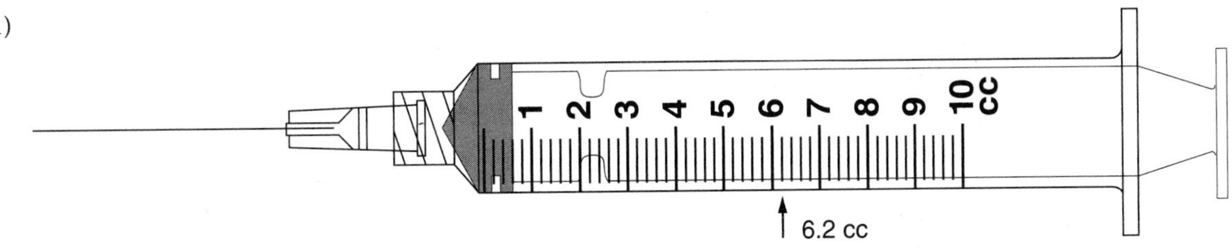

22) Critical Thinking Skill: Prevention.
This error could have been avoided by following the principle of not putting oral drugs in syringes intended for injection. Instead, place the medication in an oral syringe to which a needle cannot be attached. In addition, the medication should have been labeled for oral use only. The medication was ordered orally, not by injection. The alert nurse would have noticed the discrepancy. Finally, but just as important, a medication should be administered only by the nurse who prepared it.

Review Set 22 from pages 116 and 117.

1) Give 250 milligrams of naproxen orally 2 times a day. **2)** Give 30 units of Humulin N NPH U-100 insulin subcutaneously every day 30 minutes before breakfast. **3)** Give 500 milligrams of Ceclor orally immediately, and then give 250 milligrams every 8 hours. **4)** Give 25 micrograms of Synthroid orally once a day. **5)** Give 10 milligrams of Ativan intramuscularly every 4 hours as necessary for agitation. **6)** Give 20 milligrams of furosemide intravenously (slowly) immediately. **7)** Give 10 cubic centimeters of Gelusil orally at bedtime. **8)** Give 2 drops of 1% atropine sulfate ophthalmic in the right eye every 15 minutes for 4 applications. **9)** Give $\frac{1}{4}$ grain of morphine sulfate intramuscularly every 3 to 4 hours as needed for pain. **10)** Give 0.25 milligram of Lanoxin orally once a day. **11)** Give 250 milligrams of tetracycline orally 4 times a day. **12)** Give $\frac{1}{400}$ grain of nitroglycerin sublingually immediately. **13)** Give 2 drops of Cortisporin otic suspension in both ears 3 times a day and at bedtime. **14)** 1, 6, 8, 9, 11, 12 **15)** Contact the physician for clarification. **16)** No, q.i.d. orders are given 4 times in 24 hours, whereas q.4h orders are given 6 times in 24 hours. **17)** Determined by hospital or institutional policy. **18)** Patient, drug, dosage, route, frequency, date and time, signature of physician/writer. **19)** Parts 1–5 **20)** The right patient must receive the right drug in the right amount by the right route at the right time.

Review Set 23 from page 122.

1) 6 AM, 12 noon, 6 PM, 12 midnight **2)** 9 AM **3)** 7:30 AM, 11:30 AM, 4:30 PM, 9 PM **4)** 9 AM, 5 PM **5)** every 4 hours, as needed for severe pain. **6)** 9/7/xx at 0900 **7)** sublingual, under the tongue **8)** once a day **9)** 125 mcg **10)** nitroglycerin, Darvocet-N 100, meperidine (Demerol), promethazine (Phenergan) **11)** subcutaneous injection **12)** once (at 9 AM) **13)** Keflex **14)** before breakfast (at 7:30 AM) **15)** milliequivalent **16)** Keflex and Slow K **17)** Tylenol **18)** twice **19)** 0900 and 2100 **20)** 2400, 0600, 1200, and 1800 **21)** In the "One-Time Medication Dosage" section, lower left corner.

Practice Problems—Chapter 7 from pages 123–126.

1) ounce **2)** per rectum **3)** before meals **4)** after **5)** three times a day **6)** every four hours **7)** when necessary **8)** by mouth, orally **9)** once a day, every day **10)** right eye **11)** immediately **12)** freely, as desired **13)** hour of sleep, bedtime **14)** intramuscular **15)** without **16)** ss **17)** gtt **18)** mL **19)** gr **20)** g **21)** q.i.d. **22)** O.U. **23)** SC **24)** t **25)** b.i.d. **26)** q.3h **27)** p.c. **28)** $\bar{a}$ **29)** kg **30)** Give 60 milligrams of Toradol intramuscularly immediately and every 6 hours. **31)** Give 300,000 units of procaine penicillin G intramuscularly 4 times a day. **32)** Give 5 milliliters of Mylanta orally 1 hour before and 1 hour after meals, at bedtime, and every 2 hours as needed at night. **33)** Give 25 milligrams of Librium orally every 6 hours when necessary for agitation. **34)** Give 5,000 units of heparin subcutaneously immediately. **35)** Give 50 milligrams of Demerol intramuscularly every 3–4 hours when necessary for pain. **36)** Give 0.25 milligram of digoxin orally every day. **37)** Give 2 drops of 10% Neosynephrine to the left eye every 30 minutes for 2 applications. **38)** Give 40 milligrams of Lasix intramuscularly immediately. **39)** Give 4 milligrams of Decadron intravenously twice a day. **40)** 12:00 midnight, 8:00 AM, 4:00 PM **41)** 20 units **42)** SC, subcutaneous **43)** Give 500 milligrams of Cipro orally every 12 hours. **44)** 8:00 AM, 12:00 noon, 6:00 PM **45)** Digoxin 0.125 mg p.o. q.d. **46)** with, $\bar{c}$ **47)** Give 150 milligrams of ranitidine tablets orally twice daily with breakfast and supper. **48)** Vancomycin **49)** 12 hours **50)** Critical Thinking Skill: Prevention. This error could have been avoided by paying careful attention to the ordered frequency and by writing the frequency on the MAR.

Review Set 24 from pages 135–137.

1) B **2)** D **3)** C **4)** A **5)** E **6)** F **7)** G **8)** 1 capsule **9)** IM or IV **10)** A, C, D, E **11)** Supply dosage of Darvocet-N (100 mg/tablet) **12)** 5 mg **13)** $\frac{1}{2}$ tablet **14)** penicillin G potassium **15)** Pfizerpen **16)** 5,000,000 units per vial; reconstituted to 250,000 U/mL, 500,000 U/mL, or 1,000,000 U/mL. **17)** IM or IV **18)** 0049-0520-83 **19)** Pfizer-Roerig **20)** One vial—use half of the reconstituted volume.

Practice Problems—Chapter 8 from pages 138–141.

1) 8 mEq per tablet **2)** 57267-165-30 **3)** 600 mg per tablet **4)** ampicillin sodium/sulbactam sodium **5)** "Reconstitute with up to 100 mL of an appropriate diluent cited in the package insert." **6)** Roerig-Pfizer **7)** 10 mL **8)** 25 mg/mL **9)** 1 mL **10)** Keflin **11)** cephalothin sodium **12)** 0002-7001-01 **13)** mL, intramuscular solution **14)** 10 mL **15)** intramuscular **16)** Roche Products **17)** capsule **18)** 59° to 86°F **19)** April, 2000 **20)** 80 mg per tablet **21)** I **22)** H **23)** H **24)** oral **25)** 0666060 **26)** Critical Thinking Skill: Prevention. This error could have been prevented by carefully comparing the drug label and dosage to the MAR drug and dosage. In this instance both the incorrect drug and the incorrect dosage sent by the pharmacy should have been noted by the nurse. Further, the nurse should have asked for clarification of the order.

Section 2—Self-Evaluation from pages 142–145.

1) gr $\frac{2}{3}$ **2)** 4 t **3)** gr $\frac{1}{300}$ **4)** 0.5 mL **5)** ℥ ss **6)** four drops **7)** four hundred fifty milligrams **8)** one one-hundredth grain **9)** seven and one-half grains **10)** twenty five-hundredths liter **11)** (7.13 kg) = 7130 g = 7,130,000 mg = 7,130,000,000 mcg **12)** 0.000000925 kg = 0.000925 g = 0.925 mg = (925 mcg) **13)** 0.000125 kg = 0.125 g = (125 mg) = 125,000 mcg **14)** 0.0164 kg = (16.4 g) = 16,400 mg = 16,400,000 mcg **15)** 10 mg = 0.01 g **16)** 0.02 g = gr $\frac{1}{3}$ **17)** 12 t = 60 mL **18)** 9 L = 9000 mL **19)** 37.5 cm = 375 mm **20)** 5.62 cm = 2.25 = $2\frac{1}{4}$ in **21)** 90 kg = 90,000 g **22)** 11,590 g = 25.5 = $25\frac{1}{2}$ lb **23)** gr iii **24)** 360 mg **25)** 0.2 mg **26)** 6 L or qt vi **27)** 455 mL **28)** 2335 **29)** 6:44 PM **30)** .0417 **31)** 8:03 AM **32)** 100.4 **33)** 38.6 **34)** 99

35)

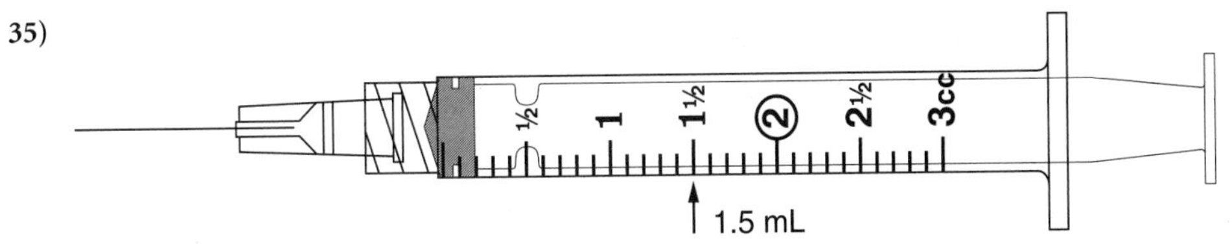

36)

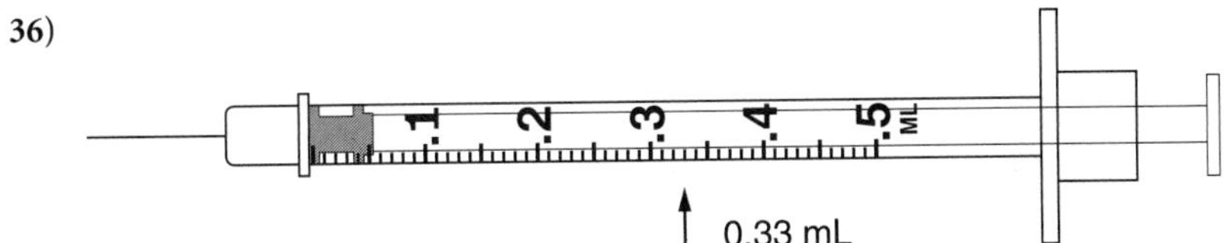

37)

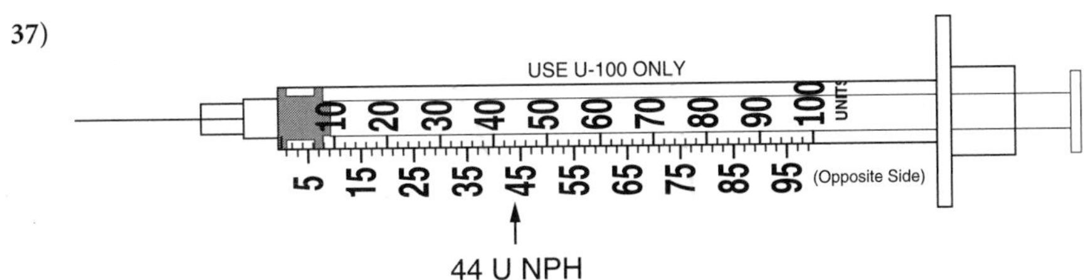

38)

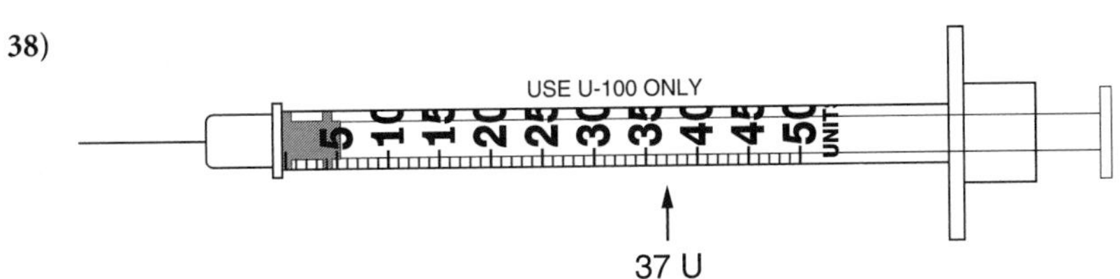

39)

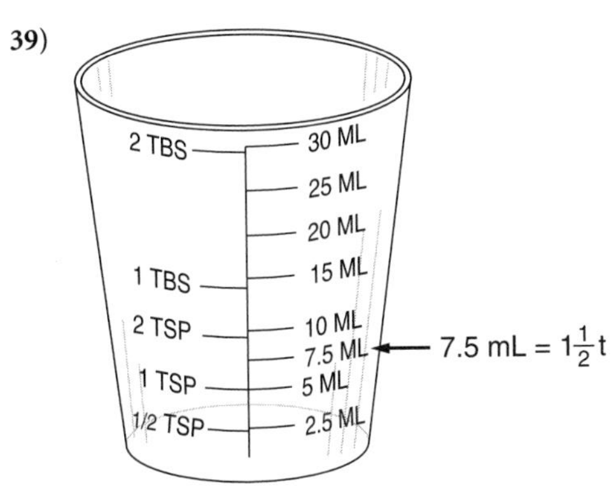

40) neomycin and polymixin B sulfates and hydrocortisone **41)** Use in ears only. **42)** 10 mL **43)** Give 2 drops of Cortisporin otic solution in both ears every 15 minutes for 3 doses **44)** 10,000 units per mL **45)** 0002-7217-01

46) Give 3750 units of heparin subcutaneously every 8 hours. **47)** Amoxil **48)** 125 mg per 5 mL

49) a. 5. b. 1

C.

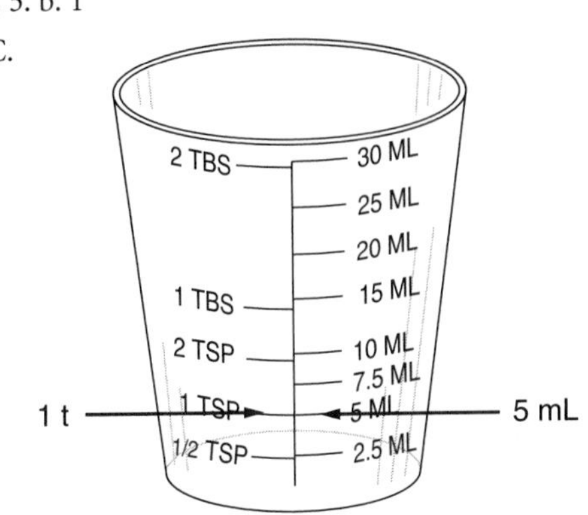

50) Give 250 mg of Amoxil by mouth 3 times per day.

Solutions—Section 2—Self-Evaluation

15) gr → mg or larger → smaller: (×);

gr $\frac{1}{6} = \frac{1}{6} \times 60 = 10$ mg

mg → g or smaller → larger: (÷)

10 mg = 10 ÷ 1000 = 0.01 g

21) lb → kg or smaller → larger: (÷)

198 lb = 198 ÷ 2.2 = 90 kg

kg → mg or larger → smaller: (×)

90 kg = 90 × 1000 = 90,000 g

24) gr → mg or larger → smaller: (×)

gr $\frac{3}{4} = \frac{3}{4} \times 60 = \frac{180}{4}$ = 45 mg; q. 3h = 8 doses/24 h;

45 mg/$\cancel{\text{dose}}$ × 8 $\cancel{\text{doses}}$ = 360 mg

27) 15 oz = 15 × 30 = 450 mL

1 t	= 5 mL
total	= 455 mL

Review Set 25 from pages 158–161.

1) 1 **2)** 1 **3)** $1\frac{1}{2}$ **4)** $\frac{1}{2}$ **5)** $\frac{1}{2}$ **6)** 2 **7)** 2 **8)** 2 **9)** $1\frac{1}{2}$ **10)** 2 **11)** 3; 6 **12)** $\frac{1}{2}$ **13)** 2 **14)** 2 **15)** 2 **16)** $1\frac{1}{2}$ **17)** 10, 1 **18)** 10 and 20; 1 of each, 4 **19)** 15, 1 **20)** 60, 1 **21)** B, 2 capsules **22)** J, 2 tablets **23)** F, 1 tablet **24)** I, 2 tablets **25)** C, 1 tablet **26)** E, 2 capsules **27)** D, 2 capsules **28)** H, 2 tablets **29)** A, 1 capsule **30)** C, 1 tablet

Solutions—Review Set 25

1) Order: 0.1 g = 0.1 × 1000 = 100 mg

Supply: 100 mg/tab

$$\frac{D}{H} \times Q = \frac{\overset{1}{\cancel{100\text{ mg}}}}{\underset{1}{\cancel{100\text{ mg}}}} \times 1 \text{ tab} = 1 \text{ tab}$$

5) Order: 0.125 mg

Supply: ~~0.25 mg/tab~~ 0.250 mg/tab

$$\frac{D}{H} \times Q = \frac{\overset{1}{\cancel{0.125\text{ mg}}}}{\underset{2}{\cancel{0.250\text{ mg}}}} \times 1 \text{ tab} = \frac{1}{2} \text{ tab}$$

10) Order: ~~5 mg~~ 5.0 mg

Supply: 2.5 mg/tab

$$\frac{D}{H} \times Q = \frac{\overset{2}{\cancel{5.0\text{ mg}}}}{\underset{1}{\cancel{2.5\text{ mg}}}} \times 1 \text{ tab} = 2 \text{ tab}$$

11) Order: 1.5 g

Supply: 0.5 g/tab

$$\frac{D}{H} \times Q = \frac{\overset{3}{\cancel{1.5\text{ g}}}}{\underset{1}{\cancel{0.5\text{ g}}}} \times 1 \text{ tablet} = 3 \text{ tab}$$

1.5 g q.i.d. = 1.5 g/$\cancel{\text{dose}}$ × 4 $\cancel{\text{doses}}$/day
= 6 g/day

14) Order: 0.1 mg = 0.1 × 1000 = 100 mcg

Supply: 50 mcg/tab

$$\frac{D}{H} \times Q = \frac{\overset{2}{\cancel{100\text{ mcg}}}}{\underset{1}{\cancel{50\text{ mcg}}}} \times 1 \text{ tab} = 2 \text{ tab}$$

17) Order: gr $\frac{1}{6} = \frac{1}{\underset{1}{\cancel{6}}} \times \overset{10}{\cancel{60}} = 10$ mg (gr i = 60 mg)

Supply: 10 mg and 2.5 mg/tab

Select 10 mg and give 1 tab

$$\frac{D}{H} \times Q = \frac{\cancel{10\text{ mg}}}{\cancel{10\text{ mg}}} \times 1 \text{ tab} = 1 \text{ tab}$$

28) Order: 0.5 mg = 0.5 × 1000 = 500 mcg

Supply: 250 mg/tab

$$\frac{D}{H} \times Q = \frac{\overset{2}{\cancel{500\text{ mg}}}}{\underset{1}{\cancel{250\text{ mg}}}} \times 1 \text{ tab} = 2 \text{ tab}$$

Review Set 26 from pages 164–168.

1) 7.5 **2)** 5 **3)** 20 **4)** 4 **5)** 1 **6)** 20 **7)** 2 **8)** 7.5 **9)** 3 **10)** 2.5 **11)** 22.5 **12)** 7.5 **13)** 2 **14)** 2.5 **15)** 5 **16)** ss **17)** $1\frac{1}{2}$ **18)** 2 **19)** 15 **20)** 1 **21)** 2 **22)** B; 2.5 mL ($\frac{1}{2}$t) **23)** C; 2 mL **24)** A; 2 mL **25)** 5 **26)** i **27)** 47 **28)** 5 **29)** 4 **30)** 0900, 1300, 1900

Solutions—Review Set 26

2) Order: gr $\frac{1}{6} = \frac{1}{\cancel{6}_{1}} \times \frac{\cancel{60}^{10}}{1} = 10$ mg (gr i = 60 mg)

Supply: 10 mg/5 mL

$$\frac{D}{H} \times Q = \frac{\cancel{10\text{ mg}}^{1}}{\cancel{10\text{ mg}}_{1}} \times 5\text{ mL} = 5\text{ mL}$$

4) Order: 100 mg

Supply: 125 mg/5 mL

$$\frac{D}{H} \times Q = \frac{\cancel{100\text{ mg}}^{4}}{\cancel{125\text{ mg}}_{5}} \times 5\text{ mL} = \frac{20}{5} = 4\text{ mL}$$

6) Order: 25 mg

Supply: 6.25 mg/t = 6.25 mg/5 mL (1 t = 5 mL)

$$\frac{D}{H} \times Q = \frac{25\ \cancel{\text{mg}}}{62.5\ \cancel{\text{mg}}} \times 5\text{ mL} = \frac{125}{6.25} = 20\text{ mL}$$

7) Order: 125 mg

Supply: 62.5 mg/5 mL

$$\frac{D}{H} \times Q = \frac{\cancel{25\text{ mg}}^{2}}{\cancel{6.25\text{ mg}}_{1}} \times 5\text{ mL} = 10\text{ mL}$$

10 mL = $\frac{10}{5}$ = 2 t (1 t = 5 mL)

11) Order: 0.24 g = 0.24 × 1000 = 240 mg

Supply: 80 mg/7.5 mL

$$\frac{D}{H} \times Q = \frac{\cancel{240\text{ mg}}^{3}}{\cancel{80\text{ mg}}_{1}} \times 7.5\text{ mL} = 22.5\text{ mL}$$

15) Order: 0.25 mg = 0.25 × 1000 = 250 mcg

Supply: 50 mcg/mL

$$\frac{D}{H} \times Q = \frac{\cancel{250\text{ mg}}^{5}}{\cancel{50\text{ mg}}_{1}} \times 1\text{ mL} = 5\text{ mL}$$

17) Order: 375 mg

Supply: 250 mg/5 mL

$$\frac{D}{H} \times Q = \frac{375\ \cancel{\text{mg}}}{\cancel{250\text{ mg}}_{50}} \times \cancel{5}^{1}\text{ mL} = \frac{375}{50} = 7.5\text{ mL}$$

7.5 mL = $\frac{7.5}{5} = 1\frac{1}{2}$ t (1 t = 5 mL)

19) Order: 1.2 g = 1.2 × 1000 = 1200 mg

Supply: 400 mg/5 mL

$$\frac{D}{H} \times Q = \frac{\cancel{1200\text{ mg}}^{3}}{\cancel{400\text{ mg}}_{1}} \times 5\text{ mL} = 15\text{ mL}$$

20) Order: 0.25 g = 0.25 × 1000 = 250 mg

Supply: 125 mg/2.5 mL

$$\frac{D}{H} \times Q = \frac{\cancel{250\text{ mg}}^{2}}{\cancel{125\text{ mg}}_{1}} \times 2.5\text{ mL} = 5\text{ mL} = 1\text{ t}$$

21) Order: 100 mg

Supply: 250 mg/5 mL

$$\frac{D}{H} \times Q = \frac{100\ \cancel{\text{mg}}}{\cancel{250\text{ mg}}_{50}} \times \cancel{5}^{1}\text{ mL} = \frac{\cancel{100}^{2}}{\cancel{50}_{1}} = 2\text{ mL}$$

Practice Problems—Chapter 9 from pages 169–179.

1) $\frac{1}{2}$ **2)** 2 **3)** $\frac{1}{2}$ **4)** 2.5 **5)** 10 **6)** 2 **7)** 8 **8)** $1\frac{1}{2}$ **9)** $1\frac{1}{2}$ **10)** $\frac{1}{2}$ **11)** $1\frac{1}{2}$ **12)** 1 **13)** $1\frac{1}{2}$ **14)** 1 **15)** 1 **16)** 5; $1\frac{1}{2}$ **17)** 7.5 **18)** $1\frac{1}{2}$ **19)** 2 **20)** 2 **21)** 0.75, 1 **22)** $\frac{1}{2}$ **23)** 2 **24)** 2 **25)** 2 **26)** 2 **27)** 15 and 30; one of each **28)** 2.4 **29)** 5 **30)** 2 **31)** D; 2 tablets **32)** A; 1 capsule **33)** C; 1 tablet **34)** B; 2 tablets **35)** I; 2 tablets **36)** G; 2 tablets **37)** F; 5 mL **38)** H; 2 tablets **39)** E; 30 mL **40)** L; 2 capsules **41)** M; 1 tablet **42)** K; 2 capsules **43)** J; 1 tablet **44)** N; 1 tablet **45)** O; 1 tablet **46)** R; 1 tablet **47)** P; 1 tablet **48)** S; 1 tablet **49)** T; 1 tablet **50)** Critical Thinking Skill: Prevention. This medication error could have been prevented if the nurse had more carefully read the physician's order as well as the medication label. The doctor's order misled the nurse by noting the volume first and then the drug dosage. If confused by the order, the nurse should have clarified the intent with the physician. By focusing on the volume, the nurse failed to follow the steps in dosage calculation. Had the nurse noted 250 mg as the desired dosage and the supply (or on-hand) dosage as 125 mg per 5 mL, the correct amount to be administered would have been clear. Slow down and take time to compare the order with the labels. Calculate each dose carefully before preparing and administering both solid and liquid form medications.

Solutions—Practice Problems—Chapter 9

2) Order: gr ss $= \frac{1}{\cancel{2}_{1}} \times \frac{\cancel{60}^{30}}{1} = 30$ mg

Supply: 15 mg/tab

$\frac{D}{H} \times Q = \frac{\cancel{30\text{ mg}}^{2}}{\cancel{15\text{ mg}}_{1}} \times 1 \text{ tab} = 2 \text{ tab}$

3) Order: 0.075 mg = 0.075 × 1000 = 75 mcg

Supply: 150 mcg/tab

$\frac{D}{H} \times Q = \frac{\cancel{75\text{ mcg}}^{1}}{\cancel{150\text{ mcg}}_{2}} \times 1 \text{ tab} = \frac{1}{2} \text{ tab}$

8) Order: 150 mg

Supply: 0.1 tab = 0.1 × 1000 = 100 mg/tab

$\frac{D}{H} \times Q = \frac{\cancel{150\text{ mg}}^{3}}{\cancel{100\text{ mg}}_{2}} \times 1 \text{ tab} = 1\frac{1}{2} \text{ tab}$

9) Order: gr $\frac{3}{4} = \frac{3}{\cancel{4}_{1}} \times \frac{\cancel{60}^{15}}{1} = 45$ mg

Supply: 30 mg/tab

$\frac{D}{H} \times Q = \frac{\cancel{45\text{ mg}}^{3}}{\cancel{30\text{ mg}}_{2}} \times 1 \text{ tab} = 1\frac{1}{2} \text{ tab}$

14) Order: gr $\frac{1}{8} = \frac{1}{\cancel{8}_{2}} \times \frac{\cancel{60}^{15}}{1} = \frac{15}{2} = 7.5$ mg

Supply: 7.5 mg/tab

$\frac{D}{H} \times Q = \frac{\cancel{7.5\text{ mg}}}{\cancel{7.5\text{ mg}}} \times 1 \text{ tab} = 1 \text{ tab}$

19) Order: 0.25 mg → 0.250

Supply: 0.125 mg/tab

$\frac{D}{H} \times Q = \frac{\cancel{0.250\text{ mg}}^{2}}{\cancel{0.125\text{ mg}}_{1}} \times 1 \text{ tab} = 2 \text{ tab}$

27) Order: gr $\frac{3}{4} = \frac{3}{\cancel{4}_{1}} \times \frac{\cancel{60}^{15}}{1} = 45$ mg

Supply: 15 mg, 30 mg, and 60 mg tablets

Select: 1 15-mg tablet and 1 30-mg tablet for 45 mg

Remember: If you have a choice, give whole tablets and as few as possible.

30) Order: gr $\frac{1}{6} = \frac{1}{\cancel{6}_{1}} \times \frac{\cancel{60}^{10}}{1} = 10$ mg

Supply: 5 mg tablets

$\frac{D}{H} \times Q = \frac{\cancel{10\text{ mg}}^{2}}{\cancel{5\text{ mg}}_{1}} \times 1 \text{ tab} = 2 \text{ tab}$

41) Order: gr x = gr 10 = 10 × 60 = 600 mg

Supply: 8 mEq = 600 mg/tab

$\frac{D}{H} \times Q = \frac{\cancel{600\text{ mg}}}{\cancel{600\text{ mg}}} \times 1 \text{ tab} = 1 \text{ tab}$

Review Set 27 from pages 188–193

1) 0.5,

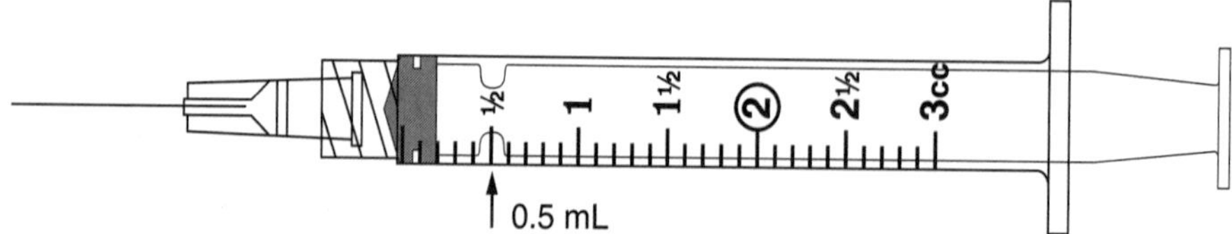

2) 4,

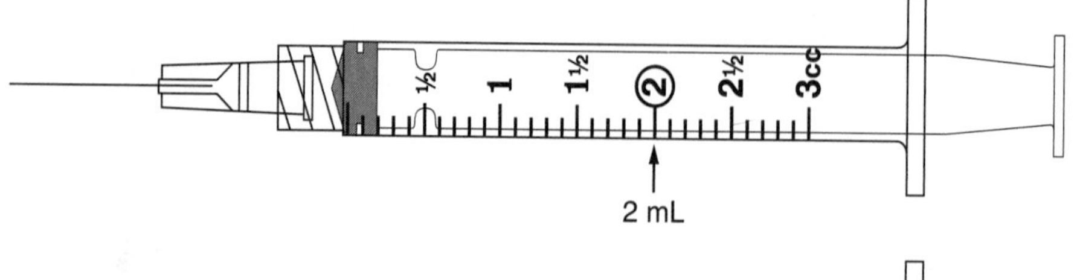

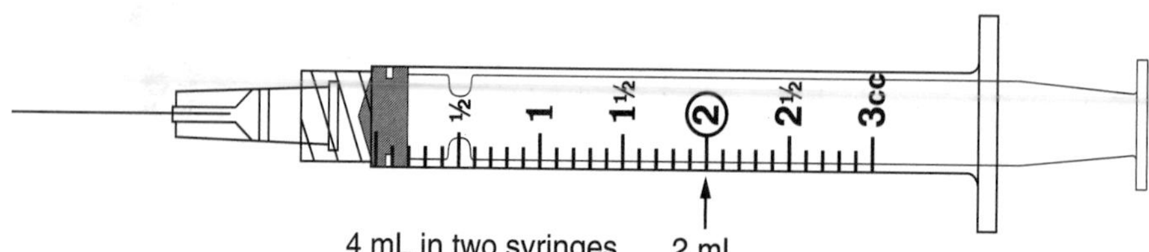

4 mL in two syringes

3) 2.4,

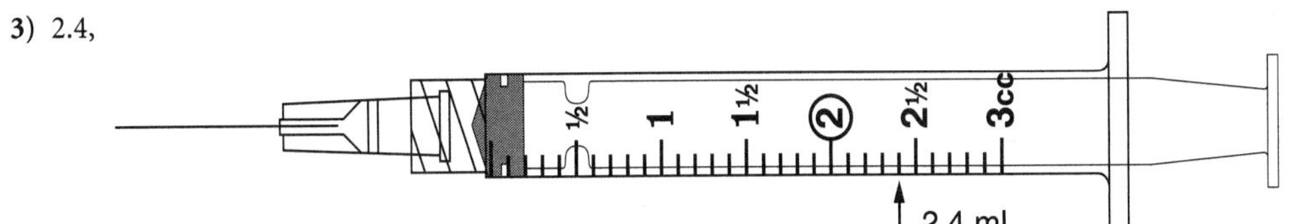

4) 2,

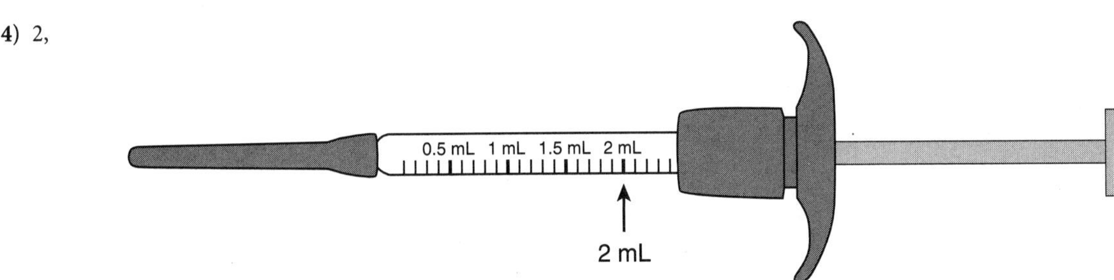

5) 2,

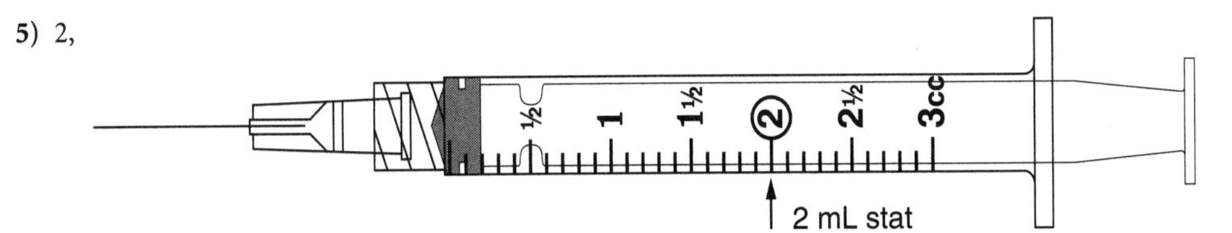

1,

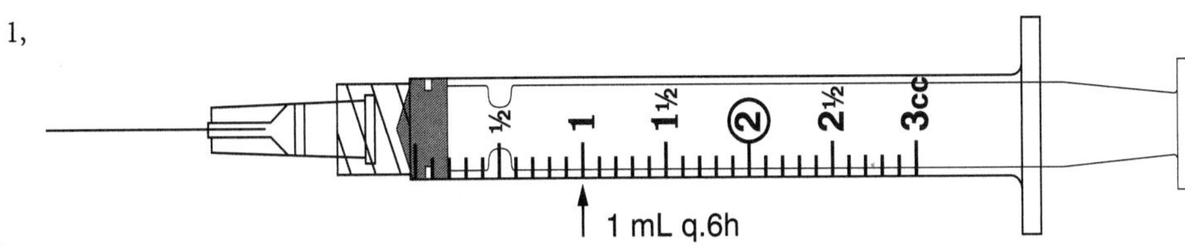

6) 0.8,

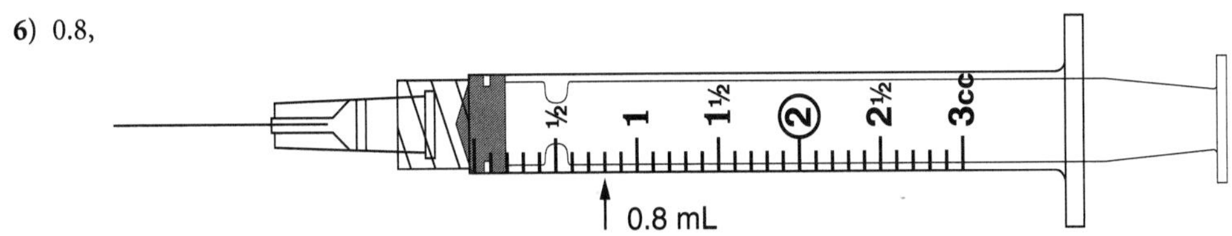

7) 7.5,

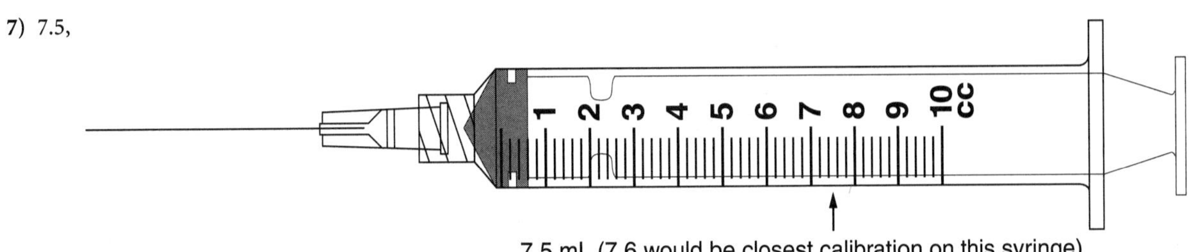

8) 1.2,

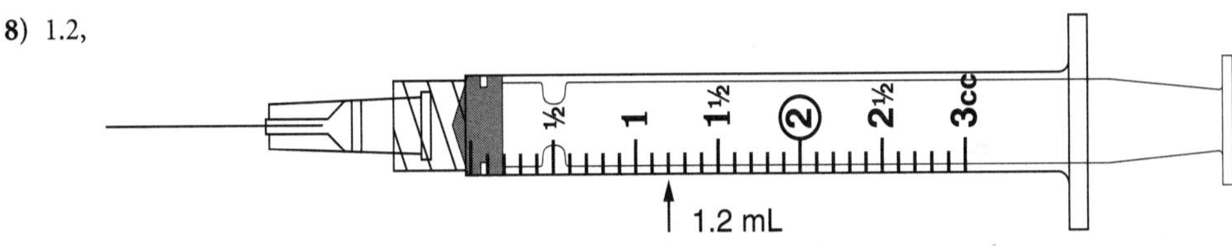

9) 1.5,

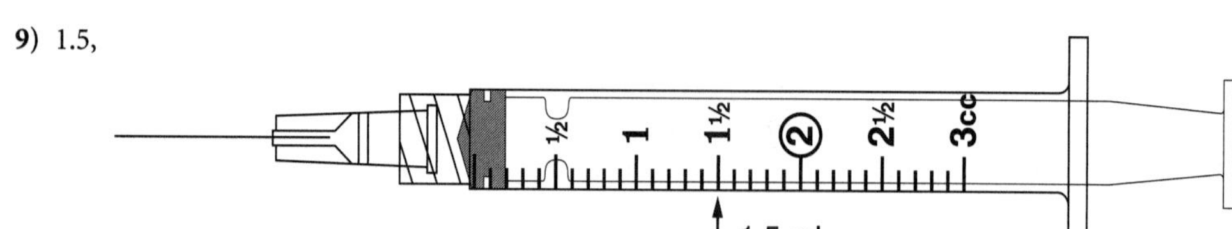

10) 1,

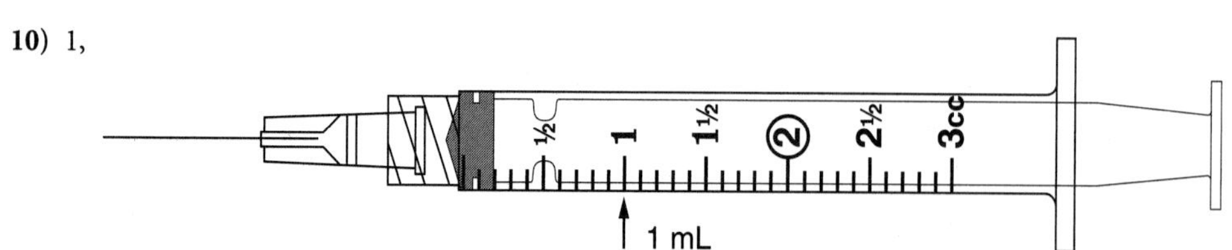

11) 1.3,

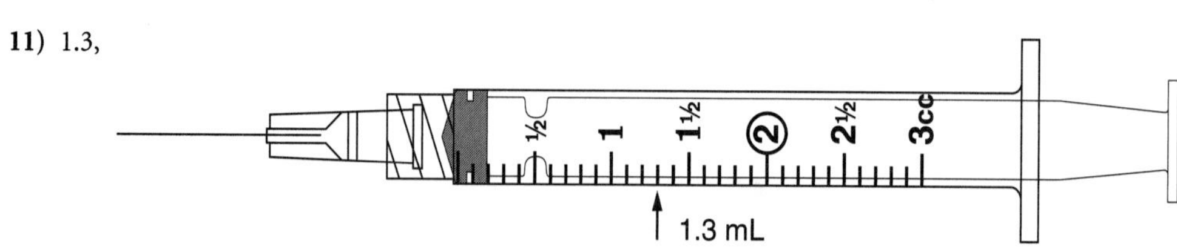

12) 0.45,

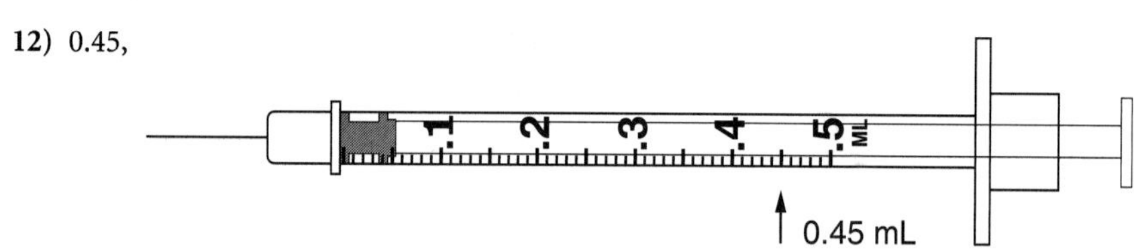

13) 1.5,

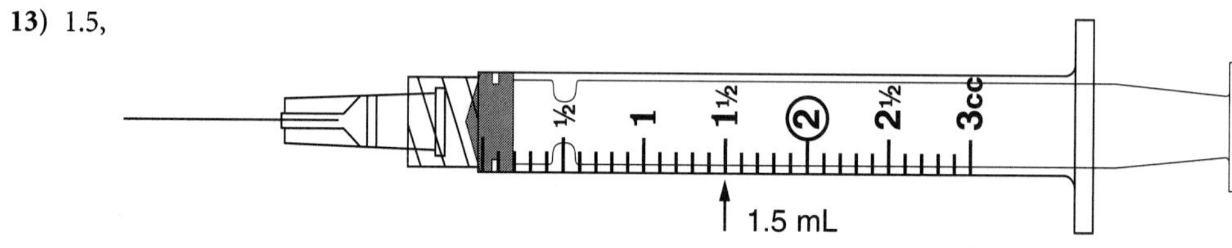

14) 0.8,

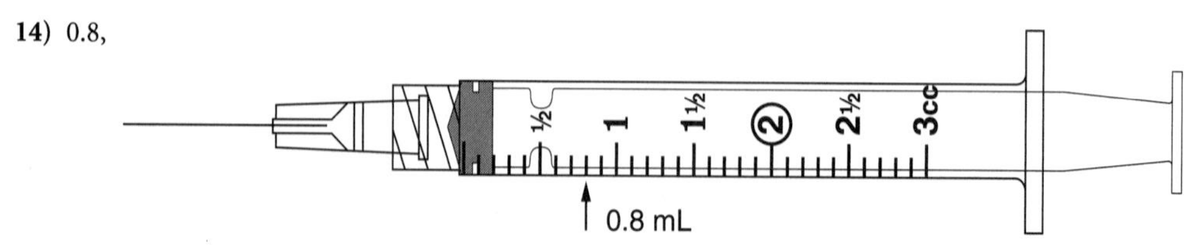

15) 1.5,

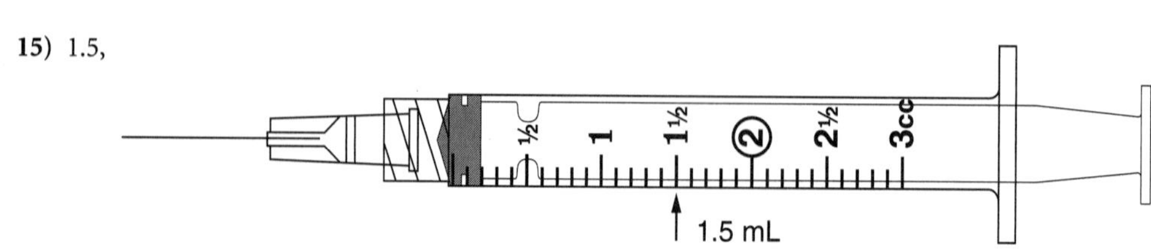

16) 1.5,

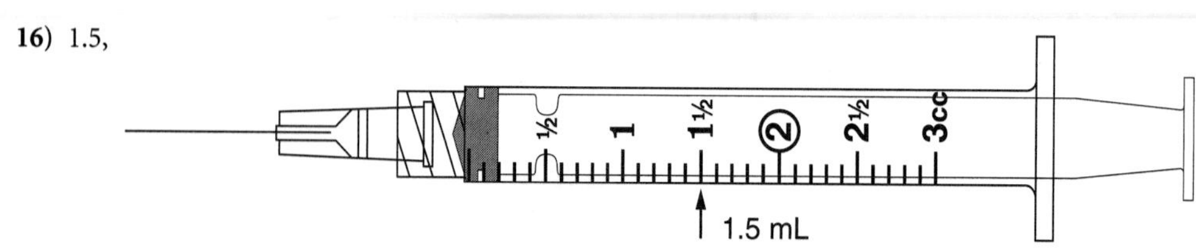

17) 0.5,

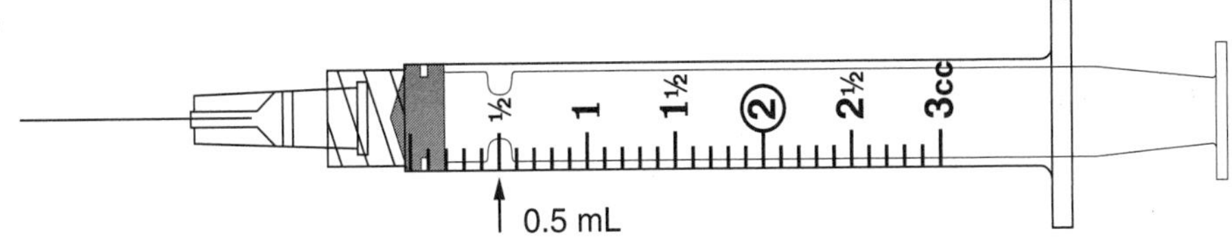

18) 0.8,

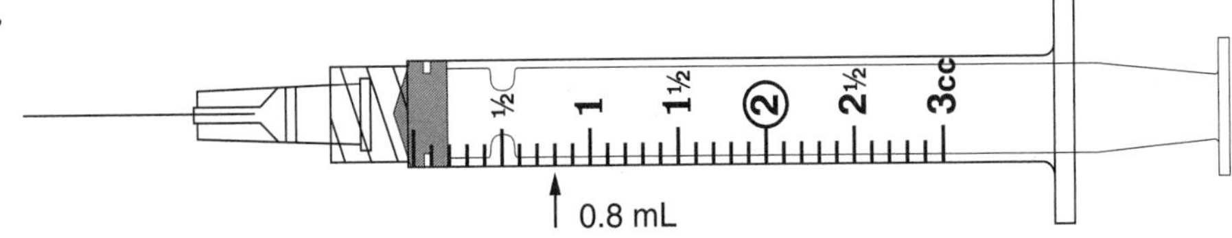

19) 0.25,

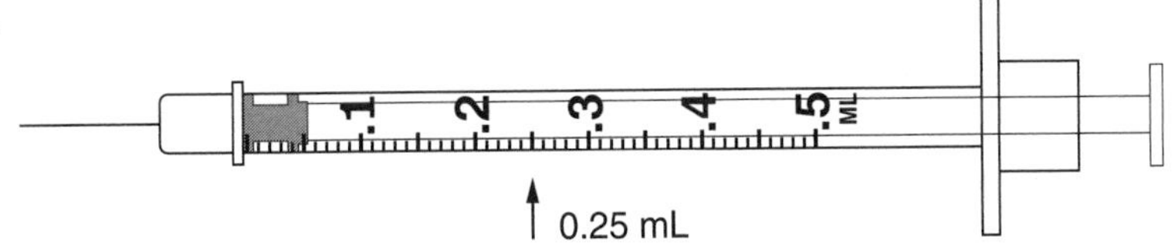

20) 1.6,

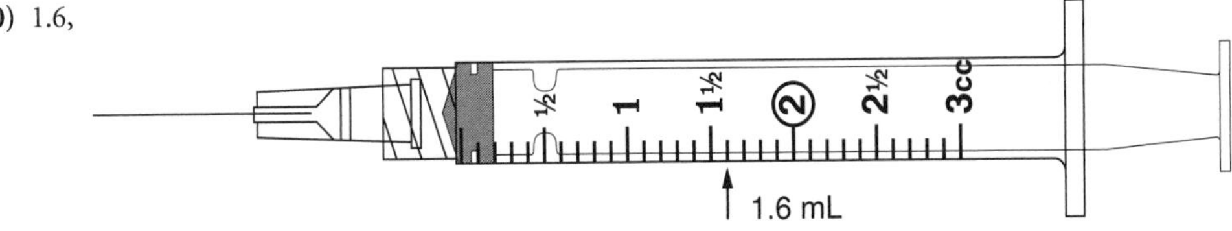

Solutions—Review Set 27

1) Order: $\text{gr}\,\frac{1}{4} = \frac{1}{\cancel{4}_{1}} \times \frac{\cancel{60}^{15}}{1} = 15\text{ mg}$

Supply: 30 mg/mL

$\frac{D}{H} \times Q = \frac{\cancel{15\text{ mg}}^{1}}{\cancel{30\text{ mg}}_{2}} \times 1\text{ mL} = 0.5\text{ mL}$

3) Order: 600 mcg

Supply: 500 mcg/2 mL

$\frac{D}{H} \times Q = \frac{\cancel{600\text{ mg}}}{\cancel{500\text{ mg}}} \times 2\text{ mL} = 2.4\text{ mL}$

6) Order: 8000 U

Supply: 10,000 U/mL

$\frac{D}{H} \times Q = \frac{\cancel{8000\text{ U}}}{\cancel{10000\text{ U}}} \times 1\text{ mL} = 0.8\text{ mL}$

8) Order: 60 mg

Supply: 75 mg/1.5 mL

$\frac{D}{H} \times Q = \frac{\cancel{60\text{ mg}}^{4}}{\cancel{75\text{ mg}}_{5}} \times 1.5\text{ mL} = \frac{6}{5} = 1.2\text{ mL}$

9) Order: $\text{gr}\,\frac{1}{100} = \frac{1}{\cancel{100}_{10}} \times \frac{\cancel{60}^{6}}{1} = 0.6\text{ mg}$

Supply: 0.4 mg/mL

$\frac{D}{H} \times Q = \frac{\cancel{0.6\text{ mg}}^{3}}{\cancel{0.4\text{ mg}}_{2}} \times 1\text{ mL} = 1.5\text{ mL}$

11) Order: 400,000 U

Supply: 300,000 U/mL

$\frac{D}{H} \times Q = \frac{\cancel{400{,}000\text{ U}}^{4}}{\cancel{300{,}000\text{ U}}_{3}} \times 1\text{ mL} = 1.33 = 1.3\text{ mL}$

19) Order: 12.5 mg

Supply: 50 mg/mL

$\frac{D}{H} \times Q = \frac{\cancel{12.5\text{ mg}}^{1}}{\cancel{50\text{ mg}}_{4}} \times 1\text{ mL} = 0.25\text{ mL}$

Review Set 28 from pages 201–206.

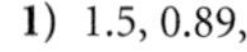

1) 1.5, 0.89,

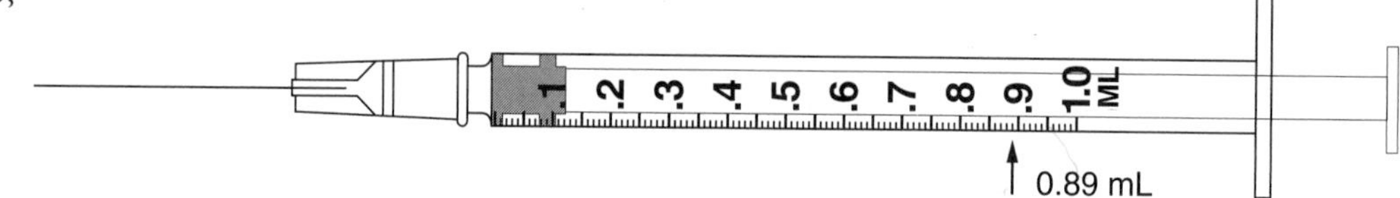

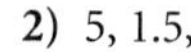

2) 5, 1.5,

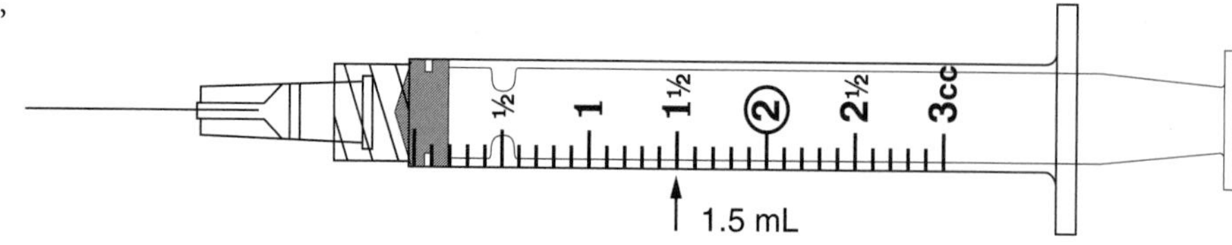

3) 2, 0.5,

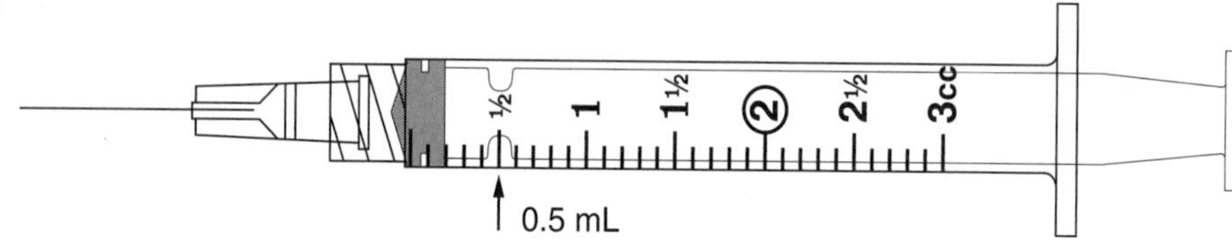

4) 50, 12.5,

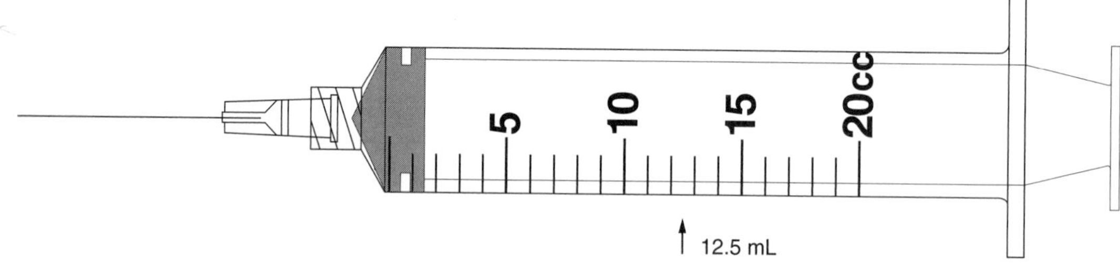

5) 50, 15,

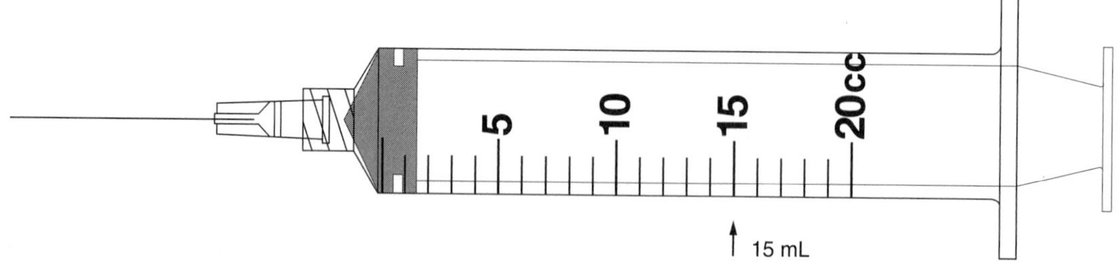

6) 3.5, 2,

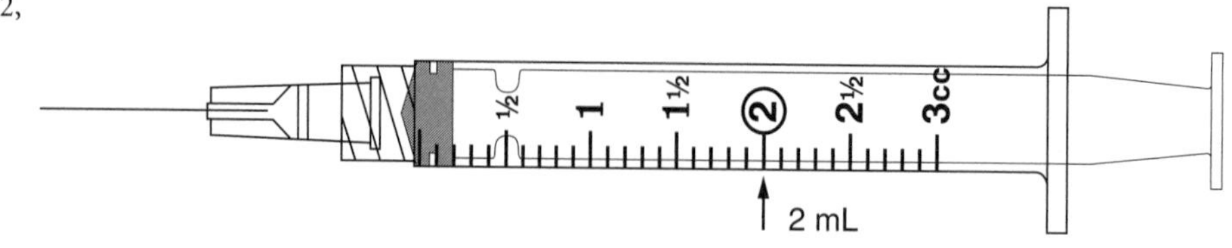

7) 8, 2.8,

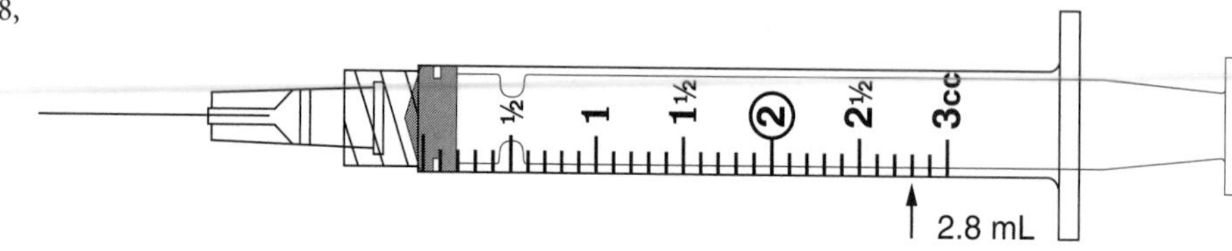

8) 4, 0.5,

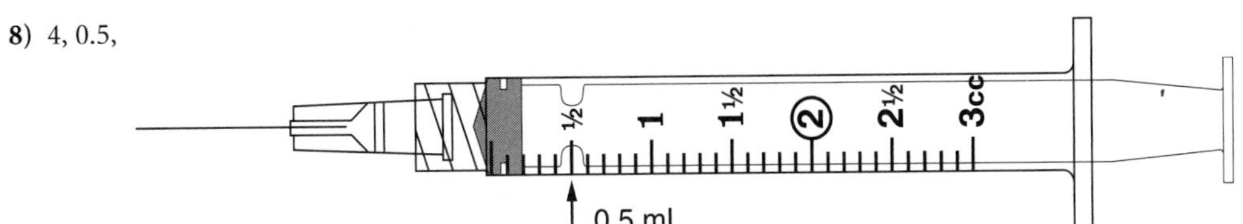

9) 1.6, 1,

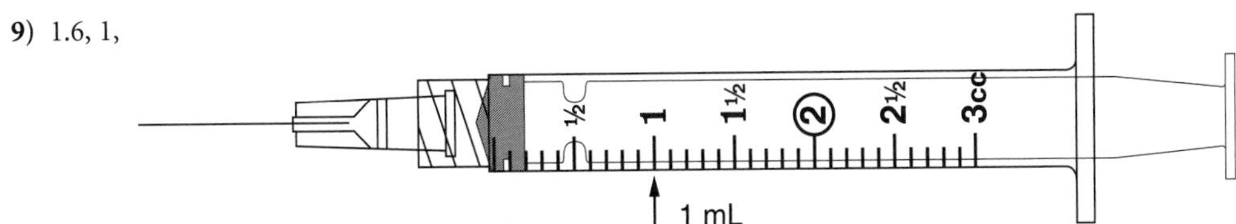

10) 1, 1.2,

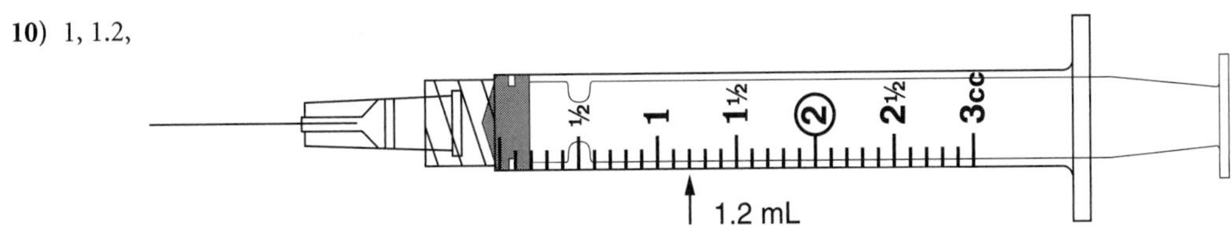

11) 1.6, 0.8,

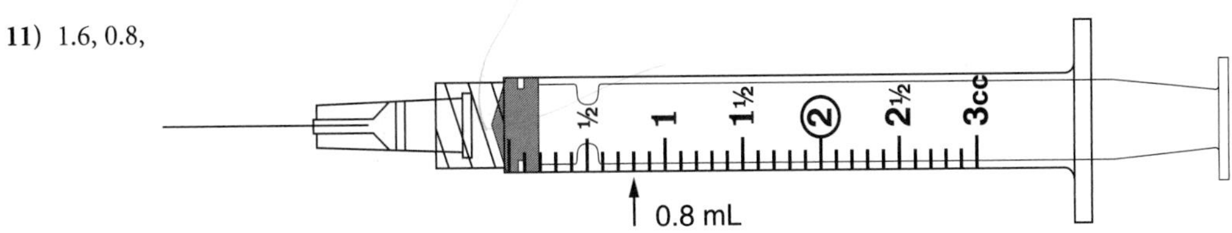

12) 2.5, 1.5,

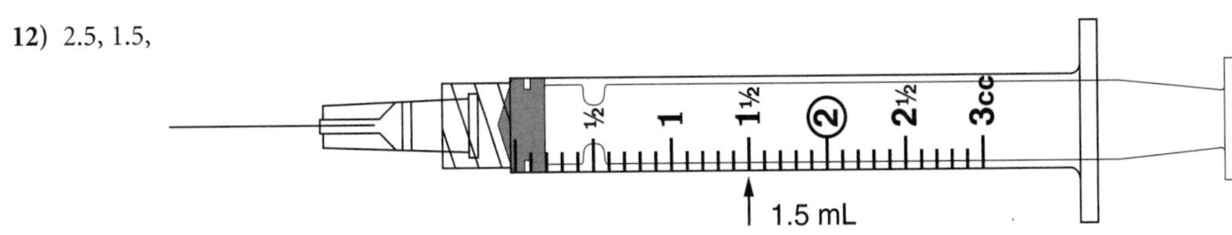

13) 6.6, 2,

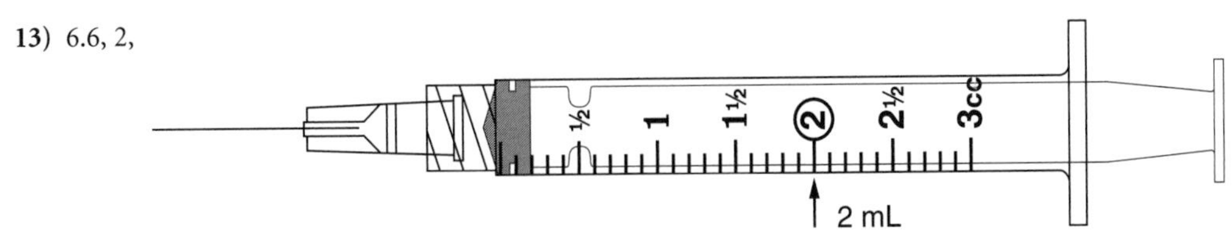

14) 10, 0.5,

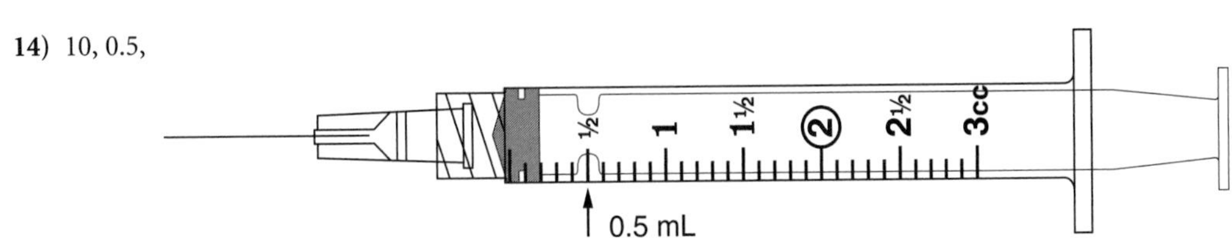

15) 2, 1.1,

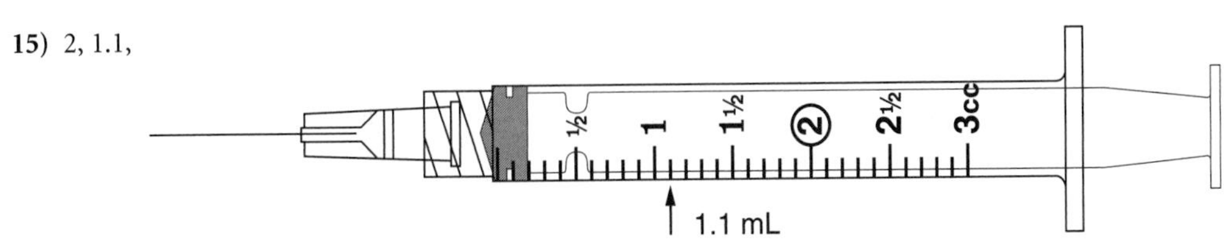

Solutions—Review Set 28

1) Order: 250 mg

Add 1.5 mL diluent

Supply: 280 mg/mL

$\frac{D}{H} \times Q = \frac{25\cancel{0} \text{ mg}}{28\cancel{0} \text{ mg}} \times 1 \text{ mL} = 0.89 \text{ mL}$

2) Select 5 mL diluent to be added to give patient smallest dosage you can measure exactly in a 3 cc syringe. If you select 4 mL, then you will have 1 g/2.5 mL. You would need to give 1.25 mL for 500 mg dose. A 3 cc syringe does not have 1.25 mL calibration. Therefore, select 5 mL diluent and you will have 1 g/3 mL. Give 1.5 mL.

$\frac{\overset{1}{\cancel{500 \text{ mg}}}}{\underset{2}{\cancel{1000 \text{ mg}}}} \times 3 \text{mL} = 1.5 \text{ mL}$

8) Order: 200 mg

Supply: 1 g/2.5 mL = 1000 mg/2.5 mL

$\frac{D}{H} \times Q = \frac{\overset{1}{\cancel{200 \text{ mg}}}}{\underset{5}{\cancel{1000 \text{ mg}}}} \times 2.5 \text{ mL} = 0.5 \text{ mL}$

15) Order: 250 mg

Supply: 225 mg/1 mL

$\frac{D}{H} \times Q = \frac{\overset{10}{\cancel{250 \text{ mg}}}}{\underset{9}{\cancel{225 \text{ mg}}}} \times 1 \text{ mL} = 1.1 \text{ mL}$

Review Set 29 from pages 214–217.

1) Humulin R Regular, Rapid-acting, Human 2) NPH Iletin II, Intermediate-acting, Pork 3) Humulin U Ultralente, Long-acting, Human 4) Protamine Zinc P & Iletin II, Long-acting, Pork 5) Humulin L, Lente, Intermediate-Acting, Human 6) Standard, dual scale 100 unit/mL U-100 syringe; Lo-dose, 50 unit/0.5 mL U-100 syringe; Lo-dose, 30 unit/0.3 mL U-100 syringe 7) Lo-dose, 30 unit U-100 syringe 8) Lo-dose, 50 unit U-100 syringe 9) 0.6 10) 0.25 11) Standard dual-scale 100 unit U-100 syringe 12) False 13) 68 14) 15 15) 23 16) 57

17)

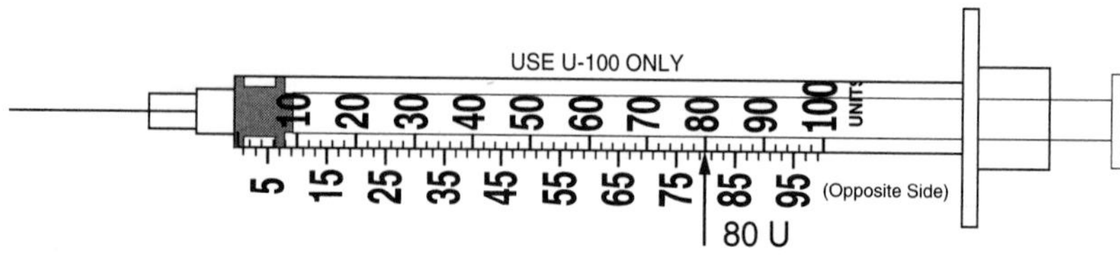

18)

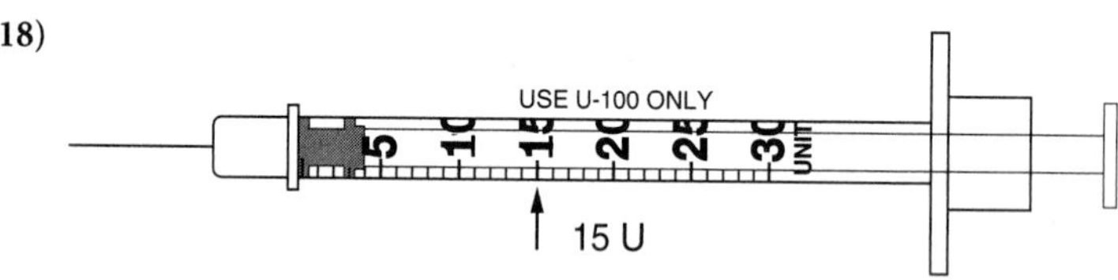

19)

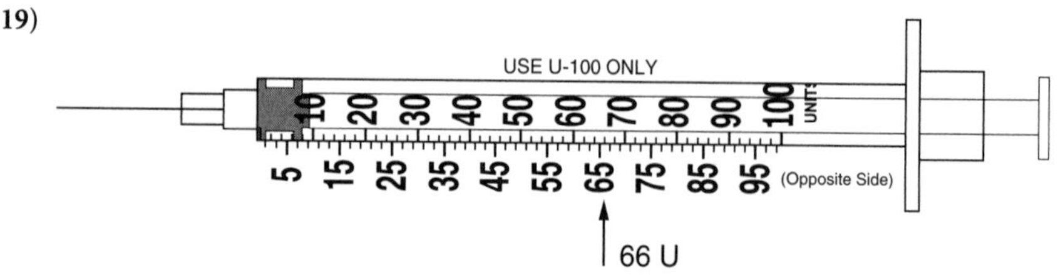

20)

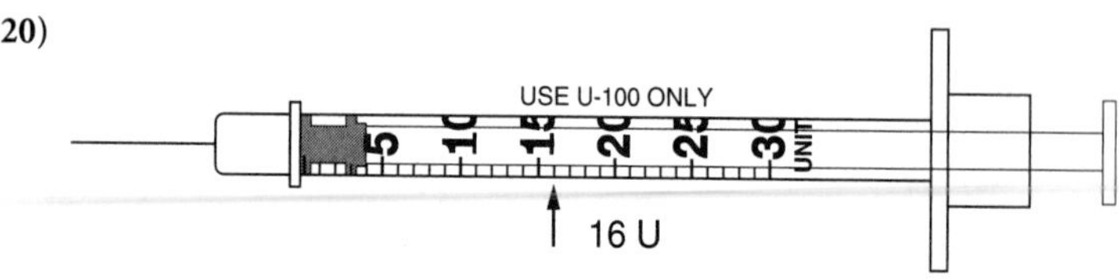

21)

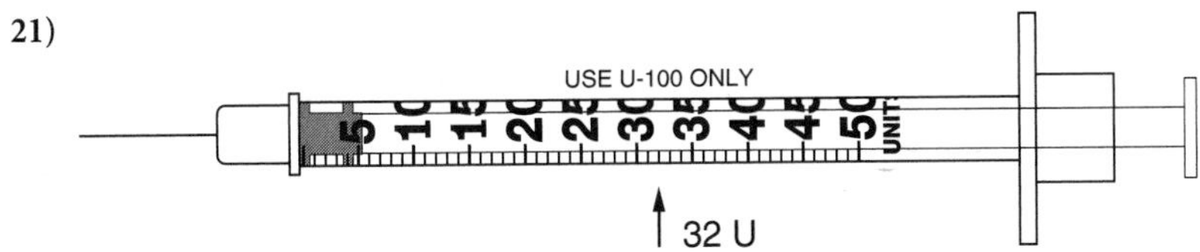

22)

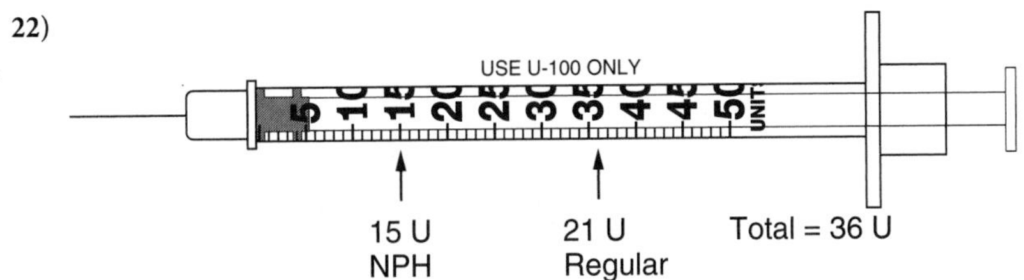

23)

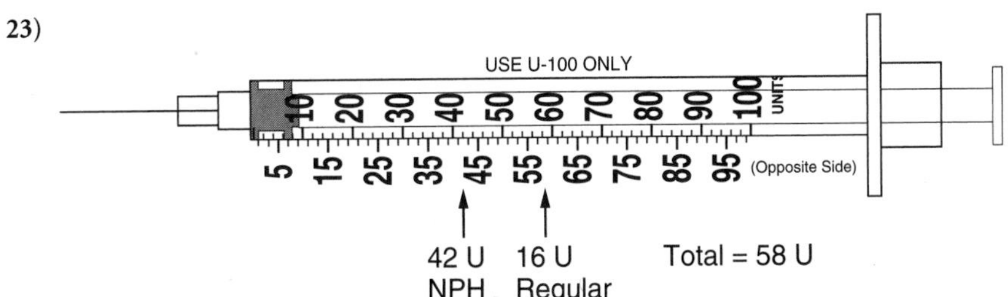

24)

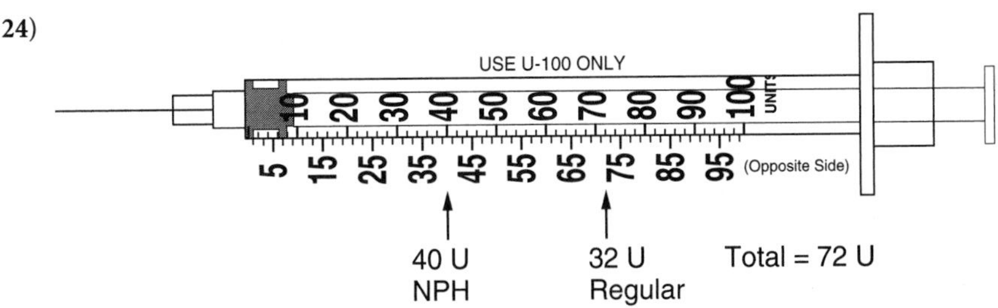

25)

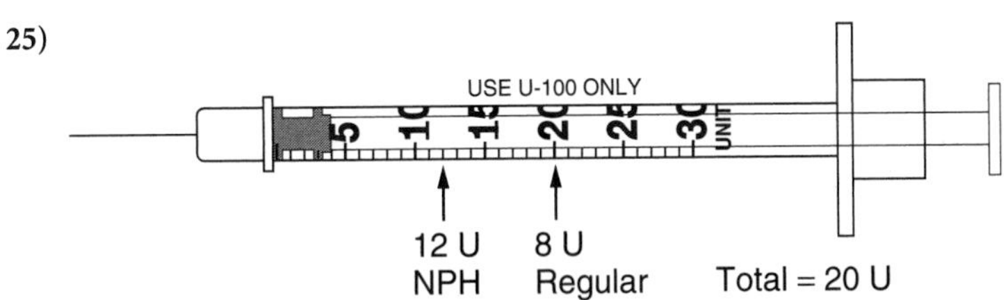

26) 0.34 **27)** 0.75 **28)** 0.22 **29)** 0.13 **30)** 0.59

Solutions—Review Set 29

26) Order: 34 U U-100 (Recall: U-100 = 100 units per mL)

$$\frac{D}{H} \times Q = \frac{34\,\cancel{U}}{100\,\cancel{U}} \times 1 \text{ mL} = 0.34 \text{ mL}$$

30) Order: 17 U + 42 U = 59 U

$$\frac{D}{H} \times Q = \frac{17\,\cancel{U}}{100\,\cancel{U}} \times 1 \text{ mL} = 0.17 \text{ mL}$$

$$\frac{D}{H} \times Q = \frac{42\,\cancel{U}}{100\,\cancel{U}} \times 1 \text{ mL} = 0.42 \text{ mL}$$

$$\begin{array}{r} 0.17 \text{ mL} \\ +\ 0.42 \text{ mL} \\ \hline 0.59 \text{ mL total} \end{array}$$

Review Set 30 from page 220.

1) 20 **2)** 1 **3)** 0.3 **4)** 0.5 **5)** 2

Solutions—Review Set 30

1) 20% = 20 g/100 mL

$\frac{D}{H} \times Q = \frac{4\,\cancel{g}}{\cancel{20}\,\cancel{g}_{1}} \times \overset{5}{\cancel{100}}\,\text{mL} = 20\text{ mL}$

3) 1:1000 = 1 g/1000 mL =

1000 mg/1000 mL =

1 mg/1 mL

$\frac{D}{H} \times Q = \frac{0.3\,\cancel{mg}}{1\,\cancel{mg}} \times 1\text{ mL} = 0.3\text{ mL}$

5) gr viiss = gr $7\frac{1}{2}$ = 7.5 ÷ 15 = 0.5 g

25% = 25 g/100 mL = $\frac{25\text{ g}}{100\text{ mL}} = \frac{.25.}{1.00.}$ =

0.25 g/1 mL

$\frac{D}{H} \times Q = \frac{\overset{2}{\cancel{0.50\,g}}}{\cancel{0.25\,g}_{1}} \times 1\text{ mL} = 2\text{ mL}$

Practice Problems—Chapter 10 from pages 222–233.

1) 0.4; 0.5 mL tuberculin
2) 1; 3 cc
3) 2.4; 3 cc
4) 0.6; 1 mL tuberculin or 3 cc
5) 2; 3 cc
6) 2; 3 cc
7) 15; 20 cc
8) 2; 3 cc
9) 15; 20 cc
10) 0.8; 1 mL tuberculin or 3 cc
11) 1; 3 cc
12) 1; 3 cc
13) 0.5; 1 mL tuberculin or 3 cc
14) 1.5; 3 cc
15) 0.6; 1 mL tuberculin or 3 cc
16) 0.6; 1 mL tuberculin or 3 cc
17) 1.9; 3 cc
18) 0.6; 1 mL tuberculin or 3 cc
19) 1; 3 cc
20) 1.2; 3 cc
21) 1.5; 3 cc
22) 1; 3 cc
23) 1.2; 3 cc
24) 0.7; 1 mL tuberculin or 3 cc
25) 0.75; 1 mL tuberculin or 3 cc
26) 1.5; 3 cc
27) 0.7; 1 mL tuberculin or 3 cc
28) 0.8; 1 mL tuberculin or 3 cc
29) 1; 3 cc
30) 3.8; 5 cc
31) 0.8; 1 mL tuberculin or 3 cc
32) 1.6; 3 cc
33) 6; 10 cc
34) 0.8; 1 mL tuberculin or 3 cc
35) 1.5; 3 cc
36) 5; 5 cc
37) 1.3; 3 cc
38) 1; 3 cc
39) 0.7; 1 mL tuberculin or 3 cc
40) 1; 3 cc
41) 30; 20 cc (2 syringes)
42) 16; Lo-Dose 30 U U-100 insulin
43) 70; standard U-100 insulin
44) 25; Lo-Dose 50 U U-100 insulin

45) 0.7,

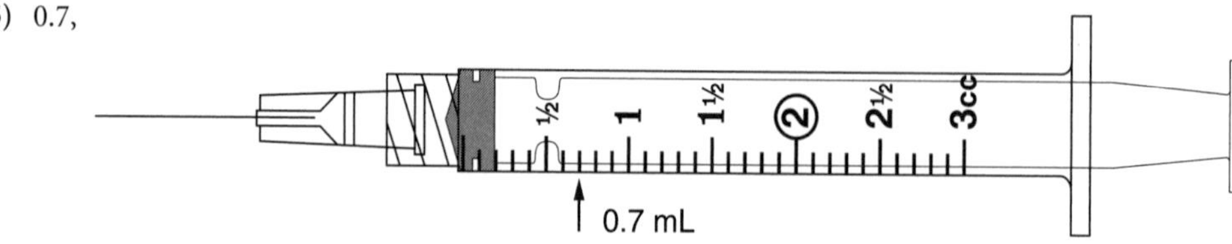

46) 2.2,

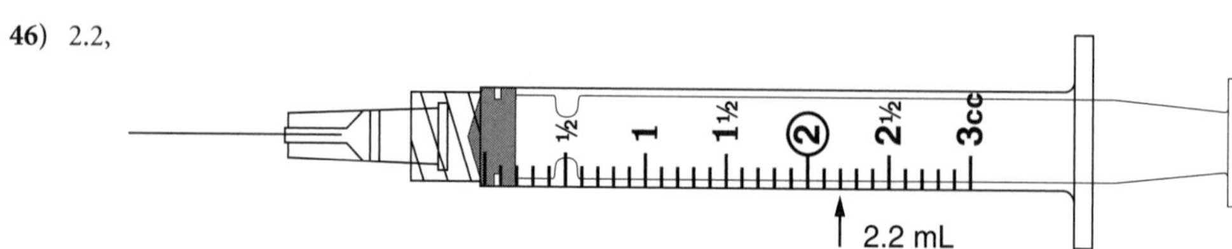

47) 1.6,

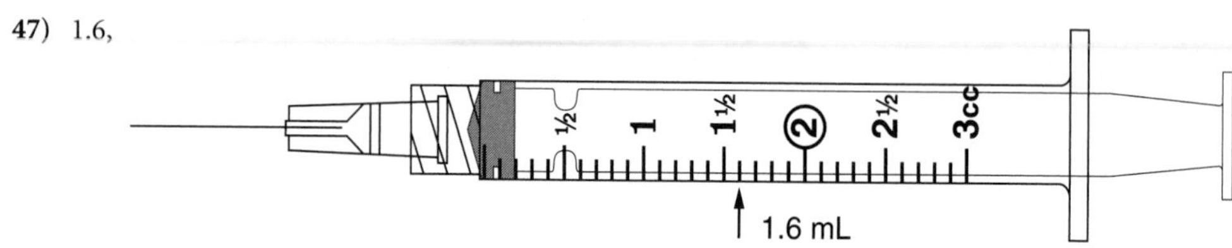

48) 5 (add 4 mL diluent),

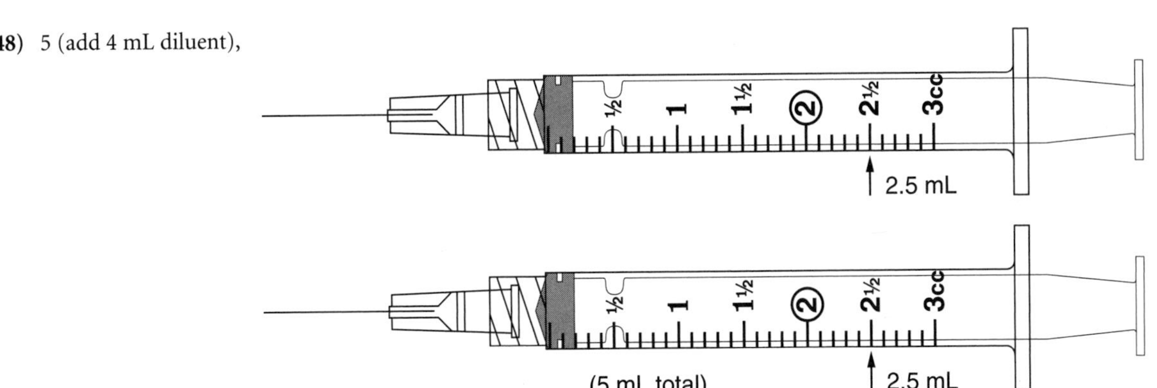

49) 0.5,

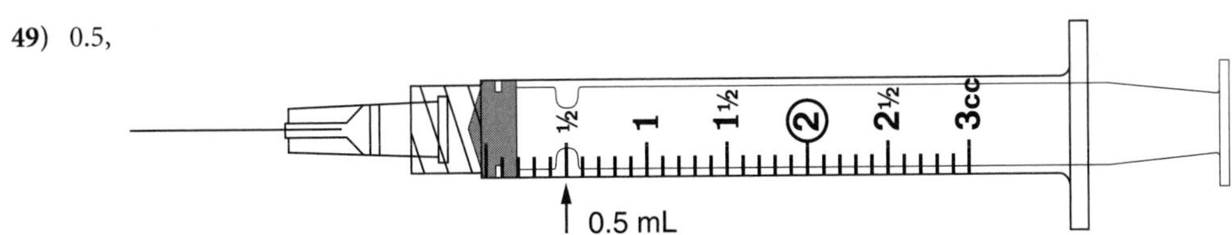

50) 1.3,

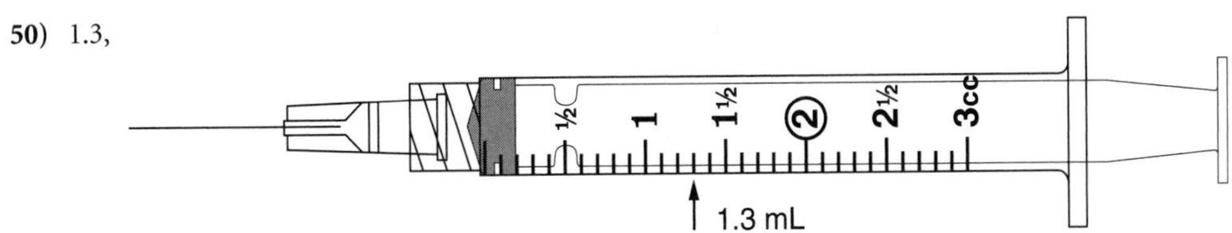

51) 22,

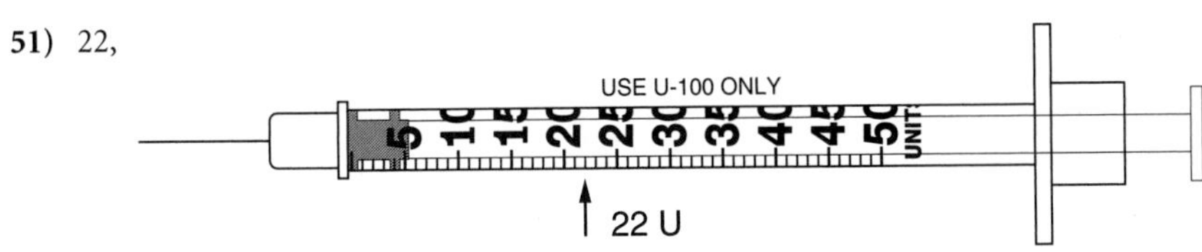

52) 1.5,

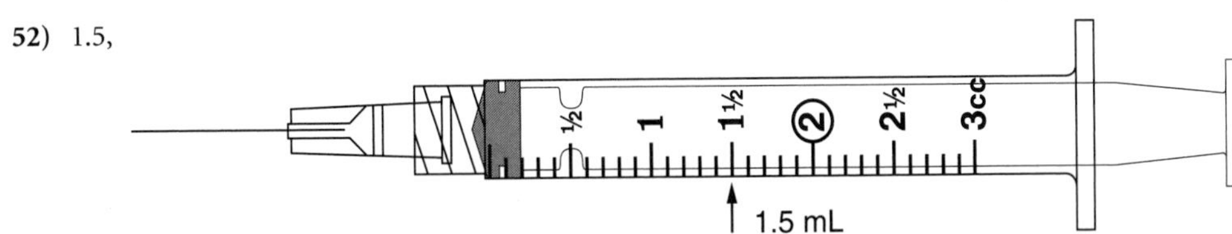

53) 0.8,

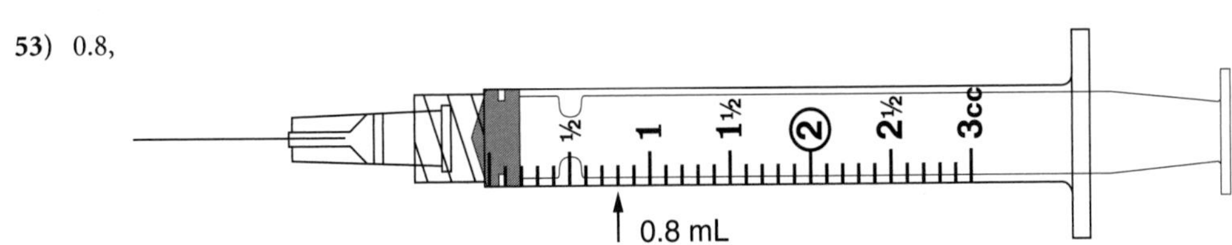

54) 1.1,

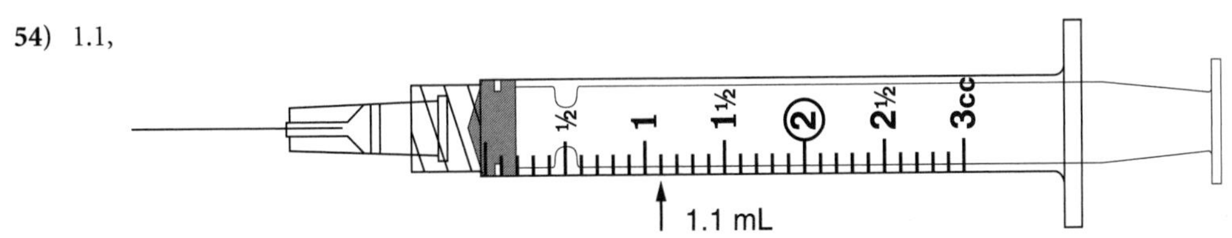

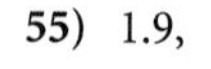

55) 1.9,

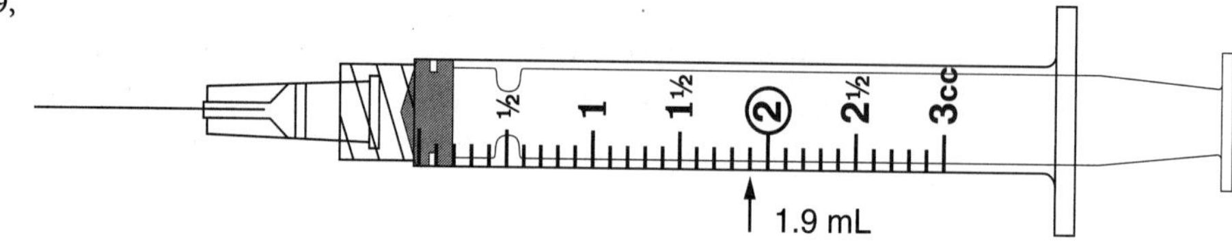

56) 1.6,

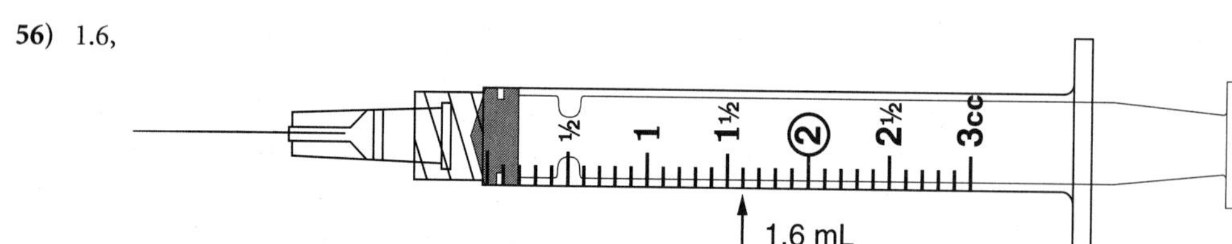

57) 2,

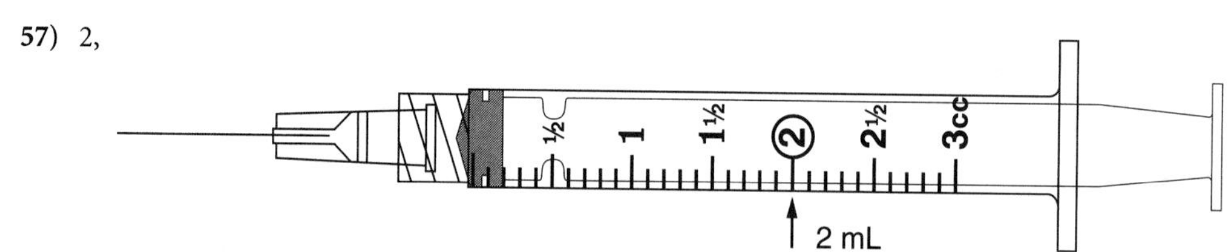

58) 0.5,

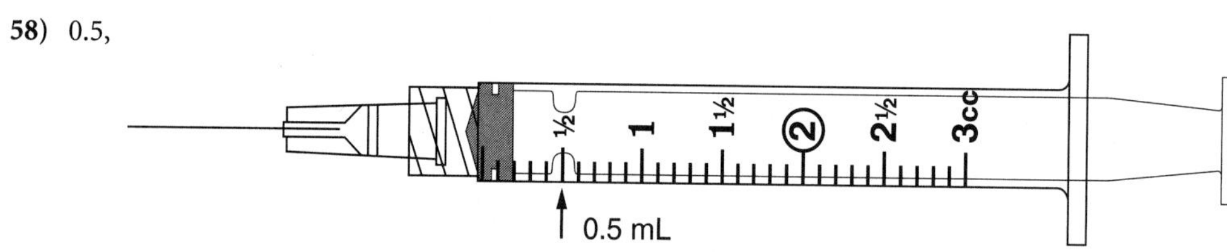

59) 1.2,

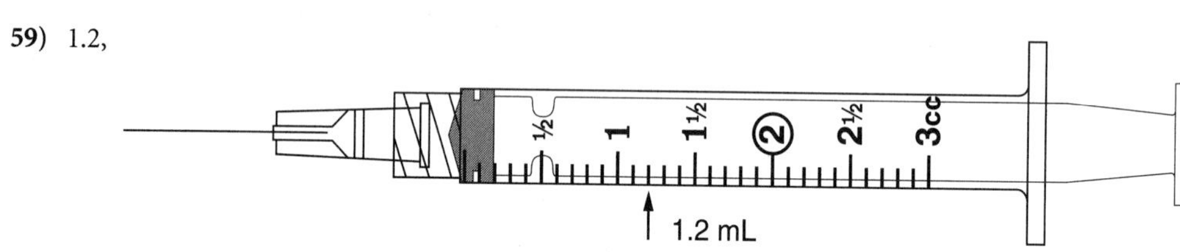

60) 0.25,

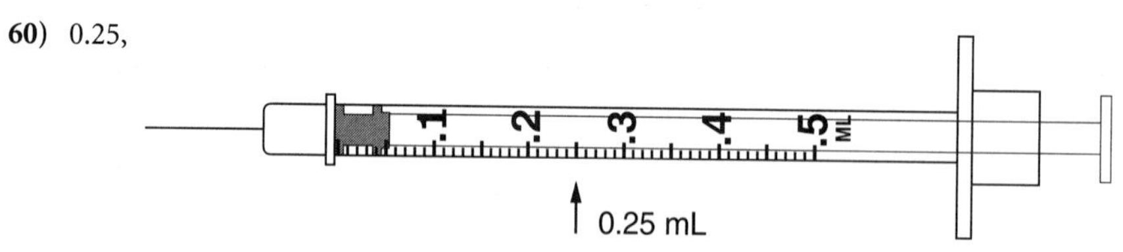

61) 86,

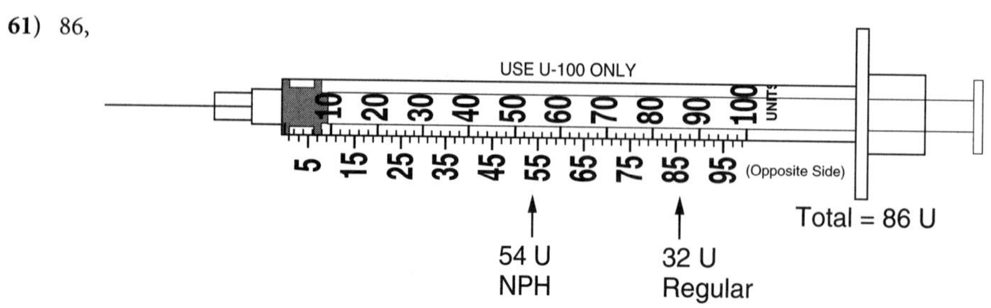

62) 46,

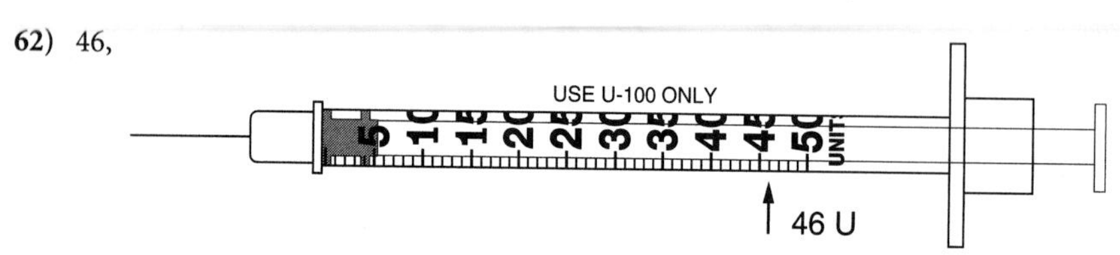

63) Critical Thinking: Prevention.
This error could have been avoided had the nurse been more careful checking the label of the insulin vial and comparing the label to the order. The nurse should have checked the label three times as taught in nursing school. In addition, the nurse should have asked another nurse to double-check her as she was drawing up the insulin, as required. Such hospital policies and procedures are written to protect the patient and the nurse.

64) Critical Thinking: Prevention.
This insulin error should never occur. It is obvious that the nurse did not use Step 2 of the three-step method. The nurse did not stop to think of the reasonable dosage. If so, the nurse would have realized that the supply dosage of U-100 insulin is 100 U/mL, not 10 U/mL.

If you are unsure of what you are doing, you need to ask before you act. Insulin should only be given in an insulin syringe. The likelihood of the nurse needing to give insulin in a tuberculin syringe because an insulin syringe was unavailable is almost nonexistent today. The nurse chose the incorrect syringe. Whenever you are in doubt, you should ask for help. Further, if the nurse had asked another nurse to double-check the dosage, as required, the error could have been found before the patient received the wrong dosage of insulin. After giving the insulin, it may be too late to rectify the error.

Solutions—Practice Problems—Chapter 10

3) Order: 0.6 mg = 0.6 × 1000 = 600 mcg

Supply: 500 mcg/2 mL

$$\frac{D}{H} \times Q = \frac{\cancel{600}\ \cancel{mcg}}{\cancel{500}\ \cancel{mcg}} \times 2\text{ mL} = \frac{12}{5} = 2.4\text{ mL}$$

7) Order: 3 mg

Supply: 1 mg/5 mL

$$\frac{D}{H} \times Q = \frac{3\ \cancel{mg}}{1\ \cancel{mg}} \times 5\text{ mL} = 15\text{ mL}$$

Note: Route is IV, so this large dose is acceptable.

14) Order: $\text{gr}\ \frac{1}{100} = \frac{1}{\cancelto{10}{100}} \times \frac{\cancelto{6}{60}}{1} = 0.6\text{ mg}$

Supply: 0.4 mg/mL

$$\frac{D}{H} \times Q = \frac{\cancelto{3}{0.6\text{ mg}}}{\cancelto{2}{0.4\text{ mg}}} \times 1\text{ mL} = 1.5\text{ mL}$$

17) Order: 75 mg

Supply: 80 mg/2 mL

$$\frac{D}{H} \times Q = \frac{75\ \cancel{mg}}{\cancelto{40}{80}\ \cancel{mg}} \times \cancelto{1}{2}\text{ mL} = \frac{75}{40} = 1.87 = 1.9\text{ mL}$$

18) $\text{gr}\ \frac{1}{10} = \frac{1}{\cancelto{1}{10}} \times \frac{\cancelto{6}{60}}{1} = 6\text{ mg}$

Supply : 10 mg/cc

$$\frac{D}{H} \times Q = \frac{6\ \cancel{mg}}{10\ \cancel{mg}} \times 1\text{ cc} = 0.6\text{ cc or } 0.6\text{ mL}$$

23) Order: 60 mg

Supply: 75 mg/1.5 mL

$$\frac{D}{H} \times Q = \frac{\cancelto{4}{60\text{ mg}}}{\cancelto{5}{75\text{ mg}}} \times 1.5\text{ mL} = \frac{6}{5} = 1.2\text{ mL}$$

30) Order: 750 mg

Supply: 1 g/5 mL = 1000 mg/5 mL

$$\frac{D}{H} \times Q = \frac{\cancelto{3}{750\text{ mg}}}{\cancelto{4}{1000\text{ mg}}} \times 5\text{ mL} = \frac{15}{4} = 3.75 = 3.8\text{ mL}$$

32) Order: 0.4 mg = 0.4 × 1000 = 400 mcg

Supply: 500 mcg/2 cc

$$\frac{D}{H} \times Q = \frac{400\ \cancel{mcg}}{500\ \cancel{mcg}} \times 2\text{ cc} = \frac{8}{5} = 1.6\text{ cc or } 1.6\text{ mL}$$

36) Order: 0.5 g

Supply: 10% = 10 g/100 mL

$$\frac{D}{H} \times Q = \frac{0.5\ \cancel{g}}{\cancelto{1}{10}\ \cancel{g}} \times \cancelto{10}{100}\text{ mL} = 5\text{ mL}$$

Note: Route is IV.

37) Order: 400,000 U

Supply: 300,000 U/mL

$$\frac{D}{H} \times Q = \frac{\cancel{400{,}000\text{ U}}}{\cancel{300{,}000\text{ U}}} \times 1\text{ mL} = \frac{4}{3} = 1.33 = 1.3\text{ mL}$$

40) Order: 0.5 mg

Supply: 1:2000 = 1 g/2000 mL =

1000 mg/2000 mL =

0.5 mg/mL

$$\frac{D}{H} \times Q = \frac{\cancel{0.5\text{ mg}}}{\cancel{0.5\text{ mg}}} \times 1\text{ mL} = 1\text{ mL}$$

47) Order: 65 mg

Supply: 80 mg/2 mL

$$\frac{D}{H} \times Q = \frac{65\ \cancel{mg}}{\cancelto{40}{80}\ \cancel{mg}} \times \cancelto{1}{2}\text{ mL} = \frac{\cancelto{13}{65}}{\cancelto{8}{40}} = 1.63 = 1.6\text{ mL}$$

Review Set 31 from pages 239 and 240.

1) 2 **2)** 2.5 **3)** 0.8 **4)** 0.7 **5)** 7.5 **6)** 0.6 **7)** $1\frac{1}{2}$ **8)** 3 **9)** 30 **10)** 1.6 **11)** 3 **12)** 0.5 **13)** 2 **14)** $\frac{1}{2}$ of 250 mg **15)** 2.4 **16)** 2 **17)** 8 **18)** 1.3 **19)** 16 **20)** 7

Solutions—Review Set 31

2) $\frac{300 \text{ mg}}{5\text{mL}} = \frac{150 \text{ mg}}{\text{X mL}}$

$300\text{X} = 750$

$\frac{300\text{X}}{300} = \frac{750}{300}$

$\text{X} = 2.5 \text{ mL}$

5) $\frac{8 \text{ mEq}}{5 \text{ mL}} = \frac{12 \text{ mEq}}{\text{X mL}}$

$8\text{X} = 60$

$\frac{8\text{ X}}{8} = \frac{60}{8}$

$\text{X} = 7.5 \text{ mL}$

6) $\frac{4 \text{ mg}}{1 \text{ mL}} = \frac{2.4 \text{ mg}}{\text{X mL}}$

$4\text{ X} = 2.4$

$\frac{4\text{ X}}{4} = \frac{2.4}{4}$

$\text{X} = 0.6 \text{ mL}$

9) $\frac{80 \text{ mg}}{15 \text{ mL}} = \frac{160 \text{ mg}}{\text{X mL}}$

$80\text{X} = 2400$

$\frac{80\text{X}}{80} = \frac{2400}{80}$

$\text{X} = 30 \text{ mL}$

13) A. Convert gr to mg: gr ss = gr $\frac{1}{2}$

$\frac{\text{gr } 1}{60 \text{ mg}} = \frac{\text{gr } \frac{1}{2}}{\text{X mg}}$

$\text{X} = 60 \times \frac{1}{2}$

$\text{X} = 30 \text{ mg}$

B. $\frac{15 \text{ mg}}{1 \text{ tab}} = \frac{30 \text{ mg}}{\text{X tab}}$

$15\text{X} = 30$

$\frac{15\text{X}}{15} = \frac{30}{15}$

$\text{X} = 2 \text{ tabs}$

16) A. Convert mcg to mg:

$\frac{1 \text{ mg}}{1000 \text{ mcg}} = \frac{0.15 \text{ mg}}{\text{X mcg}}$

$\text{X} = 150 \text{ mcg}$

B. $\frac{75 \text{ mcg}}{1 \text{ tab}} = \frac{150 \text{ mcg}}{\text{X}}$

$75\text{X} = 150$

$\frac{75\text{X}}{75} = \frac{150}{75}$

$\text{X} = 2 \text{ tabs}$

18) $\frac{80 \text{ mg}}{1 \text{ mL}} = \frac{100 \text{ mg}}{\text{X mL}}$

$80\text{ X} = 100$

$\frac{80\text{ X}}{80} = \frac{100}{80}$

$\text{X} = 1.25 = 1.3$ mL (measured in a 3 cc syringe)

19) $\frac{2.5 \text{ mg}}{5 \text{ mL}} = \frac{8 \text{ mg}}{\text{X mL}}$

$2.5\text{ X} = 40$

$\frac{2.5\text{ X}}{2.5} = \frac{40}{2.5}$

$\text{X} = 16 \text{ mL}$

Practice Problems—Chapter 11 from pages 242—244.

1) 45 **2)** 2 **3)** 2 **4)** $\frac{1}{2}$ **5)** 2.5 **6)** 16 **7)** 1.4 **8)** 0.7 **9)** 2.3 **10)** 0.13 (measured in a tuberculin syringe) **11)** 1.6 **12)** 1.5 **13)** 1.3 **14)** 2.5 **15)** 1.6 **16)** 7.5 **17)** 1.6 **18)** 2 **19)** 8 **20)** 4.5 **21)** 30 **22)** 1.4 **23)** 15 **24)** 20 **25)** 12

26) Critical Thinking: Prevention.

This type of calculation error occurred because the nurse set up the proportion incorrectly. In this instance the nurse mixed up the units with mg *and* mL in the numerators, and mg and mL in the denominators. The **mg** unit should be in both numerators of the proportion, and the **mL** unit in both denominators.

$\frac{125 \text{ mg}}{5 \text{ mL}} = \frac{50 \text{ mg}}{\text{X mL}}$

$125\text{X} = 250$

$\frac{125\text{ X}}{125} = \frac{250}{125}$

$\text{X} = 2 \text{ mL}$

In addition, **think first.** Then use ratio and proportion to calculate the dosage.

Solutions—Practice Problems—Chapter 11

1) $\frac{3.33 \text{ g}}{5 \text{ mL}} = \frac{30 \text{ g}}{X \text{ mL}}$

$3.33X = 150$

$\frac{3.33X}{3.33} = \frac{150}{3.33}$

$X = 45 \text{ mL}$

2) $\frac{5{,}000{,}000 \text{ U}}{20 \text{ mL}} = \frac{500{,}000 \text{ U}}{X \text{ mL}}$

$5{,}000{,}000X = 10{,}000{,}000$

$\frac{5{,}000{,}000X}{5{,}000{,}000} = \frac{10{,}000{,}000}{5{,}000{,}000}$

$X = 2 \text{ mL}$

6) $\frac{12.5 \text{ mg}}{5 \text{ mL}} = \frac{40 \text{ mg}}{X \text{ mL}}$

$12.5X = 200$

$\frac{12.5X}{12.5} = \frac{200}{12.5}$

$X = 16 \text{ mL}$

7) $\frac{500{,}000 \text{ U}}{2 \text{ mL}} = \frac{350{,}000 \text{ U}}{X \text{ mL}}$

$500{,}000X = 700{,}000$

$\frac{500{,}000X}{500{,}000} = \frac{700{,}000}{500{,}000}$

$X = 1.4 \text{ mL}$

8) $\frac{10 \text{ mg}}{2 \text{ mL}} = \frac{3.5 \text{ mg}}{X \text{ mL}}$

$10X = 7$

$\frac{10X}{10} = \frac{7}{10}$

$X = 0.7 \text{ mL}$

9) $\frac{80 \text{ mg}}{2 \text{ mL}} = \frac{90 \text{ mg}}{X}$

$80X = 180$

$\frac{80X}{80} = \frac{180}{80}$

$X = 2.25 \text{ mL} = 2.3 \text{ mL}$

13) A. Convert g to mg: 1g = 1000 mg

B. $\frac{1000 \text{ mg}}{2.5 \text{ mL}} = \frac{500 \text{ mg}}{X \text{ mL}}$

$1000X = 1250$

$\frac{1000X}{1000} = \frac{1250}{1000}$

$X = 1.25 \text{ mL or } 1.3 \text{ mL}$

16) $\frac{20 \text{ mEq}}{15 \text{ mL}} = \frac{10 \text{ mEq}}{X \text{ mL}}$

$20X = 150$

$\frac{20X}{20} = \frac{150}{20}$

$X = 7.5 \text{ mL}$

18) A. Convert mg to mcg:

$\frac{1000 \text{ mcg}}{1 \text{ mg}} = \frac{X \text{ mcg}}{.075 \text{ mg}}$

$X = 75 \text{ mcg}$

B. $\frac{75 \text{ mcg}}{1 \text{ tab}} = \frac{150 \text{ mcg}}{X \text{ tabs}}$

$75X = 150$

$\frac{75X}{75} = \frac{150}{75}$

$X = 2 \text{ tab}$

Review Set 32 from pages 256–258.

1) 78–313, yes **2)** 10 **3)** Yes **4)** 1.1 **5)** Yes **6)** 6; 8 **7)** 320–480; maximum; 15 **8)** Yes

9) 0.25

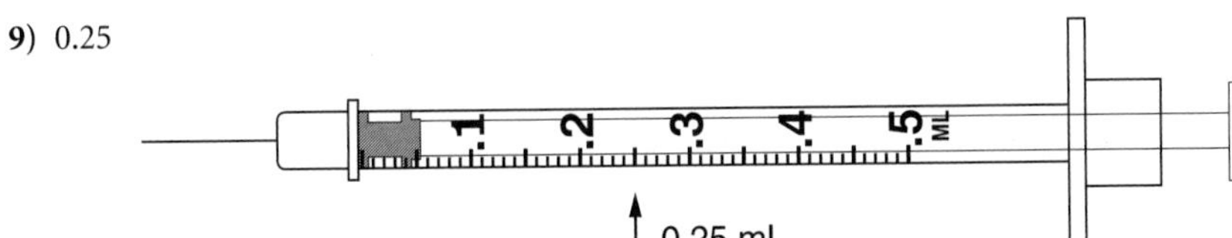

10) Yes; 2.5 **11)** 20–40 **12)** 3 **13)** Yes, for a 6.8 kg child, the dosage ordered is within the recommended dosage range of 45.3 to 90.7 mg/dose. **14)** 1.5 **15)** No. You need 30 doses and there are only 10 doses of 1.5 mL each available in the 15 mL bottle. Three bottles would be needed. **16)** 25.5 **17)** No; the dosage order is too high and too frequent. **18)** Do not administer any amount until you consult with the physician. **19)** 400 **20)** 640 **21)** 100–160 **22)** No **23)** 90–180 **24)** Yes **25)** 45 **26)** 9; 18 **27)** 17

Solutions—Review Set 32

1) 55 lb = 55 ÷ 2.2 = 25 kg

Minimum daily dosage:

$\frac{12.5 \text{ mg}}{\text{kg}} \times 25 \text{ kg} = 312.5$ mg or 313 mg/day;

$\frac{313 \text{ mg}}{4 \text{ doses}} = 78.25$ or 78 mg/dose

Maximum daily dosage:

$\frac{50 \text{ mg}}{\text{kg}} \times 25 \text{ kg} = 1250$ mg or 1250 mg/day;

$\frac{1250 \text{ mg}}{4 \text{ doses}} = 312.5$ or 313 mg/dose

Yes, dosage is safe.

2) $\frac{D}{H} \times Q = \frac{\overset{2}{\cancel{125 \text{ mg}}}}{\underset{1}{\cancel{62.5 \text{ mg}}}} \times 5 \text{ mL} = 10 \text{ mL}$

3) Convert g to kg: 2200 g = 2.2 kg

$\frac{50 \text{ mg}}{\text{kg}} \times 2.2 \text{ kg} = 110 \text{ mg}$

$\frac{110 \text{ mg}}{2 \text{ doses}} = 55$ mg/dose; yes, dosage is safe

4) $\frac{D}{H} \times Q = \frac{55 \text{ mg}}{\underset{50}{\cancel{1000 \text{ mg}}}} \times \overset{1}{\cancel{20}} \text{mL} = \frac{55}{50} = 1.1 \text{ mL}$

6) $\frac{D}{H} \times Q = \frac{\overset{6}{\cancel{120 \text{ mg}}}}{\underset{5}{\cancel{100 \text{ mg}}}} \times 5 \text{ mL} = \frac{\overset{6}{\cancel{30}}}{\underset{1}{\cancel{5}}} = 6 \text{ mL}$

$\frac{50 \text{ mL}}{6 \text{ mL/dose}} = 8.3$ doses or 8 whole doses

7) Minimum dosage: $\frac{10 \text{ mg}}{\text{kg}} \times 32 \text{ kg} = 320 \text{ mg}$

Maximum dosage: $\frac{15 \text{ mg}}{\text{kg}} \times 32 \text{ kg} = 480 \text{ mg}$

Dose is based upon *maximum* dosage, 480 mg

$\frac{D}{H} \times Q = \frac{\overset{3}{\cancel{480 \text{ mg}}}}{\underset{1}{\cancel{160 \text{ mg}}}} \times 5 \text{ mL} = 15 \text{ mL}$

16) 7 lb 8 oz = $7\frac{1}{2}$ lb = 7.5 ÷ 2.2 = 3.4 kg

$\frac{15 \text{ mg}}{\text{kg}} \times 3.4 \text{ kg} = 51 \text{ mg}$

$\frac{51 \text{ mg}}{2 \text{ doses}} = 25.5$ mg/dose

23) Minimum daily dosage:

$\frac{6 \text{ mg}}{\text{kg}} \times 15 \text{ kg} = 90 \text{ mg}$

Maximum daily dosage:

$\frac{12 \text{ mg}}{\text{kg}} \times 15 \text{ kg} = 180 \text{ mg}$

24) $\frac{D}{H} \times Q = X$

$\frac{D \text{ mg}}{16 \text{ mg}} \times 1 \text{ mL} = 6 \text{ mL}$

$\frac{D}{16} = \frac{6}{1}$

D = 96 mg per dose

Yes, the dosage is safe.

25) 66 lb = 66 ÷ 2.2 = 30 kg

Daily dosage:

450 mg AM dosage
+900 mg PM dosage
1350 mg/day

1350 mg/day ÷ 30 kg = 45 mg/kg/day

26) $\frac{D}{H} \times Q = \frac{\overset{9}{450 \text{ mg}}}{\underset{5}{250 \text{ mg}}} \times 5 \text{ mL} = 9$ mL (AM dose)

$\frac{D}{H} \times Q = \frac{\overset{18}{900 \text{ mg}}}{\underset{5}{250 \text{ mg}}} \times 5 \text{ mL} = \frac{90}{5} = 18$ mL (PM dose)

27) 9 mL + 18 mL = 27 mL given per day

$\frac{480 \text{ mL}}{27 \text{ mL/day}} = 17.7$ days or 17 full days

Practice Problems—Chapter 12 from pages 259–263.

1) 5.5 **2)** 3.8 **3)** 1.6 **4)** 2.3 **5)** 15.5 **6)** 3 **7)** 23.6 **8)** 29.1 **9)** 32.3 **10)** 0.9 **11)** 1.8 **12)** No; consult with physician or supervisor before administering any of this drug. **13)** 6.5; 13; 104 **14)** 5 **15)** 300 **16)** 150 **17)** No **18)** Consult physician or supervisor before giving this drug. **19)** Yes **20)** Yes **21)** 120 **22)** 3.8 **23)** Yes **24)** Yes **25)** 0.04; 0.08 **26)** 1.6 **27)** 187.5 **28)** 62.5 **29)** 22–44 **30)** Yes **31)** 1.3 **32)** 150–250 **33)** 75–125 **34)** Yes **35)** Yes **36)** 35 **37)** Yes **38)** 14 **39)** 420 **40)** $1\frac{1}{2}$; 7.5 **41)** 0.32 **42)** 4 **43)** 1.6 **44)** 3.5 **45)** 0.36 **46)** 1 20-mg and 1 5-mg tab; fewest to make up dose. **47)** 1.6; 1.3 **48)** 172.5; 345, Yes **49)** 3.5; 6.9

50) Critical Thinking: Prevention.

The child should have received 75 mg a day and no more than 25 mg per dose. The child received more than four times the safe dosage of tobramycin. Had the nurse calculated the safe dosage, the error would have been caught sooner, the resident consulted, and the dosage could have been adjusted before the child ever received the first dose. The pharmacist also should have caught the error but did not. In this scenario the resident, pharmacist, and nurse all committed medication errors. If the resident had not noticed the error, one can only wonder how many doses the child would have received. The nurse is the last safety net for the child when it comes to a dosage error, because the nurse administers the drug.

In addition, the nurse has to reconcile the fact that she actually gave the overdose. The nurse is responsible for whatever dosage is administered and must verify the safety of the order and the patient's 5 rights. We are all accountable for our actions. Taking shortcuts in administering medications to children can be disastrous. The time the nurse saved by not calculating the safe dosage was more than lost in the extra monitoring, not to mention the cost of follow-up to the medication error, *and most importantly*, the risk to the child.

Solutions—Practice Problems—Chapters 12

1) 1 kg = 2.2 lb; smaller → larger: (÷)

12 lb = 12 ÷ 2.2 = 5.45 = 5.5 kg

2) $8 \text{ lb } 4 \text{ oz} = 8\frac{4}{16} = 8\frac{1}{4} = 8.25 \text{ lb}$

$8.25 \text{ lb} = \frac{8.25}{2.2} = 3.75 = 3.8 \text{ kg}$

3) 1,570 g = 1570 ÷ 1000 = 1.57 = 1.6 kg

6) $6 \text{ lb } 10 \text{ oz} = 6\frac{\cancel{10}^{\,5}}{\cancel{16}_{\,8}} \text{ lb} = 6\frac{5}{8} \text{ lb} = 6.625 \text{ lb}$

$6.625 \text{ lb} = \frac{6.625}{2.2} = 3.01 = 3 \text{ kg}$

12) 66 lb = 66 ÷ 2.2 = 30 kg

$\frac{3 \text{ mg}}{\cancel{\text{kg}}} \times 30 \cancel{\text{kg}} = 90 \text{ mg};$ 105 mg is ordered per dose.

Dosage is higher than recommended amount.

Contact physician before giving medication.

13) Minimum daily dosage: $\frac{1 \text{ mg}}{\cancel{\text{kg}}} \times 13 \cancel{\text{kg}} = 13 \text{ mg}; \frac{13 \text{ mg}}{2 \text{ doses}}$

= 6.5 mg/dose

Maximum daily dosage: $\frac{2 \text{ mg}}{\cancel{\text{kg}}} \times 13 \cancel{\text{kg}} = 26 \text{ mg}; \frac{26 \text{ mg}}{2 \text{ doses}}$

= 13 mg/dose

Doctor ordered 13 mg q.12 h × 4 days.

$\frac{13 \text{ mg}}{\cancel{\text{dose}}} \times \frac{2 \cancel{\text{doses}}}{\cancel{\text{day}}} \times 4 \cancel{\text{days}} = 104 \text{ mg}$

23) Minimum daily dosage: $\frac{10 \text{ mcg}}{\cancel{\text{kg}}} \times 4 \cancel{\text{kg}} = 40 \text{ mcg}$

Maximum daily dosage: $\frac{12 \text{ mcg}}{\cancel{\text{kg}}} \times 4 \cancel{\text{kg}} = 48 \text{ mcg}$

Yes; dose is safe.

26) $\frac{D}{H} \times Q = \frac{0.08 \cancel{\text{mg}}}{0.05 \cancel{\text{mg}}} \times 1 \text{ mL} = 1.6 \text{ mL}$

30) $\frac{0.5 \text{ mg}}{\cancel{\text{kg}}} \times 40 \cancel{\text{kg}} = 20 \text{ mg}$

32) Minimum daily dosage: $\frac{6 \text{ mg}}{\cancel{\text{kg}}} \times 25 \cancel{\text{kg}} = 150 \text{ mg}$

Maximum daily dosage: $\frac{10 \text{ mg}}{\cancel{\text{kg}}} \times 25 \cancel{\text{kg}} = 250 \text{ mg}$

33) 75–150 mg q.12 h;

Minimum dosage: $\frac{150 \text{ mg}}{2 \text{ doses}} = 75 \text{ mg/dose}$

Maximum dosage: $\frac{250 \text{ mg}}{2 \text{ doses}} = 125 \text{ mg/dose}$

34) $\frac{D}{H} \times Q = X$

$\frac{D \text{ mg}}{16 \text{ mg}} \times 1 \text{ mL} = 7.5 \text{ mL}$

$\frac{D}{16} = \frac{7.5}{1}$

D = 120 mg

Yes, the dosage is safe.

36) $\frac{350 \text{ mg}}{\cancel{\text{dose}}} \times \frac{3 \cancel{\text{doses}}}{\text{day}} = 1,050 \text{ mg/day};$

$\frac{1050 \text{ mg}}{\text{day}} \div 30 \text{ kg} = 35 \text{ mg/kg/day}$

40) Order: 150 mg

Supply: 100 mg

$\frac{D}{H} \times Q = \frac{\cancel{150 \text{ mg}}^{\,3}}{\cancel{100 \text{ mg}}_{\,2}} \times 1 \text{ tab} = 1\frac{1}{2} \text{ tab}$

Supply: 150 mg/5 mL

$\frac{D}{H} \times Q = \frac{\cancel{150} \cancel{\text{mg}}^{\,3}}{\cancel{100} \cancel{\text{mg}}_{\,2}} \times 5 \text{ mL} = \frac{15}{2} = 7.5 \text{ mL}$

Section 3—Self-Evaluation from pages 264–268.

1) $\frac{1}{2}$ **2)** 360 **3)** 1 **4)** 22.5 **5)** 3 **6)** 228, 22.8 **7)** 27 **8)** $\frac{1}{2}$ **9)** $\frac{1}{2}$ **10)** 2 **11)** 2 **12)** 7.5 **13)** 2 **14)** 1 **15)** 1 **16)** 3.5 **17)** 3 **18)** 7.5; "Give $1\frac{1}{2}$ t by mouth every six hours." **19)** 2 **20)** $13\frac{1}{2}$ **21)** 0.8 **22)** 1 **23)** 1.3 **24)** 0.7 **25)** 0.5 **26)** 0.6 **27)** 2 **28)** 0.5 **29)** 1.3

30) 19,

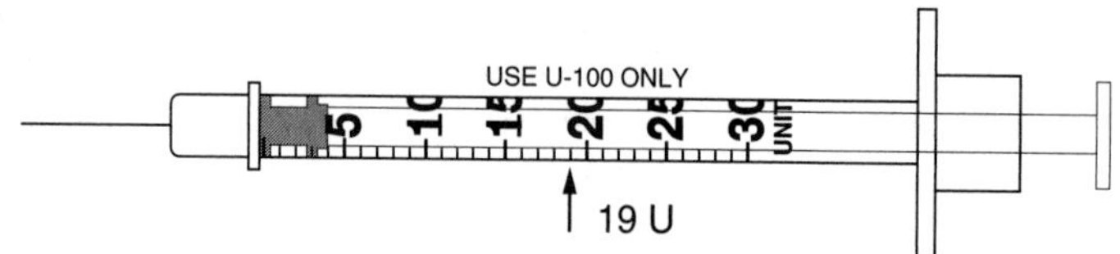

31) 53,

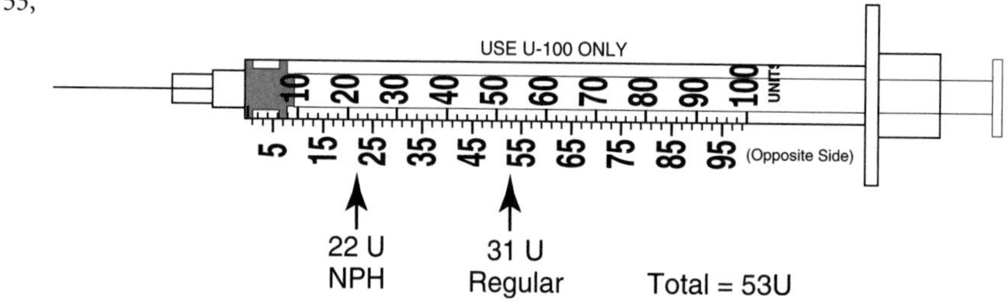

32) 18; 18; 36,

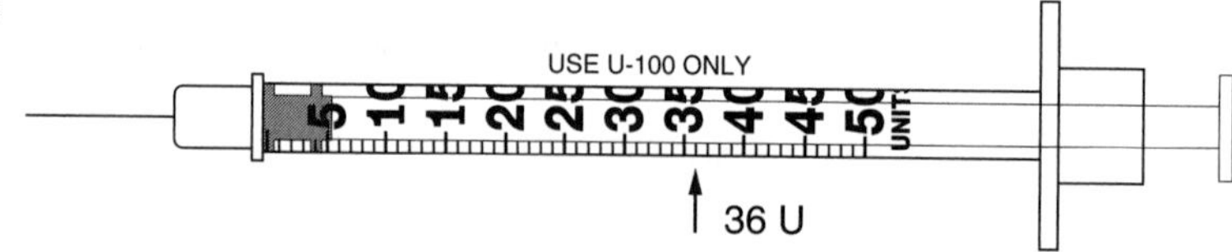

33) 2 mL,

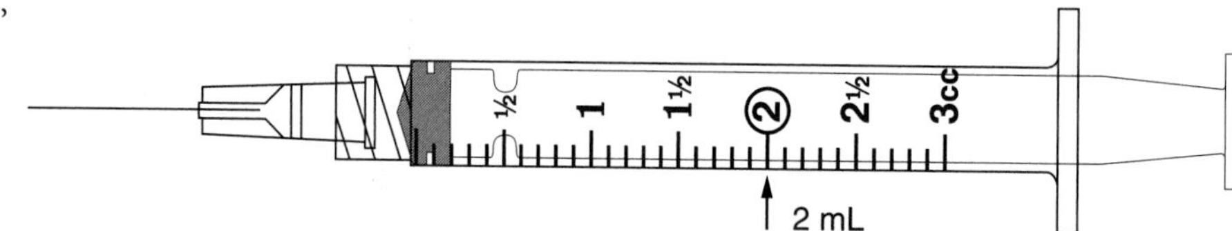

34) 3 mL,

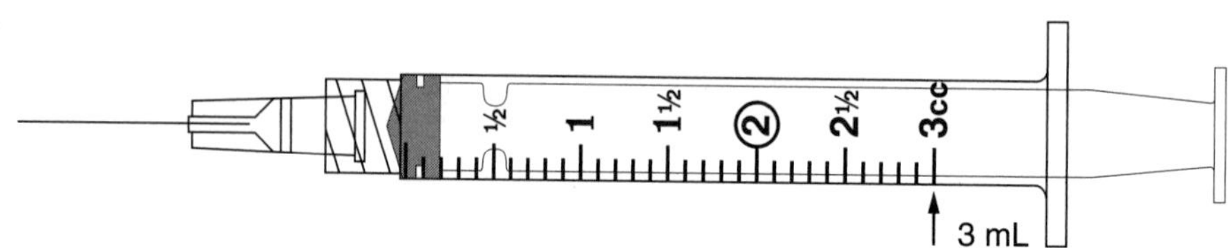

35) 0.08–0.4 **36)** 0.24 **37)** 8 **38)** 43 **39)** 4.3; 8.6 **40)** 13.5 **41)** 0.32 **42)** 1.08 **43)** 3.9 **44)** 11.4; 22.8; 0.27 **45)** 4,000,000; 40 **46)** It is excessive (too much). Do not give drug. Consult physician. **47)** It is a large underdosage; call physician to clarify before giving drug. **48)** It is safe. Recommended amount for this child is 2400 mg or 2.4 g/dose, which is the same as the ordered dosage. Daily dosage of 9.6 g is also less than the maximum allowance of 24 g/day. **49)** 0.6; 1.2 **50)** 0.45

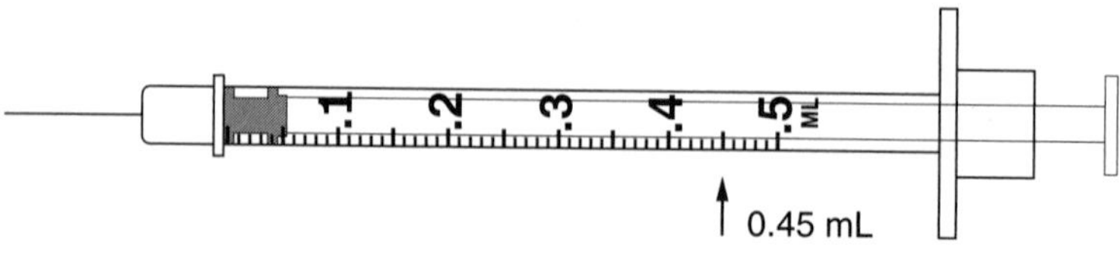

Solutions—Section 3—Self Evaluation

1) gr viss = gr $6\frac{1}{2} = 6\frac{1}{2} \times 60 = 390$ mg

$$\frac{D}{H} \times Q = \frac{\overset{1}{\cancel{195\text{ mg}}}}{\underset{2}{\cancel{390\text{ mg}}}} \times 1 \text{ tab} = \frac{1}{2} \text{ tab}$$

or

$$\frac{390\text{ mg}}{1\text{ tab}} \times \frac{195\text{ mg}}{X\text{ tab}}$$

$$390X = 195$$

$$\frac{390}{390}X = \frac{195}{390}$$

$$X = \frac{1}{2} \text{ tab}$$

3) $\text{gr } \frac{1}{300} = \frac{1}{\underset{5}{\cancel{300}}} \times \frac{\overset{1}{\cancel{60}}}{1} = \frac{1}{5} = 0.2 \text{ mg}$

Think: Now the answer is obvious. Give 1 tab.

6) Acetaminophen:

$$\frac{D}{H} \times Q = X$$

$$\frac{D\text{ mg}}{120\text{ mg}} \times 5\text{ mL} = 9.5\text{ mL}$$

$$\frac{5\text{ D}}{120} = \frac{9.5}{1}$$

$$5\text{ D} = 1140$$

$$\frac{5D}{5} = \frac{1140}{5}$$

$$D = 228\text{ mg}$$

or

$$\frac{120\text{ mg}}{5\text{ mL}} = \frac{X\text{ mg}}{9.5\text{ mL}}$$

$$5X = 1140$$

$$\frac{5X}{5} = \frac{1140}{5}$$

$$X = 228\text{ mg}$$

Codeine:

$$\frac{D}{H} \times Q = X$$

$$\frac{D\text{ mg}}{12\text{ mg}} \times 5\text{ mL} = 9.5\text{ mL}$$

$$\frac{5\text{ D}}{12} = \frac{9.5}{1}$$

$$5\text{ D} = 114$$

$$\frac{5D}{5} = \frac{114}{5}$$

$$D = 22.8\text{ mg}$$

or

$$\frac{12\text{ mg}}{5\text{ mL}} = \frac{X\text{ mg}}{9.5\text{ mL}}$$

$$5X = 114$$

$$\frac{5X}{5} = \frac{114}{5}$$

$$X = 22.8\text{ mg}$$

7) $\frac{D}{H} \times Q = \frac{4\cancel{0}\text{ }\cancel{mg}}{9\cancel{0}\text{ }\cancel{mg}} \times 5\text{ mL} = \frac{20}{9} = 2.2\text{ mL/dose};$

$$\frac{60\text{ }\cancel{mL}}{2.2\text{ }\cancel{mL}\text{/day}} = 27.2\text{ or 27 full days}$$

or $\frac{90\text{ mg}}{5\text{ mL}} = \frac{40\text{ mg}}{X\text{ mL}}$

$$90\text{ X} = 200$$

$$\frac{90\text{ X}}{90} = \frac{200}{90}$$

$$X = 2.2\text{ mL}$$

$$\frac{2.2\text{ mL}}{1\text{ day}} = \frac{60\text{ mL}}{X\text{ days}}$$

$$2.2\text{ X} = 60$$

$$\frac{2.2\text{ X}}{2.2} = \frac{60}{2.2}$$

$$X = 27.2\text{ or 27 full days}$$

10) Order: 0.3 mg = 0.3 × 1000 = 300 mcg

Supply: 150 mcg

$$\frac{D}{H} \times Q = \frac{\overset{2}{\cancel{300\text{ mcg}}}}{\underset{1}{\cancel{150\text{ mcg}}}} \times 1\text{ tab} = 2\text{ tab}$$

or

$$\frac{150\text{ mg}}{1\text{ tab}} = \frac{300\text{ mcg}}{X\text{ tab}}$$

$$150\text{ X} = 300$$

$$\frac{150\text{ X}}{150} = \frac{300}{150}$$

$$X = 2\text{ tab}$$

20)

Day 1, 2, 3 : $\frac{D}{H} \times Q = \frac{\overset{2}{\cancel{10\text{ mg}}}}{\underset{1}{\cancel{5\text{ mg}}}} \times 1\text{ tab} = 2\text{ tab}; \quad \frac{2\text{ tab}}{\cancel{day}} \times 3\text{ }\cancel{days} = 6\text{ tab}$

Day 4, 5, 6 : $\frac{D}{H} \times Q = \frac{7.5\text{ }\cancel{mg}}{5\text{ }\cancel{mg}} \times 1\text{ tab} = 1.5 = 1\frac{1}{2}\text{ tab}; \quad \frac{1\frac{1}{2}\text{ tab}}{\cancel{day}} \times 3\text{ }\cancel{days} = 4\frac{1}{2}\text{ tab}$

Day 7, 8 : $\frac{D}{H} \times Q = \frac{\cancel{5\text{ mg}}}{\cancel{5\text{ mg}}} \times 1\text{ tab} = 1\text{ tab}; \quad \frac{1\text{ tab}}{\cancel{day}} \times 2\text{ }\cancel{days} = 2\text{ tabs}$

Day 9, 10 : $\frac{D}{H} \times Q = \frac{\overset{1}{\cancel{2.5\text{ mg}}}}{\underset{2}{\cancel{5\text{ mg}}}} \times 1\text{ tab} = \frac{1}{2}\text{ tab}; \quad \frac{\frac{1}{2}\text{ tab}}{\cancel{day}} \times 2\text{ }\cancel{days} = \frac{1}{2} \times 2 = 1\text{ tab}$

6 tab
$4\frac{1}{2}$ tab
2 tab
\+ 1 tab

$13\frac{1}{2}$ tab for complete course

21) Order : 12 mg

Supply : $gr\,\frac{1}{4} = \frac{1}{4} \times \frac{60}{1} = 15$ mg

$\frac{D}{H} \times Q = \frac{12\text{ mg}}{15\text{ mg}} \times 1\text{ mL} = 0.8\text{ mL}$

29) $\frac{D}{H} \times Q = \frac{50\text{ mg}}{40\text{ mg}} \times 1\text{ mL} = 1.25 = 1.3\text{ mL}$

32) 50-50 means 50% Regular Insulin and 50% NPH insulin; 50% of 36 units = 18 units of NPH and of Regular Insulin.

35) Minimum daily dosage: $\frac{0.01\text{ mcg/day}}{\text{kg}} \times 8\text{ kg} = 0.08\text{ mcg/day}$

Maximum daily dosage: $\frac{0.05\text{ mcg/day}}{\text{kg}} \times 8\text{ kg} = 0.4\text{ mcg/day}$

36) Ordered dosage: 0.24 mcg/day. Dosage is safe.

$\frac{D}{H} \times Q = \frac{0.24\text{ mcg}}{1\text{ mcg}} \times 1\text{ mL} = 0.24\text{ mL}$

37) $\frac{1\text{ dose}}{0.24\text{ mL}} \times \frac{2\text{ mL}}{\text{vial}} = \frac{2}{0.24}$ doses/vial = 8.3 or 8 full doses/vial

38) 63 lb = 63 ÷ 2.2 = 28.63 = 28.6 kg

$\frac{30\text{ U}}{\text{kg}} \times 28.6\text{ kg} = 858$ U. Dosage is safe.

$\frac{D}{H} \times Q = \frac{858\text{ U}}{1000\text{ U}} \times 50\text{ mL} = \frac{858}{20} = 42.9 = 43\text{ mL}$

40) 23 lb 12 oz = $23\frac{12}{16} = 23\frac{3}{4} = 23.75 \div 2.2 =$

10.79 = 10.8 kg

Per dose: $\frac{0.25\text{ mmol}}{\text{kg}} \times 10.8\text{ kg} =$

2.7 mmol/dose; dosage is safe.

$\frac{D}{H} \times Q = \frac{2.7\text{ mmol}}{3\text{ mmol}} \times 15\text{ mL} = 13.5\text{ mL}$

42) Safe dosage: $\frac{0.0075\text{ mL}}{\text{kg}} \times 24\text{ kg} = 0.18\text{ mL}$

Dosage is safe.

Per day: $\frac{0.18\text{ mL}}{\text{dose}} \times \frac{6\text{ doses}}{\text{day}} = 1.08\text{ mL/day}$

45) $\frac{2\text{ mL}}{\text{dose}} \times \frac{100{,}000\text{ U}}{\text{mL}} = 200{,}000$ U/dose

$\frac{200{,}000\text{ U}}{\text{dose}} \times \frac{4\text{ doses}}{\text{day}} = 800{,}000$ U/day

$\frac{800{,}000\text{ U}}{\text{day}} \times 5\text{ days} = 4{,}000{,}000$ U

$\frac{1\text{ mL}}{100{,}000\text{ U}} \times 4{,}000{,}000\text{ U} = 40\text{ mL}$

46) Minimum daily dosage: $\frac{1\text{ mcg}}{\text{kg}} \times 9\text{ kg} = 9\text{ mcg}$

Maximum daily dosage: $\frac{10\text{ mcg}}{\text{kg}} \times 9\text{ kg} = 90\text{ mcg}$

Ordered dosage: $\frac{900\text{ mcg}}{\text{dose}} \times \frac{2\text{ doses}}{\text{day}} = 1800\text{ mcg/day}$

Too much!

Also exceeds maximum recommended dosage of 1500 mcg/day.

47) 42 lb = 42 ÷ 2.2 = 19.09 = 19.1 kg;

Minimum recommended amount per dose

$\frac{0.7\text{ mg}}{\text{kg}} \times 19.1\text{ kg} = 13.37 = 13.4\text{ mg}$

Ordered dosage is 3.8 mg/dose, which is very low. Discuss dosage with physician before administration.

Review Set 33 from page 277.

1) 160 mL hydrogen peroxide (solute) + 320 mL saline (solvent) = 480 mL $\frac{1}{3}$ strength solution **2)** 1 ounce hydrogen peroxide + 3 ounces saline = 4 ounces $\frac{1}{4}$ strength solution **3)** 180 mL hydrogen peroxide + 60 mL saline = 240 mL $\frac{3}{4}$ strength solution **4)** 8 ounces hydrogen peroxide + 8 ounces saline = 16 ounces $\frac{1}{2}$ strength solution **5)** 15; 15; 3; 500 **6)** 60; 240 **7)** 250; 250 **8)** 4; 12

Solutions—Review Set 33

1) $D \times Q = \frac{1}{3} \times 480\text{ mL} = 160$ mL solute

480 mL (quantity desired solution) – 160 mL (solute) = 320 mL (solvent)

5) $D \times Q = \frac{3\text{ g}}{100\text{ mL}} \times 500\text{ mL} = 15\text{ g} = 15$ mL salt;

(1 t = 5 mL) 15 mL salt = $\frac{15}{5}$

= 3 t salt added to 500 mL water

6) $D \times Q = \frac{20}{100} \times 300\text{ mL} = 60$ mL solute

300 mL (solution) – 60 mL (solute) = 240 mL solvent

8) Convert : 1 pt = 16 oz

$D \times Q = \frac{1}{4} \times 16\text{ oz} = 4$ oz (solute)

16 oz (solution) – 4 oz (solute) = 12 oz (solvent)

Review Set 34 from pages 280–281.

1) 300 mL Ensure + 600 mL water = 900 mL $\frac{1}{3}$ strength Ensure; use 1 12-oz can. Discard 2 oz (60 mL).
2) 6 oz (180 mL) Isomil + 18 oz (540 mL) water = 24 oz (720 mL) $\frac{1}{4}$ strength Isomil; use 1 6-oz can. No discard.
3) 800 mL Sustacal + 400 mL water = 1200 mL $\frac{2}{3}$ strength Sustacal; 3 10-oz cans. Discard 100 mL.
4) 13 ounces Ensure + 13 ounces water = 26 ounces $\frac{1}{2}$ strength Ensure; 1 12-oz can + 1 4-oz can. Discard 3 oz (180 mL).
5) 500 mL Sustacal + 500 mL water = 1000 mL $\frac{1}{2}$ strength Sustacal; 2 10-oz cans. Discard 100 mL.
6) 36 ounces Isomil + 12 ounces water = 48 ounces $\frac{3}{4}$ strength Isomil; 3 12-oz cans. No discard.
7) 4 ounces Ensure + 2 ounces water = 6 ounces $\frac{2}{3}$ strength Ensure; 1 4-oz can. No discard.
8) 4 ounces Ensure + 12 ounces water = 16 ounces (pt i) $\frac{1}{4}$ strength Ensure; 1 4-oz can. No discard.

Solutions—Review Set 34

1) $D \times Q = \frac{1}{\cancel{3}_1} \times \cancel{900}^{300}\text{ mL} = 300\text{ mL Ensure}$

900 mL (total solution) – 300 mL (Ensure) = 600 mL (water)

1 12-oz can = 30 mL × 12 = 360 mL

360 mL (full can) – 300 mL (Ensure needed) =
60 mL (discarded)

2) $4\text{ oz q.4 h} = \frac{4\text{ oz}}{\cancel{\text{feeding}}} \times 6\ \cancel{\text{feedings}} = 24\text{ oz total;}$

$D \times Q = \frac{1}{\cancel{4}_1} \times \cancel{24}^{6}\text{ oz} = 6\text{ oz (Isomil)}$

24 oz (solution) – 6 oz (Isomil) = 18 oz (water); use 1 6-oz can.

8) $D \times Q = \frac{1}{4} \times 16\text{ oz} = 4\text{ oz Ensure}$

16 oz (solution) – 4 oz (Ensure) = 12 oz (water); use 1 4-oz can Ensure. No discard.

Practice Problems—Chapter 13 from pages 281–283.

1) 120 mL hydrogen peroxide + 120 mL normal saline = 240 mL $\frac{1}{2}$ strength solution.
2) 2 ounces hydrogen peroxide + 14 ounces normal saline = 16 ounces $\frac{1}{8}$ strength solution.
3) 120 mL hydrogen peroxide + 200 mL normal saline = 320 mL $\frac{3}{8}$ strength solution.
4) 50 mL hydrogen peroxide + 30 mL normal saline = 80 mL $\frac{5}{8}$ strength solution.
5) 12 ounces hydrogen peroxide + 6 ounces normal saline = 18 ounces $\frac{2}{3}$ strength solution.
6) 7 ounces hydrogen peroxide + 1 ounce normal saline = 8 ounces $\frac{7}{8}$ strength solution.
7) $\frac{1}{2}$ ounce hydrogen peroxide + $1\frac{1}{2}$ ounces normal saline = 2 ounces $\frac{1}{4}$ strength solution.
8) 30 mL Enfamil + 90 mL water = 120 mL $\frac{1}{4}$ strength Enfamil; 1 3-oz bottle; discard 2 oz (60 mL).
9) 270 mL Sustacal + 90 mL water = 360 mL $\frac{3}{4}$ strength Sustacal; 1 10-oz can; discard 1 oz (30 mL).
10) 300 mL Ensure + 150 mL water = 450 mL $\frac{2}{3}$ strength Ensure; 2 8-oz cans; discard 6 oz (180 mL).
11) 180 mL Isomil + 108 mL water = 288 mL $\frac{5}{8}$ strength Isomil; 2 3-oz bottles; no discard.
12) 36 oz Enfamil + 60 oz water = 96 oz $\frac{3}{8}$ strength Enfamil; 6 6-oz bottles; no discard.
13) 20 mL Ensure + 140 mL water = 160 mL $\frac{1}{8}$ strength Ensure; 1 4-oz can; discard 100 mL.
14) 225 mL Ensure + 225 mL water = 550 mL $\frac{1}{2}$ strength Ensure; 1 12-oz can; discard 135 mL.
15) $1\frac{1}{2}$ cans (12 oz Enfamil)
16) 36 oz water
17) Add 18 mL (approximately 4 t) salt to 2000 mL water.
18) Add 4.5 mL (approximately 1 t) salt to 1000 mL water.
19) Add 10 mL (2 t) salt to 500 mL water.
20) 25 mL boric acid + 475 mL water.

Solutions—Practice Problems—Chapter 13

1) $D \times Q = \frac{1}{\not{2}_1} \times \overset{120}{\not{240}}\text{ mL} = 120$ mL hydrogen peroxide;

240 mL (solution) – 120 mL (hydrogen peroxide) = 120 mL (normal saline).

7) $D \times Q = \frac{1}{\not{4}_2} \times \overset{1}{\not{2}}\text{ oz} = \frac{1}{2}$ oz hydrogen peroxide;

2 oz (solution) $-\frac{1}{2}$ oz (hydrogen peroxide) = $1\frac{1}{2}$ oz (normal saline).

8) 12 mL every hour for 10 hours = 12 × 10 = 120 mL total;

$D \times Q = \frac{1}{\not{4}_1} \times \overset{30}{\not{120}}\text{ mL} = 30$ mL Enfamil;

120 mL (solution) – 30 mL (Enfamil) = 90 mL (water);
1 3-oz bottle = 90 mL.

90 mL (full bottle) – 30 mL (Enfamil needed) = 60 mL (2 oz discarded).

15) $D \times Q = \frac{1}{\not{4}_1} \times \overset{12}{\not{48}}\text{ oz} = 12$ oz Enfamil;

need $1\frac{1}{2}$ cans (8 oz each can) of Enfamil for each infant.

16) 48 oz (solution) – 12 oz (Enfamil) = 36 oz (water)

17) 0.9% = 0.9 g per 100 mL; 2 L = 2000 mL

$D \times Q = \frac{0.9\text{ g}}{\not{100}\text{ mL}_1} \times \overset{20}{\not{2000}}\text{ mL} = 18\text{ g}$

For salt this is equivalent to 18 mL or approximately 4 t, added to 2000 mL water.

20) 1:20 = $\frac{1}{20}$ strength

$D \times Q = \frac{1}{\not{20}_1} \times \overset{25}{\not{500}}\text{ mL} = 25$ mL (boric acid stock)

500 mL (solution) – 25 mL (stock) = 475 mL (water)

Review Set 35 from pages 289–291.

1) C; sodium chloride 0.9%, 0.9 g/100 mL; 308 mOsm/L; Isotonic
2) E; dextrose 5%, 5 g/100 mL; 252 mOsm/L; Isotonic
3) G; dextrose 5%, 5 g/100 mL; sodium chloride 0.9%, 0.9 g/100 mL; 560 mOsm/L; Hypertonic
4) D; dextrose 5%, 5 g/100 mL, sodium chloride 0.45%, 0.45 g/100 mL; 406 mOsm/L; Hypertonic
5) A; dextrose 5%, 5 g/100 mL, sodium chloride 0.225%, 0.225 g/100 mL; 329 mOsm/L; Isotonic
6) H, dextrose 5%, 5 g/100 mL; sodium lactate 0.31 g/100 mL, NaCl 0.6 g/100 mL; KCl 0.03 g/100 mL; CaCl 0.02 g/100 mL; 525 mOsm/L; Hypertonic
7) B; dextrose 5%, 5 g/100 mL; sodium chloride 0.45%; 0.45 g/100 mL; potassium chloride 20 mEq per liter (0.149 g/100 mL); 447 mOsm/L; Hypertonic
8) F; sodium chloride 0.45%, 0.45 g/100 mL; 154 mOsm/L; Hypotonic

Review Set 36 from pages 293.

1) 50; 9 **2)** 25; 2.25 **3)** 25 **4)** 6.75 **5)** 25; 1.65 **6)** 150; 27 **7)** 50; 1.125 **8)** 36; 2.7 **9)** 100; 4.5 **10)** 3.375

Solutions—Review Set 36

1) D_5 NS = 5 g dextrose per 100 mL and 0.9 g NaCl per 100 mL

$\frac{5\text{ g}}{100\text{ mL}} = \frac{X\text{ g}}{1000\text{ mL}}$

$100X = 5000$

$\frac{100X}{100} = \frac{5000}{100}$

$X = 50$ g (dextrose)

$\frac{0.9\text{ g}}{100\text{ mL}} = \frac{X\text{ g}}{1000\text{ mL}}$

$100X = 900$

$\frac{100X}{100} = \frac{900}{100}$

$X = 9$ g (NaCl)

7) $D_{10}\frac{1}{4}$NS = 10 g dextrose per 100 mL and 0.225 g NaCl per 100 mL

$\frac{10\text{ g}}{100\text{ mL}} = \frac{X\text{ g}}{500\text{ mL}}$

$100X = 5000$

$\frac{100X}{100} = \frac{5000}{100}$

$X = 50$ g (dextrose)

$\frac{0.225\text{ g}}{100\text{ mL}} = \frac{X\text{ g}}{500\text{ mL}}$

$100X = 112.5$

$\frac{100X}{100} = \frac{112.5}{100}$

$X = 1.125$ g (NaCl)

Review Set 37 from page 301.

1) 100 **2)** 120 **3)** 83 **4)** 200 **5)** 120 **6)** 125 **7)** 125 **8)** 200 **9)** 75 **10)** 125 **11)** 63 **12)** 24 **13)** 150 **14)** 125 **15)** 42

Solutions—Review Set 37

1) 1 L = 1000 mL

$$\frac{\text{Total mL}}{\text{Total h}} = \frac{1000\text{ mL}}{10\text{ h}} = 100\text{ mL/h}$$

3) $$\frac{\text{Total mL}}{\text{Total h}} = \frac{2000\text{ mL}}{24\text{ h}} = 83.3 = 83\text{ mL/h}$$

4) $$\frac{100\text{ mL}}{30\text{ min}} = \frac{X\text{ mL}}{60\text{ min}}$$

$$30X = 6000$$

$$\frac{30X}{30} = \frac{6000}{30}$$

$X = 200$ mL; 200 mL/60 min = 200 mL/h

5) $$\frac{30\text{ mL}}{15\text{ min}} = \frac{X\text{ mL}}{60\text{ min}}$$

$$15X = 1800$$

$$\frac{15X}{15} = \frac{1800}{15}$$

$X = 120$ mL; 120 mL/60 min = 120 mL/h

6) 2.5 L = 2500 mL

$$\frac{\text{Total mL}}{\text{Total h}} = \frac{2500\text{ mL}}{20\text{ h}} = 125\text{ mL/h}$$

Review Set 38 from page 303.

1) 15 **2)** 20 **3)** 60 **4)** 60 **5)** 10

Review Set 39 from page 306.

1) $\frac{V}{T} \times C = R$ **2)** 21 **3)** 50 **4)** 33 **5)** 25 **6)** 83 **7)** 26 **8)** 50 **9)** 50 **10)** 80 **11)** 20 **12)** 30 **13)** 17 **14)** 55 **15)** 40

Solutions—Review Set 39

1) $$\frac{\text{Volume}}{\text{Time in min}} \times \text{Drop Factor} = \text{Rate}$$

Volume in mL divided by *time* in minutes, multiplied by the *drop factor calibration* in drops per milliliter, equals the flow *rate* in drops per minute.

2) $$\frac{V}{T} \times C = \frac{125\ \cancel{\text{mL}}}{\underset{6}{\cancel{60}}\ \text{min}} \times \overset{1}{\cancel{10}}\ \text{gtt}/\cancel{\text{mL}} = \frac{125}{6} = 20.8 = 21\text{ gtt/min}$$

3) $$\frac{V}{T} \times C = \frac{50\ \cancel{\text{mL}}}{\cancel{60}\ \text{min}} \times \cancel{60}\ \text{gtt}/\cancel{\text{mL}} = 50\text{ gtt/min}$$

Recall that when drop factor is 60 mL/h, then mL/h = gtt/min.

4) $$\frac{V}{T} \times C = \frac{100\ \cancel{\text{mL}}}{\underset{3}{\cancel{60}}\ \text{min}} \times \overset{1}{\cancel{20}}\ \text{gtt}/\cancel{\text{mL}} = \frac{100}{3} = 33.3 = 33\text{ gtt/min}$$

6) Two 500 mL units of blood = 1000 mL total volume.

$$\text{mL/h} = \frac{1000\text{ mL}}{4\text{ h}} = 250\text{ mL/h}$$

$$\frac{V}{T} \times C = \frac{250\text{ mL}}{\underset{3}{\cancel{60}}\ \text{min}} \times \overset{1}{\cancel{20}}\ \text{gtt}/\cancel{\text{mL}} = \frac{250}{3} = 83.3 = 83\text{ gtt/min}$$

7) $$\frac{\text{Total mL}}{\text{Total h}} = \frac{1240\text{ mL}}{12\text{ h}} = 103\text{ mL/h}$$

$$\frac{V}{T} \times C = \frac{103\ \cancel{\text{mL}}}{\underset{4}{\cancel{60}}\ \text{min}} \times \overset{1}{\cancel{15}}\ \text{gtt}/\cancel{\text{mL}} = \frac{103}{4} = 25.7 = 26\text{ gtt/min}$$

9) $$\frac{150\ \cancel{\text{mL}}}{\underset{3}{\cancel{45}}\ \text{min}} \times \overset{1}{\cancel{15}}\ \text{gtt}/\cancel{\text{mL}} = \frac{150}{3} = 50\text{ gtt/min}$$

Review Set 40 from pages 308 and 309.

1) 60 **2)** 1 **3)** 3 **4)** 4 **5)** 6 **6)** $\frac{\text{mL / h}}{\text{drop factor constant}} = \text{gtt / min}$ **7)** 50 **8)** 42 **9)** 28 **10)** 60 **11)** 8 **12)** 31 **13)** 28 **14)** 25 **15)** 11

Solutions—Review Set 40

4) $\frac{60}{15} = 4$

7) $$\frac{\text{mL/h}}{\text{drop factor constant}} = \frac{200\text{ mL/h}}{4} = 50\text{ gtt/min}$$

8) $$\frac{\text{mL/h}}{\text{drop factor constant}} = \frac{125\text{ mL/h}}{3} = 41.6 = 42\text{ gtt/min}$$

9) $$\frac{\text{mL/h}}{\text{drop factor constant}} = \frac{165\text{ mL/h}}{6} = 27.5 = 28\text{ gtt/min}$$

10) $$\frac{\text{mL/h}}{\text{drop factor constant}} = \frac{60\text{ mL/h}}{1} = 60\text{ gtt/min}$$

(Set the flow rate at the same number of gtt/min as the number of mL/h when the drop factor is 60 gtt/mL because the drop factor constant is 1.)

14) 0.5 L = 500 mL; $\frac{500\text{ mL}}{20\text{ h}} = 25$ mL/h; since drop factor is 60 gtt/mL, then mL/h = gtt/min; so rate is 25 gtt/min.

15) 650 mL in 10 h $= \frac{650 \text{ mL}}{10 \text{ h}} = 65$ mL/h; $\frac{\text{mL/h}}{\text{drop factor constant}} = \frac{65 \text{ mL/h}}{6} =$

10.8 = 11 gtt/min

Review Set 41 from page 310.

1) 31 **2)** 100 **3)** 33 **4)** 50 **5)** 31 **6)** 125 **7)** 35 **8)** 17 **9)** 25 **10)** 125 **11)** 83 **12)** 125 **13)** 200 **14)** 150 **15)** 200 **16)** 13.5 **17)** 20; 1.8 **18)** 22.5 **19)** 32.5; 2.145 **20)** 50; 2.25

Solutions—Review Set 41

1) $\frac{\text{Total mL}}{\text{Total h}} = \frac{3000 \text{ mL}}{24 \text{ h}} = 125$ mL/h

$\frac{V}{T} \times C = \frac{125 \text{ mL}}{60 \text{ min}} \times 15 \text{ gtt/mL} = \frac{125}{4} = 31.2 = 31$ gtt/min

7) $\frac{\text{mL/h}}{\text{drop factor constant}} =$

$\frac{105 \text{ mL/h}}{3} = 35$ gtt/min

8) $\frac{\text{mL/h}}{\text{drop factor constant}} =$

$\frac{100 \text{ mL/h}}{6} = 16.6 = 17$ gtt/min

10) $\frac{\text{Total mL}}{\text{Total h}} = \frac{1000 \text{ mL}}{8 \text{ h}} = 125$ mL/h

13) $\frac{100 \text{ mL}}{30 \text{ min}} = \frac{X \text{ mL}}{60 \text{ min}}$

$30X = 6000$

$\frac{30X}{30} = \frac{6000}{30}$

$X = 200$ mL

200 mL/60 min = 200 mL/h

15) $\frac{150 \text{ mL}}{45 \text{ min}} = \frac{X \text{ mL}}{60 \text{ min}}$

$45X = 9000$

$\frac{45X}{45} = \frac{9000}{45}$

$X = 200$ mL

200 mL/60 min = 200 mL/h

16) $\frac{1}{2}$ NS = 0.45% NaCl = 0.45 g NaCl per 100 mL

$\frac{0.45 \text{ g}}{100 \text{ mL}} = \frac{X \text{ g}}{3000 \text{ mL}}$

$100X = 1350$

$\frac{100X}{100} = \frac{1350}{100}$

$X = 13.5$ g (NaCl)

17) D_{10} = 10% dextrose = 10 g dextrose per 100 mL

$\frac{10 \text{ g}}{100 \text{ mL}} = \frac{X \text{ g}}{200 \text{ mL}}$

$100X = 2000$

$\frac{100X}{100} = \frac{2000}{100}$

$X = 20$ g (dextrose)

NS = 0.9% NaCl = 0.9 g NaCl per 100 mL

$\frac{0.9 \text{ g}}{100 \text{ mL}} = \frac{X \text{ g}}{200 \text{ mL}}$

$100X = 180$

$\frac{100X}{100} = \frac{180}{100}$

$X = 1.8$ g (NaCl)

Review Set 42 from pages 313 and 314.

1) 42; reset to 47 gtt/min (12% increase is acceptable).
2) 42; reset to 45 gtt/min (7% increase is acceptable).
3) 42; recalculated rate 67 gtt/min (60% increase is unacceptable.) Consult physician.
4) 28; reset to 31 gtt/min (11% increase is acceptable.)
5) 21; recalculated rate 31 gtt/min (48% increase is unacceptable). Consult physician.
6) 31; reset to 34 gtt/min (10% increase is acceptable.)
7) 50; recalculated rate 78 gtt/min (56% increase is unacceptable). Consult physician.
8) 33; recalculated rate 28 gtt/min (–15% slower is acceptable). IV is ahead of schedule. Slow rate to 28 gtt/min, and observe patient's condition.
9) 13; reset to 15 gtt/min (15% increase is acceptable).
10) 100; IV is on time, so no adjustment is needed.

Solutions—Review Set 42

1) $\frac{V}{T} \times C = \frac{125 \text{ mL}}{60 \text{ min}} \times 20 \text{ gtt/mL} = \frac{125}{3} = 41.6 = 42$ gtt/min (ordered rate)

$\frac{\text{Remaining volume}}{\text{Remaining hours}}$ = Recalculated mL/h; $\frac{850 \text{ mL}}{6 \text{ h}} = 141.6 = 142$ mL/h

$\frac{V}{T} \times C = \frac{142 \text{ mL}}{60 \text{ min}} \times 20 \text{ gtt/mL} = 47.3 = 47$ gtt/min (adjusted rate)

$\frac{\text{Adjusted gtt/min} - \text{Ordered gtt/min}}{\text{Ordered gtt/min}}$ = % of variation; $\frac{47-42}{42} = \frac{5}{42} = 0.12 = 12\%$

(within the acceptable % or variation); reset rate to 47 gtt/min.

3) $\frac{V}{T} \times C = \frac{125 \text{ mL}}{60 \text{ min}} \times 20 \text{ gtt/mL} = \frac{125}{3} = 41.6 = 42$ gtt/min (ordered rate)

$\frac{800 \text{ mL}}{4 \text{ h}} = 200$ mL/h; $\frac{V}{T} \times C = \frac{200 \text{ mL}}{60 \text{ min}} \times 20 \text{ gtt/mL} = 66.6 = 67$ gtt/min (adjusted rate)

$\frac{\text{Adjusted gtt/min} - \text{Ordered gtt/min}}{\text{Ordered gtt/min}}$ = % of variation; $\frac{67-42}{42} = \frac{25}{42} = 0.59 = 0.6 = 60\%$ faster;

unacceptable % of variation — call physician for a revised order.

6) 2000 mL – 650 mL = 1350 mL remaining

$\frac{V}{T} \times C = \frac{125 \text{ mL}}{60 \text{ min}} \times 15 \text{ gtt/mL} = \frac{125}{4} = 31.2 = 31$ gtt/min (ordered rate)

$\frac{1350 \text{ mL}}{10 \text{ h}} = 135$ mL/h; $\frac{V}{T} \times C = \frac{135 \text{ mL}}{60 \text{ min}} \times 15 \text{ gtt/mL} = 33.7 = 34$ gtt/min

$\frac{\text{Adjusted gtt/min} - \text{Ordered gtt/min}}{\text{Ordered gtt/min}}$ = % of variation; $\frac{34-31}{31} = \frac{3}{31} = 0.096 = 0.10 = 10\%$

(within acceptable % of variation); reset rate to 34 gtt/min.

8) $\frac{V}{T} \times C = \frac{100 \text{ mL}}{60 \text{ min}} \times 20 \text{ gtt/mL} = \frac{100}{3} = 33.3 = 33$ gtt/min (ordered rate)

$\frac{250 \text{ mL}}{3 \text{ h}} = 83$ mL/h; $\frac{V}{T} \times C = \frac{83 \text{ mL}}{60 \text{ min}} \times 20 \text{ gtt/mL} = \frac{83}{3} = 27.6 = 28$ gtt/min (adjusted rate)

$\frac{\text{Adjusted gtt/min} - \text{Ordered gtt/min}}{\text{Ordered gtt/min}}$ = % of variation; $\frac{28-33}{33} = \frac{-5}{33} = -0.15 = -15\%$

(Remember the [–] sign indicates the IV is ahead of schedule and rate must be decreased.) Within the acceptable % of variation.

Slow IV to 28 gtt/min, and closely monitor patient.

Review Set 43 from pages 319 and 320.

1) 133 **2)** 133 **3)** 50 **4)** 200 **5)** 100 **6)** 25 **7)** 50 **8)** 200 **9)** 150 **10)** 167 **11)** 133 **12)** 25 **13)** 120 **14)** 56 **15)** 200 **16)** 12; 3 **17)** 3; 3 **18)** 0.6; 2, 24 **19)** To provide IV medications and supplemental fluids when continuous infusion is unnecessary. **20)** False

Solutions—Review Set 43

1) $\frac{V}{T} \times C = \frac{100 \text{ mL}}{45 \text{ min}} \times 60 \text{ gtt/mL} = \frac{400}{3} = 133.3 =$

133 gtt/min

2) $\frac{100 \text{ mL}}{45 \text{ min}} = \frac{X \text{ mL}}{60 \text{ min}}$

$45X = 6000$

$\frac{45X}{45} = \frac{6000}{45}$

$X = 133.3 = 133$ mL

133 mL/60 min = 133 mL/h

3) $\frac{V}{T} \times C = \frac{50 \text{ mL}}{15 \text{ min}} \times 15 \text{ gtt/mL} = 50$ gtt/min

4) $\frac{50 \text{ mL}}{15 \text{ min}} = \frac{X \text{ mL}}{60 \text{ min}}$

$15X = 6000$

$\frac{15X}{15} = \frac{3000}{15}$

$X = 200$ mL

200 mL/60 min = 200 mL/h

11) $\frac{V}{T} \times C = \frac{100\ \cancel{mL}}{\cancel{15}_{3}\ min} \times \overset{4}{\cancel{20}}\ gtt/\cancel{mL} = \frac{400}{3} = 133.3 = 133\ gtt/min$

16) $\frac{D}{H} \times Q = \frac{12\cancel{0}\ \cancel{mg}}{1\cancel{0}\ \cancel{mg}} \times 1\ mL = 12\ mL$

$\frac{D}{H} \times Q = \frac{\overset{3}{\cancel{120}}\ \cancel{mg}}{\underset{1}{\cancel{40}}\ \cancel{mg}} \times 1\ min = 3\ min$

Administer 12 mL over at least 3 minutes.

17) $\frac{D}{H} \times Q = \frac{150\ \cancel{mg}}{\underset{50}{\cancel{250}}\ \cancel{mg}} \times \overset{1}{\cancel{5}}\ mL = \frac{\overset{3}{\cancel{150}}}{\underset{1}{\cancel{50}}} = 3\ mL$

$\frac{D}{H} \times Q = \frac{\overset{3}{\cancel{150}}\ \cancel{mg}}{\underset{1}{\cancel{50}}\ \cancel{mg}} \times 1\ min = 3\ min$

Administer 3 mL over 3 minutes.

18) Convert : $gr\ \frac{1}{10} = \frac{1}{\underset{1}{\cancel{10}}} \times \overset{6}{\cancel{60}} = 6\ mg$

$\frac{D}{H} \times Q = \frac{6\ \cancel{mg}}{10\ \cancel{mg}} \times 1\ mL = \frac{6}{10} = 0.6\ mL$

$\frac{D}{H} \times Q = \frac{6\ \cancel{mg}}{2.5\ \cancel{mg}} \times 1\ min = 2.4\ min$

0.4 minutes $= \frac{4}{10}$ min;

$\frac{4}{10}\ min \times \frac{60\ sec}{1\ min} = 24$ seconds; 2.4 min = 2 min + 24 sec

Review Set 44 from pages 323 and 324.

1) 5 h and 33 min or $5\frac{1}{2}$ h **2)** 6 h and 40 min or $6\frac{2}{3}$ h **3)** 8 h **4)** 6 h; 20 **5)** 4 h; 20 **6)** Approximately 11 hours later or 0300 the next morning **7)** 21; approximately 16 hours later or 0730 the next morning **8)** 3000 **9)** 1152 **10)** 3024 **11)** 260 **12)** 300 **13)** 600 **14)** 320 **15)** 540

Solutions—Review Set 44

1) $\frac{V}{T} \times C = R$

$\frac{500\ mL}{T\ min} \times 20\ gtt/mL = 30\ gtt/min$

$\frac{10{,}000}{T} = \frac{30}{1}$

$30T = 10{,}000$

$\frac{30T}{30} = \frac{10{,}000}{30}$

$T = 333\ min = 5\ h$ and 33 min rounded to $5\frac{1}{2}\ h$

2) $\frac{V}{T} \times C = R$

$\frac{1000\ mL}{T} \times 10\ gtt/mL = 25\ gtt/min$

$\frac{10{,}000}{T} = \frac{25}{1}$

$25\ T = 10{,}000$

$\frac{25T}{25} = \frac{10{,}000}{25}$

$T = 400\ min = \frac{400}{60} = 6.67 = 6\frac{2}{3}\ h = 6\ h$ and 40 min

4) Time: $\frac{Total\ vol}{mL/h} = Total\ h$

$\frac{120\ \cancel{mL}}{20\ \cancel{mL}/h} = 6\ h$

$\frac{V}{T} \times C = \frac{20\ \cancel{mL}}{\cancel{60}\ min} \times \cancel{60}\ gtt/\cancel{mL} = 20\ gtt/min$

6) $\frac{V}{T} \times C = \frac{1200\ mL}{T\ min} \times 15\ gtt/mL = 27\ gtt/min$

$\frac{18000}{T} = \frac{27}{1}$

$27T = 18000$

$\frac{27T}{27} = \frac{18000}{27}$

$T = 667\ min$

$T = \frac{667}{60} = 11.1 = 11\ h$

$1600 + 1100\ (11\ h) = 2700 - 2400 = 0300$

7) Time : $\frac{Total\ vol}{mL/h} = Total\ h$

$\frac{2000\ \cancel{mL}}{125\ \cancel{mL}/h} = 16\ h$

$1530 + 1600 = 3130 - 2400 = 0730$

$16\ \cancel{h} \times 60\ min/\cancel{h} = 960\ min$

$\frac{V}{T} \times C = \frac{2000\ mL}{\underset{96}{\cancel{960}}\ min} \times \overset{1}{\cancel{10}}\ gtt/mL = \frac{2000}{96} =$

$20.83 = 21\ gtt/min$

8) Total hours × mL/h = Total volume

$24\ \cancel{h} \times 125\ mL/\cancel{h} = 3000\ mL$

9) $\frac{V}{T} \times C = \frac{V\ mL}{1440\ min} \times 15\ gtt/mL = 12\ gtt/min$

$\frac{15\ V}{1440} = \frac{12}{1}$

$15\ V = 17{,}280$

$\frac{15\ V}{15} = \frac{17{,}280}{15}$

$V = 1152\ mL$

11) $65 \text{ mL}/\cancel{h} \times 4 \cancel{h} = 260 \text{ mL}$

14) $8 \cancel{h} \times 60 \text{ min}/\cancel{h} = 480 \text{ min}$

$\frac{\text{V mL}}{480 \text{ min}} \times 60 \text{ gtt/mL} = 40 \text{ gtt/min}$

$\frac{60 \text{ V}}{480} = \frac{40}{1}$

$60 \text{ V} = 19{,}200$

$\frac{60 \text{ V}}{60} = \frac{19{,}200}{60}$

$\text{V} = 320 \text{ mL}$

15) $\frac{\text{V}}{\text{T}} \times \text{C} = \frac{\text{V mL}}{240 \text{ min}} \times 20 \text{ gtt/mL} = 45 \text{ gtt/min}$

$\frac{20\text{V}}{240} = \frac{45}{1}$

$20\text{V} = 10{,}800$

$\frac{20\text{V}}{20} = \frac{10{,}800}{20}$

$\text{V} = 540 \text{ mL}$

Practice Problems—Chapter 14 from pages 325–328.

1) 17 **2)** 42 **3)** 42 **4)** 8 **5)** 125 **6)** Assess patient. If stable, recalculate and reset to 114 mL/h; observe patient closely. **7)** 31 **8)** 42 **9)** Assess patient. If stable, recalculate and reset to 50 gtt/min. **10)** 3000 **11)** Abbott Laboratories **12)** 15 gtt/mL **13)** 4

14) $\text{mL/h} = \frac{500 \text{ mL}}{4 \text{ h}} = 125 \text{ mL/h}$

$\frac{\text{mL / h}}{\text{drop factor constant}} = \frac{125 \text{ mL/h}}{4} = 31.2 = 31 \text{ gtt/min}$

15) $\frac{\text{V}}{\text{T}} \times \text{C} = \frac{125 \cancel{\text{mL}}}{\underset{4}{\cancel{60}} \text{ min}} \times \overset{1}{\cancel{15}} \text{ gtt}/\cancel{\text{mL}} = \frac{125}{4} =$

$31.3 = 31 \text{ gtt/min}$

16) 1930 or 7:30 PM **17)** 250 **18)** Recalculate 210 mL to infuse over remaining 2 hours. Reset IV to 26 gtt/min and observe patient closely. **19)** 125 **20)** 100 **21)** Dextrose 2.5% (2.5 g/100 mL) and NaCl 0.45% (0.45 g/100 mL) **22)** 25; 4.5 **23)** A central line is a special catheter inserted to access a large vein in the chest. **24)** A primary line is the IV tubing used to set up a primary IV infusion. **25)** The purpose of a saline/heparin lock is to administer IV medications when the patient does not require continuous IV fluids. **26)** 10 **27)** The purpose of the PCA pump is to allow the patient to safely self-administer IV pain medication without having to call the nurse for a p.r.n. medication. **28)** Advantages of the syringe pump are that a small amount of medication can be delivered directly from the syringe, and a specified time can be programmed in the pump. **29)** Phlebitis and infiltration **30)** q$\frac{1}{2}$–1 h, according to hospital policy **31)** This IV tubing has 2 spikes—one for blood, the other for saline—that join at a common drip chamber or Y connection. **32)** 14 **33)** 21 **34)** 28 **35)** 83 **36)** 17 **37)** 25 **38)** 33 **39)** 100 **40)** 33 **41)** 50 **42)** 67 **43)** 200 **44)** 8 **45)** 11 **46)** 15 **47)** 45 **48)** 150. The IV will finish in 1 hour. Leave a new IV bag in case you are delayed so the relief nurse can spike the new bag and continue the infusion. **49)** 1250

50) Critical Thinking Skill: Prevention.

This error could have been prevented had the nurse carefully inspected the IV tubing package to determine the drop factor. Every IV tubing set has the drop factor printed on the package, so it is not necessary to memorize or guess the drop factor. The IV calculation should have looked like this:

$\frac{125 \cancel{\text{mL}}}{\underset{3}{\cancel{60}} \text{ min}} \times \overset{1}{\cancel{20}} \text{ gtt}/\cancel{\text{mL}} = \frac{125}{3} = 41.6 = 42 \text{ gtt/min}$

With the infusion set of 20 gtt/mL, a flow rate of 42 gtt/min would infuse 125 mL/h. At the 125 gtt/min rate the nurse calculated, the patient received three times the IV fluid ordered hourly. Thus, the patient actually received 375 mL/h of IV fluids.

Solutions—Practice Problems—Chapter 14

1) $\frac{\text{Total mL}}{\text{Total h}} = \frac{200 \text{ mL}}{2 \text{ h}} = 100 \text{ mL/h}$

$\frac{\text{V}}{\text{T}} \times \text{C} = \frac{100 \cancel{\text{mL}}}{\underset{6}{\cancel{60}} \text{ min}} \times \overset{1}{\cancel{10}} \text{ gtt}/\cancel{\text{mL}} = \frac{100}{6} \; 16.6 = 17 \text{ gtt/min}$

2) $\frac{\text{Total mL}}{\text{Total h}} = \frac{1000 \text{ mL}}{24 \text{ h}} = 41.6 = 42 \text{ mL/h}$

drop factor is 60 gtt/mL: 42 mL/h = 42 gtt/min

5) $\frac{\text{Total mL}}{\text{Total h}} = \frac{1000 \text{ mL}}{8 \text{ h}} = 125 \text{ mL/h}$

6) $\frac{\text{Total mL}}{\text{Total h}} = \frac{800 \text{ mL}}{7 \text{ h}} = 114.2 = 114 \text{ mL/h}$

$\frac{114-125}{125} = \frac{-11}{125} = -0.088 = -9\%$ (decrease); within safe limits.

Reset infusion rate to 114 mL/h.

7) $1000 \text{ mL} + 2000 \text{ mL} = 3000 \text{ mL};$

$\frac{\text{Total mL}}{\text{Total h}} = \frac{3000 \text{ mL}}{24 \text{ h}} = 125 \text{ mL/h}$

$\frac{\text{V}}{\text{T}} \times \text{C} = \frac{125 \cancel{\text{mL}}}{\underset{4}{\cancel{60}} \text{ min}} \times \overset{1}{\cancel{15}} \text{ gtt}/\cancel{\text{mL}} = 31.2 = 31 \text{ gtt/min}$

8) $\frac{V}{T} \times C = \frac{125\ \cancel{mL}}{\cancel{60}_{3}\ min} \times \cancel{20}^{1}\ gtt/\cancel{mL} = 41.6 = 42\ gtt/min$

9) $\frac{Total\ mL}{Total\ h} = \frac{1000}{6} = 166.6 = 167\ mL/h$

$\frac{V}{T} \times C = \frac{167\ \cancel{mL}}{\cancel{60}_{4}\ min} \times \cancel{15}^{1}\ gtt/\cancel{mL} = \frac{167}{4} = 41.7 = 42\ gtt/min$

$6\ h - 2\ h = 4\ h$ remaining; $\frac{Total\ mL}{Total\ h} = \frac{800\ mL}{4\ h} = 200\ mL/h$

$\frac{V}{T} \times C = \frac{200\ \cancel{mL}}{\cancel{60}_{4}\ min} \times \cancel{15}^{1}\ gtt/\cancel{mL} = \frac{200}{4} = 50\ gtt/min$

$\frac{\text{adjusted gtt/min} - \text{ordered gtt/min}}{\text{ordered gtt/min}} =$

$\frac{50-42}{42} = \frac{8}{42} = 0.19 = 19\%$ increase;

within safe limits of 25% variance.

Reset infusion rate to 50 gtt/min.

10) q.4 h = 6 times/24 h; 6 × 500 mL = 3000 mL

13) $\frac{60}{15} = 4$

16) 1530 + 4 h = 1530 + 0400 = 1930; 1930 – 1200 = 7:30 PM

17) $\frac{Total\ mL}{Total\ h} = \frac{500\ mL}{4\ h} = 125\ mL/h$

125 mL/h × 2 h = 250 mL

18) $\frac{Total\ mL}{Total\ h} = \frac{210\ mL}{2\ h} = 105\ mL/h$

$\frac{V}{T} \times C = \frac{105\ \cancel{mL}}{\cancel{60}_{4}\ min} \times \cancel{15}^{1}\ gtt/\cancel{mL} = \frac{105}{4} = 26.2 = 26\ gtt/min$

$\frac{\text{adjusted gtt/min} - \text{ordered gtt/min}}{\text{ordered gtt/min}} =$

$\frac{26-31}{31} = \frac{5}{31} = -0.16 = -16\%$ decrease; within safe limits.

Reset infusion rate to 26 gtt/min.

19) $\frac{Total\ mL}{Total\ h} = \frac{500\ mL}{4\ h} = 125\ mL/h$

20) $\frac{50\ mL}{30\ min} = \frac{X\ mL}{60\ min}$

$30X = 3000$

$\frac{30X}{30} = \frac{3000}{30}$

$X = 100\ mL/h$

22) Dextrose 5% = 5 g/100 mL NaCl 0.9% = 0.9 g/100 mL

$\frac{5\ g}{100\ mL} = \frac{X\ g}{500\ mL}$ $\frac{0.9\ g}{100\ mL} = \frac{X\ g}{500\ mL}$

$100\ X = 2500$ $100\ X = 450$

$\frac{100\ X}{100} = \frac{2500}{100}$ $\frac{100\ X}{100} = \frac{450}{100}$

$X = 25\ g$ $X = 4.5\ g$

26) $\frac{5\ mg}{1\ min} = \frac{50\ mg}{X}$

$5X = 50$

$\frac{5X}{5} = \frac{50}{5}$

$X = 10\ min$

32) $\frac{Total\ mL}{Total\ h} = \frac{1000\ mL}{12\ h} = 83.3 = 83\ mL/h;\ \frac{V}{T} \times C =$

$\frac{83\ \cancel{mL}}{\cancel{60}_{6}\ min} \times \cancel{10}^{1}\ gtt/\cancel{mL} = \frac{83}{6} = 13.8 = 14\ gtt/min$

33) $\frac{V}{T} \times C = \frac{83\ \cancel{mL}}{\cancel{60}_{4}\ min} \times \cancel{15}^{1}\ gtt/\cancel{mL} = \frac{83}{4} = 20.7 = 21\ gtt/min$

34) $\frac{V}{T} \times C = \frac{83\ \cancel{mL}}{\cancel{60}_{3}\ min} \times \cancel{20}^{1}\ gtt/\cancel{mL} = \frac{83}{3} = 27.6 = 28\ gtt/min$

35) $\frac{V}{T} \times C = \frac{83\ \cancel{mL}}{\cancel{60}_{1}\ min} \times \cancel{60}^{1}\ gtt/\cancel{mL} = 83\ gtt/min$

Remember, when drop factor is 60 gtt/mL, then mL/h = gtt/min; so 83 mL/h = 83 gtt/min.

48) $\frac{V}{T} \times C = \frac{V\ mL}{60\ min} \times 10\ gtt/mL = 25\ gtt/min$

$\frac{10V}{60} = \frac{25}{1}$

$10V = 1500$

$\frac{10V}{10} = \frac{1500}{10}$

$V = 150\ mL$

49) $\frac{400\ mL}{75\ mL/h} = 5\frac{1}{3}$ h or 5 h and 20 min

0730 + 0520 = 1250

Review Set 45 from page 333.

1) 0.68 **2)** 2.35 **3)** 0.69 **4)** 1.40 **5)** 2.03 **6)** 1 **7)** 1.66 **8)** 0.4 **9)** 1.69 **10)** 0.52 **11)** 1.11 **12)** 0.78 **13)** 0.15 **14)** 0.78 **15)** 0.39 **16)** 0.64 **17)** 0.25 **18)** 1.08 **19)** 0.5 **20)** 0.88

Solutions—Review Set 45

1) $BSA\ (m^2)\ (household) = \sqrt{\frac{ht\ (in) \times wt\ (lb)}{3131}} = \sqrt{\frac{36 \times 40}{3131}} = \sqrt{\frac{1440}{3131}} = \sqrt{0.460} = 0.68\ m^2$

2) $BSA\ (m^2)\ (metric) = \sqrt{\frac{ht\ (cm) \times wt\ (kg)}{3600}} = \sqrt{\frac{190 \times 105}{3600}} = \sqrt{\frac{19950}{3600}} = \sqrt{5.542} = 2.35\ m^2$

Review Set 46 from pages 335 and 336.

1) 1,640,000 **2)** 5.9–11.8 **3)** 735 **4)** 15.84; 63.36 **5)** 250 **6)** 2.5 **7)** 1.2 **8)** Yes **9)** Yes; 990 **10)** 2448 **11)** 8.1; 24.7 **12)** yes **13)** yes **14)** 0.82; yes; 2.7; 50 **15)** 1.62; 4050; 5.4

Solutions—Review Set 46

1) 2,000,000 units/$\cancel{m^2}$ × 0.82 $\cancel{m^2}$ = 1,640,000 units

2) 10 mg/$\cancel{m^2}$/day × 0.59 $\cancel{m^2}$ = 5.9 mg/day (minimum safe dose)

20 mg/$\cancel{m^2}$/day × 0.59 $\cancel{m^2}$ = 11.8 mg/day (maximum, safe dose)

3) 500 mg/$\cancel{m^2}$ × 1.47 $\cancel{m^2}$ = 735 mg

4) 6 mg/$\cancel{m^2}$/day × 2.64 $\cancel{m^2}$ = 15.84 mg/day

15.84 mg/$\cancel{day}$ × 4 $\cancel{days}$ = 63.36 mg

6) $\text{BSA (m}^2\text{) (household)} = \sqrt{\frac{30 \times 25}{3131}} = \sqrt{\frac{750}{3131}} =$

$\sqrt{0.240} = 0.49 \text{ m}^2$

250 mg/$\cancel{m^2}$ × 0.49 $\cancel{m^2}$ = 122.5 mg

$\frac{D}{H} \times Q = \frac{122.5 \cancel{mg}}{50 \cancel{mg}} \times 1 \text{ mL} = 2.45 = 2.5 \text{ mL}$

8) 150 mg/$\cancel{m^2}$/day × 0.44 $\cancel{m^2}$ = 66 mg/day

$\frac{66 \text{ mg}}{3 \text{ doses}} = 22$ mg/dose

9) 900 mg/$\cancel{m^2}$/day × 0.22 $\cancel{m^2}$ = 198 mg/day

198 mg/$\cancel{day}$ × 5 $\cancel{days}$ = 990 mg

10) 600 mg/$\cancel{m^2}$ × 1.02 $\cancel{m^2}$ = 612 mg, initially

300 mg/$\cancel{m^2}$ × 1.02 $\cancel{m^2}$ = 306 mg; for 2 doses: 306 mg × 2 = 612 mg

q. 12h is 2 doses/day and 2 doses/$\cancel{day}$ × 2 $\cancel{days}$ = 4 doses

306 mg × 4 = 1224 mg

612 mg + 612 mg + 1224 mg = 2448 mg total

11) 10 mg/$\cancel{m^2}$ × 0.81 $\cancel{m^2}$ = 8.1 mg bolus;

30.5 mg/$\cancel{m^2}$/day × 0.81 $\cancel{m^2}$ = 24.7 mg/day

14) $\text{BSA (m}^2\text{) metric} = \sqrt{\frac{100 \times 24}{3600}} = \sqrt{\frac{2400}{3600}} = \sqrt{0.667} = 0.82 \text{ m}^2$

2500 units/$\cancel{m^2}$ × 0.82 $\cancel{m^2}$ = 2050 units; yes, it is safe.

$\frac{D}{H} \times Q = \frac{2{,}050 \cancel{U}}{750 \cancel{U}} \times 1 \text{ mL} = 2.7 \text{ mL};$

$\frac{100 \text{ mL}}{2 \text{ h}} \times \frac{X \text{ mL}}{1 \text{ h}}$

2X = 100

$\frac{2X}{2} = \frac{100}{2}$

X = 50 mL/h

15) 128 lb = 128 ÷ 2.2 = 58.2 kg

$\text{BSA (m}^2\text{)} = \sqrt{\frac{58.2 \times 162}{3600}} = \sqrt{\frac{9428.4}{3600}} = \sqrt{2.619} = 1.62 \text{ m}^2$

2500 units/$\cancel{m^2}$ × 1.62 $\cancel{m^2}$ = 4050 mg

$\frac{D}{H} \times Q = \frac{4050 \cancel{U}}{750 \cancel{U}} \times 1 \text{ mL} = 5.4 \text{ mL}$

Review Set 47 from pages 339 and 340.

1) 87; 2; 48 **2)** 75; 3; 57 **3)** 120; 3; 22 **4)** 80; 6; 44 **5)** 60; 1; 31; 180 **6)** 2; 23 **7)** 2; 8 **8)** 12; 45 **9)** 7.2; 36.8 **10)** 7.5; 88.5

Solutions—Review Set 47

1) Total volume: 50 mL + 15 mL = 65 mL

$\frac{V}{T} \times C = \frac{65 \cancel{mL}}{\cancel{45}_3 \text{ min}} \times \cancel{60}^4 \text{ gtt}/\cancel{mL} = \frac{260}{3} = 86.6 = 87 \text{ gtt/min}$

$\frac{D}{H} \times Q = \frac{\cancel{60 \text{ mg}}}{\cancel{60 \text{ mg}}} \times 2 \text{ mL} = 2 \text{ mL (medication)}$

Volume IV fluid to add to chamber: 50 mL – 2 mL = 48 mL

4) Total volume: 50 mL + 30 mL = 80 mL

80 mL/60 min = 80 mL/h

$\frac{D}{H} \times Q = \frac{0.6 \cancel{g}}{1 \cancel{g}} \times 10 \text{ mL} = 6 \text{ mL (medication)}$

Volume IV fluid to add to chamber: 50 mL – 6 mL = 44 mL

6) $\frac{50 \text{ mL}}{60 \text{ min}} \times \frac{X \text{ mL}}{30 \text{ min}}$

60X = 1500

$\frac{60X}{60} = \frac{1500}{60}$

X = 25 mL (total volume)

$\frac{D}{H} \times Q = \frac{\cancel{250}^2 \cancel{mg}}{\cancel{125}_1 \cancel{mg}} \times 1 \text{ mL} = 2 \text{ mL (medication)}$

Volume IV fluid to add to chamber:

25 mL – 2 mL = 23 mL

8) $\frac{85 \text{ mL}}{60 \text{ min}} \times \frac{X \text{ mL}}{40 \text{ min}}$

60X = 3400

$\frac{60X}{60} = \frac{3400}{60}$

X = 56.7 = 57 mL (total volume)

$\frac{D}{H} \times Q = \frac{\cancel{600}^{12} \cancel{mg}}{\cancel{50} \cancel{mg}} \times 1 \text{ mL} = 12 \text{ mL (medication)}$

Volume IV fluid to add to chamber:

57 mL – 12 mL = 45 mL

9) $\frac{66 \text{ mL}}{60 \text{ min}} = \frac{X \text{ mL}}{40 \text{ min}}$

$60X = 2640$

$\frac{60X}{60} = \frac{2640}{60}$

$X = 44 \text{ mL (total volume)}$

$\frac{D}{H} \times Q = \frac{720 \text{ mg}}{1000 \text{ mg}} \times 10 \text{ mL} = \frac{720}{100} = 7.2 \text{ mL (medication)}$

Volume IV fluid to add to chamber:
44 mL − 7.2 mL = 36.8 mL

Hint: Add the medication to the volume control chamber, and fill with IV fluid to the 44 mL mark. The chamber measures whole (not fractional) mL.

10) $\frac{48 \text{ mL}}{\text{h}} \times 2 \text{ h} = 96 \text{ mL (total volume)}$

$\frac{D}{H} \times Q = \frac{75 \text{ mg}}{100 \text{ mg}} \times 10 \text{ mL} = 7.5 \text{ mL}$

Volume IV fluid to add to chamber:
96 mL − 7.5 mL = 88.5 mL

Review Set 48 from pages 342 and 343.

1) 5 **2)** 2.5 **3)** 0.3 **4)** 250 **5)** 10 **6)** 19 **7)** 19 **8)** Yes **9)** 4.8; 2.4 **10)** 5.2; 2.6 **11)** 18; 9 **12)** 12.8; 6.4

Solutions—Review Set 48

1) $\frac{20 \text{ mEq}}{1000 \text{ mL}} = \frac{X \text{ mEq}}{250 \text{ mL}}$

$1000X = 5000$

$\frac{1000X}{1000} = \frac{5000}{1000}$

$X = 5 \text{ mEq (per 250 mL)}$

2) $\frac{D}{H} \times Q = \frac{5 \text{ mEq}}{2 \text{ mEq}} \times 1 \text{ mL} = 2.5 \text{ mL}$

3) Total volume: 250 mL (D_5W) + 2.5 mL (KCl) = 252.5 mL

$\frac{5 \text{ mEq}}{252.5 \text{ mL}} = \frac{X \text{ mEq/h}}{15 \text{ mL/h}}$

$252.5 X = 75$

$\frac{252.5X}{252.5} = \frac{75}{252.5}$

$X = 0.29 \text{ mEq/h}$

$X = 0.3 \text{ mEq/h}$

4) $\frac{1000 \text{ mg}}{1000 \text{ mL}} = \frac{X \text{ mg}}{250 \text{ mL}}$

$1000X = 250{,}000$

$\frac{1000X}{1000} = \frac{250{,}000}{1000}$

$X = 250 \text{ mg}$

5) $\frac{D}{H} \times Q = \frac{250 \text{ mg}}{500 \text{ mg}} \times 20 \text{ mL} = \frac{20}{2} = 10 \text{ mL}$

6) Total volume: 250 mL (D_5NS) + 10 mL (aminophylline) = 250 mL

$\frac{250 \text{ mg}}{260 \text{ mL}} = \frac{X \text{ mg/h}}{20 \text{ mL/h}}$

$260X = 5000$

$\frac{260X}{260} = \frac{5000}{260}$

$X = 19 \text{ mg/h}$

7) 1 mg/kg/h × 19 kg = 19 mg/h

9) $\frac{10 \text{ mEq}}{1000 \text{ mL}} = \frac{X \text{mEq}}{480 \text{ mL}}$

$1000X = 4800$

$\frac{1000X}{1000} = \frac{4800}{1000}$

$X = 4.8 \text{ mEq}$

$\frac{D}{H} \times Q = \frac{4.8 \text{ mEq}}{2 \text{ mEq}} \times 1 \text{ mL} = 2.4 \text{ mL}$

Review Set 49 from page 347.

1) 4 **2)** 25 **3)** 67 **4)** 48 **5)** 75 **6)** 15 **7)** 3.5 or 4; 12 **8)** 2.6 or 3; 65 **9)** 2.3 or 3; 35 **10)** 716–955; 8; 24

Hint: The equipment measures whole mL; therefore, round to the next whole mL.

Solutions—Review Set 49

1) $\frac{100 \text{ mg}}{1 \text{ mL}} = \frac{400 \text{ mg}}{X \text{ mL}}$

$100X = 400$

$\frac{100X}{100} = \frac{400}{100}$

$X = 4 \text{ mL}$

3) 100 mL/kg/day × 10 kg = 1000 mL/day for first 10 kg
50 mL/kg/day × 10 kg = 500 mL/day for next 10 kg
20 mL/kg/day × 5 kg = 100 mL/day for remaining 5 kg
1600 mL/day or per 24 h

$\frac{1600 \text{ mL}}{24 \text{ h}} = 66.6 \text{ or } 67 \text{ mL/h}$

4) 100 mL/kg/day × 10 kg = 1000 mL/day for first 10 kg
50 mL/kg/day × 3 kg = 150 mL/day for next 10 kg
1150 mL/day or per 24 h

$\frac{1150 \text{ mL}}{24 \text{ h}} = 47.9 \text{ or } 48 \text{ mL/h}$

5) 77 lb = $\frac{77}{2.2}$ = 35 kg

100 mL/~~kg~~/day × 10 ~~kg~~ = 1000 mL/day for first 10 kg
50 mL/~~kg~~/day × 10 ~~kg~~ = 500 mL/day for next 10 kg
20 mL/~~kg~~/day × 15 ~~kg~~ = 300 mL/day for remaining 15 kg
1800 mL/day or per 24 h

$\frac{1800 \text{ mL}}{24 \text{ h}}$ = 75 mL/h

7) $\frac{100 \text{ mg}}{1 \text{ mL}} = \frac{350 \text{ mg}}{X \text{ mL}}$

100X = 350

$\frac{100X}{100} = \frac{350}{100}$

X = 3.5 or 4 mL (min. dilution volume)

$\frac{30 \text{ mg}}{1 \text{ mL}} = \frac{350 \text{ mg}}{X \text{ mL}}$

30X = 350

$\frac{30X}{30} = \frac{350}{30}$

X = 11.6 or 12 mL (max. dilution volume)

10) 42 lb = $\frac{42}{2.2}$ = 19.09 = 19.1 kg

150 mg/~~kg~~/day × 19.1 ~~kg~~ = 2865 mg/day

$\frac{2865 \text{ mg}}{4 \text{ doses}}$ = 716 mg/dose

200 mg/~~kg~~/day × 19.1 ~~kg~~ = 3820 mg/day

$\frac{3820 \text{ mg}}{4 \text{ doses}}$ = 955 mg/dose

Safe range is 716 – 955 mg/dose. Dosage is safe.

$\frac{D}{H} \times Q = \frac{830 \text{ mg}}{1000 \text{ mg}} \times 10 \text{ mL} = \frac{830}{100} = 8.3$ mL medication

$\frac{63 \text{ mL}}{60 \text{ min}} = \frac{X \text{ mL}}{30 \text{ min}}$

60X = 1890

$\frac{60X}{60} = \frac{1890}{60}$

X = 31.5 or 32 mL (IV fluid per 30 min)

32 mL (total IV fluid) – 8 mL (medication, KCl) =

24 mL (D_5 0.33% NaCl)

Practice Problems—Chapter 15 from pages 348–353.

1) 1.8 **2)** No; consult with the physician or your supervisor before administering any of this drug. **3)** 0.84 **4)** 108 **5)** 2.2 **6)** 350 **7)** 1 of each (1 100-mg capsule + 1 250-mg capsule) **8)** 2,000 **9)** 2.7; No **10)** 83 **11)** 6 **12)** 13 **13)** 1.69 **14)** 1.11 **15)** 0.32 **16)** 1.92 **17)** 1.63 **18)** 0.69 **19)** 1.67 **20)** 0.52 **21)** 560,000 **22)** 1,085; 109 **23)** 1.9–3.8 **24)** 8 **25)** 40 **26)** 60; 25.8 **27)** 58.8 **28)** 70; 43.1 **29)** 22.8 **30)** 10; 33 **31)** 6.2; 37.8 **32)** 10.8; 5.4 **33)** 14; 7 **34)** 3.8; 1.9 **35)** 63 **36)** 75 **37)** 52 **38)** 10 **39)** Yes; 2.75 or 2.8 **40)** 2.8; 32.2 **41)** Yes; 6.2 **42)** 6.2; 16.8 **43)** Yes; 3.3 **44)** 3.3; 21.7 **45)** No; exceeds maximum dose. Do not give dosage ordered. **46)** Consult physician before further action. **47)** 416,667–1,041,667 **48)** Yes; 2.6 **49)** 2.6; 17.4

50) Critical Thinking: Prevention

The nurse made several assumptions in trying to calculate and prepare this chemotherapy quickly. The nurse assumed that the weight notation was the same on the two units without verifying that fact. The recording of the weights as 20/.45 was very confusing. Notice the period before the 45, which later the physician stated was the calculated BSA, 0.45 m^2. Because no unit of measure was identified, it was unclear what those numbers really meant. Never assume; always ask for clarification when notation is unclear. Also, a child who weighs 20 pounds and a child who weighs 45 pounds are quite different in size, yet the nurse failed to notice such a size difference. This nurse, though, is probably not used to discriminating small children's weight differences, but should have realized that weight in lb. is approximately two times weight in kg. Additionally, the actual volume drawn up was probably very small in comparison to most adult dose volumes that this nurse prepares. The amount of 1.6 mL likely seemed reasonable to the nurse. Finally, this is an instance in which the person giving the medication, the physician, prevented a medication error by stopping and thinking what is a reasonable amount for this child and questioning the actual calculation of the dose. Remember, the person who administers the medication is the last point at which a potential error can be avoided.

Solutions—Practice Problems—Chapter 15

2) 66 lb = $\frac{66}{2.2}$ = 30 kg; 5 mg/~~kg~~ × 30 ~~kg~~ = 150 mg; ordered loading dosage exceeds recommended dosage; *not* safe. Hold med and consult with physician.

3) BSA = 0.52 m^2

80 mg/~~m²~~/day × 0.52 ~~m²~~ = 41.6 = 42 mg/day

$\frac{D}{H} \times Q = \frac{42 \text{ mg}}{50 \text{ mg}} \times 1 \text{ mL} = 0.84$ mL

4) BSA = 0.43 m^2

250 mcg/~~m²~~/day × 0.43 ~~m²~~ = 107.5 = 108 mcg/day

6) BSA = 0.7 m^2

0.5 g/~~m²~~ × 0.7 ~~m²~~ = 0.35 g; 0.35 g = 0.35 × 1000 = 350 mg

8) BSA = 0.8 m^2

2500 U/~~m²~~ × 0.8 ~~m²~~ = 2,000 U

9) $\frac{D}{H} \times Q = \frac{2000\,\cancel{U}}{750\,\cancel{U}} \times 1\text{ mL} = 2.66 = 2.7\text{ mL};$

exceeds child maximum IM volume per injection site; give in 2 injections.

12) $BSA = 1.3\text{ m}^2$

$20\text{ mg}/\cancel{m^2} \times 1.3\,\cancel{m^2} = 26\text{ mg}$

$\frac{D}{H} \times Q = \frac{\overset{13}{\cancel{26\text{ mg}}}}{\underset{1}{\cancel{2\text{ mg}}}} \times 1\text{ mL} = 13\text{ mL}$

13) 5 ft 6 in = 66 inches (12 in/ft)

$BSA = \sqrt{\frac{66 \times 136}{3131}} = \sqrt{2.867} = 1.69\text{ m}^2$

15) $BSA = \sqrt{\frac{60 \times 6}{3600}} = \sqrt{0.1} = 0.316 = 0.32\text{ m}^2$

19) 64 in = 64 × 2.5 = 160 cm (1 in = 2.5 cm)

$BSA = \sqrt{\frac{160 \times 63}{3600}} = \sqrt{2.8} = 1.67\text{ m}^2$

22) $500\text{ mg}/\cancel{m^2} \times 2.17\,\cancel{m^2} = 1085\text{ mg}$

$1085\text{ mg} \div 1000 = 1.085 = 1.09\text{ g}$

24) $6\text{ mg}/\cancel{m^2} \times 1.34\,\cancel{m^2} = 8.04 = 8\text{ mg}$

25) $8.04\text{ mg}/\cancel{day} \times 5\,\cancel{days} = 40.2 = 40\text{ mg}$

26)
30 mL IV over 30 min
+30 mL flush over 30 min
60 mL per hour

$\frac{D}{H} \times Q = \frac{420\,\cancel{mg}}{\underset{100}{\cancel{500\,mg}}} \times \overset{1}{\cancel{5}}\text{ mL} = \frac{420}{100} = 4.2\text{ mL medication}$

30 mL total solution − 4.2 mL med. = 25.8 mL D_5NS
Note: Add 4.2 mL med. to Buretol and fill with D_5NS to 30 mL.

27) $4.2\text{ mL}/\cancel{dose} \times 2\,\cancel{doses}/\text{day} = 8.4\text{ mL/day}$; $8.4\text{ mL}/\cancel{day} \times 7\,\cancel{days} = 58.8\text{ mL total}$

28) Total volume: 45 mL IV + 25 mL flush = 70 mL
Flow rate: 70 mL/60 min or 70 mL/h

$\frac{D}{H} \times Q = \frac{285\,\cancel{mg}}{75\,\cancel{mg}} \times 0.5\text{ mL} = 1.9\text{ mL (med.)}$

Volume of IV fluid: 45 mL − 1.9 mL = 43.1 mL

29) $1.9\text{ mL}/\cancel{dose} \times 3\,\cancel{doses}/\text{day} = 5.7\text{ mL/day}$

$5.7\text{ mL}/\cancel{day} \times 4\,\cancel{days} = 22.8\text{ mL total}$

30) $\frac{D}{H} \times Q = \frac{\overset{10}{\cancel{500\text{ mg}}}}{\underset{1}{\cancel{50\text{ mg}}}} \times 1\text{ mL} = 10\text{ mL med}$

$\frac{65\text{ mL}}{60\text{ min}} = \frac{X\text{ mL}}{40\text{ min}}$

$60X = 2600$

$\frac{60X}{60} = \frac{2600}{60}$

$X = 43.3 = 43\text{ mL}$

43 mL total solution − 10 mL med = 33 mL D_5 0.33% NaCl

32) $\frac{30\text{ mEq}}{1000\text{ mL}} = \frac{X\text{ mEq}}{360\text{ mL}}$

$1000X = 10{,}800$

$\frac{1000X}{1000} = \frac{10{,}800}{1000}$

$X = 10.8\text{ mEq}$

$\frac{D}{H} \times Q = \frac{10.8\,\cancel{mEq}}{2\,\cancel{mEq}} \times 1\text{ mL} = 5.4\text{ mL}$

35) $100\text{ mL}/\cancel{kg}/\text{day} \times 10\,\cancel{kg}$ = 1000 mL/day for first 10 kg
$50\text{ mL}/\cancel{kg}/\text{day} \times 10\,\cancel{kg}$ = 500 mL/day for next 10 kg
$20\text{ mL}/\cancel{kg}/\text{day} \times 1\,\cancel{kg}$ = 20 mL/day for remaining 1 kg

1520 mL/day or per 24 h

$\frac{1520\text{ mL}}{24\text{ h}} = 63.3 = 63\text{ mL/h}$

36) 78 lb = 35.45 = 35.5 kg
$100\text{ mL}/\cancel{kg}/\text{day} \times 10\,\cancel{kg}$ = 1000 mL/day for first 10 kg
$50\text{ mL}/\cancel{kg}/\text{day} \times 10\,\cancel{kg}$ = 500 mL/day for next 10 kg
$20\text{ mL}/\cancel{kg}/\text{day} \times 15.5\,\cancel{kg}$ = 310 mL/day for remaining 15.5 kg

1810 mL/day or per 24 h

$\frac{1810\text{ mL}}{24\text{ h}} = 75.4 = 75\text{ mL/h}$

38) 2400 g = 2400 ÷ 100 = 2.4 kg

$100\text{ mL}/\cancel{kg}/\text{day} \times 2.4\,\cancel{kg} = 240\text{ mL/day}$

$\frac{240\text{ mL}}{24\text{ h}} = 10\text{ mL/h}$

39) $100\text{ mg}/\cancel{kg}/\text{day} \times 15\,\cancel{kg} = 1500\text{ mg/day};$

$\frac{1500\text{ mg}}{6\text{ doses}} = 250\text{ mg/dose}$

$125\text{ mg}/\cancel{kg}/\text{day} \times 15\,\cancel{kg} = 1875\text{ mg/day};$

$\frac{1875\text{ mg}}{6\text{ doses}} = 312.5 = 313\text{ mg/dose}$

Dosage is safe; $\frac{D}{H} \times Q = \frac{275\,\cancel{mg}}{\underset{100}{\cancel{1000\,mg}}} \times \overset{1}{\cancel{10}}\text{ mL}$

$= 2.75\text{ mL or }2.8\text{ mL}$

40) IV Fluid Volume:

$\frac{53\text{ mL}}{60\text{ min}} = \frac{X\text{ mL}}{40\text{ min}}$

$60X = 2120$

$\frac{60X}{60} = \frac{2120}{60}$

$X = 35.3 = 35\text{ mL}$

35 mL total − 2.8 mL med. = 32.2 mL D_5 0.45% NaCl

45) $200\text{ mg}/\cancel{kg}/\text{day} \times 9\,\cancel{kg} = 1800\text{ mg/day};$

$\frac{1800\text{ mg}}{6\text{ doses}} = 300\text{ mg/dose}$

$300\text{ mg}/\cancel{kg}/\text{day} \times 9\,\cancel{kg} = 2700\text{ mg/day}$

$\frac{2700\text{ mg}}{6\text{ doses}} = 450\text{ mg/dose}$

Dosage is *not* safe; exceeds maximum safe dosage.

Do not give dosage ordered; consult with physician.

47) 55 lb = $\frac{55}{2.2}$ = 25 kg

100,000 U/~~kg~~/day × 25 ~~kg~~ = 2,500,000 U

$\frac{2,500,000 \text{ U}}{6 \text{ doses}} = 416,667$ U/dose

250,000 U/~~kg~~/day × 25 ~~kg~~ = 6,250,000 U

$\frac{6,250,000 \text{ U}}{6 \text{ doses}} = 1,041,667$ U/dose

48) $\frac{D}{H} \times Q = \frac{525,000 \text{ U}}{200,000 \text{ U}} \times 1 \text{ mL} = 2.62 = 2.6$ mL

49) $\frac{60 \text{ mL}}{60 \text{ min}} = \frac{X \text{ mL}}{20 \text{ min}}$

60X = 1200

$\frac{60X}{60} = \frac{1200}{60}$

X = 20 mL

20 mL total − 2.6 mL med = 17.4 mL D_5NS

Review Set 50 from pages 359 and 360.

1) 40; 24,000; yes. **2)** 14; 26,400; yes. **3)** 10; 12,000; no; consult physician **4)** 60,000; yes; no; consult physician **5)** 3,000; 72,000; no; consult physician **6)** Yes **7)** No; consult physician **8)** Yes **9)** No; consult physician **10)** No; consult physician **11)** 10 **12)** 50

Solutions—Review Set 50

1) $\frac{D}{H} \times Q = \frac{1000 \text{ U/h}}{25,000 \text{ U}} \times 1000 \text{ mL} = \frac{1,000}{25} = 40$ mL/h

or $\frac{25,000 \text{ U}}{1000 \text{ mL}} = \frac{1000 \text{ U/h}}{X \text{ mL/h}}$

25,000X = 1,000,000

$\frac{25,000X}{25,000} = \frac{1,000,000}{25,000}$

X = 40 mL/h

1000 U/~~h~~ × 24 ~~h~~ = 24,000 U

Normal adult heparinizing dosage:

20,000 – 40,000 U/24 h; yes, order is safe.

4) $\frac{D}{H} \times Q = \frac{2500 \text{ U/h}}{40,000 \text{ U}} \times 500 \text{ mL} = \frac{2500}{80} = 31.2 = 31$ mL/h

Setting is accurate for dosage ordered.

2500 U/h × 24 h = 60,000 U

However, the order is not safe. Hold med and consult with physician.

5) $\frac{25,000 \text{ U}}{1000 \text{ mL}} = \frac{X \text{ U/h}}{120 \text{ mL/h}}$

1000X = 3,000,000

$\frac{1000X}{1000} = \frac{3,000,000}{1000}$

X = 3000 U/h

3000 U/~~h~~ × 24 ~~h~~ = 72,000 U. The order is not safe. Hold med and consult physician.

6) $\frac{30,000 \text{ U}}{500 \text{ mL}} = \frac{X \text{ U/h}}{25 \text{ mL/h}}$

500X = 750,000

$\frac{500X}{500} = \frac{750,000}{500}$

X = 1500 U/h

1500 U/~~h~~ × 24 ~~h~~ = 36, 000 U

Order is safe.

9) $\frac{30,000 \text{ U}}{500 \text{ mL}} = \frac{X \text{ U/h}}{96 \text{ mL/h}}$

500X = 2,880,000 U

$\frac{500X}{500} = \frac{2,880,000}{500}$

X = 5760 U/h

5760 U/~~h~~ × 24 ~~h~~ = 138, 240 U

The order is not safe. Hold med and consult with physician.

10) $\frac{10,000 \text{ U}}{1000 \text{ mL}} = \frac{X \text{ U/h}}{80 \text{ mL/h}}$

1000X = 800, 000

$\frac{1000X}{1000} = \frac{800,000}{1000}$

X = 800 mL/h

800 mL/~~h~~ × 24 ~~h~~ = 19, 200 U

The order is too low and is not safe.
Hold med and consult with physician.

11) $\frac{D}{H} \times Q = \frac{10 \text{ U/h}}{500 \text{ U}} \times 500 \text{ mL} = 10$ mL/h or,

$\frac{500 \text{ U}}{500 \text{ mL}} = \frac{10 \text{ U/h}}{X \text{ mL/h}}$

500X = 5000

$\frac{500X}{500} = \frac{5000}{500}$

X = 10 mL/h

Review Set 51 from pages 368 and 369.

1) 120 **2)** 60 **3)** 75 **4)** 24 **5)** 40 **6)** 142 – 568 **7)** 0.14 – 0.57 **8)** Yes **9)** 4 **10)** Yes **11)** 100; 25 **12)** 1 **13)** 0.025 **14)** 25 **15)** Yes

Solutions—Review Set 51

1) $\frac{D}{H} \times Q = \frac{4\ \cancel{\text{mg}}/\text{min}}{\underset{2}{\cancel{2000}}\ \cancel{\text{mg}}} \times \overset{1}{\cancel{1000}}\ \text{mL} = 2\ \text{mL/min}$

Rate: $2\ \text{mL}/\cancel{\text{min}} \times 60\ \cancel{\text{min}}/\text{h} = 120\ \text{mL/h}$

2) $\frac{D}{H} \times Q = \frac{2\ \cancel{\text{mg}}/\text{min}}{\underset{2}{\cancel{500}}\ \cancel{\text{mg}}} \times \overset{1}{\cancel{250}}\ \text{mL} = 1\ \text{mL/min}$

Rate: $1\ \text{mL}/\cancel{\text{min}} \times 60\ \cancel{\text{min}}/\text{h} = 60\ \text{mL/h}$

3) $\frac{5\ \cancel{\text{mcg}}/\text{min}}{\underset{4}{\cancel{2000}}\ \cancel{\text{mcg}}} \times \overset{1}{\cancel{500}}\ \text{mL} = 1.25\ \text{mL/min}$

Rate: $1.25\ \text{mL}/\cancel{\text{min}} \times 60\ \cancel{\text{min}}/\text{h} = 75\ \text{mL/h}$

4) $198\ \text{lb} = \frac{198}{2.2} = 90\ \text{kg}$; $4\ \text{mcg}/\cancel{\text{kg}}/\text{min} \times 90\ \cancel{\text{kg}} = 360\ \text{mcg/min}$

$360\ \text{mcg/min} = 360 \div 1000 = 0.36\ \text{mg/min}$

$\frac{D}{H} \times Q = \frac{0.36\ \cancel{\text{mg}}/\text{min}}{\underset{9}{\cancel{450}}\ \cancel{\text{mg}}} \times \overset{10}{\cancel{500}}\ \text{mL} = \frac{3.6}{9} = 0.4\ \text{mL/min}$

Rate: $0.4\ \text{mL}/\cancel{\text{min}} \times 60\ \cancel{\text{min}}/\text{h} = 24\ \text{mL/h}$

5) $15\ \text{mcg}/\cancel{\text{kg}}/\text{min} \times 70\ \cancel{\text{kg}} = 1050\ \text{mcg/min}$

$1050\ \text{mcg/min} = 1050 \div 1000 = 1.05\ \text{mg/min}$

$\frac{1.05\ \cancel{\text{mg}}/\text{min}}{\underset{8}{\cancel{800}}\ \cancel{\text{mg}}} \times \overset{5}{\cancel{500}}\ \text{mL} = \frac{5.25}{8} = 0.656 = 0.66\ \text{mL/min}$

Rate: $0.66\ \text{mL}/\cancel{\text{min}} \times 60\ \cancel{\text{min}}/\text{h} = 39.6 = 40\ \text{mL/h}$

6) $125\ \text{lb} = \frac{125}{2.2} = 56.81 = 56.8\ \text{kg}$

$2.5\ \text{mcg}/\cancel{\text{kg}}/\text{min} \times 56.8\ \cancel{\text{kg}} = 142\ \text{mcg/min}$

$10\ \text{mcg}/\cancel{\text{kg}}/\text{min} \times 56.8\ \cancel{\text{kg}} = 568\ \text{mcg/min}$

7) $142\ \text{mcg/min} = 142 \div 1000 = 0.14\ \text{mg/min}$

$568\ \text{mcg/min} = 568 \div 1000 = 0.57\ \text{mg/min}$

8) $\frac{500\ \text{mg}}{500\ \text{mL}} = \frac{X\ \text{mg/h}}{15\ \text{mL/h}}$

$500X = 7500$

$\frac{500X}{500} = \frac{7500}{500}$

$X = 15\ \text{mg/h}$

$\frac{15\ \text{mg/h}}{60\ \text{min/h}} = 0.25\ \text{mg/min}$

Yes, the order is within the safe range.

9) $\frac{2000\ \text{mg}}{500\ \text{mL}} = \frac{X\ \text{mg/h}}{60\ \text{mL/h}}$

$500X = 120,000$

$\frac{500X}{500} = \frac{120,000}{500}$

$X = 240\ \text{mg/h}$

$\frac{240\ \text{mg}/\cancel{\text{h}}}{60\ \text{min}/\cancel{\text{h}}} = 4\ \text{mg/min}$

10) Yes, 4 mg/min is within the normal range of 2–6 mg/min.

11) Bolus:

$\frac{2\ \text{g}}{30\ \text{min}} = \frac{X\ \text{g}}{60\ \text{min}}$

$30\ X = 120$

$X = 4\ \text{g}$ (per 60 min or 4 g/h)

$\frac{20\ \text{g}}{500\ \text{mL}} = \frac{4\ \text{g/h}}{X\ \text{mL/h}}$

$20\ X = 2000$

$\frac{20\ X}{20} = \frac{2000}{20}$

$X = 100\ \text{mL/h}$

Continuous:

$\frac{20\ \text{g}}{500\ \text{mL}} = \frac{1\ \text{g/h}}{X\ \text{mL/h}}$

$20\ X = 500$

$\frac{20\ X}{20} = \frac{500}{20}$

$X = 25\ \text{mL/h}$

12) $1\ \text{mU} = 1 \div 1000 = 0.001\ \text{U}$

$\frac{D}{H} \times Q = \frac{0.001\ \cancel{\text{U}}/\text{min}}{15\ \cancel{\text{U}}} \times 250\ \text{mL} = 0.017\ \text{mL/min}$

$0.017\ \text{mL}/\cancel{\text{min}} \times 60\ \cancel{\text{min}}/\text{h} = 1.02 = 1\ \text{mL/h}$

13) $\frac{10\ \text{mg}}{1000\ \text{mL}} = \frac{X\ \text{mg/h}}{150\ \text{mL/h}}$

$1000X = 1500$

$\frac{1000X}{1000} = \frac{1500}{1000}$

$X = 1.5\ \text{mg/h}$

$\frac{1.5\ \text{mg}}{60\ \text{min}} = \frac{X\ \text{mg}}{1\ \text{min}}$

$60X = 1.5$

$\frac{60X}{60} = \frac{1.5}{60}$

$X = 0.025\ \text{mg/min}$

14) $0.025\ \text{mg/min} = 0.025 \times 1000 = 25\ \text{mcg/min}$

Review Set 52 from pages 372 and 373.

1) 33; 19 **2)** 40; 42 **3)** 25; 32 **4)** 50; 90 **5)** 50; 40 **6)** 100; 100 **7)** 200; 76 **8)** 200; 122 **9)** 17; 21 **10)** 120; 112

Solutions—Review Set 52

1) Step 1. IV PB rate : $\frac{V}{T} \times C = \frac{100 \text{ mL}}{30 \text{ min}} \times 10 \text{ gtt/mL} = \frac{100}{3} = 33.3 = 33 \text{ gtt/min}$

Step 2. Total IV PB time: q.4 h × 30 min = 6 × 30 min = 180 min = 3 h

Step 3. Total IV PB volume: 6 × 100 mL = 600 mL

Step 4. Total Regular IV volume: 3000 mL – 600 mL = 2400 mL

Step 5. Total Regular IV time: 24 h – 3 h = 21 h

Step 6. Regular IV rate: $\frac{\text{mL / h}}{\text{drop factor constant}} = \text{gtt/min}$

$\frac{2400 \text{ mL}}{21 \text{ h}} = 114 \text{ mL/h}$

$\frac{114}{6} \text{ mL/h} = 19 \text{ gtt/min}$

2) Step 1. IV PB rate: When drop factor is 60 gtt/mL, then mL/h = gtt/min. Rate is 40 gtt/min.

Step 2. Total IV PB time: q.i.d. × 1 h = 4 × 1 h = 4 h

Step 3. Total IV PB volume: 4 × 40 mL = 160 mL

Step 4. Total Regular IV volume: 1000 mL – 160 mL = 840 mL

Step 5. Total Regular IV time: 24 h – 4 h = 20 h

Step 6. Total Regular IV rate: mL/h = $\frac{840 \text{ mL}}{20 \text{ h}}$ = 42 mL/h. When drop factor is 60 gtt/mL, then mL/h = gtt/min. Rate is 42 gtt/min.

3) Step 1. IV PB rate: $\frac{V}{T} \times C = \frac{50 \text{ mL}}{30 \text{ min}} \times 15 \text{ gtt/mL} = \frac{50}{2} = 25 \text{ gtt/min}$

Step 2. Total IV PB time: q.6 h × 30 min = 4 × 30 min = 120 min = 2 h

Step 3. Total IV PB volume: 4 × 50 mL = 200 mL

Step 4. Total Regular IV volume: 3000 mL – 200 mL = 2800 mL

Step 5. Total Regular IV time: 24 h – 2 h = 22 h

Step 6. Regular IV rate: $\frac{\text{mL / h}}{\text{drop factor constant}} = \text{gtt/min}$

$\frac{2800 \text{ mL}}{22 \text{ h}} = 127 \text{ mL/h}$

$\frac{127}{4} = 31.7 = 32 \text{ gtt/min}$

4) Step 1. IV PB rate: 50 mL/h or 50 gtt/min (because drop factor is 60 gtt/mL)

Step 2. Total IV PB time: q.6 h × 1 h = 4 × 1 h = 4 h

Step 3. Total IV PB volume: 4 × 50 mL = 200 mL

Step 4. Total Regular IV volume: 2000 mL – 200 mL = 1800 mL

Step 5. Total Regular IV time: 24 h – 4 h = 20 h

Step 6. Regular IV rate: $\frac{1800 \text{ mL}}{20 \text{ h}}$ = 90 mL/h or 90 gtt/min (because drop factor is 60 gtt/mL)

5) Step 1. IV PB rate: 50 mL/h or 50 gtt/min (because drop factor is 60 gtt/mL)

Step 2. IV PB time: q.8 h × 1 h = 3 × 1 h = 3 h

Step 3. IV PB volume: 3 × 50 mL = 150 mL

Step 4. Total Regular IV volume: 1000 mL – 150 mL = 850 mL

Step 5. Total Regular IV time: 24 h – 3 h = 21 h

Step 6. Regular IV rate: $\frac{850}{21}$ = 40.4 mL/h = 40 gtt/min (because drop factor is 60 gtt/mL)

6) Step 1. IV PB rate:

$$\frac{50 \text{ mL}}{30 \text{ min}} = \frac{X \text{ mL}}{60 \text{ min}}$$

$$30X = 3000$$

$$\frac{30X}{30} = \frac{3000}{30}$$

$$X = 100 \text{ mL; } 100 \text{ mL/60 min} = 100 \text{ mL/h}$$

Step 2. IV PB time: q.6 h × 30 min = 4 × 30 min = 120 min = 2 h

Step 3. IV PB volume: 4 × 50 mL = 200 mL

Step 4. Total Regular IV volume: 2400 mL – 200 mL = 2200 mL

Step 5. Total Regular IV time: 24 h – 2 h = 22 h

Step 6. Regular IV rate: $\frac{2200 \text{ mL}}{22 \text{ h}} = 100 \text{ mL/h}$

7) Step 1. IV PB rate:

$$\frac{100 \text{ mL}}{30 \text{ min}} = \frac{X \text{ mL}}{60 \text{ min}}$$

$$30X = 6000$$

$$X = 200 \text{ mL; } 200 \text{ mL/60 min} = 200 \text{ mL/h}$$

Step 2. IV PB time: q.8 h × 30 min = 3 × 30 min = 90 min = $1\frac{1}{2}$ h

Step 3. IV PB volume: 3 × 100 mL = 300 mL

Step 4. Total Regular IV volume: 2000 mL – 300 mL = 1700 mL

Step 5. Total Regular IV time: 24 h – $1\frac{1}{2}$ h = $22\frac{1}{2}$ h

Step 6. Regular IV rate: $\frac{1700 \text{ mL}}{22.5 \text{ h}} = 75.5 = 76 \text{ mL/h}$

8) Step 1. IV PB rate

$$\frac{50 \text{ mL}}{15 \text{ min}} = \frac{X \text{ mL}}{60 \text{ min}}$$

$$15X = 3000$$

$$\frac{15X}{15} = \frac{3000}{15}$$

$$X = 200 \text{ mL; } 200 \text{ mL/60 min} = 200 \text{ mL/h}$$

Step 2. IV PB time: q.6 h × 15 min = 4 × 15 min = 60 min = 1 h

Step 3. IV PB volume: 4 × 50 mL = 200 mL

Step 4. Total Regular IV volume: 3000 mL – 200 mL = 2800 mL

Step 5. Total Regular IV time: 24 h – 1 h = 23 h

Step 6. Regular IV rate: $\frac{2800 \text{ mL}}{23 \text{ h}} = 121.7 = 122 \text{ mL/h}$

Practice Problems—Chapter 16 from pages 375–378.

1) 60 **2)** 5 **3)** 20 **4)** 50 **5)** 1 **6)** 12; 28,800; Yes **7)** 15 **8)** 63 **9)** 4000; No **10)** 6; 15 **11)** 60 **12)** 45 **13)** 60 **14)** 24 **15)** Yes **16)** 17; 22 **17)** 100; 127 **18)** 102 **19)** 8 mEq **20)** 2 **21)** 1; 40 **22)** 1932 **23)** 1536 **24)** 15 **25)** 50; 50 **26)** 75; No **27)** 7.4 **28)** 12; 18 **29)** 150; 50 **30)** 2 **31)** 35; Yes **32)** 1500; yes **33)** 8 **34)** 63 **35)** 80 **36)** 0.4 **37)** 4 **38)** 4 **39)** 200 **40)** 100 **41)** 0.2; 200 **42)** 30 **43)** 200; 50 **44)** 5 **45)** 550 **46)** 2450 **47)** 19 **48)** 129 **49)** 13; 39

50) Critical Thinking Skill: Prevention.

The nurse who prepares any IV solution with an additive should *carefully* compare the order and medication 3 times: before beginning to prepare the dose, after the dosage is prepared, and just before it is administered to the patient. Further, the nurse should verify the safety of the dosage using the 3 step method (convert, think, and calculate). It was clear that the nurse realized the error when a colleague questioned what was being prepared and the nurse verified the actual order. Also taking the time to do the calculation on paper helps the nurse to "see" the answer and avoid a potentially life-threatening error.

Solutions—Practice Problems—Chapter 16

1) Volume control sets are microdrip infusion sets calibrated for 60 gtt/mL.

3) $\frac{50 \text{ mL}}{60 \text{ min}} = \frac{X \text{ mL}}{30 \text{ min}}$

$60X = 1500$

$\frac{60X}{60} = \frac{1500}{60}$

$X = 25$ mL total volume

25 mL total – 5 mL med = 20 mL D_5W

4) $\frac{\text{mL / h}}{\text{drop factor constant}} = \frac{50 \text{ mL/h}}{1} = 50$ gtt/min;

when drop factor is 60 gtt/mL, then mL/h = gtt/min.

5) once at 1200 hours

6) $\frac{D}{H} \times Q = \frac{1200\ \cancel{\text{U}}/\text{h}}{\underset{100}{\cancel{25{,}000}\ \cancel{\text{U}}}} \times \overset{1}{\cancel{250}} \text{ mL} = \frac{1200}{100} = 12$ mL/h or,

$\frac{25{,}000 \text{ U}}{250 \text{ mL}} = \frac{1200 \text{ U/h}}{X \text{ mL/h}}$

$25{,}000X = 300{,}000$

$\frac{25{,}000X}{25{,}000} = \frac{300{,}000}{25{,}000}$

$X = 12$ mL/h

$1200 \text{ U}/\cancel{\text{h}} \times 24\ \cancel{\text{h}} = 28{,}800$ U

This is within normal range of 20,000–40,000 U/24 h.

7) $\frac{D}{H} \times Q = \frac{30\ \cancel{\text{mg}}/\text{h}}{\underset{2}{\cancel{500}\ \cancel{\text{mg}}}} \times \overset{1}{\cancel{250}} \text{ mL} = \frac{30}{2} = 15$ mL/h or,

$\frac{500 \text{ mg}}{250 \text{ mL}} = \frac{30 \text{ mg/h}}{X \text{ mL/h}}$

$500X = 7500$

$\frac{500X}{500} = \frac{7500}{500}$

$X = 15$ mL/h

8) $\frac{D}{H} \times Q = \frac{500\ \cancel{\text{mg}}/\text{h}}{\underset{8}{\cancel{4000}\ \cancel{\text{mg}}}} \times \overset{1}{\cancel{500}} \text{ mL} = 62.5 = 63$ mL/h or

$\frac{4000 \text{ mg}}{500 \text{ mL}} = \frac{500 \text{ mg/h}}{X \text{ mL/h}}$

$4000X = 250{,}000$

$\frac{4000X}{4000} = \frac{250{,}000}{4000}$

$X = 62.5 = 63$ mL/h

9) $\frac{40{,}000 \text{ U}}{1000 \text{ mL}} = \frac{X \text{ U/h}}{100 \text{ mL/h}}$

$1000X = 4{,}000{,}000$

$\frac{1000X}{1000} = \frac{4{,}000{,}000}{1000}$

$X = 4000$ U/h

$4000 \text{ U}/\cancel{\text{h}} \times 24\ \cancel{\text{h}} = 96{,}000$ U

Normal range is 20,000–40,000 U/24 h.

Dosage is too high.

10) 1.5 L = 1500 mL

$\frac{1500\ \cancel{\text{mL}}}{4\ \cancel{\text{mL}}/\text{min}} = 375$ min

375 min ÷ 60 min/h = 6.25 h = $6\frac{1}{4}$ h = 6 h 15 min

11) $\frac{D}{H} \times Q = \frac{4\ \cancel{\text{mg}}/\text{min}}{\underset{4}{\cancel{2000}\ \cancel{\text{mg}}}} \times \overset{1}{\cancel{500}} \text{ mL} = \frac{4}{4} = 1$ mL/min, which is the same as 60 mL/60 min or 60 mL/h.

12) $\frac{D}{H} \times Q = \frac{3\ \cancel{\text{mg}}/\text{min}}{\underset{4}{\cancel{1000}\ \cancel{\text{mg}}}} \times \overset{1}{\cancel{250}} \text{ mL} = \frac{3}{4} = 0.75$ mL/min

$0.75 \text{ mL}/\cancel{\text{min}} \times 60\ \cancel{\text{min}}/\text{h} = 45$ mL/h

13) $\frac{D}{H} \times Q = \frac{2\ \cancel{\text{mg}}/\text{min}}{\underset{2}{\cancel{1000}\ \cancel{\text{mg}}}} \times \overset{1}{\cancel{500}} \text{ mL} = \frac{2}{2} = 1$ mL/min which is the same as 60 mL/60 min or 60 mL/h.

14) $5 \text{ mcg}/\cancel{\text{kg}}/\text{min} \times 80\ \cancel{\text{kg}} = 400$ mcg/min

400 mcg/min = 400 ÷ 1000 = 0.4 mg/min

$\frac{D}{H} \times Q = \frac{0.4\ \cancel{\text{mg}}/\text{min}}{\underset{1}{\cancel{250}\ \cancel{\text{mg}}}} \times \overset{1}{\cancel{250}} \text{ mL} = 0.4$ mL/min

$0.4 \text{ mL}/\cancel{\text{min}} \times 60\ \cancel{\text{min}}/\text{h} = 24$ mL/h

15) $\frac{2000 \text{ mg}}{1000 \text{ mL}} = \frac{X \text{ mg/h}}{75 \text{ mL/h}}$

$1000X = 150{,}000$

$\frac{1000X}{1000} = \frac{150{,}000}{1000}$

$X = 150$ mg/h

$150 \text{ mg}/\cancel{\text{h}} \div 60 \text{ min}/\cancel{\text{h}} = 2.5$ mg/min,

within normal range of 1–4 mg/min

16) IV PB flow rate: $\frac{\text{mL / h}}{\text{drop factor constant}} = \frac{100 \text{ mL/h}}{6} =$

16.6 = 17 gtt/min

Total IV PB time: q.6 h × 1 h = 4 × 1 h = 4 h

Total IV PB volume: 4 × 100 mL = 400 mL

Total Regular IV volume: 3000 mL – 400 mL = 2600 mL

Total Regular IV time: 24 h – 4 h = 20 h

Regular IV rate: mL/h = $\frac{2600 \text{ mL}}{20 \text{ h}} = 130$ mL/h;

$\frac{\text{mL / h}}{\text{drop factor constant}} = \frac{130 \text{ mL/h}}{6} = 21.6 = 22$ gtt/min

17) IV PB Rate: $\frac{50 \text{ mL}}{30 \text{ min}} = \frac{X \text{ mL}}{60 \text{ min}}$

$30X = 3000$

$\frac{30X}{30} = \frac{3000}{30}$

$X = 100$ mL; 100 mL/60 min = 100 mL/h

Total IV PB time: q.i.d. × 30 min = 4 × 30 min = 120 min = 2 h

Total IV PB volume: 4 × 50 mL = 200 mL

Total regular IV volume: 3000 mL − 200 mL = 2800 mL

Total regular IV time: 24 h − 2 h = 22 h

Regular IV rate: $\frac{2800 \text{ mL}}{22 \text{ h}} = 127.2 = 127$ mL/h

18) 125 lb = $\frac{125}{2.2} = 56.81 = 56.8$ kg;

3 mcg/~~kg~~/min × 56.8 ~~kg~~ = 170.4 mcg/min

170.4 mcg/min = 170.4 ÷ 1000 = 0.17 mg/min

$\frac{D}{H} \times Q = \frac{0.17 \text{ mg/min}}{50 \text{ mg}_{1}} \times 500^{10} \text{ mL} = 1.7 \text{ mL/min}$

1.7 mL/~~min~~ × 60 ~~min~~/h = 102 mL/h

19) 1000 mL − 800 mL = 200 mL infused

$\frac{40 \text{ mEq}}{1000 \text{ mL}} = \frac{X \text{ mEq}}{200 \text{ mL}}$

$1000X = 8000$

$\frac{1000X}{1000} = \frac{8000}{1000}$

$X = 8$ mEq

20) $\frac{125 \text{ mL}}{60 \text{ min}} = 2.1 \text{ mL/min} = 2 \text{ mL/min}$

21) $\frac{V}{T} \times C = \frac{250 \text{ mL}}{T \text{ min}} \times 10 \text{ gtt/mL} = 25 \text{ gtt/min}$

$\frac{2500}{T} = \frac{25}{1}$

$25T = 2500$

$\frac{25T}{25} = \frac{2500}{25}$

$T = 100$ min

$\frac{100 \text{ min}}{60 \text{ min/h}} = 1.67 \text{ h} = 1\frac{2}{3} \text{ h} = 1$ h 40 min remaining

22) $\frac{100 \text{ mL}}{T \text{ min}} \times 60 \text{ gtt/mL} = 33 \text{ gtt/min}$

$\frac{6000}{T} = \frac{33}{1}$

$33T = 6000$

$\frac{33T}{33} = \frac{6000}{33}$

$T = 181.8 = 182$ min = 3 h 2 min or 0302 hours

1630 hours + 0302 hours = 1932 hours

23) $\frac{V}{T} \times C = \frac{V \text{ mL}}{480 \text{ min}} \times 15 \text{ gtt/mL} = 48 \text{ gtt/min}$

$\frac{15V}{480} = \frac{48}{1}$

$15V = 23{,}040$

$\frac{15V}{15} = \frac{23{,}040}{15}$

$V = 1536$ mL

24) $\frac{1500 \text{ mL}}{100 \text{ mL/h}} = 15$ h

25) $\frac{D}{H} \times Q = \frac{2 \text{ mEq/h}}{40 \text{ mEq}_{1}} \times 1000^{25} \text{ mL} = 50$ mL/h or

50 gtt/min, (because drop factor is 60 gtt/mL) or,

$\frac{40 \text{ mEq}}{1000 \text{ mL}} = \frac{2 \text{ mEq/h}}{X \text{ ml/h}}$

$40X = 2000$

$X = 50$ mL/h or 50 gtt/min

(because drop factor is 60 gtt/mL)

26) $\frac{D}{H} \times Q = \frac{3750 \text{ U/h}}{50{,}000 \text{ U}_{50}} \times 1000^{1} \text{ mL} = \frac{3750}{50} = 75$ mL/h or,

$\frac{50{,}000 \text{ U}}{1000 \text{ mL}} = \frac{3750 \text{ U/h}}{X \text{ mL/h}}$

$50{,}000X = 3{,}750{,}000$

$\frac{50{,}000X}{50{,}000} = \frac{3{,}750{,}000}{50{,}000}$

$X = 75$ mL/h

3750 U/~~h~~ × 24 ~~h~~ = 90,000 U

No; safe range is 20,000–40,000 U/24 h; dosage is too high.

27) $\frac{5 \text{ mg}}{1 \text{ mL}} = \frac{37 \text{ mg}}{X \text{ mL}}$

$5X = 37$

$\frac{5X}{5} = \frac{37}{5}$

$X = 7.4$ mL

28) 10 U = 10 × 1000 = 10,000 mU

$\frac{D}{H} \times Q = \frac{4 \text{ mU/min}}{10{,}000 \text{ mU}_{20}} \times 500^{1} \text{ mL} = \frac{4}{20} =$

0.2 mL/min for first 20 min

0.2 mL/~~min~~ × 60 ~~min~~/h = 12 mL/h

$\frac{D}{H} \times Q = \frac{6 \text{ mU/min}}{10{,}000 \text{ mU}_{20}} \times 500^{1} \text{ mL} = \frac{6}{20} =$

0.3 mL/min for next 20 min

0.3 mL/~~min~~ × 60 ~~min~~/h = 18 mL/h

29) Bolus:

$$\frac{3\text{ g}}{30\text{ min}} = \frac{X\text{ g}}{60\text{ min}}$$

$$\frac{30X}{30} = \frac{180}{30}$$

$X = 6$ g

6 g/60 min = 6 g/h

$$\frac{D}{H} \times Q = \frac{6\,\cancel{g}/h}{\underset{1}{\cancel{20}\,\cancel{g}}} \times \overset{25}{\cancel{500}}\text{mL} = 150\text{ mL/h}$$

Continuous infusion:

$$\frac{D}{H} \times Q = \frac{2\,\cancel{g}/h}{\underset{1}{\cancel{20}\,\cancel{g}}} \times \overset{25}{\cancel{500}}\text{mL} = 50\text{ mL/h}$$

33) $\dfrac{\overset{8}{\cancel{4000}}\text{ mg}}{\underset{1}{\cancel{500}}\text{ mL}} = 8$ mg/mL

34) $\dfrac{D}{H} \times Q = \dfrac{500\,\cancel{mg}/h}{\underset{8}{\cancel{4000}\,\cancel{mg}}} \times \overset{1}{\cancel{500}}\text{mL} = \dfrac{500}{8} = 62.5\text{ mL/h} = 63\text{ mL/h}$

35) 1 U = 1,000 mU

80 U = 8,000 mU

$\dfrac{\overset{80}{\cancel{80,000}}\text{ mU}}{\underset{1}{\cancel{1000}}\text{ mL}} = 80$ mU/mL

37) 1 mg = 1, 000 mcg

4 mg = 4, 000 mcg

$\dfrac{\overset{4}{\cancel{4000}}\text{ mcg}}{\underset{1}{\cancel{1000}}\text{ mL}} = 4$ mcg/mL

41) $\dfrac{\overset{2}{\cancel{20}}\text{ mg}}{\underset{10}{\cancel{100}}\text{ mL}} = \dfrac{2}{10} = 0.2$ mg/mL

0.2 mg/mL = 0.2 × 1000 = 200 mcg/mL

42) 1 mcg/$\cancel{kg}$/min × 100 $\cancel{kg}$ = 100 mcg/min

$$\frac{D}{H} \times Q = \frac{100\,\cancel{mcg}/\text{min}}{\underset{200}{\cancel{20,000}\,\cancel{mcg}}} \times \overset{1}{\cancel{100}}\text{ mL} = \frac{100}{200} = 0.5\text{ mL/min}$$

0.5 mL/$\cancel{min}$ × 60 $\cancel{min}$ = 30 mL/h

43) IV PB rates:

$$\frac{100\text{ mL}}{30\text{ min}} = \frac{X\text{ mL}}{60\text{ min}}$$

30X = 6000

$$\frac{30X}{30} = \frac{6000}{30}$$

X = 200 mL

200 mL/60 min = 200 mL/h ampicillin

Gentamycin is 50 mL/h.

44) Ampicillin: q.6 h × 30 min = 4 × 30 min = 120 min = 2 h

Gentamycin: q.8 h × 1 h = 3 × 1 h = 3 h

Total IV PB time: 2 h + 3 h = 5 h

45) Ampicillin: 4 $\cancel{doses}$ × 100 mL/$\cancel{dose}$ = 400 mL

Gentamycin: 3 $\cancel{doses}$ × 50 mL/$\cancel{dose}$ = 150 mL

Total IV PB volume: 400 mL + 150 mL = 550 mL

46) 3000 mL – 550 mL = 2,450 mL

47) 24 h – 5 h = 19 h

48) $\dfrac{2,450\text{ mL}}{19\text{ h}} = 128.9 = 129$ mL/h

49) 190 lb = $\frac{190}{2.2}$ = 86.36 = 86.4 kg

4 mcg/$\cancel{kg}$/min × 86.4 $\cancel{kg}$ = 345.6 mcg/min

345.6 mcg/$\cancel{min}$ × 60 $\cancel{min}$/h = 20,736 mcg/h =

20,736 mcg/h = 20,736 ÷ 1000 = 21 mg/h

$$\frac{D}{H} \times Q = \frac{21\,\cancel{mg}/h}{\underset{8}{\cancel{800}\,\cancel{mg}}} \times \overset{5}{\cancel{500}}\text{ mL} = \frac{105}{8} =$$

13.1 = 13 mL/h initial rate

12 mcg/kg/min × 86.4 kg = 1036.8 mcg/min

1036.8 mcg/$\cancel{min}$ × 60 $\cancel{min}$/h = 62,208 mcg/h

62,208 mcg/h = 62,208 ÷ 1000 = 62 mg/h

$$\frac{D}{H} \times Q = \frac{62\,\cancel{mg}/h}{\underset{8}{800\,\cancel{mg}}} \times \overset{5}{\cancel{500}}\text{ mL} = \frac{310}{8} =$$

38.7 = 39 mL/h after titration

Section 4—Self-Evaluation from pages 379–383

1) 120 **2)** 240 **3)** 20 **4)** 120 **5)** $1\frac{1}{2}$ **6)** 1 **7)** 32 **8)** 3 **9)** 540 **10)** Add 1 tsp table salt to 1 pint or 2 cups warm water. **11)** Isotonic **12)** Hypertonic **13)** Hypotonic **14)** 50 **15)** 3.3 **16)** 2.25 **17)** 75 **18)** 6.75 **19)** mL/h **20)** 21 **21)** 83 **22)** 1940 **23)** 1536 **24)** Give a total of 3000 mL IV solution per day to include 5% normal saline (0.9% NaCl) with 20 milliequivalents of potassium chloride added per liter (1000 mL) *and* a piggyback IV solution of 250 mg Kefzol added to 100 mL of normal saline (0.9% NaCl) every 8 hours. To administer the order each day, give 900 mL NS with KCl over $7\frac{1}{2}$ hours × 3 administrations and 100 mL NS with Kefzol over $\frac{1}{2}$ hour × 3 administrations. **25)** 120 **26)** 200 **27)** Reset rate to 118 gtt/min. **28)** 2.5 **29)** 59 **30)** 5 **31)** 0.48 **32)** 1.30 **33)** 0.5 **34)** 18.5–37.5 **35)** Yes; 18.5 **36)** 120 **37)** 18.5 **38)** Yes; 1.6 **39)** 18; 2 **40)** 7.5 **41)** No; under dosage. Consult physician **42)** 43 **43)** 200 **44)** 43; 200 **45)** 50 **46)** 12 **47)** 8 **48)** 80 **49)** 14 **50)** 41

Solutions—Section 4—Self-Evaluation

1) $\frac{1}{3}$ strength = $\dfrac{\text{1 part solute}}{\text{3 parts total solution}}$

$D \times Q = \frac{1}{3} \times 360 = \frac{360}{3} = 120$ mL solute

2) 360 mL (total solution volume) – 120 mL (solute) = 240 mL (solvent)

3) $D \times Q = X$

$\frac{3}{4} \times Q = 60 \text{ mL}$

$\frac{3}{4} Q = 60 \text{ mL}$

$$\frac{\frac{3}{4}Q}{\frac{3}{4}} = \frac{60}{\frac{3}{4}}$$

$$Q = \overset{20}{\cancel{60}} \times \frac{4}{\underset{1}{\cancel{3}}}$$

$Q = 80$ mL (total solution volume)

$80 \text{ mL} - 60 \text{ mL} = 20 \text{ mL}$ (solvent, normal saline)

4) $8 \text{ oz} = 8 \times 30 = 240 \text{ mL}$ (℥i = 30 mL)

$D \times Q = X$

$\frac{2}{3} \times Q = 240 \text{ mL}$

$\frac{2}{3} Q = 240 \text{ mL}$

$$\frac{\frac{2}{3}Q}{\frac{2}{3}} = \frac{240}{\frac{2}{3}}$$

$$Q = \overset{120}{\cancel{240}} \times \frac{3}{\underset{1}{\cancel{2}}} = 360 \text{ mL}$$

$360 \text{ mL} - 240 \text{ mL} = 120 \text{ mL}$ (solvent, sterile water)

5) $360 \cancel{\text{mL}} \div 240 \cancel{\text{mL}}\text{/feeding} = \frac{360}{240} = 1\frac{1}{2}$ feedings

6) $26 \text{ mL}/\cancel{\text{feeding}} \times 8 \cancel{\text{feedings}} = 208$ mL (total volume)

$$D \times Q = \frac{3}{\underset{1}{\cancel{8}}} \times \overset{26}{\cancel{208}} \text{ mL} = 78 \text{ mL (solute)}$$

$3 \text{ oz} = 3 \times 30 \text{ mL} = 90$ mL (Enfamil)

You will need 1 bottle of Enfamil.

7) $\frac{3}{8}$ strength $= \frac{\text{3 parts solute}}{\text{8 parts total solution}}$; with 5 parts solvent.

Using a 3 oz Enfamil (3 parts) + 5 oz water (5 parts) = 8 oz of $\frac{3}{8}$ strength formula;

$8 \cancel{\text{oz}} \times 30 \text{ mL}/\cancel{\text{oz}} =$ 240 mL (total sol. vol.)
− 208 mL (total feedings)
32 mL (unused reconstituted formula)

8) 9 infants require 4 oz each = $4 \text{ oz} \times 9 = 36$ oz (total)

$$D \times Q = \frac{1}{\underset{1}{\cancel{2}}} \times \overset{18}{\cancel{36}} \text{ oz} = 18 \text{ oz (Isomil)}$$

$\frac{18 \cancel{\text{oz}}}{8 \cancel{\text{oz}}\text{/can}} = \frac{18}{8} = 2\frac{1}{4}$ cans (needed for reconstitution therefore you need to open 3 cans)

9) 36 oz (total solution) − 18 oz (solute) = 18 oz (solvent or water). $18 \text{ oz} = 18 \times 30 = 540$ mL (water)

10) NS = 0.9% = 0.9 g NaCl/100 mL

$$\frac{0.9 \text{ g}}{100 \text{ mL}} = \frac{X \text{ g}}{500 \text{ mL}}$$

$100X = 450$

$$\frac{100X}{100} = \frac{450}{100}$$

$X = 4.5$ g; to make salt water, 4.5 g = 4.5 mL or 5 mL = 1 tsp table salt

Add 1 tsp. salt to 1 pint or 2 cups of water.

14) 5% dextrose = 5 g dextrose/100 mL

$$\frac{5 \text{ g}}{100 \text{ mL}} = \frac{X \text{ g}}{1000 \text{ mL}}$$

$100X = 5000$

$$\frac{100X}{100} = \frac{5000}{100}$$

$X = 50$ g

15) 0.33% = 0.33 g/100 mL

$$\frac{0.33 \text{ g}}{100 \text{ mL}} = \frac{X \text{ g}}{1000 \text{ mL}}$$

$100X = 3300$

$$\frac{100X}{100} = \frac{3300}{100}$$

$X = 3.3$ g

20) $\frac{2000 \text{ mL}}{24 \text{ h}} = 83.3 = 83 \text{ mL/h}$

$\frac{\text{mL / h}}{\text{drop factor constant}} =$

$\frac{83 \text{ mL/h}}{4} = 20.75 = 21 \text{ gtt/min}$

22) $\frac{V}{T} \times C = \frac{400 \text{ mL}}{T \text{ min}} \times 15 \text{ gtt/mL} = 24 \text{ gtt/min}$

$\frac{400}{T} \times 15 = 24$

$$\frac{6000}{T} = \frac{24}{1}$$

$24T = 6000$

$$\frac{24T}{24} = \frac{6000}{24}$$

$T = 250$ min

$250 \cancel{\text{min}} \div 60 \cancel{\text{min}}\text{/h} = 4\frac{1}{6} \text{ h} = 4 \text{ h } 10 \text{ min}$

1530 hours
+ 410 hours
1940 hours

23) $\frac{V}{T} \times C = \frac{V \text{ mL}}{60 \text{ min}} \times 10 \text{ gtt/mL} = 32 \text{ gtt/min}$

$$\frac{10V}{60} = \frac{32}{1}$$

$10V = 1920$

$$\frac{10V}{10} = \frac{1920}{10}$$

$V = 192$ mL/h; $192 \text{ mL}/\cancel{\text{h}} \times 8 \cancel{\text{h}} = 1536$ mL (administered during your 8 h shift)

25) $\frac{2700 \text{mL}}{22.5 \text{ h}} = 120 \text{ mL/h}$

26) $\frac{100 \text{ mL}}{30 \text{ min}} = \frac{X \text{ mL}}{60 \text{ min}}$

$30X = 6000$

$\frac{30X}{30} = \frac{6000}{30}$

$X = 200 \text{ mL}$

200 mL/60 min = 200 mL/h

27) $\frac{1200 \text{ mL}}{100 \text{ mL/h}} = 12 \text{ h}$ (total time to infuse 1200 mL

2200 hours
− 1530 hours
630 = 6 h 30 min

$6\frac{1}{2}\text{h} \times 100 \text{ mL/h} = 650 \text{ mL}$

1200 mL − 650 mL = 550 mL

After $6\frac{1}{2}$ h, 650 mL should have been infused, with 550 mL remaining. IV is behind schedule.

$\frac{650 \text{ mL}}{5.5 \text{ h}} = 118 \text{ mL/h}$ (adjusted rate)

$\frac{\text{Adjusted gtt/min} - \text{Ordered gtt/min}}{\text{Ordered gtt/min}} = \%$ of variation;

$\frac{118-100}{100} = \frac{18}{100} = .18. = 0.18 = 18\%$ (variance is safe)

If policy and patient's condition permit, reset rate to 118 mL/h.

28) $\frac{20 \text{ mEq}}{1000 \text{ mL}} = \frac{X \text{ mEq}}{250 \text{ mL}}$

$1000X = 5000$

$\frac{1000X}{1000} = \frac{5000}{1000}$

$X = 5 \text{ mEq}$

$\frac{D}{H} \times Q = \frac{5 \text{ mEq}}{2 \text{ mEq}} \times 1 \text{ mL} = \frac{5}{2} = 2.5 \text{ mL}$

29) $40 \text{ lb} = \frac{40}{2.2} = 18.18 = 18.2 \text{ kg}$

1st 10 kg: 100 mL/kg/day × 10 kg =	1000 mL/day
Remaining 8.2 kg: 50 mL/kg/day × 8.2 kg =	410 mL/day
	1410 mL/day

$\frac{1410 \text{ mL}}{24 \text{ h}} = 58.7 = 59 \text{ mL/h}$

30) 1185 g = 1185 ÷ 1000 = 1.185 = 1.2 kg

1st 10 kg: 100 mL/kg/day × 1.2 kg = 120 mL/day

$\frac{120 \text{ mL}}{24 \text{ h}} = 5 \text{ mL/h}$

31) $\text{BSA} = \sqrt{\frac{30 \times 24}{3131}} = \sqrt{\frac{720}{3131}} = \sqrt{0.229} = 0.479 = 0.48 \text{ m}^2$

32) $\text{BSA} = \sqrt{\frac{155 \times 39}{3600}} = \sqrt{\frac{6045}{3600}} = \sqrt{1.679} = 1.295 = 1.30 \text{ m}^2$

34) Minimum safe dosage: $37 \text{ mg/m}^2 \times 0.5 \text{ m}^2 = 18.5 \text{ mg}$

Maximum safe dosage: $75 \text{ mg/m}^2 \times 0.5 \text{ m}^2 = 37.5 \text{ mg}$

35) $\frac{D}{H} \times Q = \frac{18.5 \text{ mg}}{1 \text{ mg}} \times 1 \text{ mL} = 18.5 \text{ mL}$

36) 2 mL/mg × 18.5 mg = 37 mL

$\frac{D}{H} \times Q = \frac{1 \text{ mg/min}}{18.5 \text{ mg}} \times 37 \text{ mL} = 2 \text{ mL/min}$

$\frac{2 \text{ mL}}{\text{min}} \times \frac{60 \text{ min}}{\text{h}} = 120 \text{ mL/h}$

37) At 1 mg/min, 18.5 mg will infuse in 18.5 minutes.

$\frac{1 \text{ mg}}{1 \text{ min}} = \frac{18.5 \text{ mg}}{X \text{ min}}$

$X = 18.5 \text{ min}$

38) $\text{BSA} = 0.8\text{m}^2$

$2 \text{ mg/m}^2 \times 0.8 \text{ m}^2 = 1.6 \text{ mg}$

39) $\frac{40 \text{ mL}}{60 \text{ min}} = \frac{X \text{ mL}}{30 \text{ min}}$

$60 X = 1200$

$\frac{60 X}{60} = \frac{1200}{60}$

$X = 20 \text{ mL}$

$\frac{D}{H} \times Q = \frac{\overset{2}{250 \text{ mg}}}{\underset{1}{125 \text{ mg}}} \times 1 \text{ mL} = 2 \text{ mL}$ (Ancef)

20 mL (total IV solution) − 2 mL (Ancef) = 18 mL (NS)

40) $\frac{100 \text{ mg}}{1 \text{ mL}} = \frac{750 \text{ mg}}{X \text{ mL}}$

$100 X = 750$

$\frac{100 X}{100} = \frac{750}{100}$

$X = 7.5 \text{ mL}$

7.5 mL IV solution to be used with the 750 mg of Ticarcillin for minimal dilution

41) 750 U/h × 24 h = 18,000 U. This is not within the safe dosage range. No, order is not safe.

42) Total IV PB volume: 100 mL × 6 = 600 mL

Regular IV volume: 1500 mL − 600 mL = 900 mL

Total IV PB time of q.4 h × 30 min = 6 × 30 min = 180 min = 3 h

Total Regular IV time: 24 h − 3 h = 21 h

Regular IV rate: $\text{mL/h} = \frac{900 \text{ mL}}{21 \text{ h}} = 42.8 = 43 \text{ mL/h}$ or 43 gtt/min because mL/h = gtt min when drop factor is 60 gtt/mL.

$\frac{\text{mL / h}}{\text{Drop factor constant}} = \text{gtt/min}; \frac{43 \text{ mL/h}}{1} = 43 \text{ gtt/min}$

43) $\frac{100 \text{ mL}}{30 \text{ min}} = \frac{X \text{ mL}}{60 \text{ min}}$

$30 X = 6000$

$\frac{30 X}{30} = \frac{6000}{30}$

X = 200 mL; 200 mL/60 min = 200 mL/h or 200 gtt/min (because drop factor is 60 gtt/mL)

44) See #42, Regular IV rate calculated at 42.8 or 43 mL/h.

See #43, IVPB rate calculated at 200 mL/h.

45) $\frac{D}{H} \times Q = \frac{\overset{1}{\cancel{2\text{ mEq}}}\text{/h}}{\underset{20}{\cancel{40\text{ mEq}}}} \times 1000\text{ mL} = 50\text{ mL/h}$ or,

$$\frac{40\text{ mEq}}{1000\text{ mL}} = \frac{2\text{ mEq/h}}{X\text{ mL/h}}$$

$$40X = 2000$$

$$\frac{40X}{40} = \frac{2000}{40}$$

$$X = 50\text{ mL/h}$$

46) $\frac{25\text{ mg}}{1\text{ L}} = \frac{25.000.}{1.000.} = \frac{25{,}000\text{ mcg}}{1000\text{ mL}} = \frac{25{,}\cancel{000}\text{ mcg}}{1\cancel{000}\text{ mL}} = 25\text{ mcg/mL}$

$\frac{D}{H} \times Q = \frac{\overset{1}{\cancel{5\text{ mcg}}}\text{/min}}{\underset{5}{\cancel{25\text{ mcg}}}} \times 1\text{ mL} = 0.2\text{ mL/min}$

$\frac{0.2\text{ mL}}{\cancel{\text{min}}} \times \frac{60\text{ }\cancel{\text{min}}}{\text{h}} = 12\text{ mL/h}$

47) $\frac{15\text{ U}}{1\text{ L}} = \frac{15.000.}{1.000.} = \frac{15{,}\cancel{000}\text{ mU}}{1\cancel{000}\text{ mL}} = 15\text{ mU/mL};$

$\frac{D}{H} \times Q = \frac{2\text{ }\cancel{\text{mU}}\text{/min}}{15\text{ }\cancel{\text{mU}}} \times 1\text{ mL} = 0.13\text{ mL/min}$

$\frac{0.13\text{ mL}}{\cancel{\text{min}}} \times \frac{60\text{ }\cancel{\text{min}}}{\text{h}} = 7.8 = 8\text{ mL/h}$

48) $\frac{\overset{4}{\cancel{20}}\text{ }\cancel{\text{mU}}\text{/min}}{\underset{3}{\cancel{15}}\text{ }\cancel{\text{mU}}} \times 1\text{ mL} = 1.33\text{ mL/min}$

$\frac{1.33\text{ mL}}{\cancel{\text{min}}} \times \frac{60\text{ }\cancel{\text{min}}}{\text{h}} = 80\text{ mL/h}$

49) $150\text{ lb} = \frac{150}{2.2} = 68.18 = 68.2\text{ kg};$

$4\text{ mcg/}\cancel{\text{kg}}\text{/min} \times 68.2\text{ }\cancel{\text{kg}} = 272.8 = 273\text{ mcg/min}$

$273\text{ mcg/}\cancel{\text{min}} \times 60\text{ }\cancel{\text{min}}\text{/h} = 16{,}380\text{ mcg/h}$

$\frac{600\text{ mg}}{0.5\text{ L}} = \frac{600.000.}{0.500.} = \frac{\overset{1200}{\cancel{600{,}000}}\text{ mcg}}{\underset{1}{\cancel{500}}\text{ mL}} = 1200\text{ mcg/mL}$

$\frac{D}{H} \times Q = \frac{16{,}380\text{ }\cancel{\text{mcg}}\text{/h}}{1200\text{ }\cancel{\text{mcg}}} \times 1\text{ mL} = 13.6 = 14\text{ mL/h}$

50) $12\text{ mcg/kg/min} \times 68.2\text{ kg} = 818.4 = 818\text{ mcg/min}$

$\frac{818\text{ mcg}}{\text{min}} \times \frac{60\text{ min}}{\text{h}} = 49{,}080\text{ mcg/h}$

$\frac{D}{H} \times Q = \frac{49{,}080\text{ }\cancel{\text{mcg}}\text{/h}}{1200\text{ }\cancel{\text{mcg}}} \times 1\text{ mL} = 40.9 = 41\text{ mL/h}$

Essential Skills Evaluation from pages 385–397.

1) 1

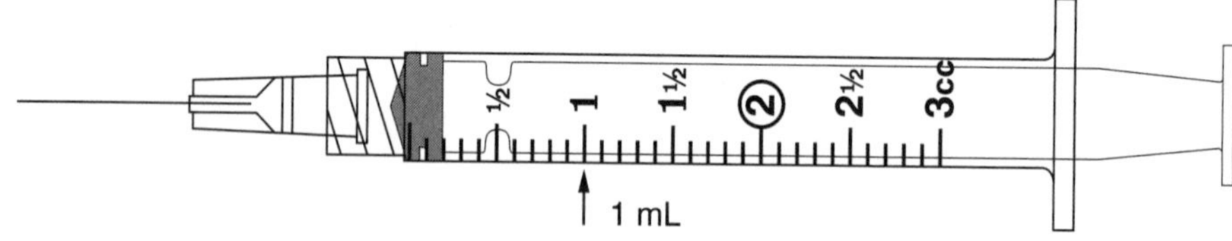

2) 0.25

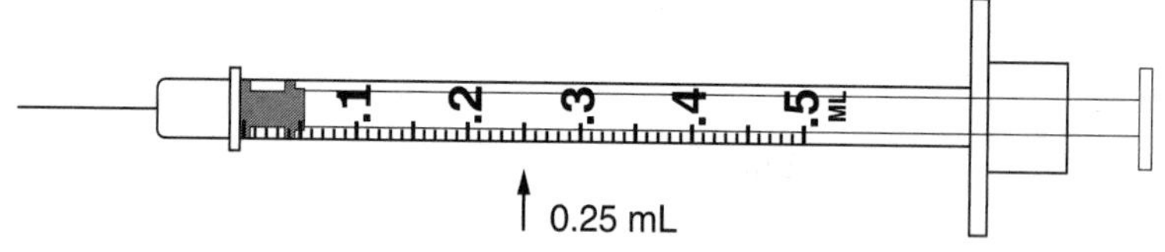

3) 1.4

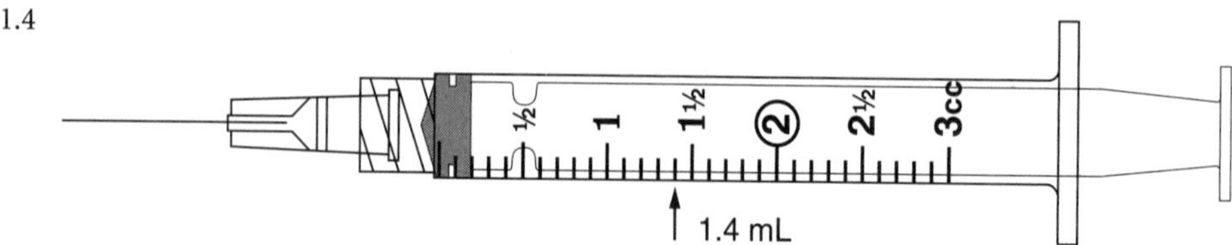

4) 2 5) $1\frac{1}{2}$

6) 0.5

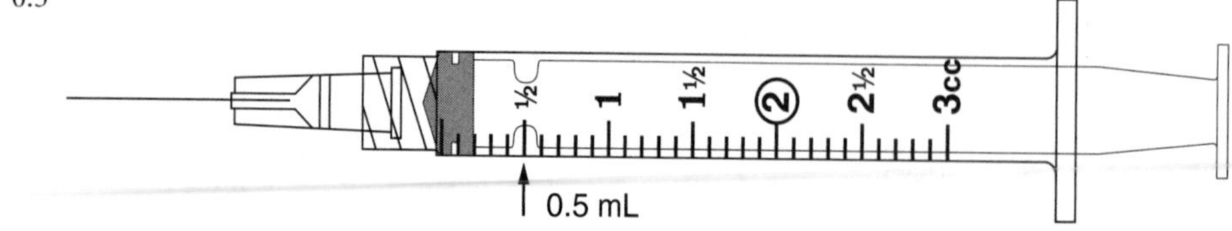

7) $\frac{1}{2}$

8) 1.4

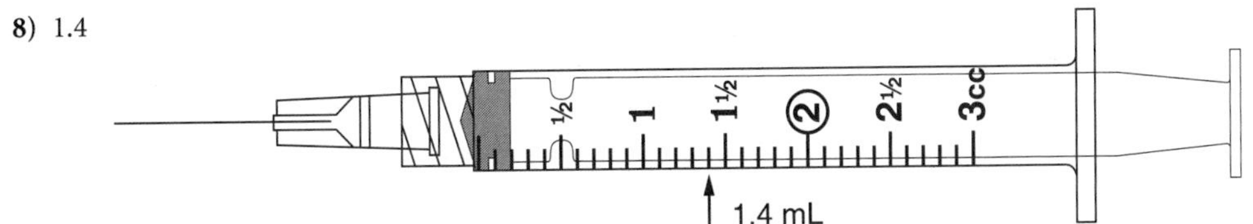

9) 68

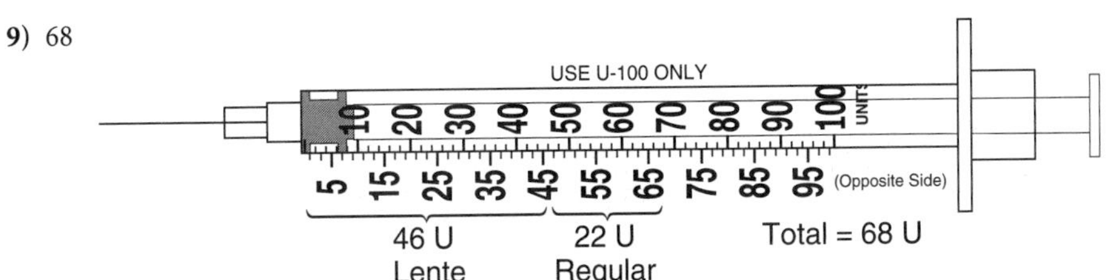

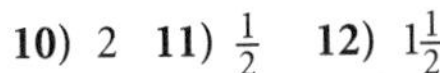

10) 2 **11)** $\frac{1}{2}$ **12)** $1\frac{1}{2}$

13) 0.8

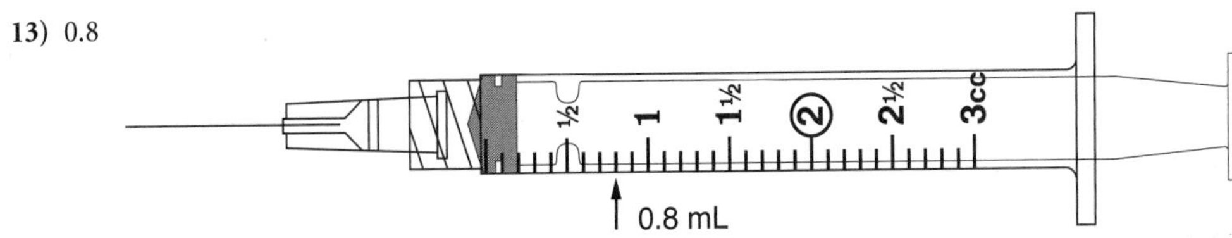

14) 1.5

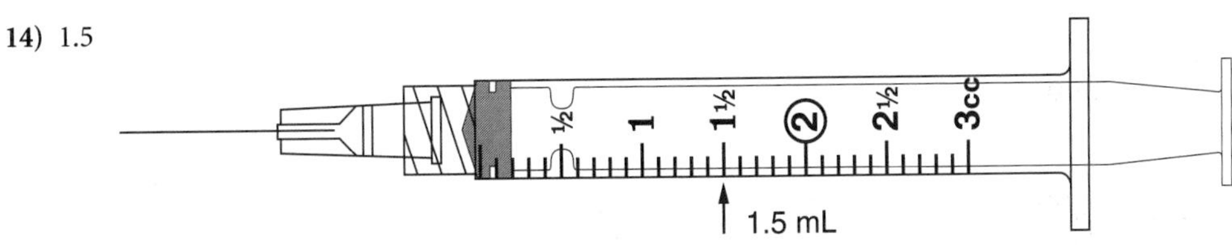

15) 4

16) 1.5

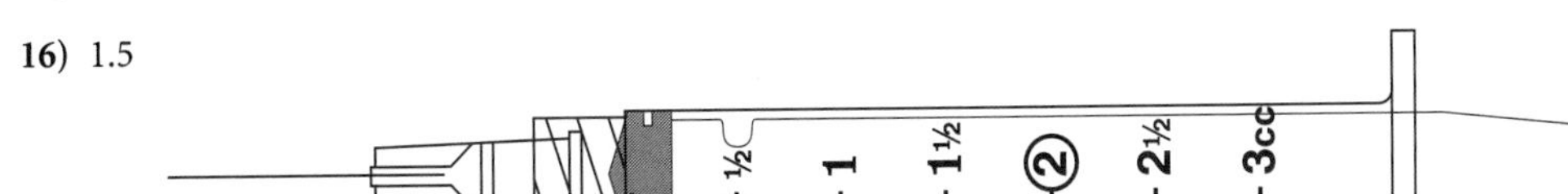

17) 2; 25

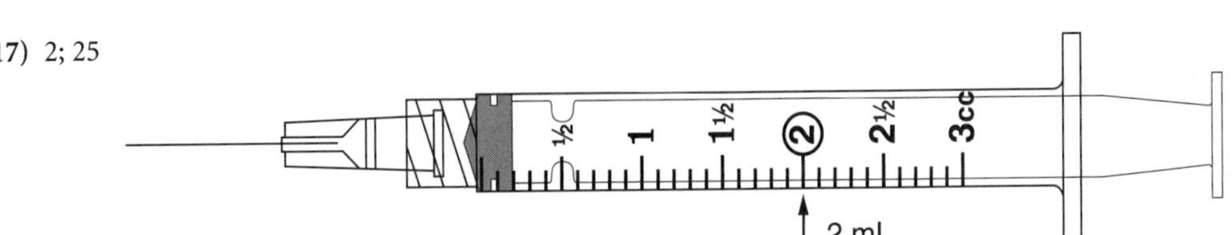

18) Yes. Her temperature is 102.2°F. Tylenol is indicated for fever > 101°F every 4 hours. It has been 5 hours and 5 minutes since her last dose. **19)** 2; 650 **20)** one-half

21) Nubain; 0.2

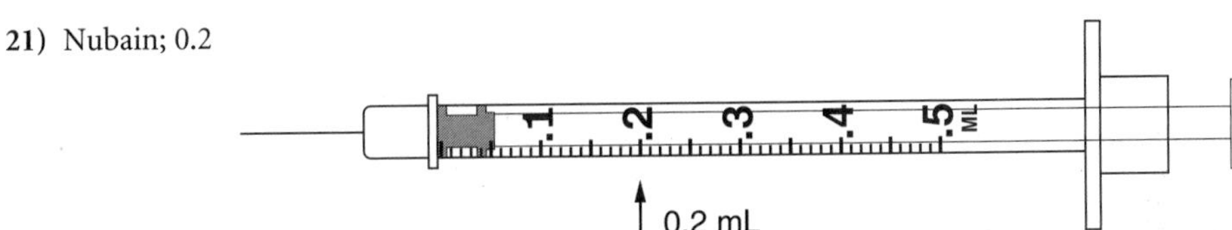

22) Narcan; 1

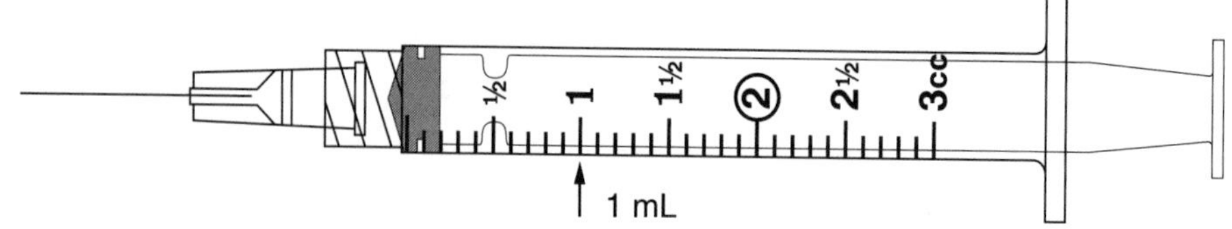

23) 6; 100 **24)** 100 **25)** 8; 2 **26)** 1; 0745, 1145, 1745, 2200

27) 18; subcutaneous

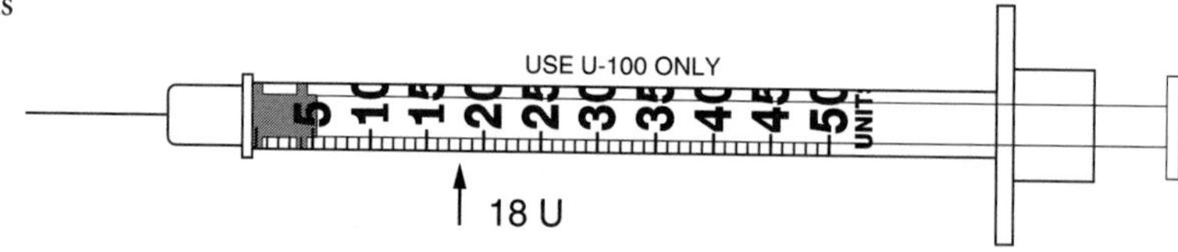

28) 9 **29)** Yes. The usual dosage is 20–40 mg/kg/day divided into 3 doses q.8 h, which is equivalent to 45 – 91 mg per dose for a 15 lb (6.8 kg) child. **30)** 1 **31)** 1; every 8 hours **32)** Yes; 1.7; 25. **33)** 1000 **34)** Yes **35)** 4.8; dosage is safe **36)** 38 **37)** 280–420 **38)** 13 **39)** Hypertonic **40)** Isotonic **41)** 30; no **42)** Do not administer; consult with physician before giving drug. **43)** 1 **44)** 50; 5 **45)** 30 **46)** 2030; 8:30 PM **47)** 200 **48)** 3; 330; 1 **49)** 1.5 **50)** "1/30/XX, 1400, reconstituted as 330 mg/mL. Expires 1/31/XX, 1400. Store at room temperature. G.D.P."

Solutions—Essential Skills Evaluation

1) $\frac{D}{H} \times Q = \frac{\overset{1}{\cancel{50}}\text{ mg}}{\underset{5}{\cancel{250}}\text{ mg}} \times 5\text{ mL} = \frac{5}{5} = 1\text{ mL}$

2) $\frac{D}{H} \times Q = \frac{12.5\cancel{\text{ mg}}}{50\cancel{\text{ mg}}} \times 1\text{ mL} = 0.25\text{ mL}$

3) $\frac{D}{H} \times Q = \frac{\overset{7}{\cancel{35\text{ mg}}}}{\underset{5}{\cancel{25\text{ mg}}}} \times 1\text{ mL} = 1.4\text{ mL}$

4) $\frac{D}{H} \times Q = \frac{\overset{2}{\cancel{400\text{ mg}}}}{\underset{1}{\cancel{200\text{ mg}}}} \times 1\text{ tab} = 2\text{ tab}$

5) $\frac{D}{H} \times Q = \frac{7.5\text{ mg}}{5\text{ mg}} \times 1\text{ tab} = 1.5 = 1\frac{1}{2}\text{ tab}$

6) $0.125\text{ mg} = 0.125 \times 1000 = 0.125. = 125\text{ mcg}$

$\frac{D}{H} \times Q = \frac{125\cancel{\text{ mcg}}}{\underset{250}{\cancel{500\text{ mcg}}}} \times \overset{1}{\cancel{2}}\text{ mL} = 0.5\text{ mL}$

7) $\text{gr}\ \frac{1}{8} = \frac{1}{8} \times \frac{60}{1} = \frac{60}{8} = 7.5\text{ mg}$

$\frac{D}{H} \times Q = \frac{7.5\cancel{\text{ mg}}}{15\cancel{\text{ mg}}} \times 1\text{ tab} = 0.5 = \frac{1}{2}\text{ tab}$

8) $\frac{D}{H} \times Q = \frac{\overset{7}{\cancel{350\text{ mg}}}}{\underset{10}{\cancel{500\text{ mg}}}} \times 2\text{ mL} = 1.4\text{ mL}$

9) 46 U + 22 U = 68 U (total)

10) $0.05\text{ mg} = 0.05 \times 1000 = 0.050. = 50\text{ mcg}$

$\frac{D}{H} \times Q = \frac{\overset{2}{\cancel{50\text{ mcg}}}}{\underset{1}{\cancel{25\text{ mcg}}}} \times 1\text{ tab} = 2\text{ tab}$

11) $\frac{D}{H} \times Q = \frac{\overset{1}{\cancel{40\text{ mg}}}}{\underset{2}{\cancel{80\text{ mg}}}} \times 1\text{ tab} = \frac{1}{2}\text{ tab}$

12) $\frac{D}{H} \times Q = \frac{\overset{3}{\cancel{375\text{ mg}}}}{\underset{2}{\cancel{250\text{ mg}}}} \times 1\text{ tab} = 1.5 = 1\frac{1}{2}\text{ tab}$

13) $\frac{D}{H} \times Q = \frac{\overset{4}{\cancel{40\text{ mg}}}}{\underset{5}{\cancel{50\text{ mg}}}} \times 1\text{ mL} = 0.8\text{ mL}$

14) $\frac{D}{H} \times Q = \frac{3\cancel{\text{ mg}}}{2\cancel{\text{ mg}}} \times 1\text{ mL} = 1.5\text{ mL}$

You will need 2 vials of the drug, because each vial contains 1 mL.

15) $\frac{D}{H} \times Q = \frac{\overset{4}{\cancel{100\text{ mg}}}}{\underset{5}{\cancel{125\text{ mg}}}} \times 5\text{ mL} = \frac{20}{5} = 4\text{ mL}$

16) $\text{gr}\ \frac{1}{100} = \frac{1}{100} \times \frac{60}{1} = \frac{60}{100} = 0.6\text{ mg}$

$\frac{D}{H} \times Q = \frac{\overset{3}{\cancel{0.6}}\text{ mg}}{\underset{2}{\cancel{0.4}}\text{ mg}} \times 1\text{ mL} = 1.5\text{ mL}$

17) $0.5\text{ g} = 0.5 \times 1000 = 0.500. = 500\text{ mg}$

$\frac{D}{H} \times Q = \frac{\overset{2}{\cancel{500\text{ mg}}}}{\underset{1}{\cancel{250\text{ mg}}}} \times 1\text{ mL} = 2\text{ mL}$

$\frac{V}{T} \times C = \frac{50\cancel{\text{ mL}}}{\underset{2}{\cancel{30}}\text{ min}} \times \overset{1}{\cancel{15}}\text{ gtt}/\cancel{\text{mL}} = \frac{50}{2} = 25\text{ gtt/min}$

18) $°F = 1.8°C + 32 = (1.8 \times 39) + 32 = 70.2 + 32 = 102.2°F$

19) $\frac{2\cancel{\text{ tab}}}{\text{dose}} \times \frac{325\text{ mg}}{\cancel{\text{tab}}} = 650\text{ mg/dose}$

20) $\frac{30\cancel{\text{ mg}}}{60\cancel{\text{ mg}}} = \frac{1}{2}$

21) $\frac{D}{H} \times Q = \frac{\overset{1}{\cancel{2\text{ mg}}}}{\underset{5}{\cancel{10\text{ mg}}}} \times 1\text{ mL} = 0.2\text{ mL}$

22) $\frac{D}{H} \times Q = \frac{\cancel{0.4\text{ mg}}}{\cancel{0.4\text{ mg}}} \times 1\text{ mL} = 1\text{ mL}$

23) $\frac{D}{H} \times Q = \frac{\overset{3}{\cancel{150\text{ mg}}}}{\underset{5}{\cancel{250\text{ mg}}}} \times 10\text{ mL} = \frac{30}{5} = 6\text{ mL}$

$\frac{V}{T} \times C = \frac{50\cancel{\text{ mL}}}{\underset{1}{\cancel{30}}\text{ min}} \times \overset{2}{\cancel{60}}\text{ gtt/}\cancel{\text{mL}} = 100\text{ gtt/min}$

24) 100 gtt/min = 100 mL/h, because

gtt/min = mL/h when drop factor is 60 gtt/mL

25) $\frac{\overset{2}{\cancel{125\text{ mg}}}}{\underset{1}{\cancel{62.5\text{ mg}}}} \times 1\text{ mL} = 2\text{ mL}$

26) $\frac{\cancel{1\text{ g}}}{\cancel{1\text{ g}}} \times 1\text{ tab} = 1\text{ tab}$

29) 15 lb $= \frac{15}{2.2} = 6.82 = 6.8$ kg

Minimum dosage: 20 mg/$\cancel{\text{kg}}$/day × 6.8 $\cancel{\text{kg}}$ = 136 mg/day

$\frac{136\text{ mg}}{3\text{ doses}} = 45.3 = 45$ mg/dose

Maximum dosage: 40 mg/$\cancel{\text{kg}}$/day × 6.8 $\cancel{\text{kg}}$ = 272 mg/day

$\frac{272\text{ mg}}{3\text{ doses}} = 90.6 = 91$ mg/dose

30) $\frac{D}{H} \times Q = \frac{\cancel{50\text{ mg}}}{\cancel{50\text{ mg}}} \times 1\text{ mL} = 1\text{ mL}$

31) 1 mL = 1 dropperful

32) 110 lb $= \frac{110}{2.2} = 50$ kg

Minimum dosage: 20 mg/$\cancel{\text{kg}}$/day × 50 $\cancel{\text{kg}}$ = 1000 mg/day

$\frac{1000\text{ mg}}{4\text{ doses}} = 250$ mg/dose

Maximum dosage: 40 mg/$\cancel{\text{kg}}$/day × 50 $\cancel{\text{kg}}$ = 2000 mg/day

$\frac{2000\text{ mg}}{4\text{ doses}} = 500$ mg/dose

$\frac{D}{H} \times Q = \frac{\overset{5}{\cancel{250\text{ mg}}}}{\underset{6}{\cancel{300\text{ mg}}}} \times 2\text{ mL} = \frac{\overset{5}{\cancel{10}}}{\underset{3}{\cancel{6}}} = \frac{5}{3} = 1.66 = 1.7\text{ mL}$

$\frac{V}{T} \times C = \frac{50\cancel{\text{ mL}}}{\underset{2}{\cancel{20}}\text{ min}} \times \overset{1}{\cancel{10}}\text{ gtt/}\cancel{\text{mL}} = \frac{50}{2} = 25\text{ gtt/min}$

33)

IV fluid =	200 mL
gelatin = ℥ iv = 4 × 30 =	120 mL
water = ℥ iii × 2 (3 × 30) × 2 = 90 × 2 =	180 mL
apple juice = pt i =	500 mL
	1, 000 mL

34) 40 lb $= \frac{40}{2.2} = 18.18 = 18.2$ kg

40 mg/$\cancel{\text{kg}}$/day × 18.2 $\cancel{\text{kg}}$ = 728 mg/day

$\frac{728\text{ mg}}{3\text{ doses}} = 242.6 = 243$ mg; close approximation to ordered dosage of 240 mg; dosage is safe.

35) $\frac{D}{H} \times Q = \frac{\cancel{240\text{ mg}}}{\underset{50}{\cancel{250\text{ mg}}}} \times \overset{1}{\cancel{5}}\text{ mL} = \frac{240}{50} = 4.8\text{ mL}$

36) $\text{mL / h} = \frac{\overset{150}{\cancel{600}}\text{ mL}}{\underset{1}{\cancel{4}}\text{ h}} = 150\text{ mL/h}$

$\frac{V}{T} \times C = \frac{150\cancel{\text{ mL}}}{\underset{4}{\cancel{60}}\text{ min}} \times \overset{1}{\cancel{15}}\text{ gtt/}\cancel{\text{mL}} = \frac{150}{4} = 37.5 = 38\text{ gtt/min}$

37) 61 lb 8 oz = 61.5 lb $= \frac{61.5}{2.2} = 27.95 = 28$ kg

Minimum dosage: 10 mg/$\cancel{\text{kg}}$ × 28 $\cancel{\text{kg}}$ = 280 mg

Maximum dosage: 15 mg/$\cancel{\text{kg}}$ × 28 $\cancel{\text{kg}}$ = 420 mg

38) $\frac{D}{H} \times Q = \frac{42\cancel{0}\cancel{\text{ mg}}}{8\cancel{0}\cancel{\text{ mg}}} \times 2.5\text{ mL} = \frac{105}{8} = 13.1 = 13\text{ mL}$

41) 52 lb $= \frac{52}{2.2} = 23.63 = 23.6$ kg

5 mg/$\cancel{\text{kg}}$/day × 23.6 $\cancel{\text{kg}}$ = 118 mg/day

$\frac{118\text{ mg}}{4\text{ doses}} = 29.5 = 30$ mg/dose; dosage is too low to be therapeutic and is not safe.

43) $\frac{D}{H} \times Q = \frac{\cancel{10\text{ mg}}}{\underset{10}{\cancel{300\text{ mg}}}} \times \overset{1}{\cancel{30}}\text{ mL}$

$= \frac{10}{10} = 1\text{ mL}$

44) 10 mg/$\cancel{\text{dose}}$ × 5 $\cancel{\text{doses}}$ = 50 mg

1 mL/$\cancel{\text{dose}}$ × 5 $\cancel{\text{doses}}$ = 5 mL

45) $\frac{\overset{30}{\cancel{300\text{ mg}}}}{\underset{1}{\cancel{10\text{ mg}}}\text{/dose}} = 30\text{ doses}$

46) $\frac{30\cancel{\text{ doses}}}{5\cancel{\text{ doses}}\text{/h}} = 6\text{ h}$

1430 h	2030
+ 600 h	− 1200
2030 h	8:30 PM

47) $\frac{100\text{ mL}}{30\text{ min}} = \frac{X\text{ mL}}{60\text{ min}}$

$30X = 6000$

$\frac{30X}{30} = \frac{6000}{30}$

$X = 200\text{ mL}$

200 mL/60 min = 200 mL/h

49) $\frac{D}{H} \times Q = \frac{50\cancel{0}\cancel{\text{ mg}}}{33\cancel{0}\cancel{\text{ mg}}} \times 1\text{ mL} = \frac{50}{33} = 1.51 = 1.5\text{ mL}$

Comprehensive Skills Evaluation from pages 399–409.

1) 2

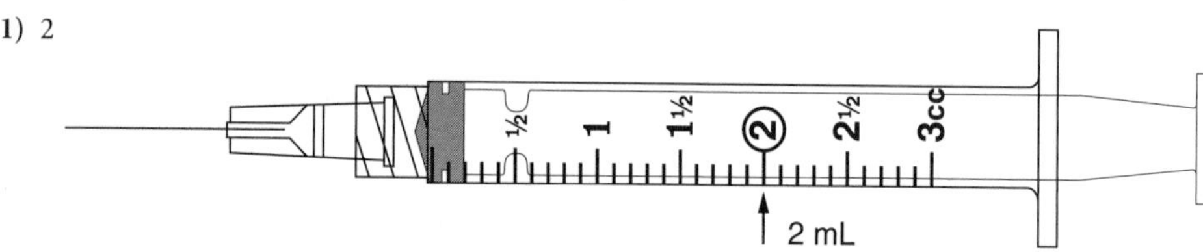

2) 1 **3)** 2 **4)** Sublingual. The medication is to be administered under the tongue.

5) 1

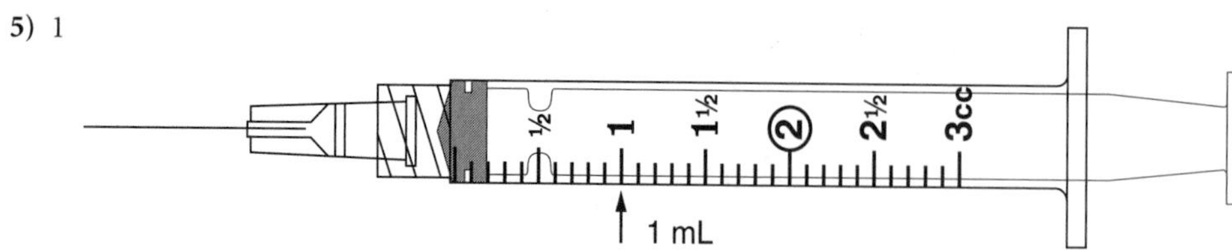

6) $\frac{1}{2}$ **7)** 80

8) 5

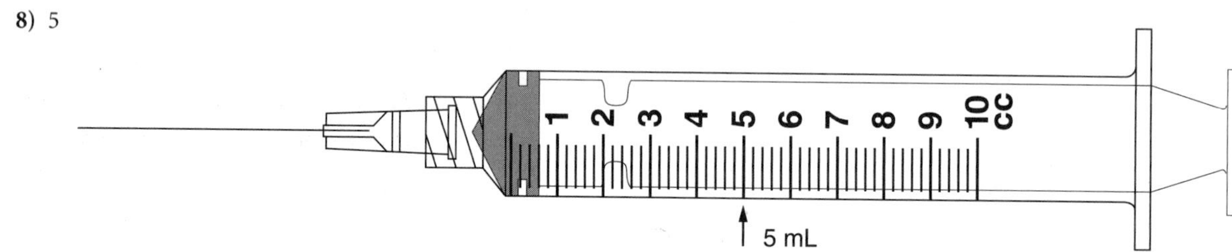

9) 0.8 **10)** 1920 **11)** 0500; 9/4/XX **12)** 2 **13)** 80 **14)** digoxin, KCl, and acetaminophen

15) 5

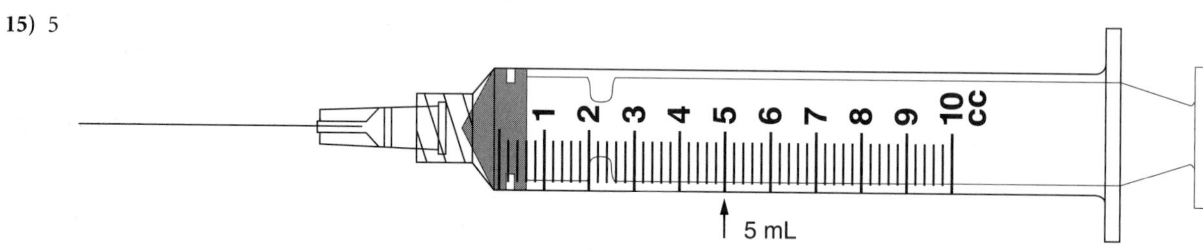

16) 30

17) 5

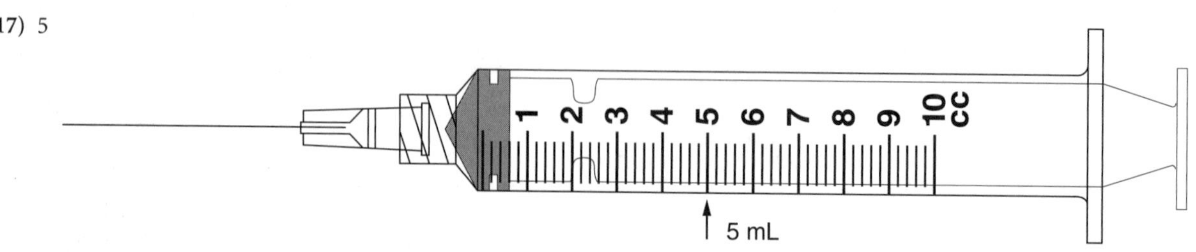

18) 19 **19)** 1 **20)** 60 **21)** Yes; 2; 23; 40 **22)** Yes **23)** 25 **24)** Yes; safe dosage is 300 mg, which is the same as the ordered dosage. **25)** 6 **26)** 44 **27)** 1200 **28)** 5 **29)** 2.5 **30)** 19

31) 5; 45

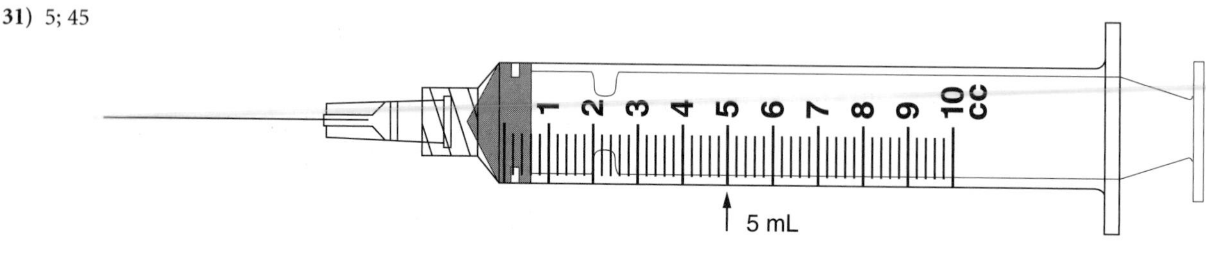

32) 50

33) Yes; 2; 60

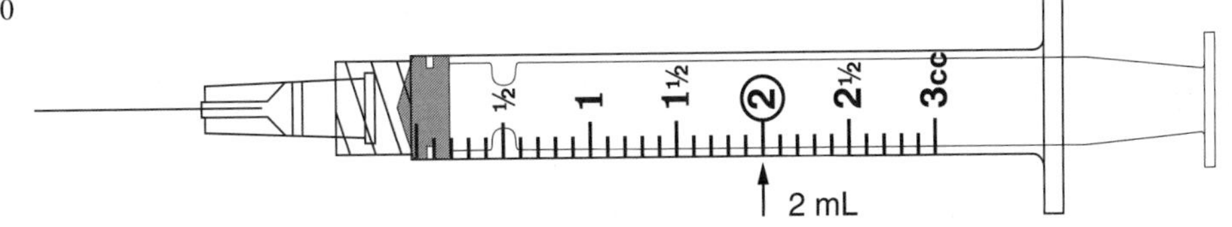

34) 8; 0.08

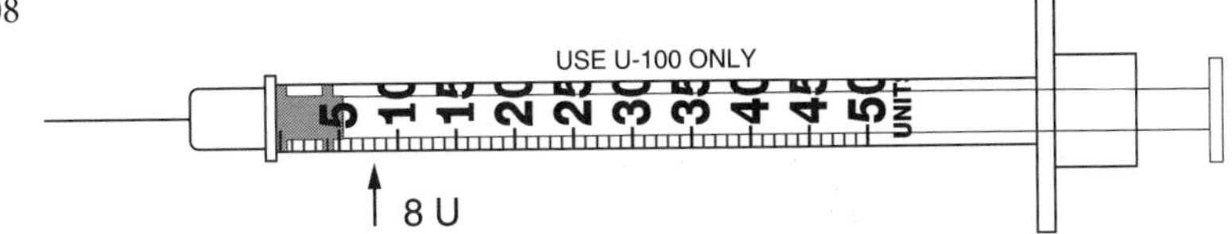

35) 60

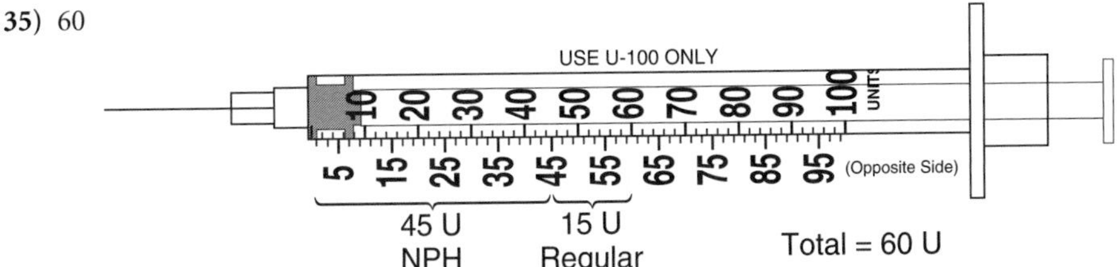

36) 20 **37)** 720; 960 **38)** 640 **39)** 730 **40)** 30 **41)** 12 **42)** 30; 1180 **43)** 49 **44)** 50; 3.3 **45)** 8; 4 **46)** 2.2 **47)** 47.8 **48)** Yes; the minimal amount of IV fluid to safely dilute this med is 13.5 mL. The order calls for 50 mL total, or 47.8, almost 48 mL of IV fluid. **49)** 2,400,000; yes **50)** 75

Solutions—Comprehensive Skills Evaluation

1) $\frac{D}{H} \times Q = \frac{\overset{2}{\cancel{20}\text{ mg}}}{\underset{1}{\cancel{10}\text{ mg}}} \times 1\text{ mL} = 2\text{ mL}$

2) $\frac{D}{H} \times Q = \frac{\cancel{20\text{ mg}}}{\cancel{20\text{ mg}}} \times 1\text{ tab} = 1\text{ tab}$

3) $\frac{D}{H} \times Q = \frac{\overset{2}{\cancel{13}\text{ mg}}}{\underset{1}{\cancel{6.5}\text{ mg}}} \times 1\text{ cap} = 2\text{ cap}$

5) 0.25 mg = 0.25 × 1000 = 0.250. = 250 mcg

$\frac{D}{H} \times Q = \frac{\overset{1}{\cancel{250}\text{ mg}}}{\underset{2}{\cancel{500}\text{ mg}}} \times 2\text{ mL} = \frac{2}{2} = 1\text{ mL}$

6) 0.125 mg = 0.125 × 1000 = 0.125. = 125 mcg

$\frac{D}{H} \times Q = \frac{\overset{1}{\cancel{125}\text{ mcg}}}{\underset{2}{\cancel{250}\text{ mcg}}} \times 1\text{ tab} = \frac{1}{2}\text{ tab}$

"q.d." means once per day; will need $\frac{1}{2}$ tab per 24 h.

7) $\frac{\text{mL/h}}{\text{drop factor constant}} = \text{gtt/min}$

$\frac{80\text{ mL/h}}{1} = 80\text{ gtt/min}$ or,

80 mL/h = 80 gtt/min (because drop factor is 60 gtt/mL)

8) $\frac{D}{H} \times Q = \frac{10\ \cancel{\text{mEq}}}{\underset{2}{\cancel{30}\ \cancel{\text{mEq}}}} \times \overset{1}{\cancel{15}}\text{ mL} = \frac{10}{2} = 5\text{ mL}$

9) The total fluid volume is:

1000 mL $D_5\ \frac{1}{2}$NS + 5 mL KCl = 1005 mL

$\frac{10\text{ mEq}}{1005\text{ mL}} = \frac{X\text{ mEq/h}}{80\text{ mL/h}}$

$1005X = 800$

$\frac{1005X}{1005} = \frac{800}{1005}$

$X = 0.8\text{ mEq/h}$

10) $80\text{ mL}/\cancel{h} \times 24\ \cancel{h} = 1920\text{ mL}$

11) $\frac{1000\ \cancel{\text{mL}}}{80\ \cancel{\text{mL}}/\text{h}} = 12.5\text{ h} = 12\text{ h }30\text{ min}$

1630 hours + 12 h 30 min later =

0500 hours the next day.

12) $\frac{D}{H} \times Q = \frac{\overset{2}{\cancel{650}\text{ mg}}}{\underset{1}{\cancel{325}\text{ mg}}} \times 1\text{ tab} = 2\text{ tab}$

13) mL/h = gtt/min when drop factor is 60 gtt/mL; order is for 80 cc/h or 80 mL/h.

15) $\frac{D}{H} \times Q = \frac{\overset{5}{\cancel{50}\text{ mg}}}{\underset{1}{\cancel{10}\text{ mg}}} \times 1\text{ mL} = 5\text{ mL}$

16) $\frac{D}{H} \times Q = \frac{2\ \cancel{\text{mg}}/\text{min}}{\underset{4}{\cancel{2000}\ \cancel{\text{mg}}}} \times \overset{1}{\cancel{500}}\text{ mL} = \frac{2}{4} = 0.5\text{ mL/min}$

$\frac{0.5\text{ mL}}{\cancel{\text{min}}} \times \frac{60\ \cancel{\text{min}}}{\text{h}} = 30\text{ mL/h}$

17) $\frac{D}{H} \times Q = \frac{\overset{5}{\cancel{400\text{ mg}}}}{\underset{1}{\cancel{80\text{ mg}}}} \times 1\text{ mL} = 5\text{ mL}$

18) $110\text{ lb} = \frac{110}{2.2} = 50\text{ kg}$

$10\text{ mcg}/\cancel{\text{kg}}/\text{min} \times 50\,\cancel{\text{kg}} = 500\text{ mcg/min}$

$500\text{ mcg/min} = 500 \div 1000 = .500. = 0.5\text{ mg/min}$

$\frac{D}{H} \times Q = \frac{0.5\,\cancel{\text{mg}}/\text{min}}{\underset{8}{\cancel{400\text{ mg}}}} \times \overset{5}{\cancel{250}}\text{ mL} = \frac{2.5}{8} = 0.312 = 0.31\text{ mL/min}$

$\frac{0.31\text{ mL}}{\cancel{\text{min}}} \times \frac{60\,\cancel{\text{min}}}{\text{h}} = 18.6 = 19\text{ mL/h}$

19) $\frac{D}{H} \times Q = \frac{20\,\cancel{\text{mEq}}}{\underset{2}{\cancel{30\text{ mEq}}}} \times \overset{1}{\cancel{15}}\text{ mL} = \frac{20}{2} = 10\text{ mL}$

The total IV volume is: 1000 mL $D_5\frac{1}{2}$NS + 10 mL KCl = 1010 mL

$\frac{20\text{ mEq}}{1010\text{ mL}} \times \frac{X\text{ mEq/h}}{50\text{ mL/h}}$

$1010X = 1000$

$\frac{1010X}{1010} = \frac{1000}{1010}$

$X = 1\text{ mEq/h}$

20) $\frac{D}{H} \times Q = \frac{4\,\cancel{\text{mg}}/\text{min}}{\underset{4}{\cancel{2000\text{ mg}}}} \times \overset{1}{\cancel{500}}\text{ mL} = \frac{4}{4} = 1\text{ mL/min}$

$\frac{1\text{ mL}}{\cancel{\text{min}}} \times \frac{60\,\cancel{\text{min}}}{\text{h}} = 60\text{ mL/h}$

21) $33\text{ lb} = \frac{33}{2.2} = 15\text{ kg}$

$15\text{ mg}/\cancel{\text{kg}}/\text{day} \times 15\,\cancel{\text{kg}} = 225\text{ mg/day}$

$\frac{225\text{ mg}}{3\text{ doses}} = 75\text{ mg/dose}$

$\frac{D}{H} \times Q = \frac{\cancel{75\text{ mg}}}{\cancel{75\text{ mg}}} \times 2\text{ mL} = 2\text{ mL Kantrex}$

25 mL total IV solution – 2 mL Kantrex = 23 mL $D_5\frac{1}{2}$NS

25 mL total solution + 15 mL flush = 40 mL total in 1 h

40 mL over 1 h is 40 mL/h.

22) $55\text{ lb} = \frac{55}{2.2} = 25\text{ kg}$

$1\text{ mg}/\cancel{\text{kg}}/\text{h} \times 25\,\cancel{\text{kg}} = 25\text{ mg/h}$

Order is for 25 mg/h; order is safe.

23) $\frac{D}{H} \times Q = \frac{25\,\cancel{\text{mg}}/\text{h}}{\cancel{250\text{ mg}}} \times \cancel{250}\text{ mL} = 25\text{ mL/h}$

24) $66\text{ lb} = \frac{66}{2.2} = 30\text{ kg}$

$40\text{ mg}/\cancel{\text{kg}}/\text{day} \times 30\,\cancel{\text{kg}} = 1200\text{ mg/day}$

$\frac{1200\text{ mg}}{4\text{ doses}} = 300\text{ mg/dose}$

25) $\frac{D}{H} \times Q = \frac{300\,\cancel{\text{mg}}}{\underset{50}{\cancel{500\text{ mg}}}} \times \overset{1}{\cancel{10}}\text{ mL} = \frac{300}{50} = 6\text{ mL}$

26) 50 mL total IV volume – 6 mL Vancocin = 44 mL $D_5\frac{1}{2}$NS

27) $50\text{ mL}/\cancel{\text{h}} \times 24\,\cancel{\text{h}} = 1200\text{ mL}$

28) $\frac{20\text{ mEq}}{1000\text{ mL}} \times \frac{X\text{ mEq}}{250\text{ mL}}$

$1000X = 5000$

$\frac{1000X}{1000} = \frac{5000}{1000}$

$X = 5\text{ mEq}$

29) $\frac{D}{H} \times Q = \frac{5\,\cancel{\text{mEq}}}{2\,\cancel{\text{mEq}}} \times 1\text{ mL} = 2.5\text{ mL}$

30) Select smallest quantity diluent (19 mL) to obtain most concentrated solution because 50 mL IV fluid is ordered for each Prostaphlin dose.

31) $\frac{D}{H} \times Q = \frac{500\,\cancel{\text{mg}}}{\underset{100}{\cancel{1000\text{ mg}}}} \times \overset{1}{\cancel{10}}\text{ mL} = \frac{\cancel{500}}{\cancel{100}} = 5\text{ mL}$

50 mL total IV volume – 5 mL Prostaphlin = 45 mL D_5W

32) 50 mL over 60 min = 50 mL/h

33) $1200\text{ U}/\cancel{\text{h}} \times 24\,\cancel{\text{h}} = 28{,}800\text{ U}$; within safe adult range.

$\frac{D}{H} \times Q = \frac{\overset{2}{\cancel{10{,}000\text{ U}}}}{\underset{1}{\cancel{5000\text{ U}}}} \times 1\text{ mL} = 2\text{ mL}$

$\frac{D}{H} \times Q = \frac{1200\,\cancel{\text{U}}/\text{h}}{\underset{20}{\cancel{10{,}000\text{ U}}}} \times \overset{1}{\cancel{500}}\text{ mL} = \frac{\overset{60}{\cancel{1200}}}{\underset{1}{\cancel{20}}} = 60\text{ mL/h}$

34) $\frac{100\text{ U}}{1\text{ mL}} \times \frac{8\text{ U}}{X\text{ mL}}$

$100X = 8$

$\frac{100X}{100} = \frac{8}{100}$

$X = 0.08\text{ mL}$

35) 15 U + 45 U = 60 U

36) U 100 insulin: 100 U/mL

$\frac{100\text{ U}}{1\text{ mL}} \times \frac{300\text{ mg}}{X\text{ mL}}$

$100X = 300$

$\frac{100X}{100} = \frac{300}{100}$

$X = 3\text{ mL}$

Total IV volume: 150 mL NS + 3 mL insulin = 153 mL

$\frac{300\text{ U}}{153\text{ mL}} \times \frac{X\text{ U/h}}{10\text{ mL/h}}$

$153X = 3000$

$\frac{153X}{153} = \frac{3000}{153}$

$X = 19.6 = 20\text{ U/h}$